Praise for *Awakening Hippocrates* and i
A Practical Guide to Global Health Servi

This comprehensive and beautifully written volume (Awakening
Hippocrates) *is essential reading for anyone who cares about global
poverty and health inequality and wants to do something about it.
All health professionals should read this book: there may be no clearer
mission for the medical profession today. In a strong and compelling
voice, Dr O'Neil explores the roots of poverty, and explains the "moral
imperative" shared by all health providers to engage directly in alleviating
global health inequalities. This book should inspire a revolution within
the health profession, in which international health becomes a staple of
every medical school. It is a clarion call for action that will ultimately
change our world.*

**Jim Yong Kim, MD, PhD, Co-Director of the Program in Infectious
Disease and Social Change, Chair of the FXB Center for Health and
Human Rights and the Division of Social Medicine and Health
Inequalities, Harvard Medical School**

Awakening Hippocrates *confronts us with the challenge of the inadequacies of health conditions in the developing world, where general poverty
adds a terrible obstacle to solutions for the many complex problems. This
book is written with impressive knowledge and with the compassion of a
medical doctor who has worked in the poorest countries of the world and
whose life has been marked by the miseries he has come across.*

*As encouragement, he presents the lives of some of his colleagues who
were able to make a notable difference, some of them well known, like
my father Albert Schweitzer, others unknown by the general public, but
achieving remarkable, beneficial improvements.*

This book is a moving and pressing appeal to all people of goodwill.

**Rhena Schweitzer Miller, former director of the Schweitzer-Bresslau
Hospital in Lambarene, Gabon, and daughter of Albert Schweitzer, MD**

*Once, visiting a graveyard in a small Massachusetts town, I came across
the seven headstones of an 18th century family, entirely wiped out by a
single measles epidemic. I remember congratulating myself on having
been born in a better age. Then Dr Paul Farmer showed me Haiti. There,
and in many other impoverished places, public health catastrophes are
at least as common today as they were in colonial America. The difference*

of course is that the health sciences have made such catastrophes unnecessary. The fact that they persist is a curse on all humanity. These two books should comprise an important tool in what I hope will be a genuine global movement both to understand and to remedy the great disparities in global health that afflict our times.

Tracy Kidder, Pulitzer-prize-winning author of *Mountains Beyond Mountains: The Quest of Dr Paul Farmer, A Man Who Would Cure the World*

Challenge – that's what Awakening Hippocrates *offers to readers from the health professions. Few books have mastered such a breadth of complex issues and done so in such clear and readily understandable prose. This book should appeal to anyone interested in global volunteerism, non-profit and governmental efforts in international medicine, and the under-lying forces that propagate poverty and ill health. The author encourages American health professionals to raise their commitments to care for the poor around the world using examples of outstanding individual efforts like those of Tom Dooley, MD, and Albert Schweitzer, MD. The companion book,* A Practical Guide to Global Health Service, *gives individuals direct opportunities to provide medical care and education in countries with large populations of the poor and medically underserved. These two books should become essential reading for every medical student and resident in the country, as well as anyone else who cares enough to address directly the health inequalities that plague so much of humanity.*

Robert Sparks, MD, Dean Emeritus Tulane University School of Medicine, President Emeritus and Senior Consultant for the W. K. Kellogg Foundation, former Chancellor of the University of Nebraska Medical Center, member Institute of Medicine.

In a world of dramatically worsening health disparities, A Practical Guide to Global Health Service *offers physicians and other health care profession-als a logical means through which they can directly improve global health through service in poor countries.*

He provides a roadmap for selecting, preparing for, and integrating a global experience into current practice or study. This book should unleash a new cadre of international health care volunteers, and, more important, shift the focus of the medical profession toward global health inequality.

**Kathryn E. Johnson
(Retired) CEO HEALTH FORUM**

AWAKENING HIPPOCRATES

A PRIMER ON HEALTH, POVERTY, AND GLOBAL SERVICE

EDWARD O'NEIL, JR, MD

FOREWORD BY PAUL FARMER, MD, PhD

AMA
AMERICAN MEDICAL ASSOCIATION

Library of Congress Cataloging-in-Publication Data

O'Neil, Edward.
   Awakening Hippocrates : a primer on health, poverty, and global service / by Edward O'Neil, Jr.
     p. cm.
   Summary: "A comprehensive overview of the current state of world poverty and health, directed to the health care provider interested in volunteering abroad"—Provided by publisher.
   Includes bibliographical references and index.
   ISBN 1-57947-772-0
   1. Poverty. 2. Public health. 3. Human rights. 4. Volunteer workers in medical care.   I. Title.
   [DNLM: 1. Poverty. 2. World Health. 3. International Cooperation. 4. Health Services Accessibility. 5. Voluntary Workers.   WA 530.1 O577a 2006]
HC79.P6O55 2006
362.1—dc22

                                          2005030364

Photos on pages 399 and 429 by Erica Anderson with permission of The Albert Schweitzer Fellowship.

ISBN 1-57947-772-0
BP08:05-P-042:02/06

To my parents, Edward Sr and Ruth, for your love and encouragement; your ethical examples were the greatest of gifts, and started me along this path.

To my brilliant wife Judy, my life partner and best friend, for supporting me every step along this path; you made this book possible.

And to our children, James, Michaela, and Sean, that you and your generation will follow the ideals depicted herein, and build a more just world than the one we are leaving you.

Contents

Acknowledgments

This book began as a concept in 1993, and evolved into a quest over the ensuing thirteen years. Its roots go back further, to my experiences as a medical student working in rural Tanzania in 1987. Because of its length, it has been rightly divided into two books, this one and its sequel, *A Practical Guide to Global Health Service*. Because this book has taken many years to write and so many people have influenced it, this might take a while, so sit back.

I will start with the group that has played the most important role: my family. I can never thank my wife, Judy, enough for her willingness to put aside her own careers, first in the FBI, and then in the law, to care for our kids at home while I pursued this quest. Judy has been a constant source of wisdom, support, and strength during this entire process. I avoid clichés whenever possible, but this one is unavoidable—without you, this book couldn't have happened. The writing of this book and its sequel has spanned the births of our three children, James, Michaela, and Sean. There is no doubt that the writing has taken me away from them far more than we had hoped, through missed vacations and years of late nights and weekends spent writing, but it is time, I hope, to make up. When my son crept downstairs to visit late at night or my daughter insisted that I draw "fishies" all over an early manuscript, they gave me reprieves from the work and brought more clearly into focus the reasons to continue.

Work in international health may seem far from work as a Boston police officer, the profession of my father and paternal grandfather. Yet both are service professions that ultimately look to the law for guidance; it's no real surprise that I ended up here. Both of my parents instilled a strong sense of justice, and the strong moral tone of this book very much reflects their influences on me. For years, they sacrificed to pay for college and help with medical school tuitions; I hope this book in some small repays that effort. My three older sisters too have always been there for me, and yes, all of those Beatles' records did make an impression. My uncle Frank became a close friend and strong supporter of this work—he knew as much about it as anyone; I was fortunate to spend his last days with him, and carry his love and support with me.

My earliest teachers in this realm were the late Dr Jack Millar at GWU and Sister/Dr Margaret Ann Meyer in Tanzania's Makiungu Hospital. Thanks for being so generous with your time and your willingness to answer scores of questions from an inquisitive student. The many poor that comprised the patients in that hospital and in Nazareth Hospital in Nairobi years later also shared valuable insights into their lives with me, insights that continue to shape my worldview. Father Dr Bill Fryda continues to inspire me and I value his friendship enormously. I count him among my most influential teachers. I hope that through this book, more people will become aware of his and his Kenyan team's extraordinary accomplishment that is St Mary's Hospital in Nairobi.

This book is inextricably linked to Omni Med, the NGO I founded in 1998. Many of the stories and people depicted herein come through Omni Med, and I will recognize many of them here. Belize became the site of the first Omni Med program and introduced me to an impressive group of people, whose stories course through this book. Loretta and Vincent Palacio have opened their home and their lives to me; I thank them for their friendship and influence over the many years we have worked together. Dr Peter Allen has been a friend and teacher since we first met in 1997. I've never met anyone who radiates such good cheer while working so hard. I greatly admire his dedication to improve the lives of all Belizeans, and value his insights into politics, aid, development, and service. Other important teachers for me in Belize include Dr Francis Smith, Dr Gil Paiz, Mr Austin Flores, Mr Bill Butcher, and the scores of physicians, nurses, and technicians throughout the hospitals in Belize that have allowed me to work among them and learn from their steadfast dedication to their work. I have long admired their ability to provide high quality medical care with such limited resources.

I came to Belize only because of an extraordinary group of individuals that came together under the banner of Rotary International. From the time I first met Richard Bridges, Sheldon Daly, Harold Lincoln, and Jim Roberts from the Hingham Rotary Club, I knew this group was special. Richard Bridges became a good friend and a model of ethical and servant leadership, while a host of other club members impressed me with their dedication to service. In Belize, a small group of people that comprised the Orange Walk Rotary Club joined up with the Hingham Rotarians to turn a small idea into a multi-million dollar service effort. I have the good fortune to count its many members among my teachers and friends in Belize, including Fred, Eduardo, and Ena Martinez, Chonita Escalante, Ms Terry (the divine "Ms T") Avila, Leslie and Javita Sharpe, Johnny Briceno, Ed Zetina, and many others. Bill and Kathy Butcher, Rod Allen, Dr Lesbia Guerra, Mr. John Waight, Joan Burke, Johnny Searle, Luis Alpuche, Pam Cardona, and Teresita Fabro have also helped considerably. Prime Minister Said Musa and many people in the Ministry of Health have supported our efforts from the start.

This book also owes an enormous debt to the people who make up Omni Med. All of this book's proceeds will go to Omni Med and directly into our programs, one of which is the maintenance of the database included in *The Practical Guide to Global Health Service*. To those who question why someone would work gratis for nearly ten years at an NGO, I can only advise them to look at our results. I am proud of those who have come into the Omni Med family and done such extraordinary things with so little funding. Dr John O'Brien has become a close friend and an indispensable part of our NGO's work in Belize and Guyana. Drs Mike Morley and Kathy Morrow joined our little effort in Belize and founded a successful program in Thailand that continues to expand. Dr James Eadie evolved from a promising student at Harvard Medical School into a seasoned physician who founded and now directs our program in Guyana. As I write this, he is serving with the US Air Force in Iraq; we all wish him health, safety, and a speedy return home. Dr John Varallo joined Omni Med and has turned a novel idea into a cervical cancer-screening program that is becoming a national model in Guyana. Peter and Nancy Mogielnicki have participated in almost all of our programs and introduced several other Dartmouth-Hitchcock physicians to Omni Med. For that and your ongoing support and involvement, thanks. None of these physicians is compensated for their time or effort; all cover their own travel expenses, and all share an ideal that we should be doing this. I can never thank each of you enough for your time, your sacrifice, and your extraordinary dedication to this cause. To the scores of health providers that have served through our various programs, I offer a heartfelt thanks.

Behind any effort like that of Omni Med's is a group that supports and sustains it. I could not have a better board of directors than the one we have, all with Kellogg Foundation roots. Dr Roger Sublett has supported my efforts from the beginning. He became the first board member, the first donor, and encouraged me from the outset to turn these ideas into a book and a functioning, living organization. Omni Med, and most likely this book, would not exist if not for the support, encouragement, friendship, and wise counsel of Dr Sublett. My study of ethical leadership offered no better example than the man who became an important mentor. Roger, thanks.

Our other board members have helped guide Omni Med and me through some turbulent times, many brought on by our dire finances. Dr Robert Sparks has always been there for me, always with the right take on any complicated situation that arises. Likewise, Kathryn Johnson has always been there personally and professionally, and has lent her great vision and strategic thinking to help plot our future course. Ambassador Harry Barnes has been a great friend and source for advice, and adds the seasoned experience that only a former US ambassador can add. I also thank all of the above for their invaluable contributions during the edits of this text, and for many valuable suggestions along the way. The late Dr Tom Durant served as a board member early on and freely provided his sage advice—always peppered with his biting commentary—during a friendship that lasted several years. Tom left a huge void when he left us and I count myself among the many who miss him and think of him often.

Many other people have supported the work of Omni Med through the years and warrant mention. Malcolm Visser has always challenged me to think more broadly and through the years has been a good friend, a teacher, a sounding board, and a generous supporter. Daren Samaweera has had the admirable tendency to back up strong beliefs with equally strong support in Omni Med and in other international programs, such as help for tsunami victims in Asia, for example. Drs Rick Foster and Thomas Bruce have also backed our efforts and have earned our eternal thanks.

During the roughly seven years of writing, a number of people contributed to this book within the context of Omni Med. Fran Wang has lent her technological expertise and her quiet competence and dedication for years. Dr Doreen Ho did some background research for a few early chapters; I am quite proud to watch her develop as a neurology resident at St Elizabeth's Hospital, and hope she will find her way back to international work. Dr Jamie McCabe first worked out of my living room before there was an Omni Med; I also expect great things from him. Many other students along the way worked on various aspects of Omni Med and this book, including Phillip Choi, Ian McClure, Maggie Zraly, Leila Strachan, David Monteiro, Ethan Merlin, Jane Humphries, Edward Chan, and Yioula Sigounas. Peter Cuomo lent his considerable legal skills to developing a glossary, editing hundreds of sources in the bibliography, and putting the final touches on the Omni Med database, which appears in the sequel to this book. Peter will no doubt make important contributions at whatever legal firm is fortunate enough to land him. Anne Lauriat brought Peter aboard and provided me with considerable help at just the right time.

A number of people generously gave of their time to read and offer important feedback on certain chapters. Rhena Schweitzer Miller was most gracious with her time and our regular phone conversations and occasional meetings offered me a trove of insight into her famous father's life and thought. She carefully edited the chapters about her father. Getting to know Rhena has been one of the true pleasures to emerge from this research, and I greatly value her friendship and support through the years. I hope this book will help in some small way to clarify her father's ideas and further his substantial contributions to forging a more just world order.

Many other people generously offered their feedback on several chapters herein. Robert Sparks read several, as did Kathryn Johnson, Harry Barnes, and Roger Sublett. Dr Ron Roskens read several chapters sent to him from a complete stranger and offered important insights. Sean, Stephen, and

Mrs. Frederica Durant all provided important feedback on the chapter about the late Dr Tom Durant. Father/Dr Bill Fryda and Dr Peter Allen were gracious in providing feedback on chapters about them, painful as it was for each. Demetria Royals read a difficult chapter on race and, as always, offered insightful feedback that I greatly value. Jim Kim offered feedback on the chapter about Paul Farmer and him, and served as a sounding board and advisor to me for all of the years of the writing of this book. Their NGO, Partners In Health, serves as an inspirational model to us all. A worldview that they have long espoused has seeped into the pages of this book, in large part because of Jim's advice and example. Dr John Ross, my colleague at St Elizabeth's Hospital, read several chapters and offered key insights and encouragement; I thank him for both.

Author William Zinsser selflessly offered his time and considerable editing skills to the earliest drafts of this manuscript. He taught me valuable lessons on the art of writing and the importance of editing. I owe him a great debt for whatever "clarity, brevity, simplicity, and humanity" comes through in the writing that follows. His classic book, *On Writing Well*, was my constant companion during most of this book's writing. Author Dr Jack Weatherford was always willing to discuss his experiences and has been a great source of advice throughout this process. Other authors, including Dr Drew Weston, Dr Wayne and Mary Sotile, and Teri Louden freely gave of their time and experience.

Suzanne Fraker, the senior acquisition editor at the American Medical Association, believed in this concept from the beginning, and pushed hard for over two years to make it become a reality. I owe her an enormous debt of gratitude for her perseverance, her strong will, her political acumen, and, most important, her basic humanity in seeing this through. I also thank the AMA for going out on a limb with this entire project. This book expresses ideas that are far from the mainstream and I am grateful that I had the editorial freedom to say things that I think need to be said, even if some may disagree. My editor, Katharine Dvorak, was patient and meticulous in her edits, and this final manuscript reflects her professional and caring touch. Best of luck to you and your husband as you embark on the incredible journey that is parenthood. Mary Kay Kozrya, who did the copyediting, also helped to iron out any grammatical errors. Together, they polished every line and made the finished product much better. Amy Postlewait Burgess came up with the intriguing cover design and has put considerable effort into making this book known; thank you. It has been a pleasure working with everyone at the AMA right from the beginning. Many thanks.

Every book has a contract making it legal and I am indebted to all of those attorneys from Kirkland and Ellis who worked for several months pro bono on behalf of Omni Med and me to see this through. Thanks to Dr Doreen and Derek Ho for making the connection and to Monica Tay for starting the ball rolling so many years ago. Rebecca Hazard and Kevin Rothman were models of patience and sage counsel, while Kate Dubin, Cristin Bolsinger, and Bradley Silver all contributed at key times. Micah Burch also gave generously of his time and modeled a professionalism and competency that I greatly admire and appreciate. All of these legal experts helped to steer this and the accompanying text to becoming Omni Med enterprises. It is right and fitting that all royalties will go to Omni Med, not me. I'd also like to thank Bill Mahony for his considerable pro bono work making Omni Med a legal entity back in 1998.

Any effort of this magnitude owes a considerable debt to those who have gone before; their voices course through this text. To paraphrase Sir Isaac Newton, I have had the good fortune to be able to stand on the shoulders of giants. Those giants are many, and warrant a brief mention. Albert Schweitzer, Paul Farmer, Jim Kim, Jeffrey Sachs, Gustavo Gutierrez, Laurie Garrett, Tom Dooley, Jonathan Mann, Jared Diamond, Randy Shilts, Greg Behrman, and Catherine Caufield all wrote articles and texts that greatly influenced core pieces of what follows here. Similarly, the scores of doctors, nurses, and other allied health personnel who have been brave enough to stake their lives firmly to a belief that the world order is imperfect and warrants fixing have influenced my writing. Further, the oft-muted voices of those who find themselves at the bottom of economic orders in societies throughout the world have greatly influenced the tone of what follows herein.

I owe a small debt to the musical and lyrical influences whose words grace the pages of the text, and have influenced me for as far back as I can remember. Bob Marley's music quite justifiably provides the background music for every developing country I've been in throughout Africa, the Caribbean, and the Americas. Similarly, Billie Holiday, the Beatles, Sting, U2, and a host of other artists inspire us all through their songs and hopeful messages. I have taken the liberty to add in musical selections in many of the chapters' introductions. I played piano in bars for years and find that music evokes a deeper feeling that is often beyond the range of even the most eloquent words. Much of what follows here may appeal to the mind but needs to be felt by the heart. Letting Billie Holiday, Marvin Gaye, or the Beatles play in the back of your mind while you read the following would not be a bad thing. Rather, it should help to set a mood, and may help to soften previously solidified feelings. Music has that effect. Each lyric has a particular message relevant to the chapter it heads. Besides, most medical professionals spend far too little time listening to music and dreaming anyway.

This text and its sequel took shape during my Kellogg fellowship in 1994 through 1997. In addition to the previous people mentioned from the Kellogg Foundation, I would like to acknowledge those Kellogg advisors, staff, and fellows who made a considerable impact on me and whose voices echo through what follows: Sanford Cloud, James Rocheleau, Patricia

Turner-Smith, Georgia Sorenson, Delores Parker, Bill Grace, Bruce Sherrick, Demetria Royals, Dan Mulhern, Elliott Gimble, Ellen Kahler, Ed DeJesus, Beth Beyer, Roger Casey, Markita Cooper, Carmen Foster, Sam Intrator, Kevin Dean, Julie Cowie, Dave Mattocks, Terry Plater, Cathy Raines, Lessa Phillips, Robert Jackson, Carlos Monteagudo, and Anna Sheppard. Steve Levitsky encouraged my original application way back when, and Ray Gotchalian was an inspirational figure whom I knew far too briefly and who left us far too soon. I'd also like to thank the W.K. Kellogg Foundation for providing me with such an incredible opportunity through the fellowship. Through that magical experience I met extraordinary, selfless leaders who share "a passion to make a difference," and ultimately, to make a better world. That collection of people and experiences influenced this text as much as any other entity, and added considerable depth. Again, my heartfelt thanks.

I divide my time between Omni Med and the emergency department at St Elizabeth's Medical Center in Boston. Before that, I worked at Lahey Clinic NorthShore; I'd like to thank the nursing staff there for their support during the early years of research and writing. At St Elizabeth's, I'd like to thank the nursing staff in the Emergency Department for your considerable support over the past six years. Your encouragement has provided me with an important source of strength during the more difficult times of this work. It has always been a pleasure and a privilege to work with you. A special thanks to Kathy Dawley for your interest and support; it has meant a lot. Three physician colleagues, Drs Sush Prusty, Howard Tarko, and Gian Corrado took an active interest and offered plenty of encouragement; for that and your friendship, thanks. Dr. Ali Tirmizi freely shared his views on Islam and gave me a copy of the Koran. Catherine Guarcello and Marybeth Edwards are librarians extraordinaire at St Elizabeth's; thanks for all of your help. I am fortunate to work with such an incredible collection of doctors, nurses, and other staff at St. Elizabeth's, where most of my family and I receive our health care.

Finally, I'd like to thank our friends and family for their patience during the writing of this book. John and Joan Stilla, Nancy, Corky, DJ, Rob and Jan, Ed D., Ed U., Joe, George, Rich, Ted, Mal, and several other close friends and neighbors, thanks for putting up with my frequent absences over these past several years. I hope the time can be made up.

Preface

On a balmy Wednesday afternoon in April 1994, an Italian surgeon named Carlo and I visited clinics in the Kariobangi and Dandora Slums in the northeast section of Nairobi, Kenya. Both were outreach clinics of Nazareth Hospital where we worked at the time. Of Greater Nairobi's 4 million people, roughly 40% live in conditions of extreme poverty, with many in slums (Fryda 2000, 10).

Within the Dandora Slum one finds the Nairobi City Dump, a place an appallingly large number of people call home. I have seen many shocking things while working in rural and urban settings in East Africa. However, I vividly recall one of the most surreal being that of people sitting in trash, picking through it for food, and having casual conversation while standing in piles of acrid smelling garbage in Dandora. Barefoot, young children played soccer just yards away from the fly-infested, rotting carcasses of several large dogs. One of the Catholic Sisters who worked at Kariobangi and assisted us that day estimated that of the 120,000 people living in the immediate slum areas, 80% were HIV positive. Her estimate, quite understandably, better reflected the dismal experiences of clinic work in Kariobangi than actual data. Current estimates place HIV positivity at 25% of Nairobi's slum-dwelling population.[1]

Of the many AIDS patients I saw that day, one remains forever fixed in my mind due to her innocent yet proud manner amid impossible circumstance. She sought our help for her progressive weakness, weight loss, and fever. Like everyone else trapped by the circumstances of life in Kariobangi, she was foremost a survivor. Being young and female limited her choices, so she did the only thing that she and many other young girls in the slums of Nairobi could do to survive—she became a prostitute. She either entertained johns or she starved; not much of a choice, really. Try to picture your mother or sister or daughter faced with the same choice. This young girl learned the oldest profession from lying under her now deceased mother's bed. In the one room shacks and huts that cover the slum landscape, the children either stay under the bed or go outside while the mother earns a living. Her mother got thirty shillings a night, the equivalent of less than one US dollar—and AIDS—as compensation. Now this girl was following in her mother's footsteps on the worn paths of Kariobangi—another AIDS orphan harshly sentenced for the crime of being born into poverty.

I interviewed her through a nun serving as interpreter, and examined her. She had large lymph nodes in her neck, under both arms and in her groin. Her mouth was filled with thrush and she was very thin.[2] She had beautiful features yet clearly bore the emaciated countenance of AIDS. Unfortunately, at the time we had nothing to offer her for the causes of her sickness—HIV and the poverty that led her to it. During the examination, she carefully avoided my eyes. I did not judge her; I understood she had no other options in how she survived. Still, she exuded shame and embarrassment, common feelings in those stigmatized by their illness. She knew the reason why she had been losing weight and having recurrent fevers. Her eyes revealed a street-born wisdom far beyond her years. Outside she was tough, inside a terrified little girl whose future was clear. As she walked away in silence, I felt the all too familiar feeling that one has in places like Kariobangi—that of my heart breaking. She was 10 years old.

How, we might ask, can it be that this young girl has no better survival option than becoming a prostitute—a profession that carries with it in places like Kariobangi the virtual certainty of acquiring AIDS? How, we might also ask, can poverty and disease devastate entire populations while the "developed" world mostly watches in silence or funnels aid dollars into elite pockets? More relevant for us, where are the doctors, nurses, and other health providers from a well-financed medical profession?

To answer these questions, we must first start by looking at our world with eyes fully open; it is a very imbalanced place. Nearly one third of the people in the least developed countries, mostly in sub-Saharan Africa, will die before reaching age 40 (United Nations Development Program [UNDP] 1997, 5), while the life expectancy gap between those in the wealthiest and poorest countries in the year 2000 was more than 25 years (UNDP 2002, 152). In poor countries each year, half a million women die in childbirth, at rates 10 to 100 times those in industrial countries (UNDP 1997, 3). The Joint United Nations Program on HIV/AIDS (UNAIDS) estimates that 40 million are now infected with HIV, including 2.5 million children.[3] Containing this epidemic—even providing basic health care—requires infrastructures that are far too often lacking in poor countries. Enormous disparities in health and health care still very much define our global order.

Such disparities have not gone unnoticed through time. A number of responses, from bilateral aid missions to multilateral World Bank efforts, have attempted to reduce global disparities in health with mixed results. But, some of the more successful ventures have come in the field of health. Albert Schweitzer and Tom Dooley elevated the status of the medical profession through their widely acclaimed work in Africa and South East Asia. Other committed individuals—William Larimer and Gwen Mellon,

Bernard Kuschner, Jonathan Mann, and Paul Farmer—have continued that tradition. Health workers from CARE, the International Committee of the Red Cross, and the United Nations (UN) have worked in some of the world's worst humanitarian crises over the past 50 years. A group of French physicians, Médecins Sans Frontières (MSF), changed the way we respond to disasters. A handful of physicians and scholars at Partners In Health changed the way the world treats tuberculosis. Teams of World Health Organization (WHO) public health officers conquered smallpox. Schweitzer, MSF, Amnesty International, and several specialized UN agencies have won the Nobel Peace Prize. All these people have placed a higher calling above personal comfort, professional advancement, or material acquisition. In so doing, they have tapped into the ethical, faith-based roots of our profession, where the art of medicine intersects with the highest aspirations of man.

Stories of people and organizations involved in this work have percolated down through the medical profession like surreal dreams. For most health providers, this realm has remained distant and seemingly inaccessible. "Mainstream" medicine has averted its gaze, concentrating on worthy but different priorities. Most individual health providers have followed suit, though not for a lack of interest. Many have expressed at least a modicum of interest in working internationally. Whether inspired by stories of Schweitzer, Farmer, or Dooley, or perhaps knowing someone who had served abroad, they have expressed to me a wish to reconnect with the ideals that first drew them to a career in health care, or to give something back in exchange for all they have derived from their work in the field.

Despite such interest, however, opportunities to serve abroad have long been hard to find, and relatively few providers have engaged. In one of the few surveys to date, Johns Hopkins' Dr Timothy Baker found that only 0.32% of physicians and 0.12% of nurses surveyed had been active in international health prior to the study's publication in *JAMA* in 1984 (Baker et al 1984, 502). While such dismal numbers have likely increased slightly over the past 20 years, it is time for a far wider swath of the medical profession to consider engaging where they are most needed, and for the ideal of international health service to move into the mainstream of the medical profession.

A logical first step is to make it easier for health providers to engage. That is the chief purpose of this book and its companion, *A Practical Guide to Global Health Service* (American Medical Association, 2006), both of which fill a void long known to those who have tried to do this work. For many people, the first step is to call the Peace Corps, then MSF or other well-known nongovernmental organizations (NGOs), where they frequently fail to find the opportunity they are looking for, and stop their search. Those who do serve abroad often do so with little advance preparation, with little research into the "critical reflections" that should inform this kind of work. Much of the literature surrounding this work describes charitable, short-term endeavors rather than justice-based work designed cooperatively with those in the host countries. The history of international health service is full of stories of people who went abroad with the best intentions but did little to help—or even harmed—those they sought to aid. This book will help you think about these issues, and its companion, *A Practical Guide to Global Health Service*, will provide the practical information you need.

Why This Book?

Three simple observations fueled this text. First, the United States and most wealthy countries have a large cadre of health care providers whose healing powers now reach unprecedented levels due to an explosion in the biomedical sciences over the last 60 years. In rich countries, it's easy to see the doctor; according to the UN, there were just 362 people for every physician in the United States during the 1990s. In other rich countries, like France and Sweden, the ratios were comparably low (UNDP 2003, 254). In many urban areas like Boston, where I live and practice, the ratio is even lower. In these advanced countries, the steady progress of medical science has made our ability to heal greater than at any time in history. We regularly perform miracles that prior generations could scarcely dream of.

Second, however, our profession has an Achilles' heel: that our knowledge and talents remain concentrated among those who can afford them. We have fallen short of the lofty ideals rooted in our profession's creed. That most of the world's poor lack adequate health care is painfully clear to anyone who works clinically in or travels to a poor country. Consider the people-to-physician ratios in sub-Saharan Africa. In the same years that the people-to-physician ratio in the United States was 362:1, the ratio in Burundi was 100,000:1; that of Ethiopia was 33,333:1; Central African Republic, 25,000:1; and Angola, 20,000:1 (UNDP 2003, 257).

Third, there is an ethical imperative that compels us to care for all who need our services. When confronted with a critically ill patient, our first impulse is not to question how this person will pay for our care, but to provide it. Such impulses stem from a shared ethic in the clinical practice of medicine, with roots that date back to the religious prophets of antiquity. Today, however, our profession has moved away from these values, increasingly consigned to the dictums of the marketplace.

How This Book Is Designed and How to Use It

This book was originally conceived as an orientation to the world of poverty and health for health providers, in the hope that more health providers would serve internationally where most needed. As such, the first version contained a comprehensive overview of the important issues, a section of inspirational biographies, a pragmatic section on the mechanics of serving overseas, and finally, an extensive database of international health service opportunities with a cross-referencing section to make all searches far easier. However, I soon realized that there was simply too much material for one text. The material was subsequently split into two books, this one and a companion, *A Practical Guide to International Health Service*, which is also published by the American Medical Association. The split was a logical and natural one, with this book covering the macro issues of poverty, health and ethics, while leaving the more practical matters of international health service to the *Guide*. This split has the advantage of fitting more cleanly into specific reader interests; the topics covered in this book should have a far broader appeal for those even outside of health care, while primarily those who are planning on travel overseas will be interested in the *Guide* and its pragmatic material and database. As constructed, this book thus serves as an introduction to the world of poverty and health in the hope that readers will be motivated to serve. Although targeted at health care providers, it is by no means restricted to them. I believe the issues covered in this book are among the most important of our time; *everyone* should understand them. In addition, although better health provides one of the keys to reducing global poverty, it will require far more than health care providers alone to accomplish this feat. We will need those from business, government, education, and many other realms.

Taken together, these books are designed both to inform and to motivate. Those who read them and then serve internationally through any of the organizations listed in the *Guide* will have fully taken advantage of what these books offer. The whole is a map and compass through which many will find their way to service. The realm of international health service has long been characterized as a charitable endeavor built on the good intentions of the medical community at large. While such notions have their basis in truth, there is far more to the story, and all who enter this realm should first reflect on the reasons why those of us from the privileged parts of the world first came to be in a position to offer assistance. Why, after all, is it that those from Sub-Saharan Africa are not sending relief supplies to Michigan in lieu of current practices? This book will provide answers to many of the jolting questions that inevitably arise during service.

This book is comprised of two parts. Part 1, "Understanding Global Disparities in Health," offers a view of the world through the lenses of health and ethics. Before entering a world of poverty and health resource scarcity, one should consider the forces at work that create and maintain such dire conditions. I start by explaining some important concepts, including health, structural violence, and poverty. Given the importance of poverty to health, I then analyze the hold that poverty has over people in rich and poor countries alike. Following a reconstruction of the history that has led to unprecedented levels of health in the industrialized world, I review how some of the knowledge in public health and biomedical science has diffused throughout the world and how some UN agencies have improved the health of the poor. Because the NGO sector comprises a core part of the rich world's response to poverty, I trace the rise of this sector through some tumultuous periods of recent world history and examine some representative groups. Because international health service falls under the larger umbrella of development, and so many mistakes have been made in this realm, I trace the history of bi- and multilateral aid and place this all in perspective. I then dissect out the "forces of disparity" that shape our world order, including racism, sexism, AIDS, inequality, governance, militarism, history, and trade, among others.

The forces of disparity will ultimately give way to ethics and the rule of law, informed by the best our civilization has thus far offered. As such, the conclusion of Part 1 brings us to the foundation of the Universal Declaration of Human Rights (UDHR), formed in the aftermath of World War II.

The UDHR offers a new paradigm of essential, guaranteed "rights" to which all people lay claim as a birthright. In tracing their evolution, we find that world religious and legal thought from all cultures created the fabric of this document, once described as a "glimmering thread in a web of power and interest" (Glendon 2001, 19). By focusing its collective efforts on human rights, the NGO community has advanced its struggle for the betterment of mankind to a higher ground, at times with the help of, and at times at odds with host governments. By reviewing the emphasis that world monotheistic religions place on relief for the poor and tracing these origins to their inclusion in the UDHR, we conclude a journey that ultimately comes full circle. We then turn our broad understanding of the forces involved to the 10-year-old girl who opened this chapter. Can we still view her struggle from a distance? The will to elevate the least fortunate among us is ultimately a challenge neither for our intellect nor our strength, but for our collective will, rooted in ethics.

In Part 2, "Icons and Inspirations," I consider the life stories of health service veterans who inspire us all through their work. Some, such as Albert Schweitzer, Tom Dooley, and Paul Farmer are more widely known. Others, however, like Father Bill Fryda, Peter Allen, Jim Kim, and Tom Durant, are people I have had the good fortune to know and work with through the years. They are all heroes to me; I have written brief biographies on each and tried to use their own words whenever possible to tell their life stories. I include this section because I find there are a lot of people who would like to do this work, but for one reason or another, never do. Sometimes a little inspiration is all that is missing.

In the end of Part 2, I review Albert Schweitzer's philosophy, termed "Reverence for Life." The reader might ask why so much time is devoted to Schweitzer and Reverence for Life. The answer is a simple one; the answers to many of the stated problems are not intellectual, they are deeper. We can read about poverty and study economics, or the negative effects of some

World Bank programs on the poor. Yet it will only be through studying ourselves and our role in the world that real transformational change can take place. Schweitzer articulated these ideals as well as anyone who has worked in this realm. His is a timeless ideal, and one that anyone entering service work in poor areas should consider. His ethic resonates well with the stated ideals of the three major monotheistic religions, liberation theology, and the UDHR, all of which I will cover.

For those who finish this text and decide to serve internationally, the companion text to this one, *A Practical Guide to International Health Service* will provide the information necessary for health providers, and anyone else interested in serving internationally, to go and serve. Briefly, the *Guide* discusses the practical aspects of how one can safely and effectively serve internationally. It covers how one can overcome the chief obstacles of fear, time and money constraints, work and family obligations, and inertia. It contains concise discussions on travel, booking cheap flights, and reducing dangers while abroad, among many others. Culture is a landmine in of itself and this is covered in depth. The bulk of the *Guide* includes the Omni Med Database of International Health Service Opportunities, which may be the most comprehensive of its kind. It includes complete information on more than 240 organizations that send health personnel abroad. A cross-referencing section allows for specific searches quickly and easily. For example, a medical student interested in short-term service in Kenya could quickly find which organizations use medical students, have short-term opportunities, and go to Kenya, simplifying searches that previously took weeks. All members of the health profession, including doctors, nurses, hospital administrators, technicians, and more can easily find the organizations that seek their services. Many of these organizations also employ non-health professionals in their overseas programs as well.

It is my sincere hope that you will use this text wisely, in a manner that will assist those who need you. We stand at the dawn of the new millennium, filled with possibility and hope. We in the health profession can be stewards of a new age of reasoned compassion. Ours is a unique position in the world and in the societies of man. I urge you to make full use of the information that follows, reflect on the critical questions, and finally, to act. Whether through the political process, any of the civil service organizations involved in these struggles, or best of all, directly through international service, there is no shortage of opportunities for you. You have only to choose.

Endnotes

1. Conversation with Father Bill Fryda, MD, in June 2002. Father Bill Fryda, a Catholic priest, physician, and veteran of 20 years in East Africa places the number closer to 25%, based on data acquired at St Mary's Hospital in Nairobi, on the edge of the Kibera Slum.

xxii Awakening Hippocrates

2. Clinically, her weight loss, chronic fever (both major signs), generalized adenopathy, and oropharyngeal candidiasis (both minor signs) qualified her for the WHO case definition of AIDS in Children (less than or equal to 12 years old). This clinical constellation of signs does not require HIV serological testing for confirmation. See *Hunter's Tropical Medicine and Emerging Infectious Diseases, 8th Edition* (W.B. Saunders, 2000).
3. For more information, go to the UNAIDS web site at www.unaids.org.

Foreword

Having worked mostly in places where to be poor means to be bereft of rights, I saw early, as a student of medicine, the panicky dead end faced by so many of the destitute sick. Most of the dead ends I witnessed early on were in rural Haiti, but these scenes are played out again and again throughout the world: a young woman who welcomes her infant into the world and a few days later is dead from a readily prevented or treated infection. A child writhing in the spasms of a terrible infectious disease for which a vaccine has existed—for over a century. A young coworker whose guts are irreparably shredded by bacteria from impure water. An 8-year-old caught in a cross-fire. Young people consumed slowly by wasting diseases such as AIDS and tuberculosis. A pregnant woman whose life, and that of another, are one day ended suddenly by malaria.

Fighting such "stupid deaths"—a Haitian term—is never the work of one person, or of even a small group. I've had the privilege of joining many others seeking to provide medical care and other basic services to people who would otherwise not enjoy them. Most of my coworkers are not physicians or nurses; they are community health workers. But the number of physicians eager to serve is impressive and growing; so is the amount that can be accomplished by tools now at our disposal, but unavailable to the destitute sick. It is impossible to count the number of medical students and physicians (and of course many others) who ask, "What is to be done?"

All of the stupid deaths mentioned above can be averted; it's been done again and again and the methods are by and large well documented. There is great satisfaction to be had in the doing, in "simply" providing competent medical care to the needy. But after many years at the task, the doing itself, even when successful on a small scale, was never quite reward enough. Seeing health care as a right *is* a worthy goal, but here the path forward has been littered with failure. Failure because, short of resources, we were forever supplicants to institutions with power, money, and the ability to decide the fates of hundreds of millions of souls. Failure because ill health, we learned (as had many before us), is caused mostly, at least in the places we've worked, by poverty and violence and inequality—and what were we doing to fight those? Failure because every premature death, witnessed or otherwise, was a rebuke. But failure in this painful undertaking brought new clarity to the second, the third, the thousandth attempt to provide health care and other basic rights for the most vulnerable.

The most vulnerable, many of whom do fight for their rights, are not often invited to write or preface books. But the destitute sick are very present in this magisterial new volume by Dr Ed O'Neil. *Magisterial* is a word that's probably much overused in forewords, but it's an apposite word to describe *Awakening Hippocrates*. We at last have, in this moving book and in a companion volume, *A Practical Guide to Global Health Service*, an authoritative overview that allows the reader to understand not only how poverty and inequality shorten lives in a time of medical miracles but also what can be done about it.

A book like this—which leads from an analysis of why things are the way they are to a consideration of what is to be done and finally to advice on how to do it—takes a long time in gestation. I remember meeting with Dr O'Neil when this project was little more than a table of contents buttressed by a great deal of conviction. He intended to offer a largely medical audience a distillation of what we need to know about the political economy of health and illness across the globe; he promised a critical review of medical ethics and an exploration of health and human rights. Dr O'Neil intended to link such a review with inspirational stories and a how-to guide that would allow concerned professionals and students (and, indeed, anyone) to become involved in efforts to remedy inequalities of access and outcome that mark modern medicine and public health. "It's too grand a project," I worried out loud. "How can you cover all that in one book?"

On one score I was correct: this will be a two-volume effort. The pragmatic how-to *Guide*, which will be invaluable to students and others seeking placements in the right projects and to faculty who seek to help them, will soon follow *Awakening Hippocrates*. Included in this first volume is a substantive—scholarly and critical but very readable—review of "global disparities in health." When O'Neil uses the word *global*, it is not simply as a gloss for *overseas*. This book looks at both local and transnational disparities of risk and outcome, giving us the numbers, which are jarring, and linking dispassionate analysis with his own personal experience as an American physician with significant clinical experience in his own country and in others. O'Neil also reviews attempts, many of them botched, to respond to the problem of health inequalities through the vast development assistance apparatus and through other forms of aid. In so doing, he offers us a critical analysis of international health, a series of object lessons that all of us need to consider as we proceed.

Part 2, "Icons and Inspirations," introduces the reader to physicians who have tried, in Dr O'Neil's view, to live up to the promise of our profession. We learn something about what inspires or inspired them. Even this book's appendices are worth close attention if you'd like to learn, for example, what the Universal Declaration of Human Rights has to say about the right to health care. Or what the Millennium Development Goals are and why they (or goals like them) are so important to attain if we're to have any hope of starting and sustaining effective medical and public-health programs. If O'Neil's analysis is sound, which I believe it is, then physicians and allied health professionals need to know how and why conventionally defined medical interventions must be linked to poverty alleviation.

I know of no other project that has been able to link such sound analysis to the pragmatic advice that all of us need as we ask and answer (sometimes without ever learning the lessons of those who've gone before us) the "what's-to-be-done" question. Many Americans who have worked among the world's poorest have read, and used, the handbook *Where There Is No Doctor*. Throughout O'Neil's book, we learn what some physicians have done in settings in which there are, in fact, very few trained medical professionals. But *Awakening Hippocrates* also asks, and answers, the question, "*Why* is there no doctor?" It asks why physicians have not done more to promote health care as a right rather than merely a commodity. O'Neil looks unflinchingly at what he terms the Achilles Heel of our profession: "that our knowledge and talents remain concentrated among those who can afford them."

And yet there is an army of medical students and physicians and nurses, young and old, now seeking to engage the problems examined so carefully in this book. If you have or might describe yourself in this way, *Awakening Hippocrates* and the companion *Guide* are the books for you. Fifteen years of teaching medical students and physicians leads me to conclude that there is a vast reservoir of untapped talent and training and enthusiasm waiting to be brought into a movement for global health equity. At Harvard Medical School, for example, half of all medical students spend time in service projects in the urban United States or abroad. At the Brigham and Women's Hospital, there was so much demand for more serious attention to health inequalities that we were called to start a special residency program in order to train physicians to address health disparities effectively in the United States and in the poorest parts of the world (similar training programs are being established at Duke, the University of Miami, and Stanford University; other teaching hospitals and universities will surely follow suit). Partners In Health, the nongovernmental organization we founded to serve as the "effector arm" that would permit health professionals to use their training on behalf of the destitute sick, has been overwhelmed with offers from volunteers.

One of the tools needed to engage such goodwill is a book, or two of them, reviewing the major problems confronting all of us who seek to promote the right to health care and also a detailed guide describing organizations and networks that can link health professionals to those who need their services most. The American Medical Association (AMA) is due thanks for publishing this massive project. It is only fitting that the AMA do its part to respond not only to the massive need for better health care, in this country as elsewhere, but also to respond to the growing demand from US physicians and medical students who wish to do their part to respond to an appalling persistence of unmet need.

I risk repeating myself in thanking Dr Ed O'Neil for keeping his promise to hold our collective feet to the fire and allow us to live up to the noble goals of medicine and public health. I'm sorry I ever doubted it could be done. *Awakening Hippocrates* may be magisterial, but it is also beautifully written and well documented. With its companion volume, *A Practical Guide to Global Health Service*, it fills a huge gap in the armamentarium of those who believe in the goodwill of so many health professionals and each day ask and answer the question, "What is to be done?"

Paul Farmer, MD, PhD
Brigham and Women's Hospital
Harvard Medical School
and
Partners In Health

Introduction

Martin Luther King, Jr, once said, "The racial problem in America will be solved to the degree that every American considers himself personally confronted with it" (Cloud 1996). We can extend a similar analogy to the problem of global health inequality. This problem too will only be solved to the degree to which each of us feels personally confronted by it—particularly those of us in the health profession. That remains difficult if the overwhelming majority of health providers remain secluded away in the relative comfort of the industrialized world.

It is only through an active engagement with the poor that our perspectives can evolve. Gustavo Gutierrez, the father of liberation theology, once advised people to forget the "head trip" of studying the problems of the poor and take a "foot trip" to work among them (Brown 1990, 50). Only through such engagement, he argued, can we begin to work with them toward solutions. Poverty remains the most important killer in the world, and the best way to understand it is to work with those who live under its yoke.

While working abroad, we may also acquire the tools needed to affect political change here at home. The forces that serve to maintain current global disparities in health are both powerful and largely invisible. Many stem directly from decisions made by governments in the United States and other industrialized countries. Yet, doctors, administrators, nurses and other workers in the profession remain widely respected. When they speak, the public usually listens. If more health providers would take a role in attacking the global inequalities in health, great change would result. Influencing the levers of power in the United States may more greatly affect change for the global poor than an army of doctors volunteering their services abroad.

In that process, we may also save the lives of some of our young soldiers. As this was being written in 2005, a steady drumbeat of killed or wounded young American soldiers returning home from Iraq echoed through the United States. It is fitting to ask whether there is anything that we, as individuals, can do to reduce such conflicts. A 1994 Central Intelligence Agency study found that "state failure"—defined as war, genocide, or disruptive regime changes—followed three common characteristics in a given country: lack of democracy, lack of "openness" of an economy, and a rising infant mortality rate (Sachs 2001a, 187). In other words, societies that fail to listen to their people, close themselves off from the world, and don't care for their most vulnerable, tend to fail, producing war or chaos. Failed states inevitably become "seedbeds of violence, terrorism, international criminality, mass migration and refugee movements, drug trafficking, and disease." This same study, which tracked 113 cases of state failure between 1957 and 1994, also found that state failure preceded every instance of US military intervention abroad since 1960. While the perpetrators of the horrific 9/11 attacks may have been wealthy Saudis, their Al Qaida associates found sanctuary in the impoverished, failed state of Afghanistan. To prevent war, we might look more closely at means to bring health and stability to poor countries abroad. We might even revisit the concept of a US International Health Service Corps, albeit one primarily focused on training and education (Baker and Quinley 1987, 2622; US Congress 1987; Kindig et al 1984, 10).

We can best do this by sharing our knowledge, our wealth, and our most valuable resource of all, our people. Perhaps nowhere is this as important as through those who care for the sick. In the Millennial Survey of 1999, people around the world rated "good health" as their number one concern, reflecting long-held patterns.[1] From my research on the rise of health in the industrialized world, it is clear that the transfer of knowledge among nations has contributed more than any other factor to steady increases in life expectancies everywhere.

In the process of addressing such global inequalities, those who undertake this work will share some great experiences. During the last 17 years, I've traveled to Africa, Central and South America, and Asia. I've hitchhiked through East Africa, played in piano bars in Europe and Asia, and scaled Mayan ruins in the jungles of Central America. Along the way, I've met some remarkable people, seen some of the wonder of the world, and come to better understand myself and the nature of man. I have been able to look back on the culture of my birth and see it clearly for the first time. Living and working abroad has enriched my life and that of my family beyond anything else I can imagine. Although I want my fellow providers to serve internationally because there is such dire need and because we are ethically compelled to do so, I also want more providers to share in a truly uplifting experience. Most who go wonder why it took them so long to get involved.

Some clinicians may ask: why should those of us who are comfortable, after years of hard work reaching a certain position in the health profession, bother with those who are suffering? We can find answers from a variety of sources. Christianity, Judaism, Islam, and almost every other faith share worldviews rooted in social justice. Each commands its adherents to care for the poor while creating a just world order. A branch of Christianity called Liberation Theology compels its adherents to follow the scriptures and *act* to free the poor from their oppression. Similarly, the expanding paradigm of human rights informs us that each person has a birthright to life, health, education, freedom, and the dignity that comes from membership in the human race.

Albert Schweitzer searched world theology and philosophy, ultimately arriving at the principle, "Reverence for Life," which compels each of us to care for all of the life around us, including people not within our traditional realm of concern. He added a message to the comfortable,

> Just as the wave cannot exist for itself, but is ever a part of the heaving surface of the ocean, so must I never live my life for life itself, but always in the experience which is going on around me. It is an uncomfortable doctrine which the true ethics [of Reverence for Life] whisper to my ear. You are happy, they say; therefore you are called upon to give much (Schweitzer 1949a, 321).

From a practical perspective, the summons is equally strong. AIDS, MDR TB, and many other infectious pathogens that arise from poverty ultimately threaten all of humanity. We ignore such lessons at our own peril. Paul Farmer has written extensively on the microbial links that still connect the poor with the affluent, "despite all the barriers our age has set up to separate them" (Kim et al 2000, xiv). Farmer also found the following passage, written well over a century ago by physician and writer William Budd, warning of the dangers of typhoid,

> This disease not seldom attacks the rich, but it thrives among the poor. But by reason of our common humanity we are all, whether rich or poor, more nearly related here than we are apt to think. The members of the great human family are, in fact, bound together by a thousand secret ties, of whose existence the world in general little dreams. And he that was never yet connected with his poorer neighbor, by deeds of charity or love, may one day find, when it is too late, that he is connected with him by a bond which may bring them both, at once, to a common grave (Budd, 1931, 174).

When we consider that MDR-TB, HIV, Ebola, and Lassa have all freely traversed international borders, we should reconsider just how "other" they are who are most commonly afflicted. The idea that one group of people can remain isolated from any other group should have long ago expired. SARS should have destroyed any remaining illusions. The next plague, the one that will inevitably follows AIDS, is just one short airplane flight away. The sooner we embrace all of humanity, the better our prospects for long-term survival will be.

There is yet one more compelling reason for this undertaking: to dispel widely held beliefs about poor people that say, "People are poor because they are lazy, stupid, or immoral. They simply need to pull themselves up by their bootstraps and get a job." One does not have to look far to find those with such beliefs. As this book will show, however, the reality is far different from the mythology surrounding poverty. People are poor for reasons that are complex and largely invisible to those of us who live in relative comfort in the wealthier countries. Most people are not, in fact, poor chiefly due to their own faults. Some are lazy, some hard working, some good and some bad, but the overwhelming majority of people are poor because the array of forces aligned against them is utterly insurmountable. For those of us venturing to work among them, it is important to try, at the outset, to understand the constraints under which they live their lives. It is far easier to find fault and abandon rather than to understand complex issues and engage, and the default mode for many through the years has been to blame the victims for the problems they face. As such, it is easier not to "waste" the money, or spend the time and energy required on those deemed somehow unworthy. One of the chief reasons for undertaking the rather daunting task of outlining the historical and modern factors that create global disparities in health and survival is to eliminate this possibility. People may find other reasons to avoid this work, but it should not be because those most in need don't warrant the effort.

Charity and Justice

Dr King once wrote, "The moral arc of the universe is long, but it bends toward justice." I picture this "moral arc" as a tangible reality, consisting of increasing degrees of righteousness, clarity of purpose, and importance to the poor as we move toward its end. Inherent within such an arc lie the ideals of both charity and justice. Charity is a core principle both in Judaism and Christianity and is one of the five pillars of Islam. It conveys a love of man for fellow man, or benevolence, often manifested through acts of kindness to those in need. Charity is also the term that best describes much of the medical literature on international health service.

Most of the medical service work that we read about is worthwhile, though constrained by a lack of perspective. In the realm of "charity," those who give to the less fortunate are, by wide agreement, doing good work. Their motives and their methods, however, are rarely questioned. Author Christopher Hitchens wrote, "The rich world likes and wishes to believe that someone, somewhere, is doing something for the Third World. For this reason it does not inquire too closely into the motives or practices of anyone who fulfills, however vicariously, this mandate" (Hitchens 1997, 49). Because the givers are doing good works, their methods remain beyond reproach. The history of charitable endeavors abroad is littered with the harm that results from well intended, though poorly informed people who undertake such work. Even the large bi- and multilateral donors have made huge errors due to a lack of perspective. Program designs often accomplish far less than they could have had the founders only thought more broadly at their inception. Further, by following subconscious "charitable" notions, we may even become trapped by a blinding self-righteousness, unable to hear criticism from the oft-muted voices of those with the greatest stakes involved. We may fail to search out deeper root causes to the harsh realities we see; even exonerate ourselves after learning that we are very much complicit in maintaining orders of inequality.

Most of the focus of charitable work remains on the giver. A typical medical mission reported in the literature describes how a group of health providers provided care in a poor setting, left, and then expressed thanks for the opportunity to call a place like the United States "home." Those they cared for remain poor, unfortunate people, unable to help themselves. The "poor" thus remain mere passive recipients of the benevolent acts of the more fortunate.

While charity has its place, it is important to reflect on our motivations for undertaking such work. We must look behind the veil of humanitarianism to understand how our own motivations might clash with the needs and desires of those whom we hope to serve. How might we turn the noble impulse of "charity" into something more powerful?

> *While charity has its place, it is important to reflect on our motivations for undertaking such work. We must look behind the veil of humanitarianism to understand how our own motivations might clash with the needs and desires of those whom we hope to serve.*

Let's take a deeper look at the point in Dr King's "moral arc" where it bends "toward justice." Justice is a fundamental concept in our worldview, defined by Merriam Webster as "the use of power and authority to uphold what is right, just, or lawful." Just such a process did occur during the framing of the Universal Declaration of Human Rights in the aftermath of World War II. (See Chapter 10.) Yet the concept of justice requires more work than that of a charitable act. Charity focuses our attention on the comfortable, familiar domain of the giver, while justice demands that we focus our attention on the unseemly and disturbing world of those on the receiving end. In charity, we can send some surplus supplies abroad, or we can give our time and skills to those in need. But, to arrive at justice, we are required to take a far more arduous journey. We need to understand the needs and desires of the poor as well as the forces that constrain their hopes or very existence. Such understanding does not come easily. Many of the answers to the most pressing questions lie buried deep under common presuppositions that we rarely challenge. The very recordings of our society preclude an honest assessment for the majority of us.

The basic question, "Why are they poor?" answers the question, "Why are they sick?" and requires that we understand the complex worlds of trade relations, history, racism, sexism, foreign aid flows, development, governance and global financial flows, among others, all of which conspire to perpetuate poverty. Only through such work can we understand what is real in the world. At such a time, many of the arguments that historically blame the victims fall away. We can then target our efforts at the forces most responsible, crafting solutions while working directly with those in poor communities.

This is a tall order for the medical profession. We have long viewed the world through the comfortable position of providing life-enhancing care on a daily basis. Ours is truly a profession that allows us to do well while doing good work. That we care for the sick, and do so with such competence, provides us with sufficient moral cover. We can hear of others responding to the ills of the world and consider ourselves involved, if only through our daily work. Yet, there is far more required of us, both abroad in poor settings, and at home in the corridors of power.

On Transformation: An Introduction to Poverty and Health in East Africa

Albert Schweitzer once said, "In influencing others, example is not the main thing, it is the only thing." As such, I share my story here—with humility—in the hope that others will see the value and power of the experience, as well as how easy it is to get involved. My experiences in East Africa, Central America, and beyond raised questions that ultimately shaped the design and content of this text. They also transformed me.

When I was a third-year medical student at George Washington University, I happened to hear a lecture given by a charismatic doctor who was just back from two years working in rural Kenya. He told stories of operating by flashlight, of baboons running off with surgical instruments, and of becoming the only means for patients in that rural part of Kenya to receive that level of medical care. He spoke of a quiet dignity in the local tribes, of people accustomed to early death but grateful for the doctor who helped them to cheat it just a little. After he finished his lecture, I sensed that something important had just happened to me. His was a world that held a strange allure, and I was soon planning my first trip abroad.

At GWU at that time, a man named Jack Millar worked as the international studies coordinator. He had been everywhere, serving the US Navy in Micronesia and other locales in the South Pacific. His office was a windowless room no larger than a prison cell, but there he painted a world of endless possibility that fired my imagination. He arranged an elective for me at Makiungu Hospital in the heart of Tanzania, East Africa. When I left in January 1987, I had little preparation for and almost no understanding of the realm I was entering.

The flights from Washington to London to Nairobi took 18 hours covering 7,200 miles. The overland trip from Nairobi, Kenya to Singida, Tanzania took 10 days, covering 500 miles. The rainy season had made a simple trip difficult. The public bus skidded along rain-slicked mountainous roads until it mercifully became stranded once the skies opened up. I then

hitchhiked from mission to mission until I finally reached Makiungu
Hospital. During those first days in Africa I entered for the first time a world
of poverty and experienced the mind-numbing realism that is so difficult at
first to comprehend. The reality of this other world soon balanced any naïve,
idealistic notions I harbored at the time. I experienced what Dr Tom Dooley
bluntly called, "the stink and misery in which idealism must rub its nose"
(Fischer 1997, 171).

The long trips by *matatu* (a small van) gave me my first views of life
as it is in Africa. At each stop, crowds swarmed over all of the foreigners,
trying to sell us carvings, wares, or fruit. Many of the people showed clear
signs of pathology, some limping, others rail thin, clearly wasting away;
others with a plethora of physical deformities. I could clearly see the pathos
in the eyes of many. Everywhere, there were hordes of such people, many
just sitting, watching, idly passing the day sheltered from the sun, or begging.

I had not previously realized the level of misery that defined existence
for so many. Seeing it was so much more powerful than reading about it, and
I recall feeling overwhelmed by the deprivation. Some might say I was experiencing the beginnings of culture shock, but it felt like more of an awakening. I settled in to the mission house in Arusha where an overwhelming
sense of despair enveloped me. I couldn't get the images of poverty out of
my mind. It was as if the images had wrapped themselves around me and
pervaded all my senses. I could smell the raw sewage, hear the dogs barking
in the village market, and see all of those thin, wretched individuals just sitting and watching, seeming to want to be anywhere else. I sat under the
omniscient gaze of an icon of Jesus in stunned silence until the last strains of
daylight faded into evening. It was several hours before I ventured outside
into the beauty and mystery of the African night. I gazed with wonder at the
curious beauty of the star-filled night sky, such a stark contrast to the misery
and the seeming hopelessness below. Those first days in Africa were powerful,
but paled in comparison to the experience of working among these people.

I went to work in Makiungu Hospital, which rises out of the grassy,
hilly terrain of central Tanzania. There, diseases infrequently seen in the
Western world scattered bodies across the ward floors and clogged the
small waiting area of the outpatient department. People slept two to a bed
and three to a floor mat. Many of the patients suffered from such "tropical"
illnesses as malaria, typhoid, polio, tuberculosis, leprosy, and schistosomiasis. The year was 1987, but we saw no AIDS in this rural area, far from
the main truck routes. I saw easily treated illnesses that had become serious
after going untreated for months or years, an all-too-common result of no
available health care. Operable tumors had grown inoperable and routine infections had progressed to osteomyelitis (infected bone) or gangrene (infected,
often dying tissue), requiring amputation as a life-saving measure. Many
children stared blankly, bearing the listlessness of those suffering from
starvation-induced diseases of merasmus or kwashiorkor. Road accidents

often caused death and serious injury. The "disease burden" of these people was overwhelming, though their grace under such adversity was admirable.

Nevertheless, I found the work immensely rewarding, largely due to the quality of the people there. I had come to offer my meager skills to these poor people and to learn medicine in a way that was not possible at home. I had naively assumed that they needed my help and would learn from my presence among them—even as a medical student. However, I gained far more from them than the reverse. Like brilliant flowers blooming from volcanic rock, I saw the beauty of a people trapped in the death grip of poverty and impossible circumstance. They always welcomed me and offered food, drink or whatever they had. These "poor people" had great insight into life and the ways of man. For many of them, all they had was each other, so they treated each other as life's most precious commodities. They cared for each other in ways that many in the "developed world" seem to have forgotten. Distant relatives prepared meals for, bathed, and generally cared for patients they hardly knew. They were related, somehow, and that was all that mattered. Many African cultures stress the importance of the extended family and for many, that belief represents the sole, wispy thread of survival.

As a medical student working in East Africa, I had the privileged position to know people well. Through the intimacy of so many clinical interactions, I gained a unique insight into their culture. I was with people when they died. I watched as pain covered the face of a young mother who lost her young son to typhoid fever. I was stunned when she momentarily cast aside her grief and wholeheartedly thanked us for trying our best. Every morning an elderly man paralyzed from the neck down greeted me with a smile. His wife did the same as she bathed him, fed him, and lifted his—and our—spirits. I recognized true Grace when a poor farmer offered me a goat for caring for his extensive burns.

I can still vividly picture the first time I walked by the male medical ward at night. The night was clear and the sky was filled with stars. As I approached the ward, I heard the sound of laughter. I recall wondering how there could be that much joy amid so much sickness and suffering. It was a question that I revisited many times while there. I briefly glimpsed the power of the human spirit while working in Makiungu.

I had learned a valuable lesson about working with the poor. I had come to see them as people first and not as objects of my own benevolence or charity. By caring for them, I had come to respect them. My relationship could no longer be one seen through the lens of charitable work. I had begun to see their problems as *our* problems. I had taken the first step. I had entered a world that I could now never leave, as long as my conscience held sway over my other desires.

Finally, however, my experiences in East Africa produced more questions than answers—questions that have followed me ever since. First, these were mostly good people. How was it possible that they suffered so horribly

I had learned a valuable lesson about working with the poor. I had come to see them as people first and not as objects of my own benevolence or charity.

and died so young? They loved their children, cared for each other, and lived with a dignity and grace that defied their circumstance. Second, why were they so poor? Tens of billions of dollars had flowed to Africa through bilateral and multilateral aid channels through the years. But none of that money had seemed to make it here. Third, why was it that so few people back in the United States seemed to understand what was going on here and other similar distressed parts of the world? Americans have always prided themselves on some of the saving roles we have played in the world. Yet here was a war we were clearly not winning. In fact, we seemed completely disengaged.

Return to Kenya and the Creation of Omni Med

Images of these admirable people stayed with me long after my brief stay ended. Something powerful had happened to me in Tanzania, and I planned to return to East Africa one day to learn more, to share my skills, and to try to answer the questions that had gnawed at me over the intervening years. After four years of residency at Boston City Hospital, and two and one half years of paying some of my medical school loans, I returned to Kenya in the winter and spring of 1994. I ran a medical ward in Nazareth Hospital, on the outskirts of Nairobi, and again found the value in service. In the people around Nazareth, I found the same strength of character, the same generosity, and the same cultural strength as the people in Tanzania.

But I also began to understand the larger forces that perpetuated their poverty. The hospital director Father Bill Fryda, the patients, and staff at Nazareth, and a host of books all served as my tutors. In lieu of helping the poorest among Kenyan society, government officials at every level seemed most intent on swelling their own wallets. The United Nations, World Bank, and International Monetary Fund seemed utterly impotent at best. Trade favored the wealthy countries primarily. Even foreign aid seemed a sham, with most of the dollars finding their way into the pockets of the elite. Meanwhile, the world stood by as neighboring Rwanda exploded in a genocidal rage with 800,000 people killed in 100 days. The larger global structures designed to help people did not appear to be working. It became increasingly clear to me that, in order to understand why so many people suffered as they did, I would need to better understand the larger forces at work upon them.

While in Nazareth Hospital I learned that I had been accepted to the W.K. Kellogg Foundation's National Leadership Program, which, over the next three and one half years, enabled me to study leadership and development on a part-time basis. As a group we also studied empowerment zones in Detroit, community development in Miami, race relations and indigenous issues in Brazil, governance and transition in China, and history and policy in Russia and Eastern Europe. The process of bringing together 45 strong-minded men and women from different walks of life, all grounded in social justice, offered tremendous opportunity for growth and a chance to address the questions I had posed in East Africa. The fellowship provided the perfect opportunity to better understand the complex issues involved, and breathed life into the idea of writing this book and founding a non-governmental organization (NGO).

In September of 1997, members of the Hingham Rotary Club invited me to Belize to advise them on their medical equipment donation program there. An impressive group of lay individuals, they had already accomplished more for the poor in their brief work than most physicians in the United States accomplish in a lifetime. I toured the country with a large group of Rotarians and a few other physicians, including Dr Tom Durant. (See his story in Chapter 15.) What became clear was the need for continuing medical education. I founded a non-profit organization called Omni Med (loosely translated from the Latin meaning *health care for all*) in February 1998, with a focus on getting more US health care providers to serve effectively in developing countries. In January 1999, we launched a program to bring American doctors to teach in Belize every other month; nearly 40 have since gone. Omni Med has since become established in several developing countries, and is an important source of continuing medical education in Belize and Guyana.

Several physicians from the Belize program, including Drs Mike Morley, Kathy Morrow, James Eadie, John O'Brien, and John Varallo have started new programs in Thailand and Guyana. Together, we have developed some innovative programs that are making a difference for the health of the poor in these and other countries. We have evolved a program model in which we work with host personnel to develop programs that *they* value, while simultaneously expanding the pool of US health care providers with international experience. Program examples include: a national cervical cancer initiative (Dr Varallo) and an HIV/AIDS education program (Drs Eadie and O'Brien) in Guyana; continuing medical education programs in Belize, Thailand, Guyana, and Kenya; and an eye-screening and treatment program (Drs Morley and Morrow) in Thailand. Our programs emphasize health volunteerism, innovative design, and ethical leadership; we encourage all of our volunteers to get more involved and provide leadership for new cooperative and sustainable ventures. Our combined experience informs our new program ventures in Jamaica and beyond. Underlying all of this work is a program philosophy that states that *all* people have a right to health and quality health care; and that all health professionals, by their very involvement in the profession, share an ethical imperative to make quality health care broadly accessible to all people, regardless of nationality or income.

A medical student recently asked me why I do this work. My immediate answer is because I like it and think it is important. On a deeper level, I respond that I am the son and grandson of Boston Police Officers. While growing up, my father and mother were both models of ethical behavior. They stressed the importance of fairness and instilled a strong sense of justice. "There but for the Grace of God go I," was a common refrain from my mother. Years later, when I arrived in Tanzania, I was shocked by what I saw. That people were forced to live in such a manner was an affront to everything I held as decent and right. I found it morally offensive. Life for these people revealed a profound injustice, and demanded some attempt at corrective action. Although I am but one small player on this stage, I continue to be a part of this fight mainly because it is, quite simply, the right thing to do. Further, while I did not start in this work for faith-based reasons, I now find considerable resonance there. The experience of seeing young innocents drowning in a sea of poverty was enough to tap into something far deeper within me. As the roots of my own faith have deepened, I have found it impossible to avert my gaze. Poverty mocks faith, and I see no other way to respond to the moral imperatives that naturally flow from true ethics—rooted in faith—than to address these problems directly.

On Transformation

If there is a moral to my story—one that I could wish for the entire medical profession—it is transformation. One of the more powerful products of working with the poor is the personal transformation that often results. Within the realm of international service work among the poor, such stories are legion. The sheer power of the experience is sufficient to change hearts and minds. We may more readily understand the concept of transformation by turning to some of our more celebrated political leaders. We know Franklin D. Roosevelt as the compassionate president who launched the New Deal, Social Security, and the Four Freedoms—the "touchstone" of the Universal Declaration of Human Rights (Glendon 2001, 176) When he contracted polio, according to biographer Doris Kearns Goodwin, he "came to empathize with the poor and the underprivileged, with people to whom fate had dealt a difficult hand" (Goodwin 1994, 16). Eleanor Roosevelt added, "Anyone who has gone through great suffering is bound to have a greater sympathy and understanding of the problems of mankind." Robert F. Kennedy underwent a similar transformation upon the assassination of his brother. Following the deep melancholy that engulfed him after the fall of "Camelot," the transformed Attorney General actively sought out the poor of America, touring shacks of the rural South, meeting with migrant workers and marginalized people of color, in the process attracting armies of the dispossessed until his untimely death at age 42.

More pertinent to our task here, Tom Dooley grew up a wealthy aristocrat in St Louis, aspiring to become a society obstetrician. However, seeing up close the misery of Vietnam's refugees tapped a faith-based wellspring within him, transforming his remaining life into a resolute struggle against poverty and illness in South East Asia. (See his story in Chapter 11.) Paul Farmer, similarly, found the suffering and premature dying of the poor in rural Haiti more than he could bear. Such injustice has driven him to work for decades in poor communities around the world, always seeking a means to improve their health and quality of life. (See his story in Chapter 13.) Poverty and the devastation wrought by AIDS have had a similar transformative effect on U2 front man Bono, US Secretary of State Colin Powell, economist Jeffrey Sachs, and others (Behrman 2004, 265). In each of these stories, the sheer power of harsh experience proved enough to transform the individual. There may be no more passionate or potent force than that unleashed by those who have been transformed.

Through the experience of service, I have no doubt that more Paul Farmers will emerge, and hundreds of people will rededicate a portion of their clinical lives. Health providers widely share the trait of compassion. It is impossible to do this work well without it. As such, health providers form the ideal cohort to reach out into the world to bring the experience of poverty home to a slumbering electorate. In the process, they can send out ripples of change that can reverberate powerfully throughout our country and our world.

Endnotes

1. For more information, see the Gallup International Association web site at www.gallupinternational.com.

Part 1

Understand-ing Global Disparities in Health

The evil that is in the world always comes out of ignorance, and good intentions may do as much harm as malevolence, if they lack under-standing.

—Albert Camus,
The Plague

So why should a busy clinician care about poor kids dying of hunger or AIDS in Africa? And why should a physician who has spent years learning the science of medicine invest precious time learning the complex fields of developmental economics and trade policy? Simply because ours is a profession dedicated to healing, and perhaps for the first time in history, we can truly heal the world. A constellation of forces has brought us to the point where we can realistically talk about the end of extreme poverty, along with the illness and premature death that inevitably accompany it (Sachs, 2005a). But to accomplish this, health providers must engage in the world—personally and politically—in far greater numbers than we ever have previously.

Most health providers have spent so much time learning the art of their craft that they have little direct exposure to or understanding of the problems of extreme poverty in our world. Nor do they realize just how great their power is should they choose to invest some of their time in a developing country. These providers could become part of something historic, something life changing, and it is my sincere hope that many more will do so.

Part 1 is written with a busy practitioner's schedule in mind. As a practicing physician, I realize that most of my colleagues do not have the time to read the many well-written books about global poverty and illness. Part 1 of this text concisely explains the forces of disparity that propagate poverty and illness, as well as the rich world's response to poverty to date. It begins with a clarification of terms, including *health*, *poverty*, and *structural violence*, and discusses the inherent designs of our societies that consign some to forever lowered expectations. By comparing the health indices of the United States and Kenya, we see just how different life is in each, and just how important one's nationality and relative place in the socioeconomic order of the respective society is to predict health and longevity. To further decipher the differences between the rich and poor countries, we then review the factors that directly contributed to the rise of good health in the West, mainly nutrition, economic growth, and the technological advances in public health and medicine that allowed a formerly sickly workforce to power the engines of industry.

Until the 1800s, the entire world was poor and virtually all people lived short, illness-ridden lives. Following the Industrial Revolution, Europe and later the United States developed rapidly, with rising incomes and longevity the result. Once these stunning advances were achieved however, just how much has the rich world helped those in poor countries? We look closely at the history of the United Nations, the World Bank, the International Monetary Fund, and the explosion of the important non-governmental organizations sector (eg, CARE, the Red Cross, and Médicines Sans Frontiéres). We think we help those in poor countries far more than we actually do, and foreign aid has historically served the needs of the donors far more than the recipients. Despite some very real progress in the amount and efficacy of bilateral and multilateral aid, there remains a yawning gap that must be filled in order to eradicate extreme poverty.

Current political discussions provide ample ammunition for those who say that time and money expended on those in poor countries is inevitably wasted. Further, those who live in the affluent West often have trouble understanding the constraints under which most of the world's people live; it therefore becomes easy to believe the many myths about poverty. To understand why the myths are wrong, we must dissect out and examine the many component forces that keep so many countries "trapped" in poverty.

Trade, global financial flows, inequality itself, and the actions of some multinational corporations all propagate global poverty. History is very much alive and repercussions from foreign conquest, colonization, and slavery still exert an enormous influence on most of the developing world. Less obvious factors, like geography, distance from navigable rivers and oceans, and disease burdens like malaria, tuberculosis and HIV/AIDS all combine to rob millions of their lives and opportunities to escape their harsh poverty. The pressures of overpopulation, environmental destruction, poor governance and militarism all conspire to add to the poor man's burden. All combined, these forces of disparity explain in real terms just why so many people in developing countries will not be able to pull themselves out of the poverty traps that engulf them. In lieu of helping them, those of us in the rich countries have simply added obstacles in their way.

Yet, the current world order stands in sharp contrast to the sentiments of virtually all world religions, and the ethical premise of the Universal Declaration of Human Rights, the seminal document drafted by a band of dreamers in the aftermath of World War II. Ultimately, the question of whether or not to intervene to stop needless suffering and dying is not one for science or technology; it is one for ethics and the collective conscience of mankind. By examining the ethical roots of the major world religions, particularly the monotheists, we will come full circle to a place where we can again take up the fundamental questions of why such things go on and why we should engage at the outset. We can then return to the questions posed in the beginning of this text, such as why a 10-like-old girl has to turn to prostitution—and the inevitable sentence of AIDS—just to survive in the new millennium.

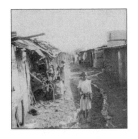

Chapter 1

Health, Poverty, and Structural Violence

The worst form of violence is poverty.

—Mahatma Gandhi

Fighting hunger and poverty and promoting development are the truly sustainable way to achieve world peace. . . . There will be no peace without development, and there will be neither peace nor development without social justice.

—Luiz Inácio Lula da Silva, President of Brazil

Imagine no possessions, I wonder if you can, No need for greed or hunger, A brotherhood of man, Imagine all the people Sharing all the world . . . You may say I'm a dreamer, but I'm not the only one, I hope some day you'll join us, And the world will live as one.

—John Lennon

Humans have long viewed health as foremost among their concerns. In this chapter we review basic definitions of health and how these definitions have evolved over time. We then take an in-depth look at the most determined and important foe of good health—poverty—and the structural components that fuel its propagation. The differences of life expectancy, health, and life quality that separate those at the top from those at the bottom are encompassed in the phrase structural violence. We take an in-depth view of the impact of structural violence on both poor and rich countries. Although most can see the destructive potential of poor nutrition, poor sanitation, and lack of public health and health care, there are less visible factors that add to poverty's destructive power, particularly in developed countries. We review these factors, with a focus on their history in the United States and Great Britain. By understanding health, poverty, and structural violence, we take an important first step to understanding the world as it is.

Health

Health has always held a prominent position among human concerns. Its importance to both individuals and societies is obvious. Good health fosters productive workers and growing economies—it allows people to pursue that which they value in life. Poor health prematurely shortens lives, crumples nations, and precipitates wars (Sachs 2001b, 191). Those of us in the clinical realm of the medical profession see the importance of good health every day. We understand the emotional, physical, and economic costs that those afflicted with poor health must bear.

The World Health Organization (WHO) defines *health* as a positive state of complete physical, social, and mental well-being. According to the WHO, health is "a resource for everyday life, not the objective of living: it is a positive concept emphasizing social and personal resources as well as physical capabilities" (Whitehead 1992, 223). Maintaining such a state and staving off illness has rightly evolved as a central concern of all governments. All but three of 29 industrialized nations—the United States, Mexico, and Turkey—covered health care costs for all of their citizens in 1997 (Anderson 1997, 6). Indeed, Article 25 of the Universal Declaration of Human Rights maintains that everyone around the world has a right to good health and well-being through a sufficient standard of living and adequate food, clothing, housing, medical care, and social services (Mann et al 1999, 456).

In 1999, the Gallup Institute undertook history's largest opinion poll, interviewing 50,000 people from 60 countries.[1] Pollsters asked the simple question, "What matters most in life?" and offered respondents choices of a job, an education, good health, freedom, religion, a good standard of living, a happy family life, or living in a country without war, violence or corruption. Across lines of faith, race, gender, and nationality, people valued their health most, as they always have.

In my reading of the Gospels, there are 65 occasions (with some repetition among the four authors) when Jesus Christ heals the blind, the lame, the sick, or exorcizes demons—considered the cause of seizures and other maladies in the ancient world. Christ's healing power over all types of illnesses, including infections, attracted followers who then heard his message. Some have cited the importance of his healings and exorcisms in establishing his ministry, a crude reflection on the importance of health to those living during that time (Crossan 1989, 93). Infectious illness continued to play an important role long after Christ's death, and early Christianity no doubt benefited from the massive conversions that occurred after each successive wave of bubonic plague or smallpox (Zinsser 1934, 139).

Lacking the curative powers of modern biomedical science, mankind was utterly defenseless against the pestilence of biblical times. Plagues borne by Roman armies returning from the Far East and Africa wiped out whole cities. Afflicted with mysterious illnesses in strange, distant places, soldiers fled home, inadvertently carrying with them the devastation of plague, typhus, smallpox, tuberculosis, and a host of other diseases. Lacking the revelations of science, people assigned the blame for infectious disease to spirits, the retribution of an enemy, or an angry god. Many Greeks attributed the Plague of Cyprian, a devastating global epidemic of bubonic plague from AD 250 to 260, to punishment for a failure to honor properly the god Jupiter (Zinsser 1934, 139). Others searched their souls for moral error or looked for anyone sufficiently "other" to blame for their maladies—a leading factor in the long history of Jewish persecution in Europe.

Potential devastation from disease dominated the outlook of people of ancient times. Disease was to be feared above all else. As Hans Zinsser wrote in 1934, mankind suffered from, "the dreadful affliction of inescapable, mysterious, and deadly disease. Mankind stood helpless as though trapped in a world of terror and peril against which there was no defense. . . . During the first centuries after Christ, disease was unopposed by any barriers. And when it came, as though carried on storm clouds, all other things gave way, and men crouched in terror, abandoning all their quarrels, undertakings, and ambitions, until the tempest had blown over" (Zinsser 1934, 80, 134).

In their wake, those pestilences reduced entire civilizations to "uncontrolled savagery," continuing their destructive effects long after they had passed. They shaped human history far more than we appreciate. "The epidemics get the blame for defeat; the generals get the credit for victory" (Zinsser 1934, 153).

Historical examples abound. In the fifth century B.C., the "plague of Athens," probably smallpox, devastated armies and civilians on both sides and influenced the result of the Peloponnesian War (Zinsser 1934, 119). The Plague of Justinian, probably bubonic plague, contributed directly to the fall of Rome (145). The Crusades repeatedly were turned back by disease more than by armed resistance (155). "The pestilence," as the Black Plague was known before 1800, wiped out one third of Europe's population between 1347 and 1350, roughly 20 million people (Cantor 2002, 7). Napoleon's army succumbed more to disease than to Russia's troops or cold winters (Zinsser 1934, 164). The trend continued into the 19th century. Two thirds of the 660,000 deaths during America's Civil War came from infectious disease—a dramatic improvement when we compare the ratios of infectious disease related deaths to combat-related deaths in the Mexican-American War (7:1) and the Napoleonic Wars (8:1). Haiti became a free nation in 1804 chiefly because 22,000 of Napoleon's 25,000 troops, who were sent to quell the revolt, succumbed to yellow fever (Zinsser 1934, 160).

The Evolution of Medicine as a Science

Our views of health have evolved considerably over time, as have the abilities of those who venture to restore it. Before the Industrial Revolution, most people lived short lives dominated by poverty and infectious disease. Health meant not having any of the infectious or nutritional diseases against which there was no defense. Moral, religious, and mystical views held sway in disease causality, and doctors who tried to heal generally failed miserably, as they did on the fateful day in 1685 when Britain's King Charles II suddenly fell ill:

> With a cry, he fell. Dr. King, who, fortunately happened to be present, bled him with a pocket knife. Fourteen physicians were quickly in attendance. They bled him more thoroughly; they scarified and cupped him; they shaved and blistered his head; they gave him an emetic, a clyster (an enema) and two pills. During the next eight days, they threw in fifty-seven separate drugs; and toward the end, a cordial containing forty more . . . and as a final remedy, the distillate of human skull. In the case report it is recorded that the emetic and purge worked so mightily well that it was a wonder the patient died (Kleinman et al 1997, 359).

Such practices continued for another 200 years. It was not until the 19th century that medicine evolved into a science and with it the capacity to intervene effectively. Such capacities, along with advances in nutrition, public health, and technology, have largely shaped our modern world. Today's industrialized countries could not have risen to their current prominence with the sickly and malnourished workforce that characterized the world preceding the Industrial Revolution. A healthier workforce with increased stamina was required to drive industry. The Industrial Revolution both spawned and benefited from improvements in health, which have been unprecedented globally, with none more impressive than in the past half century.

According to a 1993 World Bank report, "Health conditions around the world have improved more in the past 40 years than in all previous human history" (World Bank Group 1993, 21). "The 20th century," added the WHO a few years later, "has seen a global transformation in human health unmatched in history," representing, "arguably, humankind's most dramatic achievement" (World Health Organization [WHO] 1999, 1, 7). By any measurement, the gains in life expectancy and general health in recent decades are astounding, achieving levels only dreamed of by our ancestors.

From 1960 to 1993, life expectancy increased by more than one third in developing countries–from 46 years to 62 years (United Nations Development Programme [UNDP] 1996, 18). During the same period, infant mortality fell by more than half–from 150 per thousand live births to 70 (19). In 1955, 21 million children died before attaining their fifth birthday; in 1997, "only" 11 million children suffered a similar fate. Current projections reduce this number to 5 million by 2025 (WHO 1999, 3). We can trace such dramatic improvements directly back to economic growth, better nutrition, and advances in biomedical science and public health. Aggressive campaigns for basic immunization in recent years have saved the lives of roughly 3 million children per year (UNDP 1996, 4). Roughly 80% of the world's children now receive vaccinations against the primary infectious diseases of childhood (World Bank Group 1993, 35). At the same time, low-cost oral rehydration is now widely practiced, saving the lives of 1 million children per year (UNDP 1997, 111).

Health Disparities Remain

Nevertheless, enormous disparities in health remain. The gap between the richest and poorest countries remains close to 30 years (UNDP 2002, 152). Even though more than 80% of the world's children are immunized, infant mortality rates (IMR), defined as the probability of dying between birth and age 1, are nearly 17 times higher in the least developed countries than in the most developed countries (UNDP 2001, 168).[2] These disparities between the poor and those better off remain disturbingly present—a challenge unmet.

The sources of poor health are less readily apparent. Poor genes, bad lifestyle choices, and capricious visitations by debilitating illness all play important roles in health. But these account for only part of the story. We cannot fully understand global disparities of health without first looking at the single entity that most utterly destroys it. That entity has plagued mankind since the earliest recorded history. That entity, of course, is poverty.

Poverty

From time immemorial, the poor have lived shorter and sicker lives than the rich. It has always been so, with statistical evidence dating back 200 years and anecdotes from two millennia before that. Although conditions have improved for most people in recent decades, for the bulk of the world's poor, the classic axiom of Thomas Hobbes remains painfully accurate, "Life is nasty, brutish, and short." The WHO's International Classification of Diseases codifies extreme poverty as an illness, not unlike cancer or dysentery:

> [Poverty is] the world's most ruthless killer and the greatest cause of suffering on earth . . . [wielding] its destructive influence at every stage of human life from the moment of conception to the grave. It conspires with the most deadly and painful diseases to bring a wretched existence to all who suffer from it. . . . Poverty is the main reason why babies are not vaccinated, clean water and sanitation are not provided, and curative drugs and other treatments are unavailable, and why mothers die in childbirth. Poverty is the main cause of reduced life expectancy, of handicap and disability, and of starvation. Poverty is a main contributor to mental illness, stress, suicide, family disintegration and substance abuse (WHO 1995, 1).

Kofi Annan, the secretary-general of the United Nations (UN), has long targeted poverty as the UN's number one concern, citing the war on poverty as even more important than the war on terrorism (National Public Radio 2003a). Dr Jonathan Fine, the founder of Physicians for Human Rights, summed it up succinctly at a Physicians for Human Rights' conference in 1997, "The poorer you are, the sicker you are, the sooner you die."

It is difficult for those living in the affluent Western world to comprehend poverty—the inhuman, backbreaking existence that is life's only option for many of the world's people. But what does it mean to be truly poor? For those who are the worst off, it means constantly fighting losing battles with hunger and disease, living a far shorter life over which you have little control, and holding your young children as they die, ravaged by treatable illness. To be poor means getting by without the basic necessities that the more affluent take for granted: clean water, basic sanitation, shelter, education, health care, material possessions, and the hope that your children may one day lead better lives. To be poor is to be invisible or, if noticed at all, to be blamed for your circumstances and then "erased" by history after you're gone. Regarded as less than human in the eyes of the more fortunate, countless poor people lose faith in the governments and multilateral organizations that so often fail them. Ultimately, and most tragically, many lose faith in themselves. Iracema da Silva, a slum dweller in Brazil, poignantly expressed the plight of the poor when he said, "Sometimes I think, 'If I die, I won't have to see my children suffering as they are.' So often I see them crying, hungry; and there I am, without a cent to buy them some bread. I think, 'My God, I can't face it! I'll end my life. I don't want to look anymore!'" (Sider 1997, 1).

Another Brazilian, the acclaimed educator Paulo Freire, knew hunger and poverty from his childhood. After the stock market crash of 1929, his family descended into the depths of poverty inhabited by what he called the "wretched of the earth" (Freire 1970, 13). Subsequently, he dedicated his life to helping others escape from poverty and oppression. Freire died in 1997 following a lifetime of teaching the poor how to liberate themselves from the shackles that bind them. In his classic book, the *Pedagogy of the Oppressed*, written in 1970, Freire noted that many people in Latin America are "living corpses, shadows of human beings, hopeless men, women, and children victimized by an endless invisible war in which their remnants of life are devoured by tuberculosis, schistosomiasis, infant diarrhea, [and other] diseases of poverty" (Freire 1970, 152).

Clarifying Poverty

But what is poverty? Traditional indexes have focused on available wealth, with the world's poor falling into three broad categories: extreme (also called absolute), moderate, and relative poverty. According to the World Bank, anyone earning less than $1 per day is absolutely poor. Because

$1 will purchase much more in a poor country like Kenya than in a rich country like the United States, economists compare countries through the "purchasing power parity" of the dollar, meaning how much will $1 purchase in an given country. This enables economists to assess degrees of poverty in markedly differing economies. "Extreme" or "absolute" poverty occurs only in developing countries and means that people lack the income necessary to meet their basic survival needs. These people, often called the "poorest of the poor," are chronically hungry and ravished by illness. They lack health care, clean water, sanitation, basic education and reliable shelter; many die prematurely. In essence, they are "trapped" by their poverty. According to the World Bank, in 2001 there were 1.1 billion people living in extreme poverty, roughly one sixth of humanity. The overwhelming majority of these people (93%) live in three regions: East Asia, South Asia, and sub-Saharan Africa. Since 1981, the number of people living in extreme poverty has fallen from 1.5 billion to 1.1 billion, chiefly due to rapid economic growth in China and India. In sub-Saharan Africa, the numbers of extreme poor have continued to rise (Sachs 2005a).

The next category is "moderate" poverty, which included roughly 1.5 billion people in 2001. These people, known simply as "the poor," live on $1 to $2 dollars per day. They often lack clean water and sanitation, and struggle just to make ends meet. Any setback like an economic downturn or serious illness can plunge them into extreme poverty. Together, the extreme and moderate poor account for roughly 40% of humanity. The final category, "relative poverty," includes those who fall below a given percent of national income, including those in rich countries, making data harder to come by (Sachs 2005a).

For perspective, we can classify the world's roughly 6 billion people into four categories: the extreme poor (1.1 billion); the moderate poor (1.5 billion); the middle-income (2.5 billion), ie, those who live in cities in the developing world with jobs and comfortable housing, though would be considered poor by rich world standards; and the rich (1 billion), ie, those who live in the rich world or comprise the affluent classes in urban centers in middle-income countries.

In recent years, the definition of poverty has expanded beyond material deprivation alone. In 1997, the UN developed a human poverty index (HPI) that focused more on human "capabilities" and the deficiencies that stem from poverty. If people have some funds but no education, their opportunities to "live the lives they value" will be constrained. Similar restrictions will result from poor health, unsafe water, or lack of access to medical care and a host of other deprivations that might not be captured by viewing poverty only through available finances. Recognizing that poverty "is too complex to be reduced to a single dimension of human life" (UNDP 1997, 15), the HPI incorporated indices of longevity, knowledge, and a decent standard of living. Thus, *human poverty*, with its multiple parameters, is distinguished from *income poverty*. According to this more accurate measurement, one fourth of the developing world's people are poor and a third are income poor. The difference reflects the various approaches taken by governments to address the needs of their people. Some developing countries, such as Cuba, Singapore, and Costa Rica, have considerably reduced human poverty despite persistent income poverty. Other countries, like Egypt and Morocco, have reduced income poverty far more than human poverty (UNDP 1997, 22).

Historical Examples

While there will never be a controlled clinical trial to measure the impact of impoverishing one group of people while leaving a "control" group alone, history offers many close parallels. In countries throughout history, indicators of human welfare have always worsened after their economies soured and more people became poor. Virtually any country in recession with high unemployment or internal conflict sees the life expectancies and health indices of its people plummet.

A study from the United States found that a 1% rise in unemployment increased the mortality rate by 2%, the infant mortality rate by 5%, and rates of homicides and imprisonments by 6%.

A study from the United States found that a 1% rise in unemployment increased the mortality rate by 2%, the infant mortality rate by 5%, and rates of homicides and imprisonments by 6% (Gilligan 1996, 192).

Following the demise of the Soviet Union and the free-fall of the Russian economy, deep recession and hyperinflation caused unemployment and poverty for many Russians. Health indicators reflected the results of the new-found deprivation. From 1990 to 1995, life expectancy decreased by almost seven years in men and four years in women. Infant mortality rates rose to four times that of the United States and fertility rates fell to the point where the population began shrinking (UNDP 1996, 84). During a visit in 1996, I saw elderly pensioners and soldier amputees begging in the streets and subway stations—a new and harsh experience for people accustomed to having all basic needs met by their government.

A more dramatic example occurred in Bataan, the southernmost region of Luzon in the Philippines, in the early 1940s (Sides 2002). Young and healthy American and Filipino soldiers became prisoners of the Imperial Japanese Army after their supply lines were cut. Following the 75-mile trek known as the Bataan Death March, during which 24,000 men died, these imprisoned soldiers suffered from starvation and untreated medical illness at Camp O'Donnell and Camp Cabanatuan. Of roughly 9,000 American prisoners to pass through these camps, nearly one third died and many more became seriously ill (Sides 2002, 134). While some succumbed to beheadings or the sequelae of torture, most died from conditions that afflict poor people all over the world today: chiefly; starvation and infectious disease. Many developed nutritional deficiencies such as beriberi, scurvy, and pellagra, while some went blind. Infectious diseases such as typhus, malaria, dysentery, dengue, diphtheria, typhoid, tuberculosis, and gangrene, decimated people who had been made more vulnerable through starvation-induced immunodeficiency, a common affliction among the poor.

As the writer Hampton Sides put it, "[Camp] O'Donnell was less a prison than it was an incubatorium for disease, a study in what happens when thousands of starving, ill men are brought together in close proximity in the tropics" (Sides 2002, 108). That description could also apply to the conditions of extreme poverty that exist in urban slums in many poor countries today. If young American soldiers at the peak of their physical prowess succumb in droves to the conditions that mimic severe poverty, it should be no surprise that the poor of our world suffer as they do. Unlike the prisoners of war who returned from Bataan and were given a huge welcoming ceremony in San Francisco, those who routinely bear many of the same burdens see no relief on the horizon. Instead, they are blamed for their poverty and remain prisoners of a different sort.

Much of the Western response to the poor has been characterized by avoidance. "A wall between the rich and poor countries is being built," writes the Chilean theologian Pablo Richard, "so that poverty does not annoy the powerful and the poor are obliged to die in the silence of history" (Kleinman et al 1997, 280).

Structural Violence

The fact that poor people around the world have shorter and harder lives is the result of human design. This phenomenon is called "structural violence." The increased rates of death and disability among those who occupy the lowest rungs of the class systems in unequal societies are not caused by acts of nature or individual will. They result from the choices made both by individual countries and the world community regarding allocation of resources. The forces that contribute to structural violence are complex and largely invisible. As such, they receive only a smattering of attention from world leaders and our rather undiscerning populace. We will explore these forces throughout the remainder of this section.

Many researchers have tried to assess the damage inflicted by structural violence. Eckhardt and Young (1977), for example, wrote that between 1948 and 1967, structural violence claimed over 300 times the number of lives lost to "civil conflict." Another study, published by a Canadian group in 1976 (Kohler and Alcock 1976), postulated that if all the world's countries had similar resources and allocated them in similar fashion, structural violence—and its resulting higher mortality for the poor—would disappear. Taking the year 1965 as a model, the researchers used Sweden as the society closest to ideal resource allocation and compared Swedish life expectancy with that of one of the world's poorest countries, Guinea. Life expectancy for the two countries was 74.7 years and 27.0 years, respectively. The author concluded that 83,000 deaths in Guinea could have been avoided if life expectancies were identical in the two countries. By expanding the model to all countries, the author concluded that 18 million people died as the result of structural violence in 1965, more than all of World War II's battlefield casualties and 150 times more than in all of 1965s armed conflicts. Although the study has its limitations, its chief points are both compelling and correct. Poverty kills and it does so relentlessly, invisibly (at least to those of us on the wealthier side of the equation), and in far greater numbers than the armed conflicts that understandably command our attention.

The system most widely adopted for estimating the global burden of disease, which stems largely from structural violence, comes from the World Bank. In its 1993 World Development Report, the Bank proposed a system to quantify disability adjusted life years (DALYs) to account for the effects of structural violence (World Bank Group 1993, 26). The report noted that 12.4 million children under age five in the developing world had died in 1990—34,000 deaths per day. If those children had life expectancies similar to those in "established market economies," there would have only been 1.1 million deaths (3,014 deaths per day), a reduction of almost 90%.

Poverty and Health: A Closer Look

What is it about poverty that makes it so virulent? There is a sizable literature looking at this question, both in poor and in rich countries. It is easy enough to understand that living without proper nutrition, clean water, sanitation, shelter, education, stable parenting, medical care, and many other factors exposes poor people to illnesses that most people in rich countries never experience. But it is a surprise to learn how much is unknown about how relative poverty wields its destructive effects even in developed countries like the United States and the United Kingdom. There is far more to the equation than basic deprivation alone.

Health and Wealth Gradients Between Countries: the United States, Kenya, and the World

The two most important predictors for one's health are the country of one's birth and where one falls in that country's class structure. This book opened with a story of a young girl living in extreme poverty in Nairobi's Kariobangi slum. To better understand why nationality and one's place on the national economic ladder are so important, we'll compare the health indices of her country, Kenya, with the health indices of the country of her treating physician, the United States. Kenya is poor with many of its citizens ill, while the United States is rich with most of its citizens healthy. To begin to understand why, we'll start with some background information on Kenya.

Kenya is a democratic nation of 31 million located along the Indian Ocean in East Africa. As currents of change swept the world after World War II, Kenya achieved its independence from Great Britain in 1963. The visionary Jomo Kenyatta became the first prime minister of Kenya in 1964 and ruled over a poor but reasonably well-governed country until his death in 1978. Daniel Arap Moi replaced Kenyatta and presided over a declining state ruled by corruption and ineffectual governance.

Most in the developed world focus erroneously on corruption when trying to understand why poor countries remain poor. While this focus diverts attention from other more substantive causes, in Kenya at least, corruption certainly plays a role. Transparency International, a nonprofit organization that ranks corruption in governments, found only five countries in the world that were more corrupt than Kenya (2003). Daniel Arap Moi's ability to manipulate the ancient tribal animosities kept him and his corrupt regime in place until the constitution required him to abdicate power. His designated successor, Uhuru Kenyatta, the son of Jomo Kenyatta, lost in a landslide to Mwai Kibaki in a historic election that saw power shift from the Kenya African National Union (KANU) party to the rival National Rainbow Coalition in January 2003 (Makua 2003). By comparison, the United States, despite its business scandals, was just 16 places from the top of the corruption survey as one of the world's least corrupt countries (Transparency International 2003).

Although corruption in Kenya and other poor countries receives huge coverage in the world media, it is important to recognize that it is just one of many factors contributing to poverty in that country, and certainly not the most important. Corruption is more destructive in Kenya than in rich countries because there is so much less money to go around. It is far more visible when a head of state like Moi builds private airports and palaces and protects corrupt friends, while millions of his countrymen suffer ("Moi, Lord of Kenya's Empty Dance" 1999). People in rich countries just don't suffer to the same degree when their leaders rob the store. Consider the $1.3 *trillion* dollars lost in the US savings and loan scandals of the 1980s. Such a loss would cripple most world economies but it did not phase the US economy.

Kenyans have been poor for generations because of many complex and interwoven factors, including: the population explosion; the social and economic costs of illnesses such as AIDS, malaria, and tuberculosis;[3] a relatively short time to recover from decades of colonial exploitation; ineffective governance modeled after colonialist practices; lack of basic infrastructure; unfair global trade practices; debt repayments that rob vital social services ("Mired in Poverty" 1999); lack of foreign capital infusion ("Nairobbery" 2002); subjugation to global powers like the World Bank and the International Monetary Fund; ineffective and occasionally destructive "foreign aid"

(Randel et al 2002); and so on. Mostly, however, Kenyans remain poor because they are caught in a "poverty trap," formed by all of the above. Overwhelmed by disease, hunger and the extreme deprivation that rules their lives, most Kenyans simply try to survive, unable to achieve the universal dream of providing better lives for their children. The government lacks the tax revenues to provide even basic amenities like health, education, clean water and sanitation, virtually guaranteeing that the process continues unabated. A comparison with the United States highlights the glaring disparities in the most basic of health measures—survival. The average American in 2000 could expect to live nearly 25 years longer than the average Kenyan (UNDP 2002, 174). And that difference has widened since, chiefly due to AIDS. A baby born in Kenya today has a better than one in three chance of not surviving until age 40 (158).

The disparities hold true for virtually any aspect of health or quality of life. Infant mortality rates are 11 times higher in Kenya than they are in the United States. Children under age five die at rates 15 times higher than their American counterparts. Almost as dangerous a trial as that of childhood in Kenya is that of giving birth. A woman in Kenya is more than 74 times more likely to die in labor than a woman in America (UNDP 2002, 174).

Nevertheless, Kenyan women continue to produce babies at an alarmingly fast rate. The average Kenyan woman has 4.6 children over her lifetime, compared with 2.0 for the average American woman. This means that while the American population grows incrementally at 1% per year, Kenya's is growing at 3.3% per year—the 10th highest in the world (UNDP 2002, 162). Recognizing the desperation that rural life holds for them, many Kenyans move to the cities, crowding into squalid slums like Kibera that serve as incubators for disease and pessimism. Between 1975 and 2000, Kenya's urban population increased from one tenth of the national population to one third (164). Kenyans regularly succumb to the malnutrition and disease that dominate their lives. It is no wonder that so many Kenyan children don't survive—nearly half are malnourished and a quarter to a third are severely malnourished (UNDP 2002, 170). Poor nutrition leaves millions susceptible to infectious disease, which is rampant in Kenya. Judging by my experience there in 1994, most Kenyans have malaria and fully expect a recurrence with any new infection or trauma. They just take their chloroquine and hunker down, waiting for the fevers to break. Ironically, those in the United States spend almost $2.4 billion more on the common cold and sinusitis than Kenyans spend on life-threatening malaria, AIDS, and tuberculosis combined (Osguthorpe and Hadley 1999, 27). In fact, those in the United States spent more on colds and sinus infections than Kenyans spent on all health care costs combined in 2000 (UNDP 2002, 164, 168).[4] The United States, by contrast, had few cases of malaria and only six cases of tuberculosis per 100,000 people (17,000 cases) (170).

While the United States pours billions of dollars into research and treatment for its people infected with HIV and AIDS, Kenya puts almost no money toward AIDS, which now affects 15% of its population (UNDP 2002, 170). The epidemic has dealt a crushing blow to the economy through the constant illness and death of Kenyan workers and by taxing sparse government health services. The emotional and social impact has also been enormous, wiping out entire villages and producing more then 1 million AIDS orphans (BBC News 2001).

Kenyans and Americans can expect drastically different experiences from their health systems. The United States spends more than any other country in the world on health care, averaging $4,200 per person per year. By contrast, Kenya spends on average only $31 per person per year (UNDP 2002, 166). In the United States there is 1 doctor for every 358 people, in Kenya there is just 1 doctor for every 7,692 people. Less than half of the births in Kenya receive attention from skilled health care providers (166).

Nearly two thirds of Kenya's population lives on less than $2 a day, while more than a quarter live on less than $1 a day. Nearly half live below the poverty line (UNDP 2002, 158). Other indices reveal larger differentials in earned income. On average, Americans earn more than 33 times as much as Kenyans do (149). A dollar will go farther in Kenya but not far enough to make up for this differential. The lack of available safety nets, like Medicare and Medicaid in the United States, drives Kenyans to have large families, so the children can take care of their parents later on. This, in turn, merely feeds the cycles of poverty and ill health.

Such glaring disparities between the United States and Kenya reflect the larger world around us. Researchers have been tracking development data for decades, with some of the most widely quoted coming from the UN and its multiple agencies. In 1990, the UN developed a human development index (HDI), replacing earlier attempts to measure human development solely with economic indicators such as a country's annual gross domestic product. Reflecting the beliefs of scholars such as Nobel laureate Amartya Sen and others, consensus emerged that development needed to focus more on human "capabilities" than solely on economic growth, the definitive gauge for years. The HDI combines life expectancy, educational achievement, and gross domestic product to reflect a given country's human development. The data is published annually in a compendium called the *Human Development Report* (HDR).

The health and human development profile of the United States is typical of rich, industrialized countries. The United States' rank of sixth in the HDI places it near the top, while Kenya's rank of 134 places it just above the "low human development" group at the bottom, which includes most countries in sub-Saharan Africa (UNDP 2002, 149).

The countries of sub-Saharan Africa comprise many of the world's poorest.[5] The disparities between the United States and Kenya are even greater when the sub-Saharan Africa region as a whole is compared to the world's wealthiest countries, which are organized together under the rubric of "high-income OECD" (ie, the Organization for Economic Co-operation and Development, which is made up of 23 countries including the United States, Japan, Germany, the United Kingdom, and France) (271).[6] The resulting comparison between rich and poor nations provides still more evidence of the devastation caused chiefly by poverty. Life expectancy differs by 30 years. Infant mortality is nearly 20 times higher and the mortality for children under age five is nearly 30 times higher in sub-Saharan Africa (149). More than one third of those in sub-Saharan Africa are malnourished; more than half are illiterate; and, on average, they earn 1/16 as much income as their wealthy counterparts in the West. While the wealthy OECD countries include just 1.6 million AIDS patients among them, or 4% of the world total, countries in sub-Saharan Africa include 25.4 million, some two thirds of the world total at the end of 2004 (UNAIDS 2004). Despite such impending misery, women in sub-Saharan Africa continue to produce, on average, nearly six children during their lifetimes, while women in the rich countries produce less than two. In OECD countries, there is 1 physician available to treat every 450 people, while in sub-Saharan Africa, there is 1 physician for every 3704 (UNDP 2000, 193).[7]

These numbers provide the starkest evidence of the huge differences in wealth and general health between countries, yet we need to remember that hidden within the numbers are individual lives ruined by disabilities and the premature deaths of loved ones. Each incremental bump in the infant mortality rate represents thousands of mothers crying over the loss of their infants. Years of life expectancy subtracted from the norm of those in wealthier countries represents someone's needlessly lost father, mother, child, or sibling. Just as the young girl whose story opened this book prematurely lost her mother to AIDS, she too became a victim of the same plague now rioting through sub-Saharan Africa. The numbers provide compelling evidence of a world gone awry; but there is more to the story.

Health and Wealth Gradients within Countries

Poverty's effects on the health of those who live in poor countries are both obvious and intuitive. Yet, when we look at health between different classes within industrialized, wealthy countries, something unexpected happens—the health and wealth gradients persist. Long after the point where the perceived effects of poverty would be expected to cease, we find remarkably consistent health gradients across class lines. Those with more wealth have better health and live longer, even in the world's wealthiest countries. After examining the data, we find a universal truth—those on the bottom rungs in most human populations have the highest rates of morbidity and mortality (Adler et al 1999, 194).

Anyone who has worked in an inner city hospital has seen illnesses typically absent or far less common in more affluent locations. AIDS, drug addiction, alcoholism, homelessness, and violence all factored heavily into our caseload during my four years at the Boston Medical Center (O'Neil and Reardon 1992). Pockets of poverty define modern America just as they define other countries with steep class divisions. Much has been made of the study that found that black men in Harlem have a lower life expectancy than men living in Bangladesh, one of the world's poorest countries (McCord 1990, 173). Other studies show similar disparities. While white men in the 10 "healthiest" US counties have a life expectancy of 76.4 years, black men living in the 10 "least healthy" counties have a life expectancy of far less, for example, 61 years in Philadelphia, 60 years in Baltimore and New York, and 57.9 years in the District of Columbia (Marmot 2000, 134).

> *Pockets of poverty define modern America just as they define other countries with steep class divisions.*

The homeless population provides another window into the striking health disparities that exist in the United States. While the average American lived roughly until age 75 during the late 1980s and early 1990s, studies from the same period show that homeless people survived on average to age 44 in Atlanta, 41 in San Francisco, and 47 in Boston (Hwang et al 1997, 625). The homeless in Boston died chiefly of AIDS, homicide, traumatic injuries, poisonings, and pneumonia. The authors of the Boston study attributed the high death rates from homicide and accidental injury to "poverty, substance abuse, and living on the streets" (628). The homeless in Philadelphia had an age-adjusted mortality nearly four times higher than that of the general population (Hibbs 1994, 304). Those in Boston were more fortunate than their peers elsewhere in the United States, surviving until age 47 on average, roughly the same life expectancy as someone then living in Chad, Mozambique, or the Central African Republic (World Bank Group 1993, 238). Obviously, many factors selectively reduce longevity in homeless adults in the United States, including mental illness, addictions, and violence. However, as these studies make clear, not all of those living in wealthy countries share equally in the benefits.

When we look back through time, we find similar patterns. Around the 5th century B.C., Hippocrates noted how peasants and slaves could not expect healthy lives because they lacked the resources necessary to "live right." Galen made similar observations around the time of Christ. "But whoever is completely free," he wrote, "both by fortune and by choice, for him it is possible to suggest how he may enjoy the most health, suffer the least sickness, and grow old most comfortably" (Krieger et al 1993, 92).

In one of the largest reviews ever done on the subject, Aaron Antonovsky concluded simply, "the time at which one dies is related to one's class" (Antonovsky 1967, 31). Antonovsky found more than 30 studies that traced class and longevity from the earliest recorded data in the 17th century to the mid-20th century. Almost every study showed conclusively that class differentials correlate directly with longevity (66). British studies dating back to the 17th century showed that London "gentlemen" lived twice as long as the men who performed manual labor (Fein 1995, 577). A century later, researchers found similar patterns among Britain's professionals, tradesmen, and laborers (Antonovsky 1967, 34). Such patterns have persisted through time, and no country has shown more interest in these patterns than Great Britain.

The British Experience

The issue of social class and health is of such importance in the United Kingdom that the government funded the two largest studies ever done on the subject: the *Black Report* in 1980 and the *Health Divide* in 1987 (Whitehead et al 1992). Both reports received widespread media attention and generated considerable political controversy, chiefly because they each offered clear proof that socioeconomic status, even in a wealthy industrialized country like Britain, greatly affects health. It is, in fact, more of a pathogenic force. Of course, poverty and class-based inequalities cause deaths in far-off places. But in Britain? The idea that income differentials were actually killing people, and had been since the 1930s, was sheer political dynamite, precipitating fights on the floor of Parliament, page-one news coverage throughout the country, and scores of debates in newspapers and prominent medical journals. The reverberations continue to the present day.

The British preoccupation with health and class dates back to 1911, when the registrar general of the United Kingdom developed a system to codify social class into five categories based on occupation. This information was recorded on every death certificate. Despite occasional minor changes, the system persisted, affording researchers the opportunity to study long-term trends in mortality data by class. The five classes include: professionals like physicians and lawyers in class I; administrators, managers, and teachers in class II; nonmanual skilled people like clerks and secretaries in class III; partly skilled people like postal workers and bus drivers in class IV; and unskilled people like porters and manual laborers in class V.

The *Black Report* presented the data compiled from 1930 to 1970. The authors found significant mortality differences between those at the top of the class system and those at the bottom. Based on the figures from the last years studied, the report notes, "On the basis of the figures drawn from the early 1970s, . . . men and women in occupational class V had a two-and-one-half times greater chance of dying before reaching retirement age than their professional counterparts in occupational class I" (Whitehead et al 1992, 43). Further, the risk of death at birth and during the first month

of life was two times higher in class V than class I. Those in class III had
a 1.5 times increased risk (43). One of the most striking aspects of the data
is how consistent it is. Among infants, children, and adults, mortality
rates clearly and consistently increase from class I through class V.
Something important is going on. Still more concerning, trends showed
that from 1930 to 1970, mortality gaps between rich and poor widened
(Fein 1995, 579).

The *Health Divide* followed up on the findings of the *Black Report*
and showed that class and health disparities continued to worsen during the
1980s, a finding reported by others (Davey and Egger 1993, 1085). The
researchers concluded that the findings in the *Black Report* were real and
"cannot be explained away as artefact" (Whitehead et al 1992, 336). Further,
they wrote, "The weight of evidence continues to point to explanations
which suggest that socio-economic circumstances play the major part in
subsequent health differences" (336). In the report summary, the authors
reviewed much of the literature on health and class differentials to date, concluding the following:

> Those at the bottom of the social scale have much higher death rates than those
> at the top. This applies at every stage of life from birth through to adulthood and
> well into old age. Neither is it just a few specific conditions which account for
> these higher death rates. All the major killers now affect the poor more than the
> rich (and so do most of the less common ones). The less favoured occupational
> classes also experience higher rates of chronic sickness and their children tend
> to have lower birth-weights, shorter stature and other indicators suggesting
> poorer health status (Whitehead et al 1992, 394).

Several other British studies came to similar conclusions. In the
Whitehall Study, researchers followed 10,000 male civil service workers for
nearly 20 years, and found that the mortality rate for those in manual and
clerical jobs was 3½ times that of those in senior administrative positions
(Fein 1995, 584). Even more striking, none of the civil workers were materially deprived, lived in inadequate housing, ate poorly, or had exposure to
environmental toxins. The study sample was fairly homogeneous and had full
access to the same nationalized health care (Adler et al 1999, 182). In addition,
all of the workers lived in or around London and worked in the same offices.
A second large study, Whitehall II, followed another cohort of 10,000 civil
servants and found that absence rates due to sickness followed similar gradients regarding class. Those at the bottom grade had significantly more
absences than those at the top, with a progressive gradient in between
(North et al 1993, 361). From these and other studies, it is clear that, just as
morbidity and mortality differentials follow wealth gradients between countries, the same trends follow relative wealth disparities within countries.
Richard Wilkinson rightly concluded from the above data that, "the scale of
the excess mortality associated with lower social status dwarfs almost every
other health problem" (1994a, 1113). The widespread attention afforded

this issue in Great Britain matches the importance of the issue itself, something decidedly lacking in the United States.

The American Experience

This issue generates much less interest in the United States, as evidenced by a review of the medical literature. My search under "poverty" and "health" in 2002 turned up scores of articles and editorials in the *Lancet* and *British Medical Journal* but only a small number in mainstream US journals. Noting the growing mortality differentials between the classes in the United States, Navarro wrote, "in the US there is a deafening silence on this topic" (Navarro 1990, 1238). Krieger and Fee called social class the "missing link" in US health data, pointing out that the United States is the only advanced capitalist country that does not report vital statistics by class and income. Only since 1991 has the National Center for Health Statistics advised states to collect data on "years of educational attainment" to serve as a proxy for class (Fein 1995, 582).

Research in the United States, unique among industrialized countries, focuses more on health differences by race than socioeconomic class (Adler et al 1999, 196). This has long been the case, despite considerable evidence showing that differences in life expectancy are far more closely correlated to class than race (Navarro 1990, 1238). "It is likely," Navarro writes, "that mortality rates for white service workers, for example, are closer to those of black service workers than to those of white professionals" (1239). Haan showed that in Alameda County, California, people living in poverty had a nearly twofold increased risk of death, even after controlling for race and other potentially mitigating factors (Haan et al 1987, 989). Blacks still have worse health indices when compared to whites at the same income levels (Fein 1995, 582), though this is not as significant a factor as the poverty that rules so many of their lives. The worst indices occur because many people of color occupy the lowest classes in the United States. Many remain trapped in the poorest communities, where high unemployment, poor schools, and a toxic social environment stifle efforts to break free and foster a gnawing sense of nihilism. The Institute of Medicine produced a 2001 landmark report demonstrating race bias in medicine (Smedley et al 2001), and Senator Bill Frist introduced legislation in 2004 to "close the health care gap" between whites and minorities (Physicians for Human Rights, 2004).

Aaron Antonovsky found 16 American studies done between 1865 and 1960 that correlated life expectancy and overall mortality with various substitute markers for class. In every study, mortality gradients directly and consistently tracked socioeconomic class, with those in the upper classes surviving the longest (Antonovsky 1967, 31). Kitagawa and Hauser reached a similar conclusion in 1973 after exhaustively matching 340,000 death certificates with 1960 census data on occupation, education, and income (Kitagawa and Hauser 1973). The lower the occupational status, educational attainment, or income level, the higher the mortality rate. The authors found that level of educational attainment was the single best indicator of socio-economic status; this is now recorded on most US death certificates and used as a less accurate substitute for class (Fein, 1995, 582).

In 1986, Pappas and colleagues reproduced the Kitagawa and Hauser study and found that the same trends not only continued after 1960 but worsened, just as they had in the United Kingdom (Pappas et al 1993, 103). During the 26 years between the two studies, inequalities in mortality increased by 20% in women and 100% in men. And, although death rates declined nationally from 1960 to 1986, the authors noted that "poor and less educated people" had not shared in the benefits to the same degree as those who were wealthier or better educated (108). The authors concluded, "The results of this study raise serious questions about disparities in opportunity and equity in our nation" (103).

The United States experience reflects that of the United Kingdom, though presented through less exact indicators of economic status such as race and educational attainment. Other countries, including Ireland, Denmark, Hungary, France, Finland, Germany, Norway, and Sweden, have similar, though less marked, gradients, particularly the latter two (Antonovsky 1967, 31). For those interested in why people in poor coun-tries die so much earlier than those in rich countries, this might seem a tan-gential discussion. However, these same forces operate in both rich and poor countries, and it is important that we fully understand the forces at work at the outset. The key question now is, why do such disparities persist in all countries? It is clear how detrimental poverty, and even comparative poverty, is to health. But why? How do we explain the results of the Whitehall study in which a homogeneous population, all living in and around London, all with the same access to clean water, sanitation, and competent health care, had consistently worsening health gradients as their occupational class lessened? There is something far more pervasive at work.

Possible Mechanisms

Researchers have long tried to understand the mechanisms through which lower class status causes poorer health for those in industrialized countries. Surprisingly, most of the data point away from that which we would intuitively assume most causative: certain behaviors, lack of access to health care, and environmental risks. Although these factors do contribute some, the most significant factors lie in the deep recesses of the mind, where various psychological stressors are turned into significant illnesses of all types. Of note, it is not just one or two illnesses that comprise the chief means through which those in lower classes prematurely die, it is most forms of disease. Whitehall found a higher mortality in lower classes for cancer, heart disease, cerebrovascular disease, chronic bronchitis, other respiratory diseases, accidents, and violence (Marmot 1993, 205). Adler found a correlation between lower educational levels (a proxy for lower social class) and an increasing incidence of 32 of 37 conditions surveyed (Adler et al 1999, 184).

It is clear from considerable research that the association is not spurious (Fein 1995, 583); that poverty causes illness, much more than illness causes poverty (Adler et al 1999, 185; Lynch et al 1997, 1889); and that illness is not due to destructive, health-related behaviors, like smoking or poor diet, as we might intuitively think (Fein 1995, 583; Marmot 1993, 208). The large Whitehall II study found that health-related behaviors accounted for only a small part of the six fold differential in absences due to sickness between those in the highest and lowest employment grades (North et al 1993, 361). Another researcher, Ana Diez Roux found that the incidence of coronary heart disease was three times higher in low-income neighborhoods than high-income neighborhoods, despite controlling for known coronary artery disease risk factors (Diez Roux et al 2001, 99).

It is also clear that the association is not due to material or structural deficiencies alone, which so often comprise the primary reasons for poor health in developing countries. Recall that the Whitehall Study found clear health gradients that tracked along economic class, despite the fact that this homogeneous population all worked in the same offices, lived in the greater London area, had similar access to health care, and suffered no material deprivations of any kind (Fein 1995, 584). This study essentially refutes the idea that material deprivation is the main culprit in the United Kingdom. In addition, Wilkinson conclusively demonstrated that once countries attain a certain degree of wealth, health gradients no longer correlate with rising prosperity (1992a, 1082). Those inclined to attribute health and class differentials to available health care will do well to recall that mortality gradients in Britain, with its Universal Health Service, are similar to those of the United States, which lacks universal health coverage. (Marmot 2000, 134).

The most significant causative factor is that which at first seems the least likely—stress—and the way stress causes the mind to affect the body. For example, individuals who have little control over the daily activities in the workplace have more stress and, consequently, more illness, such as coronary heart disease and depression (Marmot 2000, 134). The same two illnesses were increased in those who felt they had little control over home and life circumstances (Marmot 2000, 134; Adler et al 1999, 188). Those who reported that talking to their closest relative or friend usually made things worse and those who had financial difficulties also came more frequently from lower classes and had higher rates of sickness and periods of absences (North et al 1993, 361).

The Alameda County Study showed that, compared to individuals with no economic hardship, those individuals with economic hardship between the years 1965 to 1994 had 4.5 times higher levels of depression, 5 times higher likelihood of being "cynically hostile," 5.7 times higher likelihood of lacking optimism, and 4.6 times greater difficulty with cognitive functions (Lynch et al 1997, 1891). As such, poverty, or even relative poverty as described in industrialized countries, leads to a lack of control, which produces a significant detriment to health (Marmot 1993, 212).

Hostility, described as "a disposition prone to anger; a cynical, distrusting view of others; and antagonistic behavior," increases with declining socioeconomic status and shows direct correlation with risk of coronary heart disease and premature mortality (Adler 1999, 189). Stress, characterized as that emanating from such life events as divorce, spousal death, and unemployment or as the state that occurs when people perceive that "demands exceed their ability to cope," has been linked to a range of clinical disorders including gastrointestinal disease, heart attacks, menstrual disorders, and susceptibility to infectious pathogens (189). Stress likely affects bodily function through neuroendocrine and immune responses. A study from Bristol, England, showed that those whose homes were flooded in 1969 had a 50% higher mortality rate than a similarly matched control group over the next year (Wilkinson 1994b, 71). Stress increases noticeably in those of lower socioeconomic status, given increased concerns over finances, work and life control, social ordering, neighborhood of residence, crime, difficult relationships, and lowered life satisfaction. Stress is a major factor contributing to the overall decreased life expectancy of those at the bottom of the economic ladder.

Hierarchical positioning also has both direct and indirect effects on health. Adler points out in her review that several animal studies have shown a causal link between social positioning and health status (Adler et al 1999, 191). Subordinate baboons have lower levels of protective HDL cholesterol, with a consequential increased risk of coronary heart disease. And socially dominant macaques have less coronary atherosclerosis than their subordinates. Adler concludes, "Hierarchical position may have direct effects on physiological processes and neuroanatomical structures, which may in turn influence an individual's biological vulnerability to agents of disease" (189).

To put the psychological effects of relative poverty into perspective, it is instructive to draw from direct clinical experience, the point where the academic meets everyday reality. I have worked for a number of years in hospitals that treat large numbers of indigent people. In the emergency departments of Boston Medical Center and St Elizabeth's Medical Center there are times when the hallways are filled with the accursed, those who have surrendered to a hard life. It is obvious that many of these people are dying prematurely. One can almost feel the weight of their psychological burden, sense their quiet—and not so quiet—desperation resulting from their place in a society that has so clearly and convincingly overwhelmed them. Such clinical experience tells us that the factors that reside in the mind must contribute significantly to health and class differentials. As Michael Marmot concludes, "The mind is a crucial gateway through which social influences affect physiology to cause disease" (Marmot 2000, 134).

> The best way for a wealthy country to increase the health and life expectancy of its citizens is to minimize the number of people living in relative poverty.

The degree to which these psychological effects take hold depends on the extent of income disparity within a society. Richard Wilkinson has shown that the degree to which mortality differentials exist in developed countries depends more on the relative income disparity within the country than on the overall per capita income (1992a, 1082). Once per capita gross domestic product (GDP) exceeds $5,000.00 per year, increases in wealth make no difference in health indices (Wilkinson 1994b, 63). Instead, what appears to correlate most clearly and consistently is the degree to which that wealth is equitably distributed throughout the population. Countries like Japan, which have narrow income differentials, have the highest life expectancies. Those countries with wider income differentials, such as the United States, United Kingdom, France, Germany, and Spain, all have lower life expectancies (67). The United Kingdom experienced widening income differentials during the 1980s with subsequent rising mortality rates (Wilkinson 1992a, 1082). As such, the best way for a wealthy country to increase the health and life expectancy of its citizens is to minimize the number of people living in relative poverty. Decreasing the distance between those at the top and those at the bottom may well comprise the most effective public health intervention possible.

Following the recommendations of the *Black Report*, the *Health Divide*, and others, we can conclude that those societies that credibly address the needs of their most vulnerable citizens are destined to succeed, while those who ignore them do so at their own peril. As Kawachi said, "Societies that permit large disparities in income to develop also tend to be the ones that under invest in human capital (eg, education), health care, and other factors that promote health" (Kawachi et al 1997, 1491). Amartya Sen has shown that the most rapid improvements in life expectancy in the United Kingdom occurred during the two decades of war, (excluding direct war-related mortality) 1911–1921 and 1940–1951, despite the fact that both were slow periods of economic growth (Sen 1999, 49). He concludes that health improvements occurred because of the increase in "the extent of social sharing during the war decades, and the sharp increases in public support for social services (including nutritional support and health care) that went with this" (49). Governments ultimately hold the key to decreasing health and class differentials.

Conclusions

Although health is the most valued human commodity, it still eludes a significant portion of humanity. Similarly, the greatest enemy of good health remains that which has stalked it since antiquity—poverty and the structural violence that perpetuates it. In poor countries, poverty reigns supreme; in wealthy countries, it exerts an equally powerful influence, though operating by stealth through relative deprivation. The solution is better allocation of resources, particularly from wealthy countries to poor ones, where less goes a lot farther.

We can only assume that the psychological factors that affect most health and class differentials in wealthy countries are also at work in poor countries. These countries are simply overwhelmed by the enormity of the material deprivation that is the order of the day.

The comparison between rich and poor countries remains instructive. The fact that the abundant good health available to most people in rich countries is the envy of those in poor countries is an understatement. But what lessons can we learn from how the rich countries attained such previously unimaginable levels of good health? In the next chapter, we track the rise of good health in the developed world.

Endnotes

1. For more information, see the Gallup International Association web site at www.gallupinternational.com.
2. Note that the "wealthy" countries used here represent the "high-income OECD countries" in UNDP data.
3. For a complete discussion of this topic, see Jeffrey Sachs, *Macroeconomics and Health: Investing in Health for Economic Development, Report of the Commission on Macroeconomics and Health*, from the World Health Organization, 2001.
4. In Kenya, 30.7 million people spending $31.00 per person annually comes to $951.7 million in annual health care costs. Still, just a fraction of what we spend in the United States for minor infections.
5. This grouping comprises 44 countries, covering just south of the Sahara Desert to and including South Africa. Eritrea and Ethiopia are considered part of Sub-Saharan Africa whereas Sudan and Somalia are not.
6. The high-income OECD countries are 23 countries mostly in Europe, but also include the United States, Australia, New Zealand, Japan, and Canada. The OECD countries not included in the "high-income OECD countries" grouping are Czech Republic, Hungary, the Republic of Korea, Mexico, Slovakia, and Turkey.
7. This number is for OECD countries, not high-income OECD countries. The number of people per physician would likely be lower if high-income OECD countries.

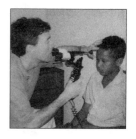

Chapter 2

The Rise of Health in the Industrialized World

Massive poverty and obscene inequality are such terrible scourges of our times—times in which the world boasts of breathtaking advances in science, technology, and wealth accumulation—that they have to rank alongside slavery and apartheid as social evils.

—Nelson Mandela

The spectacular successes of biomedicine have in many instances further entrenched medical inequalities. This necessarily happens whenever new and effective therapies—from antituberculous drugs to protease inhibitors—are not made readily available to those in need. Perhaps it was in anticipation of late-twentieth-century technology that Virchow argued that physicians must be the "natural attorneys of the poor."

—Paul Farmer, MD, PhD

When viewed through a historical lens, the health of today's poor shows haunting similarities to the abysmal health that those in "developed" countries considered the norm well over a century ago. In this chapter, we review how developed countries achieved such unprecedented levels of good health by looking at the four factors chiefly responsible: better nutrition, economic growth, the rise of public health measures, and better and more widely available medical care. We contrast each area to some of the remaining disparities that exist in poor countries. By furthering our understanding of just how the industrialized world achieved good health, we will have a better understanding of the challenges that lie ahead when we try to improve the health of those who live in poor countries.

Historical Perspective

For most of human history, people lived short, disease-ridden lives that were mere fractions of longevity today. From the time of the Roman Empire through the 19th century, the average life span was only 20 to 35 years. Then, as now, much of the excess mortality came at the expense of the youngest and most vulnerable, markedly skewing the average life expectancy downward. In one study from Vienna in the mid-18th century, more than 40% of infants died during their first year and 60% died by their fifth year (Antonovsky 1967, 32). Such trends have improved though not disappeared. As of 2000, 23 countries—all in sub-Saharan Africa—still see at least 10% of their newborns die during their first year, at rates 14 to 25 times that of the United States (United Nations Development Program [UNDP] 2002, 174). Quite expectedly, this contributes substantially to their respectively low life expectancy rates. Naturally, poverty has long played the most important role in keeping life expectancies short.

History teaches that there have been two great ascents from poverty and its associated poor health. The Industrial Revolution triggered the first in the late 19th and early 20th centuries in Europe and the United States. Better nutrition and some early public health interventions dramatically improved the health of the working class, thereby powering the engines of industry. The subsequent improvements in health have rightly been called "one of the great triumphs in human history" (Frank and Mustard 1994, 1). The second occurred in developing countries, Eastern Europe, and the former Soviet Union after World War II. Countries took advantage of technological breakthroughs made in the West and simultaneously developed poverty-reduction strategies for their people. Although far from equitably distributed, the gains are real and millions have risen out of extreme poverty (UNDP 1997, 2, 25). Global poverty has fallen more in the past 50 years than in the previous 500 years (UNDP 2001, 2).

Some of the most impressive recent gains have occurred in Asia, where the "big five" (China, India, Indonesia, Pakistan, and Bangladesh), comprising three fifths of the world's people, have all significantly reduced the percentage of "income poor" people (UNDP 1997, 33). Between 1949 and 1995, China doubled the life expectancy of its people while cutting its infant mortality rate to one fifth of what it was originally (49). Likewise, from 1961 to 1991, India nearly doubled the life expectancy of its people while cutting its infant mortality rate in half (25).

At the core of this extraordinary worldwide rise in life expectancies is the steady diffusion of knowledge, of which the four most important factors were: (1) better nutrition, (2) improved standards of living through economic growth, (3) a rise in public health measures, and (4) better and more widely available medical care (Frank and Mustard 1994). These advances have all diffused in varying degrees to poor countries, such that changes that took hundreds of years in industrialized countries may take but a generation or two today. As a 2001 United Nations (UN) report concluded, "The rapid gains [in life expectancies] of the 20th century were propelled by medical technology—antibiotics and vaccines—while the gains of the 19th century depended on slower social and economic changes, such as better sanitation and diets" (UNDP 2001, 2).

Nutrition

From the earliest times, people have advanced only as far as their nutritional resources have allowed. The earliest hunter-gatherers lived short lives tethered to an unreliable food supply. However, human history advanced appreciably around 8500 B.C., following the discovery and cultivation of wheat and other edible plants in the Fertile Crescent, the area roughly encompassing modern Jordan, Israel, Iraq, Iran, Syria, and Turkey (Diamond 1999, 99). Because 1 acre of cultivated crops can feed 10 to 100 times more people than 1 acre left alone to feed hunter-gatherers, human populations subsequently increased and the first agrarian societies were born (88).

By the 18th century, technological advances such as crop rotation, the animal-drawn plow, and fertilizer created the Agricultural Revolution, allowing Europeans and Americans to feed more people. Shortly thereafter, the Industrial Revolution spawned a rapidly growing urban population that required ever-increasing amounts of food to sustain it. These population pressures prompted technological advances such as higher-yielding crops that led to more efficient use of available land. More available food created a more productive workforce that in turn created wealth and power.

Those with inadequate nutrition suffer a form of immune deficiency, making them far more vulnerable to all microbial pathogens.

There is significant evidence that a well-fed and nutritionally sound workforce can improve the economic output of a society. Nobel prize winning economist Robert Fogel wrote that "the efficiency of the human engine" increased by 60% between 1790 and 1980, largely due to improvements in nutrition (Rosenberg 1994). This in turn fostered continued economic growth. In fact, better nutrition has accounted for more than half of Britain's economic growth since the Industrial Revolution (Frank and Mustard 1994, 15). The situation persists today. More recent studies have shown that workers are far more productive when their diets have more calories, vitamins, and minerals (UNDP 1996, 76).

Thomas McKeown, the author of *The Modern Rise of Populations* (1976), concluded that the dramatic decline in deaths due to infectious diseases in the United Kingdom from 1838 to 1970 was not due to improvements in public health or medical interventions but to the "nutritional improvement associated with rising levels of per capita income" (Rosenberg 1994, 137). Historically, a starving peasant class produced high mortality rates and slowed productivity through chronic fatigue. Those with inadequate nutrition suffer a form of immune deficiency, making them far more vulnerable to all microbial pathogens. Globally, malnutrition causes more immunodeficiency than AIDS by a wide margin (UNICEF 1998, 71).[1] Improved basic nutrition arms the immune system to fight off illness, comprising the best protection against disease, far better than any public health or medical intervention.

Most recent advances in nutrition have come through better agricultural techniques and better understanding of the nutritional causes of poor health. For example, by understanding how iodine deficiency causes mental retardation, we can now take steps to ensure adequate iodine in pregnant women's diets, like adding iodine to salt. By breeding drought-resistant plant strains, we can combat hunger. The huge reduction in malnutrition in South Asia—from 40% in the 1970s to 20% in 1997—resulted from technological advances in fertilizers, pesticides, and plant breeding made in the 1960s that doubled the yields of world cereal crops in just 40 years. By contrast, it took the English 1,000 years to quadruple wheat yields from 0.5 to 2.0 tons per hectare. Another advance helpful to poor countries is transgenics, the science through which genes are shared between different crops to produce "super crops" that have higher yields and insect and drought resistance. Genetically modified (GM) rice has increased crop yields by 15% in China (UNDP 2001, 2). Although considerable resistance to genetically modified crops remains in Europe and some developing countries (GM crops cover only 5% of global farm acreage), it still holds promise for the future ("Genetically Modified Food" 2003).

Nevertheless, significant challenges remain. There are 826 million undernourished people in the developing world today (UNDP 2001, 2), even though enough food is produced in the world to feed everyone (World Health Organization [WHO], 1998). Poor nutrition early in life may also lead to chronic diseases later in life, such as coronary artery disease, hypertension, and diabetes (UNICEF 1998, 10).

The major impact of malnutrition is, as always, on infants and children. Each day 27,000 children die of treatable illness, often spurred by malnutrition. In fact, the WHO estimated that more than half of all child deaths in developing countries in 1995 were associated with malnutrition (UNICEF 1998, 11). WHO further estimates that roughly one third of the world's children are affected by protein-energy malnutrition (PEM). These are the kids with bloated bellies and thinning hair that we see on late-night television ads. Of these, 76% live in Asia, 21% live in Africa, and 3% in Latin America (WHO 1998, 69). Globally, malnutrition causes stunted growth in 226 million poor children and causes 183 million children to weigh less than they should for their age (UNICEF 1998, 15). In addition, nutritional deficiencies during the first few years of life produce mental slowness that robs children of their future.

> *Globally, malnutrition causes stunted growth in 226 million poor children and causes 183 million children to weigh less than they should for their age (UNICEF 1998, 15).*

But not all of the danger of malnutrition comes from a mere lack of food. Many of the vitamin and mineral deficiencies described in classic literature continue apace, exacting an enormous toll on the world's poor. Vitamin A deficiency affects 100 million young children worldwide, causing blindness and, even in mild forms, immune deficiency that leaves children susceptible to diarrhea (2.2 million deaths per year) and measles (1 million deaths per year). Anemia is one factor in pregnancy complications that kills 585,000 women annually (UNICEF 1998, 10). It also produces psychomotor deficiency and markedly drops IQ scores (11). Folate deficiency during pregnancy leads to spina bifida and vitamin D deficiency causes poor bone formation and rickets. Iodine deficiency is the world's most significant cause of preventable brain damage and mental retardation (WHO 1998, 69).

Nutrition is likely the most important determinant of health (Kim et al 2000, 112); and improvements in nutrition—and thus health—have allowed both rich and poor countries to advance through healthier workforces. As we consider our roles in developing countries, it is wise to consider the toll of malnutrition and nutritional deficiencies. For example, where is the wisdom of funding expensive anti-tuberculosis drugs when people so afflicted are starving and unable to adequately mount an immune response? Similarly, is it wise to spend money on tertiary medical care when programs to enhance basic nutrition would go so much farther? Clearly, attention to nutrition should remain a core concern for those who will work abroad.

Economic Growth and Equity

Economic growth may seem a distant concern for those in clinical practice, even those who venture abroad to improve health.[2] When introducing a text on the harmful effects of some economic policies on the poor (*Dying for Growth*), the physician and anthropologist Dr Paul Farmer told a Cambridge audience that none of the doctors, activists, or scholars who had done the research had really wanted to learn about the economics. But, after years of observing the effects of economic policies on the poor, they concluded that they could avoid it no longer. In the book's preface, Farmer wrote, "Even if we had balked at making the connection between economic policy and illness experience, our patients have been quick to point out these links. When the sick in El Salvador or Haiti insist, 'I'm sick because I lost my land,' is it far-fetched to discern in such claims the impact of ill-advised decisions about land tenure and agricultural policy?' All those who participated in the writing of this volume have been forced to consider health and sickness as economic outcomes" (Kim et al 2000, xii). And so it was in the United States, Europe, and other industrialized countries a century ago. An understanding of the linkage between economic policies and health is crucial to understanding why disparities in health remain.

An understanding of the linkage between economic policies and health is crucial to understanding why disparities in health remain.

First, however, we need to clarify some basic concepts, starting with GNP and GDP, similar terms often used interchangeably. A country's *gross domestic product* (GDP) is defined as the annual amount of goods and services it produces. *Gross national product* (GNP) is similar but includes offshore production, like that of a US citizen based in the Caribbean. Put differently, GDP measures all production within the United States by everyone working there; GNP measures the production of Americans wherever they are in the world (Moneychimp, 2004). Economic growth is simply the annual change of a country's real (inflation-adjusted) GDP. Growth is more easily understood as the percent increase in a country's net economic output in one year, as compared to the prior year. Rates of 3% to 4% per year are considered healthy for developed countries and 5% to 7% targeted for developing countries (Kim et al 2000, 60). The US economy grew at a rate of 2.2% in 2002, 3.1% in 2003, and 4.4% in 2004 (US Bureau of Economic Analysis, 2004). In recent years, China and India have grown at rates of 6% to 9% per year, propelling millions out of poverty and markedly improving the health indices of their people.

The "Miracle" of Growth

Through history economic growth has propelled millions of people out of poverty and ill health. In fact, differing economic growth rates among various countries and regions have led directly to current disparities in income, and therefore in health and longevity. For example, in 1820, the gap between the world's richest economy, the United Kingdom, and its poorest region, Africa, was 4:1. By 1998, the gap between the richest economy, the United States, and the poorest region, Africa, had widened to 20:1 (Sachs 2005a, 28). Some countries grew while others did not, and our current world order primarily reflects two centuries of greatly uneven patterns of economic growth.

The Industrial Revolution (1790–1850) elevated millions out of perpetual poverty, though it came at a price. Thousands of small farmers were forced off their lands and into the poor shantytowns to work as laborers for burgeoning industry (Werner and Sanders 1997, 77). While some made vast fortunes, many more became trapped in urban squalor, as graphically portrayed by Charles Dickens. In 1870s England, schoolchildren in working class schools were malnourished and sickly, averaging 3 to 5 inches shorter than their upper-class counterparts (77). It was only in the later stages of the Industrial Revolution that real progress was made. As a reaction to the abhorrent conditions of the crowded slums of Europe, social movements, unions, and cooperatives spurred advances in public education, housing, sanitation, and public health. Similar movements occurred in the 1930s in the United States, with the advent of the Roosevelt Administration and its many social welfare programs, such as Social Security (UNDP 1997, 25). The benefits of growth became more widely shared.

It is easy to find those who tout the virtues of economic growth. Consider the following from British academician Richard Wilkinson, "While it is possible to argue the relative historical contributions of better nutrition, sewers, clean water supplies, improved housing, and eventually, immunization to the long decline in mortality rates, there can be no doubt that the enabling and sustaining power of economic growth was behind them all" (Wilkinson 1994b, 62).

The United Nations Development Program (UNDP) adds, "Sustained national GDP growth, combined with rising wages and productivity, was an important part of the historic ascent from poverty in the industrialized countries—and in the past thirty years in such countries as China, Indonesia, and Malaysia, which have dramatically reduced poverty in income and other critical dimensions" (UNDP 1997, 71). As people earn more, they live longer, have a better standard of living, and more of them become literate (UNDP 1996, 67). The UN has shown that a 1% increase in GDP per capita correlates with a 0.13% rise in life expectancy and a 1% reduction in child mortality (114). Consider an example: If Bangladesh can maintain current economic growth rates of 5% per year for the next five years, it should see the average life expectancy of its people rise by more than two years, and its infant mortality rate fall by more than 25%, impressive changes by historical standards.[3]

The World Bank (discussed further in Chapter 5) has encouraged growth-oriented policies in poor countries for decades. In its seminal World Development Report in 1993, *Investing in Health*, the Bank cited data showing child mortality rates falling by 60% during the 1980s in countries where average incomes rose by more than 1% per year. Following this and other evidence, it concluded, "Economic policies conducive to sustained economic growth are thus among the most important measures governments can take to improve their citizens' health" (World Bank Group 1993, 7). This became known as the "Washington Consensus," or "neoliberal" economic theory, and it has ruled supreme for decades (Kim et al 2000, 7).

Other data make an equally compelling case. When plotted together from 1970 to 1990, the GNP per capita and life expectancy rates show a remarkably consistent correlation, rising together at least for low-income levels (Wilkinson 1994b, 62). Put another way, as incomes rise, people live longer. There are no wealthy countries with low levels of human development, though some poor countries have been able to achieve high levels of human development. Growth certainly can be the engine that lifts people out of backbreaking poverty and its consequential ill health. Even those who have documented the damage that ruthless pro-growth governmental policies have had on the poor acknowledge that the situation faced by poor people "would almost certainly get worse without it" (Kim et al 2000, 61). The UN adds, "having no economic growth is almost entirely bad for poor people" (UNDP 1997, 71).

The Limits of Growth

Yet there are limitations to the idea that a rising tide lifts all boats. First is the effect growth has on the health of those in developed countries. Wilkinson has shown that once countries achieved a $5,000 GDP per capita in 1990 dollars, life expectancies, on average, ceased to rise (Wilkinson 1994b, 63). Beyond that level, increasing income produces radically diminished returns on improvements in health. As such, we can conclude that in the later stages of industrial development, growth has little influence on health. As we have seen, relative deprivation then becomes paramount. Where one fits into the socioeconomic tiers of industrialized societies determines how long one will live. The United States, United Kingdom, and New Zealand all experienced good average growth between 1975 and 1995, yet saw their percentage of poor rise (UNDP 1997, 7).

Second, it is far from certain that poor countries will necessarily benefit a great deal from economic growth (Wilkinson 1992b, 168). The WHO assessed the marked decline in mortality from 1960 to 1990 in 115 low- and middle-income countries and found that rising levels of income explained only 20% of the gains (WHO 1999, 5). Most gains came from advances in technology and social spending by the government. The report concludes, "The effects of economic growth on health, while real, are relatively weak and likely to be slow in coming" (7).

Finally—and most important—it is questionable just how much the benefits of growth actually "trickle down" to the poor. Certain power circles have always believed that the benefits from economic growth eventually spread to all members of a society. In the 1970s and early 1980s, however, growth slowed and many poor countries went deeply into debt. The World Bank and the International Monetary Fund (IMF) responded by pushing poor countries toward "export-oriented" growth strategies, which allowed them to generate dollars with which they could repay their debt to the wealthy lending countries. However, the economic realignment came at a price: governments had to cut social services like health, education, and nutritional programs for the poor. For most poor people life just got harder—and shorter.

Many poor people are now worse off following decades of neoliberal economic practices, with more than 1.6 billion people worse off economically in the late 1990s than they were in the early 1980s and per capita incomes in 100 countries lower in 2000 than they were 15 years earlier. Case studies from Haiti, Peru, Mexico, El Salvador, Russia, and sub-Saharan Africa show how these policies, often imposed by the IMF and World Bank, have frequently benefited the few at the expense of the many (Kim et al 2000). Policies that have supported unbridled growth—often through harshly imposed economic belt-tightening by the poor—have actually worsened the health of millions. As such, the UN concludes that although there is a general correlation between GDP per capita and increasing human development, it is "far from an automatic link" (UNDP 1996, 67).

"Pro-Poor" Growth

Although economic growth can be a powerful engine of better health and longer life for the poor, it is only when governments—prompted by their citizenry—follow strategies of growth that are more equitable that all benefit. This pattern of growth has been appropriately called *pro-poor growth* (UNDP 1996, 7). A UN reports states, "Growth should be judged not by the abundance of commodities it produces, but by how it enriches people's lives" (43).

Economist Amartya Sen has written extensively about the Indian state of Kerala (Sen 1993, 45). This state of 29 million is considerably poorer than most other states in India, which in 2000 had a per capita GDP of $2538.00 (UNDP 2002, 151). By contrast, the United States had a per capita GDP of $34,142.00 in 2000 (149). Despite low income, this region has been able to achieve a life expectancy of over age 70, largely by emphasizing public education, subsidized nutrition, and enhanced medical resources and social services (Sen 1993, 45). Sen has rightly stressed that it is not only the level of income of a society that gives quality to the lives of its inhabitants. Rather it is people's "capabilities to lead the lives they value" that matters (UNDP 1996, 49). Governments play crucial roles in creating these "capabilities" by investing in their people (Frank and Mustard 1994).

Countries show wide variations in their income distribution and relative degrees of health equality. Those with less concentrated wealth tend to derive more productivity from their citizens and more rapid growth (Wilkinson 1994b, 74). Hong Kong, Indonesia, Malaysia, the Republic of Korea, Singapore, Taiwan, and Thailand have all seen remarkable growth in recent decades (7.6% annual per capita growth from 1960 to 1993) with relatively low levels of inequality (UNDP 1996, 52). This serves to challenge the more traditional assumption that it is better economically to channel income to the rich who will invest and save more. Other countries, such as the United States, United Kingdom, and Brazil, have seen greater levels of inequality and less rapid growth. One UN study concluded that if the Republic of Korea had Brazil's level of inequality in 1960, its GDP 25 years later would have been 15% lower (53).

From 1955 to 1970, Japan achieved annual growth rates of 10%, partly because it has the narrowest income differentials in the developed world (53). Japan is also the country with the highest per capita expenditures on education and health. Life expectancy rose by a full decade between 1958 and 1993 in that country. China has similarly achieved high rates of growth with equity, albeit with far less resources than Japan. Following land reform and other poverty-reduction strategies, China reduced its rural poor population from 260 million in 1978 to 65 million in 1995 (UNDP 1997, 49). India, too, has made impressive gains over the past 50 years by sharing more widely the benefits of its economic growth (51).

Although Guinea and Sri Lanka have nearly identical GDPs per capita of $600 per year, their governments have pursued vastly different policies—Sri Lanka's human development index (HDI) is far higher than that of Guinea (UNDP 1996, 67). Ecuador and Morocco had similar GNPs per capita in 1993, yet Ecuadorians live 10 years longer with 50% more of them literate (31). Costa Rica, with a 1993 GNP per capita of only $2,150, had HDIs that placed it firmly in the company of industrialized countries with average per capita incomes as much as four times higher than Costa Rica's (30, 135).

In sum, economic growth is an important factor in improving the health of the poor. Though not the panacea it was once touted to be, it must be a component of any real poverty-reduction strategy. When governments spread the benefits of growth broadly throughout a population, health indices invariably rise. Those countries with the good sense to combine strong economic growth with large public financial outlays that improve human development stand to reap the most benefits (UNDP 1996, 82). In unequal societies where elite groups have all the power and control the resources, some benefit while many others fail. As those wealth disparities widen, so too do the respective health and longevity differentials of the class components within that society. Such has been the history of economic growth through time. Investments in health, education, and nutrition for the bulk of their population represents perhaps the best expenditure a country can make, allowing many more people to become healthy and productive citizens.

Public Health and Medical Care

Early Years in the United States and Europe

Since the late 1800s, the applications of biomedical science accounted for enormous improvements in the health and longevity of people in all countries. Whether the benefits of this science flow more through public health initiatives, direct clinical care, or legislation is a matter of considerable debate. There is no question that basic sanitation, clean water, and vaccination programs have far greater impact on the health of a country than building tertiary care hospitals (Werner and Sanders 1997, 15). However, the lines between public health, direct health care, and legislation have become increasingly blurred. Physicians now counsel patients to avoid tobacco, and local laws limit the places where people can smoke. Both of these actions originated in the realm of public health. Health providers counsel patients on family planning, treat them for hypertension, advise women to take folate during pregnancy, vaccinate children, and suggest ways to reduce violence and car injuries. All of these strategies began from public health initiatives. What is indisputable is the impact that biomedical science has had on human health.

We can best appreciate this impact by tracing its evolution and reflecting on how it has caused people to reconsider where illness comes from. It was not that long ago that people in the United States and Europe attributed illness in all forms to anything but the factors that we now understand are causative. Similar patterns have occurred in more recent times in poor countries with little or no exposure to modern medical care. Albert Schweitzer noted that his patients in Gabon in the early 1900s attributed all forms of disease to a "worm" (Schweitzer 1948a, 24). In Southeast Asia in the 1950s, American physician and popular icon Tom Dooley constantly negotiated with witch doctors and their unusual concepts of illness causation, as Paul Farmer still does today in Haiti. I treated wounds in Kenya in 1994 that were made far worse by the common practice of smearing cow dung on them. In settings of entrenched poverty, such beliefs persist.

In the early history of the United States, medieval concepts of witchcraft gradually gave way to the idea that moral deficiency was the root cause of disease. After the Reformation, Protestantism banished the supernatural from healing, replacing it with "a moral view of misfortune" (Starr 1982, 35). Paul Starr writes, "In sixteenth and seventeenth century England . . . the proper reaction to an accident or illness was to search one's soul for moral error" (35). These ideas persisted well into the 19th century on both sides of the Atlantic. In the 1830s, American ministers believed that cholera was "sent by God to punish sin." One minister warned, "The cholera is not caused by intemperance and filth, but it is a scourge, a rod in the hand of God. . . ." (36).

If the American colonists turned to religion instead of to the medical profession for relief in times of illness, they had good reason. Early medical practices lacked a scientific basis and tended to follow idiosyncratic beliefs. One prominent physician from the University of Pennsylvania told his students in 1796, "There is but one disease in the world . . . a moribund excitement induced by capillary tension" (Starr 1982, 42). That one disease had just one heroic cure: to reduce capillary tension "by letting blood with a lancet and emptying out the stomach and bowels with the use of powerful emetics and cathartics" (42). Because this regimen could produce a state of unconsciousness, the practitioners had to pursue these cures "with courage." Such practices continued through the middle of the 19th century. No wonder the medical profession was poorly regarded (47).

In 1835, Harvard physician James Bigelow acknowledged that it was "the unbiased opinion of most medical men of sound judgment and long experience [that] the amount of death and disaster in the world would be less if all disease were left to itself" (Starr 1982, 55). Gradually, less aggressive forms of therapy replaced the violent purging and bloodletting and doctors came to accept a more humble role, allowing that most cures came through natural means rather than medical interventions.

The Golden Age of Public Health

Throughout the 19th century, however, things began to change. Great advances were made in basic science and public health. French physicians correlated clinical aspects of disease with pathological changes found on autopsies. In 1816 Laennec introduced the stethoscope, which enabled physicians examining patients to correlate sounds with clinical symptoms. Other diagnostic instruments soon followed, including the ophthalmoscope and laryngoscope, x-rays, spirometers, electrocardiographs, microscopes, and machines to perform chemical and bacteriological tests (Starr 1982, 136). Increasingly secure in their claims to legitimacy, doctors no longer needed to mystify their patients with prescriptions written in Latin. Now they had a gamut of scientific tests beyond the comprehension of the average person.

Physicians in Paris began to study the effectiveness of standard treatments of the day by using the scientific method. As Starr noted, "Empirical evidence rather than dogmatic assertions of personal or traditional authority became the grounds for assessing truth" (Starr 1982, 55). As such, a core principle of clinical medicine emerged. However, most of the early "evidence" showed that the accepted therapeutic techniques of the day had no value or were harmful. Medical science had evolved a method of assessing clinical truths that, when turned on itself, had shown how wholly inadequate the standard practices really were. Nevertheless, the thinking had changed, opening the door for the important discoveries that rapidly followed.

In the mid-19th century, physicians in Europe and the United States began to stress the "social conditions in the causation of disease" (Starr 1982, 55). In one of the early success stories of public health, Dr John Snow hypothesized that something in the London water supply was the cause of the massive cholera epidemic of 1854. By removing the handle from the Broad Street water pump, Snow brought the epidemic to a halt. Although the bacteria *Vibrio cholera* was unknown at the time, Dr Snow had demonstrated that something in the water had been making people sick. When authorities changed the source of public drinking water to an area that was uncontaminated by sewage from the Thames, cholera rates fell precipitously.[4] Subsequent improvements to water supplies and sanitation markedly improved health. Sand filtration of water supplies, begun in the 1890s, proved more effective at eliminating typhoid than earlier sanitary reform (Starr 1982, 135). Chlorination of public drinking water supplies in the early 1900s further decreased the amount of waterborne illness (Centers for Disease Control and Prevention [CDC] 1999a).

The second half of the 19th century saw key breakthroughs in bacteriology through the work of Pasteur and Koch. Long before antibiotics and vaccines became available, the incidence of food and waterborne diseases such as typhoid, cholera, and salmonella fell sharply because of public health interventions as basic as hand-washing, sanitation, refrigeration, and the use of pesticides (CDC 1999b). Pasteurization of milk, widely adopted in the early 20th century, "dramatically" lowered infant mortality by eliminating an important pathogenic vector of food borne disease (Starr 1982, 135; CDC 1999b). Lister's introduction of "antiseptic" surgical technique in 1867 paved the way for dramatic improvements in surgery, with pioneer surgeons like the Mayo brothers operating on appendicitis, gallbladder disease, and stomach ulcers (Starr 1982, 156). Combating the various infectious pathogens contributed to the evolution of public health surveillance agencies, eg, Britain's National Health System (Epstein 1992, 264).

The 20th century opened to a dizzying series of public health successes, spurred on by new insights from epidemiology and biomedical science. Advances in the removal of solid waste and development of standards for housing and food quality improved the health of all people, particularly the poor. Advances in the nutritional sciences led to an understanding of the underlying causality of diseases long thought to be infectious in origin, including rickets, scurvy, beriberi, and pellagra. In 1921, 75% of infants in New York City had rickets, now rarely seen in the United States because milk has been fortified with vitamin D since the 1940s (CDC 1999b). Between

1906 and 1940 in the United States, roughly 3 million cases and 100,000 deaths were attributed to pellagra, a disease caused by niacin deficiency. It had long been associated with poverty and the poor diet that accompanies it. Following an improved diet and flour enrichment with niacin in the 1940s, pellagra became rare in developed countries (CDC 1999b).

By the 1930s, these miracles in public health had become routine in industrialized countries. Hugely successful programs had become integrated into the fabric of society. Worker safety, family planning, and food and water regulations all became part of a legislative arsenal ensuring better health for all citizens. As America moved into the 1950s, an era in which public health ruled the day had passed (Thomas 1983, 137). Energies and funding shifted increasingly toward hospitals and doctors, where the potential seemed limitless.

Medical Practice and the Broader Integration of "Health" into Society

During the 19th and early 20th centuries, doctors were members of a profession considered neither honorable nor having much to do with science. An 1870 entry in a medical journal commented that when a young man (and they were all men at the time) decided to become a physician, "the feeling among the majority of his cultivated friends is that he has thrown himself away" (Starr 1982, 83). Practice required long hours for little pay. Many physicians kept additional non-medical jobs to make ends meet—one robbed stagecoaches on the side until captured and imprisoned in 1855.

With time, medicine became a more respectable vocation, though it could still offer little in the form of curative therapies. The great writer and physician Lewis Thomas recalled going on house calls with his father in the 1920s:

> I'm quite sure my father always hoped I would want to become a doctor, and that must have been part of the reason for taking me along on his visits. But the general drift of his conversation was intended to make clear to me, early on, the aspect of medicine that troubled him most through his professional life; that there were so many people needing help, and so little that he could do for any of them. It was necessary for him to be available, and to make all these calls at their homes, but I was not to have the idea that he could do anything much to change the course of their illnesses (Thomas 1983, 13).

Thomas' observation held true for nearly two more decades, though vaccines for smallpox, rabies, typhoid, cholera, and plague gave physicians something to offer (CDC, 1999c). On the wards of Boston City Hospital during his residency in the 1930s, Thomas observed, "Whether you survived or not depended on the natural history of the disease itself. Medicine made little or no difference" (Thomas 1983, 40). The physician's role in the early

20th century was principally to diagnose, explain, and offer distraught patients some prognosis as to what was going to happen.

But the landscape was about to permanently change. In 1937 the first antibiotic, sulfanilamide, triggered a "revolution" in medicine (Thomas 1983, 35). As Thomas recalls, "I remember with astonishment when the first cases of pneumonia and streptococcal septicemia [blood-borne bacterial infection] were treated in Boston in 1937. The phenomenon was almost beyond belief. Here were moribund patients, who would surely have died without treatment, improving in their appearance within a matter of hours of being given the medicine and feeling entirely well within the next day or so" (35). For the medical profession, these biomedical advancements signaled the beginning of a revolution that would forever alter health care. Overnight, everything had changed. "Medicine," Thomas wrote, "was off and running" (35).

In March 1942, a 33-year-old woman, running fevers of up to 107°F and suffering from delirium, was hospitalized for a life-threatening streptococcal infection in a Connecticut hospital. Having failed with conventional treatments of sulfa drugs, surgery, and blood transfusions, her doctors injected her with an experimental drug as a last-ditch effort to save her. The drug was penicillin. Overnight, her temperature dropped and her delirium cleared. She survived her illness and lived to age 90 (CDC 1999a). Sir Alexander Fleming and two others later received the Nobel Prize for Physiology and Medicine for their discovery of this life-changing drug (CDC 1999a). Soon other antibiotics followed and one infectious disease after another fell under the advance of modern medical prowess.

Today, infectious disease no longer heads the list of killers in the United States and other developed countries. Despite a proliferation of antibiotic-resistant pathogens, most people living in the United States no longer worry much about infectious causes of death. In 2001, the leading causes of death in the United States were heart disease, cancer, and stroke.[5] By contrast, in 1900 the leading causes had been pneumonia, tuberculosis, and diarrhea/enteritis. These conditions, combined with diphtheria, accounted for nearly one third of all deaths that year (CDC 1999a, 621). This "epidemiological transition" represents one of the great public health and medical achievements in US history.

Yet infectious disease comprised only one of many fronts on which modern medicine advanced. Researchers uncovered the cause and cure for cardiovascular disease and the risks associated with cigarette smoking. CT and MRI scans, ultrasound, dialysis, laparoscopic and endoscopic techniques, general anesthesia, and invasive surgical techniques all represent technological advances of great importance. Advances in maternal-child care and workplace and automotive safety all resulted from a new understanding of the causes of illness and all contributed to falling mortality rates.

According to the CDC, one of the most important public health achievements has been the dramatic reduction in deaths from cardiovascular disease, which has decreased 60% since 1950 (CDC 1999d).[6] Heart disease has been the leading cause of death in the United States since 1921. Together with stroke, the third leading cause since 1938, they account for roughly 40% of all US deaths (CDC 1999d). The Framingham Heart Study, started in 1949, identified such causative factors as smoking, hypertension, diabetes, and high cholesterol, prompting dramatic lifestyle changes throughout the US public, endorsed by physicians, public health specialists, legislative action, and nonprofit groups such as the American Heart Association. Kowenhouven's closed cardiac massage launched the era of advanced cardiac life support (ACLS) and emergency medical systems (EMS) (Blackhall 1987).[7] Subsequent development of thrombolytic therapy (clot-busting medication), angioplasty, stenting of acutely closed vessels, cardiac surgery, and other advances have caused mortality rates to plummet. Coronary artery bypass and grafting (CABG) techniques are commonplace today, with patient discharge from the hospital reduced to three days after surgery. As an enduring legacy of 20th century science, many Americans have stopped smoking. A World War II poster that hung in the Boston City Hospital medical library depicted a war-weary GI smiling after his buddy offers him a cigarette. The caption read, "Give him an infusion . . . give him a Lucky Strike." Before the 1960s, tobacco manufacturers touted their product as beneficial and smoking became wildly popular; by 1965, 42.4% of the US adult population smoked. As a result, lung cancer, which had been rare in the early 1900s, became epidemic, increasing fifteen fold between 1930 and 1990 (CDC 1999e). Heart disease, lung disease, other cancers, and peripheral vascular disease also proliferated with increased smoking rates.

> *Because smoking is implicated in 20% of all deaths in the United States each year and costs $100 billion in medical and indirect costs, anti-smoking efforts represent one of the most significant—and cost-effective—public health achievements in US history.*

Then in 1964, the US Surgeon General issued a warning on the relationship between cigarette smoking and illness (citing data from more than 7,000 articles). Public health efforts targeting smoking cessation began shortly thereafter, preventing 1.6 million deaths over the next 30 years. The net effect has been to cut smoking rates almost in half in the United States. Because smoking is implicated in 20% of all deaths in the United States each year and costs $100 billion in medical and indirect costs, anti-smoking efforts represent one of the most significant—and cost-effective—public health achievements in US history (CDC 1999e).

Following medical advances in maternal care, including antibiotics, use of oxytocin to induce labor, safer blood products, and better treatment for toxemia, maternal mortality fell by 71% between the years 1939 and 1948 alone (CDC 1999f). Further advances in ob-gyn surgery and management have caused mortality rates to plummet by 99% since 1900 (CDC 1999g). Today, a woman in an Organization for Economic Co-operation and Development (OECD) country has only a 1 in 4085 chance of dying during pregnancy or childbirth, a far cry from the same woman in sub-Saharan Africa who has a 1 in 13 chance (UNDP 2002, 27). The legalization of abortion in the 1960s in the United States, while still controversial, did contribute an 89% decrease in maternal deaths from septic illegal abortions between 1950 and 1973 (CDC 1999f). In addition, combinations of clinical, public health, and legislative actions have produced benefits in various areas. Fluoridation of public drinking water dramatically reduced dental caries (CDC 1999g). Federal statutes like the Occupational Safety and Health Act of 1970 dramatically cut workplace injuries and deaths (CDC 1999h). Improvements in car safety and road design and legislation requiring the use of seatbelts and child seats caused the annual death rate from car crashes to plummet (CDC 1999i). Universal vaccination, antibiotics, and legislative mandates such as Medicaid and WIC (Women, Infants, and Children) that improved access to health care for poor kids all caused childhood mortality to fall sharply (Dowell et al 2000, 1402).

Public health officials and health providers brought these advances directly to the public and legislators turned them into laws. And others have played key roles as well. Foundations such as those founded by John D. Rockefeller, Bill Gates, W.K. Kellogg, and Robert Wood Johnson put billions into health initiatives. Nonprofit groups such as the March of Dimes, Rotary International, the American Heart Association, the American Cancer Society, Mothers Against Drunk Driving, the American Medical Association, the American Dental Association, and the American Red Cross have improved health by raising awareness and implementing specific programs.

From legislation to the establishment of state departments of public health in the late 1800s to the creation of Social Security in the 1930s to Medicare and Medicaid in the 1960s, the US government has exerted a push to bestow the benefits of health to more of its citizens. Federal agencies cover everything from ensuring access to health care to funding research in molecular biology. Agencies such as the National Institutes of Health, Federal Drug Administration, CDC, Occupational Safety and Health Administration, and US Environmental Protection Agency, which yield an enormous impact on general health, operate largely out of public view. Only an occasional crisis, such as the Ebola outbreak in Reston, Virginia, in 1989 or the SARS (severe acute respiratory syndrome) outbreak in 2002–2003, briefly raises the public visibility of these organizations. Perhaps the true test of their value is to look at countries in which their equivalent does not exist. Their influence is clear (CDC, 1999j).

The net result of these advances throughout the 20th century to Americans has been huge increases in life expectancy. In 2001, the average person in the United States could expect to live to 77.2 years, nearly *30 years* longer than someone living in 1900 (47.6 years) (CDC 1999j).[8] As incredible as these advances have been, particularly for those of us who work with them on a daily basis, it is clear that these later advances in public health and medical care do not equal the survival differences afforded by earlier rising levels of prosperity and advances in nutrition and basic water and sanitation efforts. Still, the clear efficacy of public health and medical care remains. We should recall that the life expectancy of Americans living in 1900 is similar to that of people living in sub-Saharan Africa today. Hence our most relevant question remains, how have some of these health gains spread to the developing world, while others have not? This is the question that we will explore fully in the following chapters.

Endnotes

1. "Globally, malnutrition impairs the immune systems of at least 100 million young children and several million pregnant women" (UNICEF 1998, 71). By comparison, UNAIDS estimated in December 2004 that 40 million people are infected with HIV.
2. For more in-depth discussions on growth and its impact on people's health in modern times and through history, see the 1993 World Development Report of the World Bank; the Human Development Report of 1996; several of the articles in the Fall 1994 issues of *Daedalus*, the "Health and Wealth" issue; and Kim et al's *Dying For Growth* (Common Courage Press, 2000).
3. Data from the Central Intelligence Agency *World Fact Book*, available online at www.cia.gov.
4. Data from the Supercourse: The History of Public Health web site at www.pitt.edu/~super1/lecture/lec4171/012.htm.
5. Data from the Centers for Disease Control, National Center for Health Statistics Deaths—Leading Causes web page, available at www.cdc.gov/nchs/fastats/lcod.htm.
6. For more information, see Evolution of the Joint National Committee Reports, 1988–1997. Evolution of the science of treating hypertension. *Archives of Internal Medicine*. 1997;157:2413.
7. Kouwenhoven first reported a 70% survival rate in patients with cardiac arrest undergoing closed cardiac message, a rate that has never since been duplicated. See WB Kouwenhoven et al. Closed-cardiac chest massage. *JAMA*. 1960;173:1064–1067.
8. For more information, see the Centers for Disease Control, National Center for Health Statistics Life Expectancy web page, available at www.cdc.gov/nchs/fastats/lifexpec.htm.

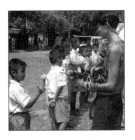

Chapter 3

Global Repercussions: Diffusion, the United Nations, and Nongovernmental Organizations

We, heads of State and Government, have gathered at United Nations Headquarters in New York from 6 to 8 September 2000, at the dawn of a new millennium, to reaffirm our faith in the Organization and its Charter as indispensable foundations of a more peaceful, prosperous and just world. We recognize that, in addition to our separate responsibilities to our individual societies, we have a collective responsibility to uphold the principles of human dignity, equality and equity at the global level. As leaders we have a duty therefore to all the world's people, especially the most vulnerable and, in particular, the children of the world, to whom the future belongs. . . . We will spare no effort to make the United Nations a more effective instrument for pursuing all of these priorities: the fight for development for all the peoples of the world, the fight against poverty, ignorance and disease; the fight against injustice; the fight against violence, terror and crime; and the fight against the degradation and destruction of our common home.

—Millennium Declaration 2000

As I walk through this wicked world Searchin' for light in the darkness of insanity. I ask myself is all hope lost? Is there only pain and hatred and misery? And each time I feel like this inside, There's one thing I wanna know: What's so funny 'bout peace love and understanding?

—Elvis Costello

In the next several chapters, we review the relationship between rich and poor countries, progressing from the most positive to the most destructive aspects. After rich countries achieve health and prosperity for most of their citizens, how much do they share these benefits with the global poor? In this chapter we review the historically important process of knowledge diffusion, through which poor countries have taken advantage of gains made by wealthier countries. Then, we look at the United Nations (UN) and the World Health Organization (WHO) in particular. The UN and its specialized agencies have done enormous good in the world but are not without their faults—we examine both perspectives.

The rest of this chapter tracks the growth and achievements of the nongovernmental organization (NGO) sector (sometimes called the nonprofit or independent sector), a movement that has grown rapidly over the past few decades. Despite its comparatively small size, this sector has made great strides in poor countries through direct programming and an increasingly powerful grip on the world's conscience, through which it has influenced government and multilateral policies. Like the UN, the NGO sector has its faults and has committed its share of harmful actions behind the veil of humanitarianism— we also cover the good and the bad in this important sector.

Diffusion of Knowledge and Technology

Accompanying the prodigious improvement in the health of those in industrialized countries is the possibility that people in all countries could enjoy longer and healthier lives. Although the possibility remains, the will to do so has long been lacking—good health remains largely sequestered among those who can afford it. In 1997, the UN calculated that for a total of $40 billion per year rich countries could cover the following for *all* the world's people: basic health care and nutrition—$13 billion; water and sanitation—$9 billion; basic education—$6 billion; and reproductive health for women—$12 billion (United Nations Development Program (UNDP) 1998, 37). Although such expenditures have not been forthcoming, poor countries have seen life expectancies increase and general health indices improve. However, most of these gains have come unintentionally from rich countries—through the diffusion of knowledge and technology.

By the second half of the 20th century, gains in agriculture, public health, biomedical science, medical care, economics, governance, and a host of other fields had spread to the developing world. This knowledge diffusion came through foundations, universities, emigration, NGOs, UN agencies, and advances in telecommunications. The effects were profound, as life expectancies in developing countries skyrocketed, infant mortality rates plummeted, and quality of life improved dramatically everywhere. From 1930 to 1960, Latin America and East Asia increased life expectancy to more than 60 years; it took Europe 150 years, starting in the 1800s, to achieve such an increase (UNDP 2001, 28).

At first it might seem counterintuitive that a mere diffusion of knowledge is responsible for such impressive gains. After all, for decades rich countries have channeled billions of dollars annually to poor countries through bilateral and multilateral aid channels. Yet such is the conclusion of many who have studied the question. "Half the gains in health between 1952 and 1992," the WHO wrote, "result from access to better technology" (WHO 1999, 6). This "better technology" includes many of the advances just covered, eg, clean water, sanitation, better diets, vaccines, and antibiotics. The World Bank reached a similar conclusion; nearly half the mortality reductions in the 20th century came through "technical progress" (UNDP 2001, 29).

Changes that once took hundreds of years in industrialized countries may take only a generation or two today.

Poor countries often benefit from technological advances in multiple fields simultaneously. For example, while one sector develops safer water sources, another initiates a vaccination program, while still another helps physicians improve their knowledge bases. Changes that once took hundreds of years in industrialized countries may take only a generation or two today. Although many medical interventions like hemodialysis or cardiac surgery remain trapped behind steep gradients of wealth, training, and technology, other medical advances have gone directly out into the world. Common surgical, delivery, and primary care techniques have become widely available, even in poor communities worldwide. Antibiotics save millions of lives annually. Such advances in basic science and clinical practice have spread through various channels. Family planning initiatives are responsible for slowing world population growth, which itself feeds cycles of poverty and illness (Robey et al 1993, 60).

In the 1950s, researchers found that those suffering from diarrheal illness improved dramatically when their rehydration solutions included both sugars and salts, leading to the development of cheap, universally reproducible oral rehydration solutions (ORS).

The Lancet hailed ORS as "possibly the most important medical discovery of the twentieth century" (UNDP 2001, 28). Despite considerable controversy regarding the best way to get this knowledge into the hands of the poor,[1] ORS is now widespread, saving 1 million lives per year—mostly children (UNDP 1997, 111). When combined with basic childhood vaccinations, ORS use helped cut the mortality rates for children under the age of five by half between 1970 and 1999 (UNDP 2001, 29).

Vaccination also has greatly benefited those in poor countries. The WHO calls immunization "the greatest public health success story in history" (WHO 1999, 23), a claim supported by a large body of evidence. In the early 1900s, more than 1 million Americans annually suffered through bouts of smallpox, diphtheria, pertussis, tetanus, polio, measles, mumps, rubella, and *Haemophilus* influenza type b—and many died. Vaccine developments throughout the century resulted in substantial reductions in their morbidity. By 1998, most illness rates had decreased by or near 100%. Vaccine initiatives in the United States eradicated smallpox by 1949 and reduced the incidence of measles from 469,924 cases and 7,575 deaths in 1920 to 89 cases and no deaths in 1998 (CDC 1999c).

Hepatitis B chronically infects more than 200 million people worldwide, including 10% of children in Africa and Southeast Asia, increasing the lifetime risk of hepatocellular carcinoma (liver cancer), the world's most frequent nonskin cancer (Bloom et al 1993, 1; Crum 2002). More than 80% of the 440,000 annual occurrences of these cancers occur in developing countries (Strickland 2000, 99). As such, vaccination against hepatitis B holds tremendous promise for the world's poor. Following intensive hepatitis B vaccination in Thailand, researchers projected a 99% reduction in the hepatitis B carrier rate and a similarly expected result in the rate of the subsequent cancer (Crum 2002). Affordability remains the largest barrier to more widespread use. Cervical cancer is currently the second most common cause of cancer death in women worldwide, with 450,000 new diagnoses and 250,000 deaths annually. In November 2002, doctors reported early results of a promising vaccine against the human papillomaviruses (HPVs) known to be causative (Koutsky et al 2002, 1645).

Many available vaccines could pay great health dividends if only funding were available to get them to more people in poor countries. In 1999, the Gates Foundation announced a $750 million contribution to the Global Alliance for Vaccines and Immunizations (GAVI), an alliance of UN bodies, private industry, and foundations, in an effort to increase worldwide vaccination rates. The Gates Foundation projects 2 million lives saved per year at a cost of $30 per child with full immunization.[2] In January 2005, the Gates Foundation doubled its original donation, giving $750 million more to GAVI, calling its original contribution "the best investment we've made" (Strom, 2005).

Of all the vaccine initiatives to date, none have been more important than those for smallpox and polio. By themselves, the vaccines would not have stopped these plagues. Eradication requires a global effort, with teams working simultaneously in all countries with active cases. Without a large coordinating global body, it is quite possible that both efforts would have failed. Only one world body had the capacity to achieve smallpox eradication and dramatically curtail polio: the WHO.

United Nations and Its Agencies

The UN has been a key contributor to global health since its founding in 1945. The UN brings many Western health improvements such as vaccines and antibiotics directly to those in poor countries, while leading efforts to help victims of wars, disasters, and refugee movements. UN peacekeeping troops have long served where no one else will, most recently in Liberia, Kosovo, East Timor, Congo, and Sierra Leone. The UN fosters economic stability through the Economic and Social Council (ECOSOC) and the International Monetary Fund (IMF) and it fosters development through the United Nations Development Program (UNDP) and World Bank. The UN High Commission for Refugees (UNHCR) oversees refugee movements and helps coordinate relief efforts. The International Court of Justice in The Hague has begun to enforce UN conventions and charters.[3] The UN has also given us one of the world's most important documents, the Universal Declaration of Human Rights (UDHR), which is reviewed in Chapter 10.

Many UN agencies focus their efforts on health and human rights. The UNHCR, the UNDP, the United Nations Children's Fund (UNICEF, formerly the United Nations International Children's Emergency Fund), the Joint United Nations Programme on HIV/AIDS (UNAIDS), the United Nations Population Fund (UNPF), and the Office of the United Nations High Commissioner for Human Rights (OHCHR) all play important roles. Because the ultimate determinants of health rest chiefly in the hands of governments, the UN's role remains important. Many of its representative agencies work directly with host governments and private organizations to coordinate health initiatives, collect data, and form policy. The global vaccine initiatives outlined previously comprise just one example of these agencies in action.

World Health Organization

Founded in 1948, the WHO formulates policy through representatives of 192 member states in the World Health Assembly and serves as the main directing and coordinating authority on international health.[4] The WHO helps local governments to fulfill their responsibilities. When governments refuse to cooperate, such as Iraq before the fall of Saddam Hussein, there is little the WHO can do. Noting the WHO's importance to global health, one author wrote, "If it were to be abolished today, it would have to be reinvented tomorrow" (Morrison 1984, 102).

Increasingly, the WHO fosters public and private partnerships to address specific diseases or problems. In efforts to eradicate smallpox, polio, and onchocerciasis, the WHO partnered with pharmaceutical companies, foundations, NGOs, other UN organizations, and host governments. Future initiatives will depend on WHO leadership and coordination.

Smallpox, Polio, and Other Eradication Efforts

One of history's great biomedical success stories is that of the eradication of smallpox, the lethal and disfiguring illness caused by the viruses variola major and variola minor. Thought to have first appeared around 1600 B.C., this scourge decimated humanity for centuries and shaped history (UNDP 1997, 51). From A.D. 165 to 180, the Roman Empire suffered a smallpox epidemic that killed up to 35% of regional populations. China, Japan, Europe, and the Americas all lost millions to subsequent pandemics (Garrett 1994, 41). Smallpox played a key role in the Spanish decimation of the indigenous peoples of the Americas, killing half of the Aztecs and most of the Incas and reducing Mexico's population from around 20 million in 1520 to 1.6 million 100 years later (Diamond 1999, 210).

In 1958, the Soviet Union went before the WHO's World Health Assembly and won broad international support for a campaign to eradicate smallpox. At the time, smallpox claimed 2 million lives per year in 33 countries, while blinding 500,000 and permanently disfiguring more than 10 million more. As recently as the early 1950s, smallpox had claimed as many as 5 million lives per year (World Bank Group 1993). Formally launched in 1967, the campaign required more than 250 million doses of vaccine annually, along with more than 100 WHO staff members and thousands of local health workers. Over an 11-year period, WHO teams faced war, natural disasters, and a host of geographic and logistical nightmares to end the threat of smallpox. In November 1975, a three-year-old girl named Rahima Banu became the last case of wild variola major in human history. Two years later, Ali Maow Maalin in Merka, Somalia, was cured of the world's last case of variola minor (Garrett 1994, 45). On May 8, 1980, the World Health Assembly formally declared the end of smallpox (47). The Centers for Disease Control and Prevention (CDC) reports that the United States recoups its $32 million investment in smallpox eradication every 26 days (CDC 1999c).

Urged on by the success of the smallpox campaign, the World Health Assembly launched the Global Polio Eradication Initiative in 1988, a year in which an estimated 350,000 cases of poliomyelitis occurred worldwide.[5] In 1997, the WHO estimated that as many as 10 to 20 million people of all ages were living with paralysis caused by polio (WHO 1997). I saw polio cases on the wards in Tanzania in 1987, and today visitors to Nairobi and other African capital cities still see people dragging themselves along the streets on cardboard boxes, the local equivalent of wheelchairs. Lacking the social safety nets of northern welfare states, like Medicare and Social Security in the United States, many polio victims in poor areas rely on extended family or become beggars to stay alive.

Jonas Salk's miraculous 1955 polio vaccine, which he refused to patent, reduced polio cases in North America and western Europe from 76,000 in 1955 to less than 1,000 just 12 years later ("Helping the Poorest" 1999; Garrett 1994, 30). Dr Albert Sabin's oral polio vaccine, the form most widely used today, followed in 1963 (Strickland 2000, 215). Following aggressive global immunization campaigns since 1988, polio incidence has fallen dramatically. The WHO certified the Western Hemisphere as polio-free in 1994 and the Western Pacific region, including China, in 1997 (220). Europe, including Eastern Europe, soon followed in June 2002. The worldwide incidence of polio decreased from 350,000 confirmed cases in 125 countries in 1988 to fewer than 800 cases in 15 countries in 2003.[6] Following a number of setbacks to the eradication campaign, including wars, natural disasters, and mistrusting religious and government leaders in the Middle East and Africa, the total case count by mid-2005 was already 857. All 13 remaining countries are in sub-Saharan Africa, the Middle East, and Asia, with India, Pakistan, and Nigeria holding the largest reservoirs. With such setbacks, it will take longer to eradicate polio, though the goal remains within reach.

The UN is currently leading massive campaigns against other serious infectious illnesses as well, including onchocerciasis, a debilitating and oft-blinding worm-mediated disease in Africa. To date, the campaign has prevented 60,00 cases of blindness and protected 18 million vulnerable children (UNDP 2005, 83). Another massive UN effort targets Dracunculiasis, or Guinea worm disease, a disease also endemic to Africa in which worms emerging through painful blisters on the feet and legs disable millions of victims annually. People have long removed the Guinea worm by slowly, painfully winding the emerging worm around a stick, a practice that many believe gave rise to the caduceus, the traditional symbol of medicine. The WHO has long tackled illnesses like these that have been ignored by the developed world's collective medical establishment.

The UN and its agencies prove invaluable to the global poor because they are often the key players in eradication efforts.

Other WHO disease targets include African trypanosomiasis (sleeping sickness), Chagas' disease, dengue, leishmaniasis, leprosy, tetanus, and schistosomiasis.[7] Many of these diseases are common in poor countries but rare in rich countries, which explains why treatments are so often slow in coming. As such, the UN and its agencies prove invaluable to the global poor because they are often the key players in eradication efforts. The UN does, however, help both those in the wealthy and poor countries alike through many of its efforts, like the WHO's Tobacco Free Initiative, for example. The WHO also maintains a large cadre of disease experts who maintain a vigil watching for new and emerging disease outbreaks. The agency rightly received praise for helping to control the severe acute respiratory syndrome (SARS) outbreak in 2003. On July 21, 2003, Dr Lee Jong-Wook assumed the position of director-general of the WHO and control over its $2 billion annual budget. At the time of his confirmation, he assumed the lead of an organization viewed as "under funded, over committed, and burdened by bureaucracy," according to the journal *Science* (Vogel 2003). A storied and essential fixture in global health, the WHO continues to serve the world's most vulnerable. Nevertheless, the organization has attracted its share of critics.

UN Critics

Many of the UN's most vocal critics reside in the United States. Amidst cries of poor management and excessive waste in the UN system, the US government remained seriously delinquent in its UN dues for many years. US unilateralism poses an even greater threat to the UN's long-term viability and relevance. Frustrated by UN intransigence over Iraq, President George W. Bush warned that the UN was "fading into history as an ineffective, irrelevant debating society" ("The United Nations" 2004). Despite more than a dozen Security Council resolutions passed against Saddam Hussein in the years before the US-led invasion, none were fully enforced ("Special Report" 2004). Still others decry the slow and plodding manner in which the UN conducts its operations. Writing in the journal, *Health Affairs*, A. B. Morrison, a former WHO consultant for 20 years, described working with individual agencies as a frustrating and "exasperating" process (Morrison 1984). In my dealings with WHO representatives in Central America, I found an overly political and bureaucratic organization that tends to funnel funds and contracts to favored consultants. One friend working in East Africa for more than 20 years has remained highly critical of UN programs, citing the expensive consultants who stay in pricey hotels, tour facilities in rented top-of-the-line vehicles, and then leave, with the poor none the better for all the money spent. I watched the local UN campus spread out on my regular excursions into Nairobi in 1994. Nothing in the area matched the UN's lavish and expansive compound. Others have been critical of the UN for consistently bowing to pressures from the United States and other wealthy donor countries (Werner and Sanders 1997, 171).

Author Graham Hancock cited a number of UN failings, including the large, tax-free salaries and perks of its employees and budgets devoted far more to employee travel and meetings than the needs of the poor (Hancock 1989, 79).

When you subtract from the "achievements" of the UN all the silly conferences, all the ineffectual meetings, all the inane committees and subcommittees, all the reports produced by learned groups recommending that more learned groups be convened to produce more reports, all the coordination mechanisms that have only complicated things further, and all the reform measures that have left things as they were—then what remains? Specifically, what remains to justify the billions of dollars that taxpayers all over the world continue to plough into the United Nations and its agencies year in and year out? (Hancock 1989, 107)

Such criticisms are harsh though justifiable. What impact might there have been if just a fraction of the enormous funds spent on flights, hotels, meals, and salaries for the millions of delegates who have attended UN conferences through the years were diverted to the global poor? The UN employees' salaries rank many times larger than those for people who do comparable work in the NGO sector, generating some friction in the field. Further, although UN conferences often dominate world headlines, they tend to produce more documents than results. In fairness to the UN, however, several of its most ambitious undertakings have failed because they required large cash infusions, and the UN's largest donors simply have not honored their financial commitments. In March 2004, reports of the UN's largest-ever scandal hit the news.

In 1996, the UN launched the Oil-for-Food Program in which Saddam Hussein was allowed to sell oil to purchase food and medicine for his people. UN-imposed economic sanctions put in place after the 1991 Gulf War had crippled the Iraq economy, producing widespread starvation and plummeting health indices. During the program's run from 1996 to 2003, 24 million Iraqis received food, medicines, and services (Sachs and Miller 2004). However, Hussein siphoned off more than $10 billion by illicitly trading oil, while UN officials turned a blind eye. Moneys designated for starving kids instead built palaces for Hussein and rewarded Baath party loyalists. Although a host of corporations in Europe, Russia, China, and the Middle East were all complicit in the illegal trading schemes, the UN, charged with policing it, came under fire for allowing it to go so far astray. Even worse, Secretary-General Kofi Annan's son Kojo received more than $120,000 in salary payments from one of the involved companies (Safire 2004). Though not illegal, it reeked of nepotism and provided grist for the chorus of UN bashers. UN supporters have pointed out that all contracts in the oil-for-food program received Security Council—and hence United States and United Kingdom approval—and that the US turned a blind eye to the considerably larger sums involved in Saddam's illegal oil sales to US allies Jordan and Turkey ("Corruption at the Heart of the United Nations" 2005). Former Federal Reserve chairman Paul Volcker headed up a commission charged with uncovering the truth, ultimately spending $3 million in an exhaustive search. In March 2005, the commission exonerated Kofi Annan, though it found Annan's son Kojo less than forthcoming about his business dealings (Hoge 2005). In August 2005 the commission reported that the UN's director of the oil-for-food program in Iraq, Benon Sevan, had "corruptly benefited" from kickbacks from the program he oversaw; another UN official had also accepted bribes ("Corruption at the Heart of the United Nations" 2005). Reaction to the Volcker Reports among US-elected representatives reflected long-standing, polarized views of the UN—conservatives called for Annan to resign while liberals celebrated his exoneration. The UN will no doubt continue to inspire passionate debate in US power circles, with its future relevance likely hanging in the balance.

Alma-Ata, the Millennium Development Goals, and the Global Fund: The Future and Relevance of the UN

In 1978, the WHO, UNICEF, and representative members of 134 countries launched a "Health for All by the Year 2000" initiative in Alma-Ata, Kazakhstan, of the former USSR. Rooted in the successes of community-based health programs of China (the Barefoot Doctors), the Philippines, and Latin America (influenced by Paulo Freire), the Alma-Ata Declaration proposed a revolutionary approach to health care (Werner and Sanders 1997, 171). The declaration recognized the larger social, economic, and political factors that compromise health and prodded governments to address the gross disparities in health between "rich and poor countries." Alma-Ata called on all governments to provide universal health care through community-based efforts in which people participated directly in the programs' design and function. These efforts were to focus on education, clean water, sanitation, immunization, family planning, nutrition, and provision of basic health services to all.

Alma-Ata may serve best as a symbol of the UN as a whole—grand in vision, indispensable in function, yet painfully short in fulfilling its promise.

To the disappointment of most, Alma-Ata failed to achieve its ambitious objectives. Lack of donor support from wealthy countries, lack of sufficient political will and basic resources from poor governments, the debt crisis of the 1980s, the increasingly strong role played by the World Bank in formulating health policies, privatization of health systems, and structural adjustment programs all contributed to the demise of this primary health care initiative (Werner and Sanders 1997, 171). The WHO, UNICEF, and other UN agencies still work with governments to foster primary health care for all, though with markedly scaled-back targets. The WHO claims that the world has made great progress toward health for all and that the vision of Alma-Ata contributed significantly to health gains since 1978 (WHO 1999, viii). However, even the UN concedes that they fell far short of their goals. The Declaration of Alma-Ata still stands as a beacon for many in poor countries. It is tragic that such a powerful vision has become so impotent in practice.

Alma-Ata may serve best as a symbol of the UN as a whole—grand in vision, indispensable in function, yet painfully short in fulfilling its promise.

One of the UN's more ambitious efforts in recent years emerged amidst the optimism and uncertainty of the millennium. Leaders from 189 countries, comprising the largest gathering of world leaders in history, gathered at the UN headquarters in New York in September 2000, and agreed on a series of eight specific millennium development goals (MDGs), all of which impact health and target their results for the year 2015.[8] The first goal, to eradicate extreme poverty and hunger, seeks to reduce by half both the number of people who suffer from hunger and the number of people whose income is less than $1/day. The second and third goals seek to provide universal primary education and to promote gender equality. The fourth seeks to reduce the mortality rate for children under five by two thirds, while the fifth seeks to reduce the maternal mortality rate by three quarters. The sixth MDG seeks to halt and reverse the spread of HIV/AIDS, malaria, tuberculosis, and other major diseases. The seventh and eighth MDGs call for improving the environment and strengthening the global partnership for development.[9] The UN proclaimed the importance of these MDGs as follows:

> This represents an unprecedented consensus by world leaders on the major global challenges of the 21st century as well as a common commitment to meet these challenges. The [Millennial] Declaration and MDGs thus provide a road map and vision of a world free from poverty and hunger, with universal education, better health, environmental sustainability, freedom, justice and equality for all.[10]

The MDGs may represent the best vehicle yet for the rich world to correct the ills of those in poor countries by taking aim at the root causes of illness through carefully constructed, clear and achievable targets. Specific numeric reductions and timelines accompanied the lofty rhetoric that has always been a core feature of major UN initiatives. Since the year 2005 began a 10-year "countdown" to the MDGs endpoint in 2015, it was widely viewed as a pivotal referendum on the progress achieved to date. The results were disheartening at best. The 2005 UNDP *Human Development Report* proclaimed, rather dourly, "There is little cause for celebration . . . the overall report card on progress makes for depressing reading. Most countries are off track for most of the MDGs. Human development is faltering in some key areas, and already deep inequalities are widening . . . the promise to the world's poor is being broken" (UNDP, 2005, 1).

There are a number of reasons why these goals are not being met; chief among them being the lack of donor support. The Organization for Economic Co-Operation and Development (OECD) estimated that the total foreign aid (official development assistance [ODA]) from rich countries in 2004 was $78 billion, a modest increase over funding levels in recent years. However, to meet the MDG targets, the rich world would have to increase ODA to $135 billion by 2006 and $195 billion by 2015 (UNDP 2005, 88). Almost no one expects the major donors, led by the United States, to meet these targets. To do so, the

United States would have had to spend $75 billion (0.7% of GNP) on ODA in 2004, not the $15 billion (0.14% of GNP) the United States actually spent that year (Sachs, 2005a, 218). Without the world's wealthiest country willing to pay its share of the cost, the MDGs will likely fail, triggering yet another round of UN bashing. An apt analogy would be for Michael Jordan, in his heyday with the Chicago Bulls, to sit out most of the NBA season, and then blame the team for its failure to achieve.

Whether or not the UN and its constituents can achieve any of these stated goals remains to be seen. History does not offer much encouragement, particularly given long-standing US opposition. On August 1 2005, President George W. Bush appointed longtime UN critic John Bolton as US ambassador to the United Nations (Williams, 2005). Bush made the controversial appointment during the Congressional summer recess, thwarting a probable democratic filibuster and avoiding a continuation of confirmation hearings during which senators from both parties had voiced significant concerns. The Bolton appointment was another in a long series of conservative actions demonstrating mistrust in, even open disdain for the UN, from Senator Jesse Helms' longstanding, biting criticisms to Republican-led cuts in UN funding.

The uneasy relationship between the UN and its largest donor—the United States—poses the gravest risk to the UN's future.

As the year 2000 approached, the United States was dangerously close to losing its vote in the UN General Assembly because of its substantial dues in arrears. The UN calculates each country's dues by estimating the country's gross national product (GNP) as a percent of the global economy. Because the US economy comprises nearly 31% of the world total, it benefits from the UN's dues ceiling of 25%. Led by sharp criticism from conservatives in Congress, the US government had been behind in its UN dues for years.[11] According to *The Economist*, the US debt stood at $1.7 billion at the end of 2000 ("Irrelevant, Illegitimate, or Indispensable" 2003). With help from a $1 billion gift from Ted Turner and negotiations to reduce the US burden from 25% to 22% of the UN administrative budget and from 31% to 27% of the UN peacekeeping budget, the United States agreed to pay most of its debt, which it did in September 2002, while simultaneously agreeing to move its payment timetable forward to avoid its traditional, annual delays ("Turner Pays US Dues" 2000). The uneasy relationship between the UN and its largest donor—the United States—poses the gravest risk to the UN's future.

In January 2000, then WHO director-general Gro Harmel Brundtland established the Commission on Macroeconomics and Health to assess the relationship between health and economics. Economist Jeffrey Sachs chaired the commission, which released its report on December 20, 2001 (Sachs 2001b). The authors noted that the world would not be able to meet the MDG targets without considerable funding from the world's wealthy nations.

Specifically, the authors called for rich countries to contribute $27 billion per year by 2007 and $38 billion per year by 2015 to poor countries for health needs, far above the current spending level of $6 billion per year for health. The commission estimated that the increased funding would save an astounding 8 million lives per year by 2010 (Sachs 2001b). Because the total GNP of donor countries was $25 trillion per year in 2001, the projections are relatively small, given the potential number of lives saved. Jeffrey Sachs said, "It will shame our generation if we don't do more" (Banta 2002). Because so many of the avoidable deaths each year are caused by three diseases, the commission called for the creation of the Global Fund to Fight AIDS, Tuberculosis, and Malaria (GFATM), which would consume $8 billion of the $27 billion per year total by 2007 (Sachs 2001b). In the end, as is true with other health issues, it all comes down to money.

Like other grand UN plans, the commission's report gained little acceptance in US power circles. The Bush administration at first pledged $300 million to the Global Fund for 2002, with a drop to $200 million in 2003. The United States has pledged an average of $300 million annually through 2008, though Congress may well scale this amount back.[12] While currying favor at the UN and in world opinion for support for a war on Iraq, President Bush announced in his State of the Union speech on January 28, 2003, that he planned to commit $15 billion over five years to combat AIDS in Africa and the Caribbean (Stolberg 2002). Of this, $1 billion would go through the GFATM, the rest unilaterally distributed ("The Other War" 2003). Jeffrey Sachs hailed it as a "historic breakthrough" but chided the president for his stubborn unilateral approach, snubbing the GFATM. "The United States," Professor Sachs said, "has got to get off its unilateralism on this issue" ("A Buildup Against AIDS" 2003). *The Economist* called Bush's disregard for the GFATM "a pity," noting, "Mr Bush clearly prefers America to decide for itself how American money is spent" ("The Other War" 2003). Greater support from the United States could radically alter the terrain against these three diseases, which claim roughly 10,000 African lives every day (Sachs, 2005a, 215).

This unilateralist approach weakens large institutions like the UN and its respective agencies (Kickbush 2000, 139). It also adds administrative burdens to inadequately staffed, poor recipient governments that have to accommodate procedural differences and wade through the reams of paperwork required by each donor. As in most areas, streamlining similar functions saves administrative time and better focuses scant funding resources. Just days after Bush's announcement, the Global Fund was, according to the *Boston Globe*, "on the verge of going broke" (Donnelly 2002a). Five months later, Global AIDS Alliance Executive Director Paul Zeitz thought the fund was "doomed" by the Bush administration's decision to seek its own unilateral response to AIDS (Donnelly 2003). During the September 2005 "replenishment" conference in London (ie, the conference in which donors decide on funding levels), the Global Fund received pledges of $3.7 billion, just over half of what

Although flawed, the UN remains the main body through which global improvements in health can become a reality. The MDGs comprise the blueprint through which the rich countries can eradicate extreme poverty—but only if those countries summon the will to pay for them.

it needed ($7.1 billion) to fund projects approved for 2006-2007 ("The Global Fund" 2005). The Global Fund seems destined to chronic insufficient funding. Given the anti-UN and unilateralist approach favored by the Bush administration, it is unlikely that the UN will gain US favor any time soon. Without US funding, many other donor nations will abstain and it is unlikely that GFATM and the other Commission recommendations will bear much fruit.

Despite conservative calls of UN "irrelevance," the world very much needs the UN—now as much as ever and regarding matters of health in particular. No other coordinating body could have defeated smallpox or assembled the forces necessary to fight polio, AIDS, malaria, and tuberculosis. Jeffrey Sachs and others have argued that the specialized UN agencies have more expertise and hands-on experience than any other organization in the world (Sachs 2002). No bilateral donor or NGO can possibly match them. The resources that come out of UN agencies form the bulk of the factual basis for this book and many others. Although flawed, the UN remains the main body through which global improvements in health can become a reality. The MDGs comprise the blueprint through which the rich countries can eradicate extreme poverty—but only if those countries summon the will to pay for them. In the larger realm, the UN still holds the promise envisioned by its founders in 1945. According to one Singaporean official, "Distance has disappeared. The world has shrunk to a global village. Every village needs a village council. The UN represents the only real village council we have" ("Irrelevant, Illegitimate, or Indispensable" 2003).

Nongovernmental Organizations

Doctors and NGOs: An Overview

When we turn our attention to the medical profession, we find a decidedly mixed picture. It is clear that doctors, nurses, and other allied health workers have not sufficiently shared their knowledge, skill, and resources with those in poor countries (Baker et al 1984, 502). Despite this, NGOs have made a considerable impact on global health and continue to do vital work. Although no entity can replace the role of nation-states in improving the health of their populations, those in NGO communities have prodded governments to action and served as the eyes and ears for the global community in remote corners of the world. Most feel that NGO contributions are critical. I have worked in the NGO community long enough to plant myself firmly in that camp. Many people in this sector are truly inspiring and their work exemplary. Even small groups of people have made considerable impact while serving in poor countries.

To get a better idea of NGO contributions, we need to consider indirect measures and briefly look at the history and impact of a noteworthy few. It is important to remember that health stems from a large set of forces acting inconspicuously and simultaneously. It may still remain somewhat foreign for clinically oriented people to presume someone working solely in human rights will directly affect health and history, yet a considerable amount of data prove otherwise. In fact, some of the most important historical contributions to health have come from nonclinical people.

Consider first, the contributions of individual health providers serving through established NGOs. Ophthalmologists serving through Project Orbis, orthopedic physicians serving through Orthopedics Overseas, and maxillo-facial/reconstructive surgeons serving through Operation Smile each provide unique skills to those in need. Through their collective efforts, they perform millions of much needed surgical procedures annually. Through other programs, nurses, physical therapists, medical and allied health students, hospital administrators, and virtually all members of the health profession contribute their skills. Virtually any member of the health profession can find opportunities to serve in the sequel to this book, *A Practical Guide to Global Health Service* (AMA 2006). Though specific data on the efficacy of such work is decidedly lacking, scores of testimonials support the rationale.

Some groups are religiously motivated, some revolve around direct service, and others are more training oriented. I have been running one such training program for seven years and can testify to the efficacy of such an approach. We have another program that combines training with direct service. Although training, direct service, and relief-oriented work each have their own merits, what is abundantly clear is the overwhelming need for all of them.

Judging Efficacy

When we look for studies that show the efficacy of NGOs and the people who serve through them, we find surprisingly little. Partners In Health, Physicians for Human Rights, and a few other groups have proven the efficacy of their work through many publications in peer-reviewed journals. However, in general, there is a paucity of data allowing us to independently judge which organizations are most effective, which approach work best, and where resources are best allocated. Much of what appears in US medical journals are self-congratulatory travel logs that gloss over efficacy and deeper issues of illness causation. Large groups such as the National Charities Rating Bureau (NCRB) do provide ratings on NGOs, though they rate only the largest organizations, leaving the vast majority still under the radar. Further, the NCRB bases its evaluations primarily on budgets submitted by NGOs. As Enron and Price-Waterhouse made all too clear in 2002 and 2003, budgets can be altered. Even humanitarian NGOs are not above altering budgets to make the bottom line look better.[13] To understand efficacy, we are forced to rely on imperfect measures.

Consider first the number of Nobel Peace Prizes awarded to individuals or groups committed to improving health. This is an indirect measure, yet it offers a window through which we can gauge the relative importance given this work by one prestigious world body. Working backward through time, we find the following winners: Médecins Sans Frontières (MSF) (1999); UNICEF (1965); the International Committee of the Red Cross (ICRC) (1963, 1944, and 1917); and Albert Schweitzer (1952).

Although the above list is impressive, it misses most of the awards that have impacted global health. If we broaden the list to include those who have contributed to health through peaceful resolution of conflict, we have a near-comprehensive list of Nobel Peace Prize winners. However, if we restrict our focus to those operating under the broad umbrella of human rights over the past 50 years, thereby improving health, we find at least 20 additional awards, including Wangari Maathai, (Kenya) (2004), Jimmy Carter (2002); United Nations, Kofi Annan (2001); International Campaign to Ban Land Mines, founder Jody Williams (1997); Carlos Filipe Ximenes Belo and Jose Ramos-Horta (East Timor) (1996); Nelson Mandella and Frederik W. de Klerk (South Africa) (1993); Aung San Suu Kyi (Burma) (1991); International Physicians for the Prevention of Nuclear War (1985); Desmond Tutu (South Africa) (1984); UNHCR (1981, 1954); Mother Theresa (India) (1979); Amnesty International (1977); René Cassin (France) (1968); and Martin Luther King Jr. (1963).

That so many prominent people devoted their lives to human rights—and the improvements in health that inevitably follow improvements in human rights—should reinforce the importance of this work. It is also striking how easily one can imagine Martin Luther King working alongside the Campaign to Ban Land Mines or Albert Schweitzer voicing support for the work of Amnesty International. There is something about this work that inspires all, something the Nobel Committee recognizes.

A second indirect measure of the efficacy of NGOs is the increasing amounts of faith—and funding—that world governments place in them. During the 1980s alone, large, multilateral donors increased the funding of NGOs by a factor of 10, and in 1993 the World Bank encouraged governments to contract with NGOs to improve efficiency in health care delivery (Kim et al 2000, 359). NGO funding has nearly doubled in the past decade, from $6.4 billion in 1995 to an estimated $12.3 billion by 2002 OECD 2004, 134). In the United States, more than 70% of funds from the Office of US Foreign Disaster Assistance goes to NGOs as does nearly 40% of the US Agency for International Development (USAID) budget (Overseas Development Institute 2002; Radelet 2003, 8). Further, just five large

NGOs—CARE, Catholic Relief Services, the International Rescue Committee, Save the Children, and World Vision—account for a full 30% of US government NGO funding, reflecting the government's strong support for these agencies. Other countries reflect these trends. Such funding levels would have been unheard of a mere 25 years ago.

A third broad reflection of the efficacy of NGOs comes from stories from the NGOs, which I divide into two groups: those who work directly in health and those who work in the realm of human rights. First, however, we will look at the limitations and problems within the sector.

Limitations and Problems of NGOs

Although the NGO sector can boast that organizations like MSF, Amnesty International, the ICRC, Health Volunteers Overseas (HVO), and CARE are among its ranks, it must also deal with those who blemish its otherwise solid reputation. In fact, the well-meaning but poorly informed, as well as the mal-intentioned, have caused considerable harm working in unsupervised settings in poor communities, as I have seen through my international work. One group traveled to southern Belize in the late 1990s and pulled teeth in a number of poor, mostly indigenous communities. Had they spent any time at all in the country first, they would have learned that full dental and medical services were available already—pulling teeth was unnecessary. Another group immunized a large group of kids near the Guatemala border of Belize, not realizing they were fully immunized already. A third group fronted an NGO while buying up citrus tracts in the south of Belize. Their "humanitarian" NGO had been nothing more than a scam. I now fully understand why the director of Health Services for Belize at the time, Dr Michael Pitts, was so reluctant to work with our group—he'd been burned before by promises from afar.

Some programs provide what I call "tailgate medicine," in which groups of well-meaning but poorly informed people visit a poor country for the first time, briefly open up a mobile clinic in a church or school, see a large volume of patients, and leave. I separate these from the invaluable short-term surgical, dental, and ophthalmologic programs that come and effectively treat hundreds of patients over a short period of time. The first type of short-term excursion harms many poor people, even though the volunteers usually go home feeling good about themselves. Expectations are raised, people line up for hours or days to see the Western doctor—who might only be a medical student—and, after doing so, their illnesses remain unchanged, making it harder for a more responsible group to subsequently gain the people's trust.

I once received an e-mail from a group of medical students who were planning a trip to Belize in six weeks to offer their services to "poor people." They requested my assistance in pointing them in the direction of needy people, helping them find preceptors in the country, and helping them clear any medical licensing requirements. I pointed out to this well-meaning group of students that it was quite a bold assumption for them to think that there were in fact poor people in Belize who needed them; that they, as medical students, were more qualified than the large number of well-qualified Belizean providers already at work; that these extremely busy practitioners could find the time or desire to precept them; or that they could possibly learn the culture and illnesses endemic to Belize in such a short period of time to actually offer any real clinical help. I applauded their motives but urged them to look more deeply into the real issues at hand, allow more time to prepare, and offer their services more responsibly in the future.

A good friend in Kenya had a love-hate relationship with the Flying Doctors of East Africa for years. The Flying Doctors are a near mythical group of surgeons who fly all over East Africa performing surgeries in remote hospitals. He recognized that the Flying Doctors provided an invaluable service to his hospital, but staff voiced concerns. No surgeon was around for the inevitable postoperative complications, which at times proved quite dangerous to the patients. The visits also required plenty of administrative scheduling and intense postoperative monitoring by the hospital staff. Similar problems arise near the Mexican border of Belize, where a local surgeon rails against the "invaders," the surgical team that comes from the United States every year to perform surgery in his operating suites. He typically plans vacation time when they arrive. This group does provide an essential and unmet service for the poor in the area, though it comes at a price.

> *NGOs frequently don't have to answer for the consequences of their actions, a luxury that governments and world bodies like the UN and World Bank do not share.*

Another problem with NGOs is what *The Economist* calls their lack of accountability. Many NGOs and civil society groups stake out their moral territory and issue proclamations, often needed but occasionally with unintended consequences. Many groups like Oxfam and 50 Years is Enough have rightly railed against global trade inequalities, which we cover in Chapter 6. When trade negotiations broke down in Mexico in 2003, the NGO community claimed victory, even though the failure to progress ultimately hurt poor countries more than it helped them (Bhagwati 2002). NGOs frequently don't have to answer for the consequences of their actions, a luxury that governments and world bodies like the UN and World Bank do not share ("Sins of the Secular Missions" 2000). During a June 2004 meeting, Leslie Ramsammy, the minister of health in Guyana, told our group, "NGOs and civic groups are unaccountable. They can just pack up and leave. The government will always be there. In those places where corruption is high and governments fail, the NGOs are even worse."

Occasional articles appear in the *New York Times* or other media that talk of shabby practices by one NGO or another (Abelson and Rosenthal 1999). Books detailing the failings of the NGO community and aid industry as a whole include Graham Hancock's *The Lords of Poverty: The Power, Prestige, and Corruption of the International Aid Business* (Atlantic Monthly Press, 1989), Michael Maren's *The Road to Hell: The Ravaging Effects of Foreign Aid and International Charity* (The Free Press, 1997), and David Rieff's *A Bed for the Night: Humanitarianism in Crisis* (Simon & Schuster, 2003). Whether one agrees or disagrees with these authors, one thing is certain—for the most part, no one is monitoring this work. Those who comprise the bulk of the recipient communities are typically poor, voiceless, and unable to get anyone to listen when things go wrong.

In his 1997 book, *The Road to Hell,* Michael Maren shares experiences from the NGO Save the Children (STC), one of the largest and most success-ful NGOs today. Maren pointed out that the late night appeals for viewers to donate money to save one child were, in fact, false advertising. STC pooled its resources and made block donations to communities, after covering their large administrative and fund-raising expenses (Maren 1997, 136). In 1985, "not particularly needy" parents in Arkansas filed a $21 million lawsuit after learning that their children had been "sold" to STC sponsors for $16 per month. The fact that their children had been used in STC advertising with-out either their knowledge or permission was a source of "embarrassment and shame" according to the suit (50). In 1986, *Forbes* reported that STC donations did not go directly to a specific child as depicted in the late night ads. A subsequent exposé by NBC television prompted the attorney general of Connecticut to threaten a lawsuit, which finally forced STC to change its advertising.

Far too often, such appeals depict the "victims" as helpless individuals incapable of fending for themselves—only the benevolent donor can step in and save them. One angry African delegate said in a conference, "The more desperate our conditions are portrayed in the US media, the more money you American organizations seem to raise for your own overhead and projects" (Maren 1997, 158). A famous photograph portrayed a starving Sudanese famine victim—a mere toddler—slumped forward while a "grimly patient" vulture watched her. STC used the photo in its fund-raising literature, not at all bothered by its blatant opportunism or insensitivity. The troubled photo-grapher, 33-year-old Kevin Carter, won the 1994 Pulitzer Prize for taking that picture, following a life of photographing some of the world's darkest moments. He recalled chasing off the vulture and remaining at the scene for hours, "smoking cigarettes and crying" ("Milestones" 1994). Haunted by depression, alcohol, and vivid memories of the dark side of humanity, Carter committed suicide only two months after receiving his prize (MacLeod 1994, 70). Perhaps the only good that came from Carter's death was that he did not live long enough to see his moving photograph used in such shameless exploitation.

Like other forms of assistance, humanitarian aid designated for relief efforts is not without its share of abuses, logistical disasters, and unintended harmful consequences.[14] AmeriCares, the US-based charity founded by Bush family friend Bob McCauley and funded largely by USAID, has had some notorious tax write-offs for large US corporations. In respective emergencies, AmeriCares sent 2 million Mars candy bars to Russia, 17 tons of Pop Tarts to Bosnia, and 12,000 Maidenform bras to Japan, prompting an official at the UNHCR to call the NGO, "an irresponsible, publicity hungry organization capable of making grandiose offers of assistance and providing planeloads of highly questionable 'relief supplies'" (Maren 1997, 264). Similarly, Pat Robertson's Operation Blessing sent more evangelists than medical workers to Goma, Zaire, during the cholera outbreak in 1994 (265).

At times, the important work of saving souls has interfered with the equally important work of saving lives. One International Christian Aid worker resigned in disgust after finding that some involved in the organization "appeared to place a higher priority on evangelizing than on administering to refugees' physical needs" (Hancock 1989, 9). NGO giant World Vision was accused of threatening to withhold food to coerce Salvadoran refugees into attending Protestant worship services, a charge it denied. Former President Ted Engstrom responded to other similar accusations by saying, "We cannot feed individuals and then let them go to hell" (9). Unfortunately, some of those who are gifted at proselytizing are not similarly gifted at healing. This should take nothing away from the many religious health providers dedicated to this work. However, when the prime mission is evangelism, the secondary missions, including health care, may suffer.

Many well-intentioned groups collect all sorts of supplies with little regard as to how they might actually ship them and still less regard as to what is actually needed.

Disaster relief efforts seem to bring out both the best and worst in the NGO community. Although heroic efforts by MSF, CARE, Oxfam, the Red Cross, and others save millions of lives, other efforts are less than helpful. Many well-intentioned groups collect all sorts of supplies with little regard as to how they might actually ship them and still less regard as to what is actually needed. A Detroit newscaster collected a variety of pharmaceuticals, foods, and blankets for Somalia famine victims in the 1980s. Unfortunately, the medicines were expired and useless, the electric blankets were not needed near the equator, and the soups and chocolate-flavored drinks for dieters were far from ideal (Hancock 1989, 12). Oxfam-America's Larry Simon said, "During a disaster, all sorts of junk keeps rolling in."

Like their larger bilateral and multilateral partners in aid, NGOs are often guilty of spending considerable sums on fund-raising, salaries, and overhead.

Minister Ramsammy in Guyana recalls one group that spent $13 million to council 54 people on HIV; $100,000 per year went for the director's salary. In Kenya, Father Bill Fryda notes how little of US AIDS funds (PEPFAR) actually makes it to those afflicted with AIDS. Most of it, he says, is spent before it leaves US territory, largely on "baseball caps and conferences." Like Father Fryda, many people I have met in developing countries have long noted the disparity between the funds allocated to many NGOs and the funds that actually make it into programs. Many NGOs hire professional telemarketers to solicit funds, draining money away from programs (Mohl 2004). Of course, not all NGOs are guilty of such actions, my own included. Yet it is a large enough problem to considerably hamper efforts abroad.

One final concern about NGOs is their involvement with food aid, which consists of surplus foods purchased by the US government and distributed to developing countries. Food aid grew out of US agricultural surpluses in the 1950s, following the stabilization of European agriculture in the aftermath of the Marshall Plan. Farmers and the wealthy agribusinesses that purchased and distributed their grains had far too much political muscle to tolerate the falling prices that surpluses would cause. So they pressured Congress to subsidize farmers through the 1954 passage of Public Law (PL) 480. Under this law, the government buys surplus grain and pays NGOs to distribute it to third world countries. In 2003, PL 480 accounted for $1.74 billion of food aid to developing countries.[15] In reality, this law directs US "foreign aid" dollars into US farming communities in the form of subsidies. Its real beneficiaries are US farmers, agribusinesses, and shipping companies that wield such enormous influence over Congress. It also sustains a number of NGOs that sell the grain cheaply overseas in return for profits they can then use to subsidize their programs.

Although food aid can provide much needed relief to victims of famine and humanitarian emergencies, only 10% of such food is designated for emergencies. Much more goes through intermediaries for long-term efforts, where it can prove enormously destabilizing. In Somalia in the late 1980s, food aid provided a ready means for enterprising people to trade food for arms, contributing to political unrest and violence. Somalia was the largest US aid recipient in sub-Saharan Africa from 1982 to 1992 and at times third overall behind Egypt and Israel (Maren 1997, 24). Much of the aid came in the form of surplus food. One Somali exclaimed, "We were made crazy with food. I became rich with food. I was able to marry another woman, a second wife who I call CARE wife" (110).

Although the NGO sector has its share of problems, it remains vital and the most accessible vehicle through which interested health providers can serve internationally. Our world would be considerably worse off without it. We will now look at representative NGOs to better understand this growing sector.

Health NGOs

Health NGOs seek all members of the health profession to teach and or clinically care for patients at home and abroad. There are hundreds of such organizations, many of which are run by one or two committed individuals who bear most or all of the burden. When interest wanes or funds run out, the organizations fail. However, just as quickly as several fade from view, others spring up.

Let me first share some impressions gleaned over 10 years from brochures, web sites, and questionnaire responses while developing our database of international health service opportunities, as reproduced in the *A Practical Guide to Global Health Service*. First, the most striking feature of the NGOs depicted in that text is the humanity that shines through their mission statements. There are a lot of good people trying to do good work, in many cases at great personal expense. Judging by their program depictions, most are succeeding. That a world of poor people should forge connections with the world's most talented and privileged health care providers seems a predetermined fait accompli. Nearly one third of the organizations in our database have religious underpinnings; most welcome practitioners of any faith. The NGO I run is secular, as are most involved in this work. Yet most organizations follow an ethical premise that clearly resonates with faith-based values, even when not overtly stated.

Second, the breadth of the NGOs in operation is striking. Some send surgical teams to operate on cleft palates. Others offer dental care. Still others send medical supplies. Some focus all of their efforts on training, others entirely on direct service. Many combine health service work with environmental, agricultural, or economic activities. Several see health work as part of their ministerial outreach. And others perform clinical services while operating chiefly in the policy or human rights realm. Anyone interested in international health service can now easily find an opportunity.

Finally, it is easy to admire the heroic efforts I read about in the organizational literature we have compiled through the years. Few in the NGO community earn high wages for doing this work. Many people volunteer their time and, despite the usual pressures from jobs, tuitions, mortgages, and family obligations, still make this happen. Through the years, I have talked with many such people and derive great pride through the affiliations. They are the beating heart of the medical profession and offer the truest moral direction for our future. Their actions should inspire those who hesitate for any reason.

Because there really is no "typical" organization in this line of work, let me summarize a few examples. Some I know from personal experience, others from research. I have selected some of the larger and more successful NGOs. However, keep in mind that most are small with missions in one or more select locales.

Surgical Eye Expeditions International   Surgical Eye Expeditions (S.E.E.) International sends surgical teams to provide eye care to those in developing countries, usually closely working with a host ophthalmologist. The founder, Dr Harry Brown, attended George Washington University School of Medicine, as I did. I met him at an alumni meeting in 2000. Harry and his wife, Bailey, who serves as chief executive officer, are humble, dedicated people who found an ophthalmologic niche in the world of need and have put most of their energies into meeting that need. Their success and the success of those who have joined them at S.E.E. International has been extraordinary. S.E.E. ophthalmologists performed over 13,000 sight-restoring surgeries in 2004 and over 74,000 sight-restoring surgeries in the past five years. All ophthalmologists volunteered their services and covered their own travel expenses to 36 developing countries. S.E.E. provided over $23 million worth of services and supplies in 2004. What began as Dr Brown's small project in 1974 has blossomed into a sight-saving enterprise, serving more than a quarter million people from 1994 to 2001.[16] Cited by *Forbes* as a "lean and inspiring" charity group that can restore one person's sight for a mere $40, S.E.E. International has an army of devoted ophthalmologists and support staff who ensure it will continue to offer sight-restoring surgery for years to come ("Investment Guide" 2001).

Project Hope   Project Hope began as a widely recognizable hospital ship in 1958 and has since expanded its teaching, training, and service mission to countries all over the world. It has sent more than 5,000 medical volunteers to 70 countries on 5 continents and currently sends more than $100 million in resources to 20 to 30 countries per year. In addition to health training and service, Project Hope founder Dr William Walsh created the Center for Health Affairs in 1981, which publishes one of the most influential health policy journals, *Health Affairs*.[17]

Health Volunteers Overseas   Founded in 1986, HVO has sent thousands of volunteers to countries around the globe. In 1994, I interviewed founder Nancy Kelly as the first step in developing this book. Nancy is gracious and dedicated, and HVO has become a fixture in a number of developing countries. It is one of the best NGOs for those interested in short-term service missions. Dedicated to health training in a culturally and regionally sensitive manner, HVO has emerged as one of the largest NGOs that sends doctors and other health personnel to serve internationally on short-term missions. According to a recent annual report, 352 HVO volunteers trained more than 2,530 health workers in 65 programs in 21 developing countries in 2004 (Health Volunteers Overseas 2005).

Operation Smile   Dr William Magee, a plastic surgeon, and his wife, Kathleen, a nurse and clinical social worker, founded Operation Smile in 1982. Following a 1981 trip to the Philippines to repair cleft lips and palates, the Magees saw hundreds left behind and vowed to return. Over the next 20 years, Operation Smile provided free reconstructive surgery for tens of thousands of children in 20 developing countries and the United States. Neither William nor Kathleen received income from their work at Operation Smile during that time (Abelson and Rosenthal 1999). Operation Smile conducts extensive training, offering a training manual and CD-ROM for use overseas. It has brought more than 460 surgeons to the United States for specialized training and provides a fellowship for physicians from mission countries, 18 since 1992. The group also brings children back to the United States for more complicated surgeries. Operation Smile is 1 of the 200 largest charities in the United States, based on *Forbes* 2002 rankings ("What's the Charity Doing with Your Money" 2002). Despite a highly critical 1999 *New York Times* article that reported several operative deaths, "lost innocence" of the organization, and complaints from host countries (Abelson and Rosenthal 1999), Operation Smile continues to garner national awards and perform thousands of cranio-facial surgeries—more than 50,000 since 1984.[18]

There are 250 similar organizations in our database, reproduced in *A Practical Guide to Global Health Service.* Within these organizations, thousands of doctors, nurses, and other allied health personnel regularly devote a part of their lives to service. We will look more closely at several of them, including their motivations, in Part 2 of this book. We now turn our attention to the organizations that have staked themselves to the most current and, perhaps most important of paradigms, that of "human rights."

Human Rights and Health Policy NGOs

Although not commonly perceived as being "health" concerns, it is impossible to deny the enormous health-related costs imposed by man-made or natural disasters, conflicts, ethnic cleansings, and other abuses of essential human rights. As Drs Geiger and Cook-Deegan have so well summarized,

> Many human rights violations [have] significant health consequences. These include the physical and psychological trauma of individual victims of violence, torture, rape, but also stem from breaches of medical neutrality, forced deportations, the use of indiscriminate weapons, mass executions, and other violent actions that affect entire populations. The purposeful destruction of health facilities and essential civilian infrastructures also leads to slower forms of death—from epidemic infectious disease, untreated chronic disease, or starvation (1993, 616).

NGOs that deal primarily with refugees (International Rescue Committee [IRC]), prisoners of war (Amnesty International), forensic evidence (Physicians for Human Rights [PHR]), and many others have sprung up. Recent decades have seen large shifts in the NGO community's approach to this work, reflecting larger changes in their working environments. In the years following World War II, the ICRC along with CARE and a few other NGOs defined the operating paradigm. They remained neutral and conducted their work with the tacit complicity of warring factions, who were typically nation-states. During earlier times, that paradigm worked reasonably well.

However, the nature of conflict has changed over the past 50 years. First, the number of conflicts has increased over time, from 10 in 1960 to 62 in 2001 (Duffield 1994, 37; Center for Defense Information 2002, 43). Second, since 1945, the overwhelming majority of war casualties has shifted from military to civilian (Bruderlein and Leaning 1999, 430). In some modern conflicts, civilians have served as human shields against air and artillery attacks, been used as pawns for political leverage, and become primary targets through "ethnic cleansing." In just three recent conflicts, civilian groups in Bosnia-Herzegovina (1992–1994), Rwanda (1994), and Kosovo (1998–1999) became prime military targets, with more than 1 million deaths, far exceeding military casualties (430). Prompted by the crimes of the Nazis, the world responded to such collective affronts to humanity by drafting a UN Convention on the Prevention and Punishment of Genocide. The convention, which came into force in 1951, led to creation of the International Criminal Court of the UN in 1998 (WHO 2002a, 215).

Almost every other week, media outlets report another aid worker killed in a zone of conflict, natural disaster, or refugee movement.

The changing nature of war has been accompanied by a more aggressive stance regarding treatment of its victims, both by UN agencies and the NGO community. As a result, the work has become far more dangerous. Almost every other week, media outlets report another aid worker killed in a zone of conflict, natural disaster, or refugee movement. Between 1985 and 1998, more than 380 humanitarian workers died in zones of conflict alone (WHO 2002a, 218). More UN civilian personnel were killed than UN peacekeeping troops. At times, humanitarian aid workers have become targets of violence and reprisal (Whitelaw 1997, 34). US physician Martha Myers, MD, who dedicated her career to caring for the poor of Yemen, died under a hail of bullets from a politically motivated assassin in 2001 (Elliott 2003, 1). CARE worker Margaret Hassan had spent 30 years in Iraq and met a similar fate in October 2004 ("More Dangerous Work" 2004). Their tragic deaths reveal the ever-increasing dangers that await those who serve in high-risk areas. Iraq has proved so dangerous that MSF, Oxfam and CARE have all left ("More Dangerous Work" 2004).

After 1945, conflicts within states became more prevalent than those between states. Coups, internal armed conflicts, and repression of opposition have often fallen outside the protections of international humanitarian law (Geiger and Cook-Deegan 1993, 616). Because the Geneva Convention of 1949 and the Additional Protocols of 1977 regulate primarily state-on-state conflicts, monsters like Iraq's Saddam Hussein and Uganda's Idi Amin ravaged their own people under the protective cover of "sovereignty." Other internally displaced peoples, such as those in Srebrenica in 1995, have suffered some of the worst war-related assaults (Bruderlein and Leaning 1999, 430). As internally displaced peoples, they too had the misfortune of having to rely on their own states for protection.

The past 50 years have also witnessed huge shifts in the global political landscape. The Cold War between the United States and the USSR dominated third world politics for more than four decades after World War II. Both powers infused massive amounts of aid and arms into the developing world in an effort to court influence and gain strategic advantage. In an attempt to halt the real and perceived advance of communism, the United States strategically forged relationships with corrupt and often brutal dictatorships in Central America, Africa, the Middle East, and Asia; many of these relationships have since come back to haunt the United States (Tisch and Wallace 1994, 47). The fact that the United States found it difficult to round up Middle Eastern support for a war on Iraq in 2003 was at least partly due to its long-standing support of corrupt regimes throughout the region (Lewis 2002).

The case of shifting alliances in the Horn of Africa during the late 1970s is particularly instructive. In a Cold War face-off, for years the United States supported Ethiopia while the USSR supported neighboring Somalia. Following a 1969 coup, the Soviets supplied Somalia's massive arms buildup under its victor, Mohamed Siyad Barre. The United States countered by supplying arms to Ethiopia. When a 1974 coup replaced Ethiopia's Emperor Haile Selassie with a socialist government, the Russians switched allegiances and began supplying arms to Ethiopia. Recognizing the importance of the Horn of Africa both to the Middle East and Kenya, the United States poured billions of arms and aid into Somalia, significantly contributing to its collapse. Such massive infusion of arms and aid by both superpowers destabilized the region and contributed to ongoing violence and bloodshed in the following decades. Arms from Somalia continue to trickle down into Kenya, infusing an epidemic rise in gun violence in Nairobi ("Nairobbery" 2000).

The Cold War's end reverberated throughout the third world, as strategic alliances suddenly lost value and political transformations occurred worldwide. US strategic interests moved from propping up corrupt third world dictators to disarming Russian nuclear arsenals. Human rights, advanced by the Carter administration (Mann et al 1999, 404), became more important after the long ideological shadow of the Cold War receded (Fidler 2000). Because the liberal political theories embraced by many NGOs were on the "winning" side of the Cold War, the NGO brand of political activism could now find resonance in a much larger public forum (Fidler 2000).

Consequently, many NGOs expanded their activities and incorporated human rights perspectives into their work during the 1980s and 1990s, though they did not find a similar mind-set in the key power centers. The conservative administrations in the United States and United Kingdom during the 1980s paid little attention to human rights, even while they rewarded repressive regimes in El Salvador, the Philippines, and South Korea for their anticommunist stances (Mann et al. 1999, 404). Still, far larger forces had been set in motion. As governments and large UN agencies found it difficult to engage in the "complex humanitarian emergencies" that define modern conflict, NGOs became increasingly sought after, playing ever-larger roles on the world stage. Some have called the growing importance of NGOs over the past 30 years an "NGO revolution." Given the long history of NGO activities, it would be more accurate to recognize the growing importance of NGOs as a reflection of the changing global landscape (Fidler 2000). There is simply a far greater need for their services and better technologies, such as the Internet, through which they can function. Yet this "revolution" is a mixed blessing at best. As David Fidler writes, "The increased opportunities for NGOs are often connected with worsening political, social, economic, health and environmental problems around the world and with the decreasing ability of governments and international organizations to deal with such problems" (Fidler 2000).

> *As governments and large UN agencies found it difficult to engage in the "complex humanitarian emergencies" that define modern conflict, NGOs became increasingly sought after, playing ever-larger roles on the world stage.*

The NGO community has expanded its scope and breadth as a result of this changing landscape. The International Red Cross is always present when disaster strikes and, seemingly, always has been. For years, MSF has combined provision of care with forceful statements against oppression and injustice, often at great risk to its members. Transparency International, which has focused a spotlight on governmental corruption, has become widely quoted and followed. Amnesty International has elevated the plight of prisoners to international attention. And Physicians for Human Rights, Physicians for Social Responsibility, the American Refugee Committee, Oxfam, Care, Human Rights Watch, and others have raised global consciousness and forced abusive governments to take heed, even curtail their worst activities. It is indeed a different era. It has become far more difficult for the Pol Pots and Saddam Hussein's of the world to operate in secrecy. Even the United States has had to increasingly justify its actions on the global stage. Someone from the NGO community is always watching.

The global push for information and access, led by NGOs, may be one of the most powerful forces able to bring down the walls of totalitarianism and oppression. The voices of Amnesty International, Human Rights Watch, and others forced the "civilized" world to confront Bosnia, long after it decreed it was just "ethnic hatred," not the genocide it was.[19] PHR unearthed evidence of mass murder in Argentina, Guatemala, and the former Yugoslavia; documented evidence of rape and torture in Iraq, Kurdistan, Haiti, and Kuwait; and discovered use of chemical weapons in the former Soviet Union and Iraq (Geiger and Cook-Deegan 1993, 616). These actions forced the world community to take notice and subsequently turn up international pressure on leaders in these countries. The end of South Africa's apartheid state stemmed in part from the actions of those in the NGO community. It is readily apparent to those who have been paying attention that the NGO community has changed the world. It is hard to imagine a world without them.

International Committee of the Red Cross

In the beginning, there was the Red Cross, "the mother of all humanitarian organizations," according to writer Adam Shatz (Shatz 2002). In 1859, Swiss businessman Henry Dunant witnessed the horrors of war when the warring powers of Austria and France left thousands of dead and dying men on a battlefield in Solferino, Italy. Dunant tried in vain to organize help for the wounded men and later resolved to develop a mechanism to care for those wounded in battle. In 1863, he and five other Swiss citizens proposed mechanisms for protecting volunteer groups caring for the wounded. From such beginnings the ICRC formed in Geneva in 1864 (Baccino-Astrada 1982, 15).

The group convened representatives of 16 nations and drafted a convention of 10 articles that stipulated that medical personnel are neutral and protected during combat; citizens assisting the wounded are likewise protected; wounded or ill combatants are to be cared for during a conflict; and the symbol of the red cross would serve to protect medical personnel, equipment, and facilities.[20] Known as the Geneva Convention, these first articles became the foundation of international humanitarian law. In 1949, diplomats expanded earlier treaties to establish four conventions with 429 articles of law that were signed by most nations; two additional protocols were added in 1977. The Geneva Conventions comprise the world's best effort to protect people during times of conflict between nations. The ICRC remains the "guardian" of the Geneva Conventions and still works to get warring countries to comply.

As an organization, the International Red Cross is widely respected and remains a fixed presence during war, internal conflict, and natural disasters. During its storied history, it has won the Nobel Peace Prize in 1917, 1944, and 1963—no other international health organization has been so honored. The organization's founding principles are humanity, impartiality, and neutrality. As such, the Red Cross does not make pronouncements about the horrors its personnel witness. Its neutrality affords it access to combatants, prisoners of war, and citizens caught in the cross fire. This principle of neutrality still fosters considerable debate in international health circles.

Médecins Sans Frontières/Médecins Du Monde

The principle of neutrality also served as a launching point for the more maverick MSF. One of the most admired NGOs today, MSF has fully used the heritage of an honored profession to stand with the victims of conflict and persecution while publicly speaking out against their oppressors. In 1971, a group of young French physicians, led by Dr Bernard Kouchner, became frustrated with the ICRC's policy of silence and neutrality while observing the Nigerian government's campaign to exterminate the Ibo people in then Biafra (Shatz 2002). The ICRC had maintained a determined silence decades earlier while its members delivered food and medicine to Nazi concentration camp internees (Mann et al 1999, 417). The ICRC had been slow to mobilize to the Biafran war and unable to provide sufficient resources given the internal nature of the conflict. More than 1 million people died before the war ended in 1970. This was completely unacceptable to the fiery young French physicians, who publicly denounced the political sources of the "Biafran genocide," stating, "medical action should not be turned into a blind and dumb instrument" (Brauman and Tanguy 1998). In their eyes, the ICRC's methods had simply become "obsolete."

The nature of war had changed; decolonization had spawned internal conflicts all over Africa and Asia; advanced telecommunications had brought a world of strife into immediacy for those in developed nations; and French citizens felt too much guilt over their own history of colonialism to watch passively or enjoin confused efforts at emergency assistance (Brauman and Tanguy 1998). A new approach was needed. Because illness and injury did not respect international borders, the founders argued, why should medical interventions? Kouchner and others split from the ICRC and founded MSF, championing a "right to interfere" and, eventually, a "duty to interfere" in conflicts and emergencies (Mann et al 1999, 417). MSF biographer Renée Fox summarized this "duty" as follows,

> Mandatory interference is anchored in the belief that there is an "ardent obligation to act" to alleviate the suffering of people urgently in need of medical care and succor, whenever on the face of the earth that suffering exists, particularly when it is a consequence of violence, torture, persecution, warfare, disenfranchisement, oppression, abandonment, exile or exodus (Mann et al 1999, 417).

With governments and multilateral organizations unable or unwilling to cope with an ever-increasing demand, MSF has grown in size and stature, becoming the world's largest independent organization for emergency medical relief. MSF personnel, mostly volunteers, have provided emergency relief in more than 70 countries to innocents trapped in war, natural disasters, and refugee movements. The so-called "smoke jumper" of the aid agencies, MSF has shown a knack for quickly setting up and delivering assistance at the onset of a disaster "when it counts," long before other relief organizations are on the ground (Leyton and Locke 1998, 195). An MSF vice president once said that the MSF doctrine calls for "plunging into the arena . . . dashing headlong into the midst of wars . . . being in the fray . . . in order to reach the victims . . . breaking whatever rules are used against [them and] humankind" (Mann et al 1999, 417). It also calls for MSF participants to make enough noise in the process to be heard while explicitly voicing opposition to the atrocities and crimes they witness. "Care for and testify" has become the operational motto.

Along the way, MSF has experienced some difficulties. Internal disagreements over a response to the "boat people" of Vietnam led to the splintering of MSF into MSF and MDM, or Médecins Du Monde, in 1979. (The US autonomous counterpart of MDM is Doctors of the World). Though both MSF and MDM continue to share the same goals (Mann et al 1999, 417), MDM does less emergency work and, unlike MSF, has operations in each of its host countries.[21] Members of both groups have been attacked, taken hostage, and killed while working in some of the most appalling and dangerous conditions the world has seen in the past 30 years.

By the late 1990s, MSF had grown to control a $250 million budget and 2500 annual volunteer departures to the field (Brauman and Tanguy 1998). In addition to its response to conflict and natural disasters, the organization has become a chief caretaker of refugees and has branched out in a number of other medical activities, including multidrug-resistant tuberculosis, AIDS, a campaign to increase the availability of essential medicines, and increasing health access for the poor. For its extraordinary efforts, the Nobel Commission awarded MSF the Nobel Peace Prize in 1999. More recently, MSF took the unusual step of refusing excess donations following the December 2004 tsunami disaster. Once they had accepted what they felt they could use responsibly, they encouraged the public to give to other NGOs, particularly Oxfam. If only more NGOs were so noble. Given the ongoing conflicts and increased tensions in the world today, MSF and Doctors Without Borders (DWB) will be around for years to come.

Physicians for Human Rights

In 1986, Dr Jonathan Fine and others founded PHR (Mann et al 1999, 404). Realizing the unique contribution that physicians, forensic scientists, and other health workers could provide to investigations of human rights' abuses worldwide, PHR has sent teams to conduct investigations in more than 50 countries since 1986.[22] Following a strict policy of impartiality, PHR teams have exhumed mass graves in the former Yugoslavia; demonstrated the use of torture in Haiti, Iraqi, Kurdistan, Kuwait, and Chile; and documented the use of chemical agents in Iraq (Geiger and Cook-Deegan 1993, 616). PHR was a corecipient of the 1997 Nobel Peace Prize for its work in banning land mines. Following the Gulf War, PHR provided testimony of ongoing atrocities against Kurdish refugees, which ultimately prompted the United States and United Nations to create a no-fly zone in northern Iraq. The organizational motto reads, "Promoting health by protecting human rights."[22] PHR strives to ally science with conscience. Writing on the first five years of PHR's extraordinary history, Drs Geiger and Cook-Deegan concluded, "In a world in which profound violations [of human rights] are likely to continue, the participation of physicians and other health workers in human rights work may be viewed as an increasingly necessary extension of the traditional professional responsibilities" (1993, 616).

Many other NGOs such as Partners In Health, International Physicians for the Prevention of Nuclear War, CARE, Amnesty International, Oxfam, and others have equally worthy histories. However, the stories thus far should emphasize the point that the more traditional role of the physician or allied health provider as solely providing clinical care will no longer suffice. Torture in Haiti, cholera in Zaire, genocide in Bosnia, chemical weapons in Iraq, and the killings of humanitarian aid workers in Somalia all call for health providers to expand their roles beyond traditional boundaries. Information comes too quickly for the noble profession of medicine to avert its collective gaze. Although aid in the larger context remains problematic, even detrimental, there are a host of individual NGOs operating effective programs that require regular infusions of health providers. In the end, getting there becomes the necessary first step. Whether that first step occurs through the relative safety of a brief teaching experience or the whole-scale devastation of conflict or refugee work, the lessons remain readily available and critically important. The image of the healing profession as inherently ethical affords health providers an opportunity to influence the decisions of governments and multilateral institutions. PHR and others offer testimony to this fact.

Conclusions

Before proceeding with the story of what has gone wrong in the aid sector, we reviewed what has gone mostly right in the world and why. The developing world has seen unprecedented gains in human development in recent years; our knowledge and technological advancement may well comprise our most important gifts to the developing world. The UN and the NGO communities have also contributed to global improvements in health. Despite some failings, the UN still represents a promise of improved health for millions of poor people. The MDGs offer the most realistic blueprint to date for the rich world to eradicate extreme poverty and its accompanying illnesses everywhere. Despite their own failings, NGOs are widely regarded as the most effective players in the development game. Most NGOs have well-motivated staffs; depend on funds from the general public, which ensures accountability; and often do great good. The chief limitation of NGOs remains their comparatively "minuscule" resources, which leave them utterly incapable of making up for the failings of the well-financed bi- and multilateral donors (Kim et al 2000, 52).

In the next two chapters, we review the history and impact of foreign aid, both in the form of country-to-country aid and the other multilateral donors including the World Bank and the IMF. It is not sufficient to understand pieces of the aid picture, as NGOs and UN organizations comprise. This industry, with fluctuating aid levels of $50 to $80 billion in recent decades, dominates the international development landscape, casting a huge shadow over all who seek to labor in this realm. In first reviewing the mostly positive accomplishments of these actors, we have already hit the highlights of the world's responses to poverty. Unfortunately, from the standpoint of the poor, it only gets worse. As we begin to review the process of how countries "aid" the poorer nations, we begin our descent into the shadowy world of the forces that serve to keep the poor just as they are. These "forces of disparity" dominate the lives of the poor everywhere. Such forces include racism, sexism, war, and trade, yet our starting point is, ironically, the very institutions that widely proclaim that they are solving the problems of the world's poor. Foreign aid, it must be said, has been a far greater force in propagating the disparities that exist in the world than in helping to alleviate them. One can only hope that the massive paradigm shifts now occurring within most donor and recipient governments toward larger and more effective aid—focused on the MDGs—will succeed, unlike so many earlier attempts.

Endnotes

1. For a detailed discussion on the ORS controversy, see Werner D, David S. *Questioning the Solution: The Politics of Primary Health Care and Child Survival, With an In-Depth Critique of Oral Rehydration Therapy.* Palo Alto, Calif: HealthRights Press; 1997:31–72.

2. Information from the Bill and Melinda Gates Foundation web site at www.gatesfoundation.org/connectedpostings/vaccinesgavi.htm.

3. For more information, see the International Court of Justice web site at www.icj-cij.org/icjwww/icj002.htm.

4. The WHO and the entire UN system has excellent Internet resources. For more information see the World Health Organization web site at www.who.int/about/overview/en.

5. Information from the WHO Poliomyelitis Fact Sheet on the World Health Organization web site at www.who.int/inf-fs/en/fact114.html.

6. Information from the Global Polio Eradication Initiative web site at www.polioeradication.org/content/fixed/casecount.shtml.

7. Information from the World Health Organization Health Topics web site at www.who.int/health-topics/idindex.htm.

8. Information from the United Nations Statistics Division web site at http://millenniumindicators.un.org/unsd/mi/mi_goals.asp.

9. The UN MDGs are widely publicized and can be readily obtained by writing to the UN if no Internet connection is available. For more information see the United Nations Millennium Development Goals web site at www.un.org/millenniumgoals/index.html.

10. Information from the United Nations Millennium Development Goals web site at www.un.org/millenniumgoals/index.html.

11. Some US conservatives claim the UN actually owes the United States money, because the United States has paid for troops in UN-sanctioned peacekeeping operations. Most, however, feel that only troops sent by the UN come under UN budgets.

12. Information from *The Global Fund to Fight AIDS, Tuberculosis and Malaria*, available at www.theglobalfund.org/en/files/pledges&contributions.xls.

13. For more information, see Maren M. *The Road to Hell: The Ravaging Effects of Foreign Aid and International Charity*. New York: The Free Press; 1997:23,138–142. Also see "Charges of Shoddy Practices Taint Gifts of Plastic Surgery," in *The New York Times*, November 24, 1999.

14. Authors Michael Maren in *The Road to Hell*, and Graham Hancock in *The Lords of Poverty*, both graphically describe the ravages of aid in humanitarian relief efforts.

15. Information from the Congressional Budget Office web site at www.cbo.gov.

16. Information from the Surgical Eye Expeditions International web site at www.seeintl.org.

17. For more information see the Project Hope web site at www.projecthope.org/walsh.htm.

18. For more information see the Operation Smile web site at www.operationsmile.org.

19. For a more compete discussion of the world's painful acquiescence to genocide, see Powers S. *A Problem from Hell: America in the Age of Genocide*. New York: Perennial; 2003.

20. Information from the American Red Cross "Fact Sheet: Summary of the Geneva Conventions of 1949 and their Additional Protocols of 1977."

21. Dr Edward O'Neil, Thomas Dougherty (Deputy Executive Director of Doctors of the World), personal communication, 2003.

22. For more information, see the Physicians for Human Rights web site at www.phrusa.org/research/index.html.

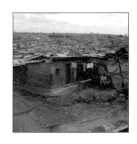

Chapter 4

Development and Foreign Aid: Perceptions and Realities of Our Beneficence, Part I Bilateral Aid

All domination involves invasion—at times physical and overt, at times camouflaged, with the invader assuming the role of a helping friend.

—Paulo Freire, *Pedagogy of the Oppressed*

But whatever the failings of the past, today there are now opportunities for reshaping development assistance. For the first time in history there is an international consensus that human development should be the primary objective of aid.

—United Nations Development Program, 2005

In this chapter, we look at the complex and controversial subjects of development and bilateral (between countries) foreign aid. For more than a half century the rich world has attempted to "help" the poor world, though most efforts have failed. We start by looking at what Americans think about aid, opening up a window into a paradoxical American psyche regarding all things foreign. We then define development, clarify the terms used in foreign aid, explain who the various players are, and focus on the history of foreign aid in the United States and other developed countries. We also look briefly at the other half of the aid question: the host countries and their role in compounding the problems of aid. Although foreign aid may seem a remote interest to health providers interested in serving abroad, it is not. All who venture into this realm will labor under the enormous shadow of aid. It is important to understand both the bilateral and multilateral spheres: why it has failed and why it has generated such resentment among those who most need real help. Finally, we review some major recent developments in aid that offer hope for current and future generations.

Foreign aid is a complex subject that evokes strong emotions, though few people understand its history or rationale. Since its origins in the aftermath of World War II, wealthy countries have transferred roughly $1 trillion to poor countries through the various intermediaries of aid ("How to Make Aid Work" 1999). Although some larger agencies such as the United Nations (UN), the World Bank, and US Agency for International Development (USAID) widely trump their successes and lobby for aid expansion, not all share their enthusiasm. Large protests, at times violent, have come to dominate meetings of the world donor community. In rich and poor countries alike, grassroots organizations have sprung up, seeking to awaken an apathetic and uninformed public. The "lords of poverty" they argue, have done quite enough damage—it is time for change.

Whichever side of the argument one takes, it is imperative that we understand the aid industry for a number of reasons. As health providers interested in service, we may well become targets of anger directed at larger forces at work in the aid industry. Many failed aid programs have colored the "recipients" in ways that hamper service endeavors that follow. During my time in East Africa, I learned that some there still question whether visiting Americans—even those involved with missionary organizations—worked for the Central Intelligence Agency.

A review of foreign aid also provides the best window into the somewhat peculiar American psyche regarding foreign affairs. Many volunteers, raised on a steady diet of newsreel clips showing American benevolence in the world, are shocked to learn just how deep the resentment is toward our government in many areas of the world. The failure of host nationals to greet visiting Americans with open arms dissuades many, contributing to the culture shock that causes some to return home early and disillusioned.

Most important, however, popular beliefs strongly influence behaviors. Many people still believe that the United States, UN, World Bank, and others are already taking care of the poor—so why should they get involved? After all, foreign aid is a multibillion dollar industry, with armies of economists, development experts, and public health officials working on the assorted problems affecting the poor. Given the experience gained from more than a half century, one would think that aid agencies would be reasonably good at solving these problems by now.

Yet, experience offers anything but assurance that all is well with aid. *The Economist* concluded that the $1 trillion flow of aid from rich to poor over the past half century has, "failed spectacularly to improve the lot of its intended beneficiaries" ("How to Make Aid Work" 1999). A congressional study of the World Bank and International Monetary Fund (IMF) in March 2000 came to the same conclusion (Lancaster 2000, 2). If our mission is to improve the health of the poor, history teaches that we need to reexamine our beliefs about foreign aid and development and seek to influence those who would make those decisions on our behalf. Foreign aid can work, and may well comprise one of the best ways for millions to break out of poverty. But it will require considerable reform. It will also require that citizens in all countries—particularly the United States—develop a far greater understanding of the complex issues involved in aid.

What We Think

Through the years, a number of polls have shed light on Americans' views toward foreign assistance and the broad issues that surround it. In brief, we are poorly informed about issues in developing countries; we feel that we have a moral obligation to help those less fortunate; and we think we do far more than we actually do. People in other developed countries generally have a better grasp of global issues but still echo many of the views held by Americans.

Knowledge about the "Third World"

Americans who venture abroad quickly realize how little we know about the world compared to those in other countries. The 1950s bestseller *The Ugly American* shocked the American public with its depictions of arrogant, culturally insensitive Americans at work in a fictitious country in Southeast Asia. Although our standing may have improved somewhat since then, many still view us in a similar fashion. The combination of an ignorance of all things not American and a foreign policy dominated by American concerns proves our undoing. A 1987 poll by the nongovernmental organizations (NGOs) Interaction and the Overseas Development Council showed that the US public is poorly informed about issues in developing countries, a finding supported by other studies and even passing observations of the US public (Contee 1987). Less than one third of the studies' respondents were able to correctly respond to questions about US membership in the North Atlantic Treaty Organisation (NATO), the Strategic Arms Limitation Talks (SALT) talks, and US policy in Nicaragua, all issues that received wide media coverage at the time.

The report concluded that this "thinness of the American knowledge base" includes all policy issues, both domestic and international. Developing countries seemed "physically and culturally remote" to survey respondents who had traveled primarily to Mexico and the Caribbean, not elsewhere in the third world. This lack of personal experience and knowledge, the study authors wrote, "undoubtedly affects Americans' perceptions about the people and governments of developing countries, as well as the economic, social and political relationships of those countries with the US" (Contee 1987). This lack of understanding reflects that of prior generations. Although the Internet and improvements in telecommunications have improved the public's knowledge of foreign policy, it is unlikely that we have improved enough—even after the terrorist attacks on September 11, 2001—to sufficiently close the knowledge gap. A RAND study found that only 14% of Americans could correctly estimate the year 2000 world population of 6 billion (RAND Corporation 2000).

Moral Obligation

Most Americans think that the United States should help the poor in other countries. In 1995, the University of Maryland's Program on International Policy Attitudes (PIPA) found that more than 80% of Americans polled—Democrats and Republicans alike—agreed that the United States should share some of its wealth with the global poor (Kull 1995a). In the same poll, more than two-thirds agreed that the United States had a "moral responsibility" to help poor countries develop economically and improve their people's lives. More than three quarters agreed with the statement, "We should send aid to starving people irrespective of whether it will promote the national interest." By contrast, the majority of respondents rejected the idea of maintaining or increasing military aid or giving aid for strategic reasons (Kull 1995b).

These attitudes have persisted through time. In 2000, close to 90% of respondents to a PIPA survey supported foreign aid that would provide food and health care to people in poor countries. This option scored highest among a list of reasons posed for giving aid. In the same poll, close to three fourths supported increasing aid to Africa and the same percent wanted to help pay for multilateral efforts to cut world hunger in half by 2015 (one of the UN's millennium development goals [MDGs])—even if it cost the average taxpayer an additional $50.00 per year (Kull 2001). In fact, three quarters of respondents to the 1995 survey were willing to pay an additional $100 per year for five years to eliminate world hunger (Kull 1995a).

People in other industrialized countries share these sentiments. Studies from Europe, Canada, and Australia all show support for aid on humanitarian grounds (Contee 1987). Despite concerns over the effectiveness of aid, most people around the world want to help those less fortunate. However, it is mainly the Scandinavian countries that provide aid to the poorest countries for primarily humanitarian reasons. The rest, as we will see, have far different incentives.

According to Us: How We Help the World

An interesting paradox has characterized American public opinion on foreign aid for years. Most people feel the foreign aid budget should be cut—often drastically; but they base their assumption on erroneous, wildly inflated dollar amounts that they think their government spends on aid. In the previously mentioned 1995 study, respondents estimated that 15% of the federal budget goes to foreign aid; more than 80% thought the United States directed a larger percentage of its budget to foreign aid than other developed countries (Kull 1995b). Other polls have found similar inflated estimates of US foreign aid spending.[1] A 2004 University of Maryland poll found that Americans thought 24% of the US budget went to foreign aid (Council on Foreign Relations 2004). One participant in a PIPA focus group spoke for many when he said, "I think the numbers are kind of mind-boggling and out of reach" (Kull 1995a). Americans remain convinced that their government gives huge amounts of money abroad and gives far more than other countries, yet are wrong on both counts.

When comparing generosity among countries, standard conventions hold that one must first level the playing field by weighing the relative sizes of national economies (by comparing their gross domestic products [GDPs]) and then viewing aid as a percentage of that size. Just as one cannot realistically expect division III football teams like Bates to compete against division I teams like Notre Dame, one cannot expect similar levels of giving from countries of vastly different economic sizes. That is why the Organization for Economic Co-Operation and Development (OECD) and most groups studying foreign aid rely on comparative data using aid as a percentage of GDP.

In 2002, the United States contributed just 23% of total world aid, far less than its 32% share of the world economy would allow.

Consider a comparison between the United States and the world's most generous donor country in percentage terms, Denmark. In 2000, the GDP of the US economy was $9.837 *trillion,* nearly one third of the world total and 60 times more than that of Denmark with its GDP of $162 *billion* (The *Economist* 2003, 24, 40). In 2000, the United States gave 0.10% of its GDP ($10 billion) in aid while Denmark gave 1.06% of its GDP ($1.7 billion). Such comparisons make clear that, while the United States gave a larger dollar amount, Denmark gave more than 10 times the level of the United States in percentage terms. People use this data to support widely disparate claims. For years, conservatives have cited the US total dollar contribution to support claims of US generosity. By contrast, liberals have used standard comparisons of aid as a percent of GDP to claim that the United States is the least generous of the 22 members of the OECD, a position it held for years. At 0.10% of GDP, the United States in 2000 fell well below the international mean of 0.22% (OECD 2002). Although both arguments are factual, logic dictates that the latter argument is more realistic, and many around the world have long viewed the United States as stingy given its overall economic might. Perhaps others see in us the potential to do so much more. In 2002, the United States contributed just 23% of total world aid, far less than its 32% share of the world economy would allow (OECD 2004, 136; *The Economist* 2005, 26).

When asked whether foreign aid levels should be kept constant or cut, US respondents have traditionally preferred cuts. This again is based on erroneous, inflated estimates of the amount of aid given. Respondents who thought the aid amount was highest were the ones most inclined to want to cut it, while those closest to the real amount were the most likely to want to increase it. Once the actual amount was clarified, almost all wanted to increase it (PIPA 2001). When 1995 survey respondents were asked what percentage of the US federal budget should go toward foreign aid, they replied "5%." Five years later, they replied "10%."

Although this subject receives sporadic attention here in the United States, it receives a lot of attention in other countries. While riding a bus in Copenhagen in 1996, I noticed the first of several signs boasting that Denmark had again committed a full 1% of its GDP to foreign aid. The sign read, "1% again. Denmark leads the world in aid!" I can't imagine a similar sign on one of Boston's public buses or anywhere else in the United States given the widespread disdain Americans feel toward perceived levels of foreign aid spending.

This overestimation of aid spending has greatly affected US policy. The 104th Congress, led by Newt Gingrich, fervently opposed foreign aid programs and succeeded in cutting back US aid spending, which Senator Jesse Helms once likened to money disappearing down "foreign rat holes" ("What the President Giveth" 2002). Because the public has long supported cuts in foreign aid, it is little wonder that aid budgets fell steadily in the 1990s. Between 1991 and 1997, the United States decreased its foreign aid by 8%, the second sharpest decline in the OECD (Kim et al 2000, 50).

Why do so many Americans erroneously think the United States leads the world in kindness? Focus group discussions have shed some light on this question (Kull 1995a). First, foreign aid receives a lot of media attention; therefore, people assume it must be a large budgetary item. Second, some public figures have misrepresented the amount spent. Foreign aid has long been a favorite target of some right-wing Republicans. In 1994, Senator Jesse Helms said, "The foreign aid program has spent an estimated $2 trillion of the American taxpayer's money," which roughly doubles the actual dollars spent on aid since World War II by the *entire* world (Kull 1995a). Third, many people confuse foreign aid with military spending. Even before the Iraq War, the US military budget, which accounts for roughly one half of the world's total military expenditures, consumed nearly a fifth of the overall federal budget (Lobe, 2004) and more than half of the nonentitle-ment spending in recent years (Center for Defense Information 1997, 26). It is little wonder that those who confuse the two think aid spending is so high.

Finally, and most important, there is within the US citizenry a collective memory of Americans as the world's saviors in two world wars and the Cold War. There is simply no way of separating military expenditures from foreign aid in the view of the average American, even though military spending is roughly *30* times larger (Sachs, 2005a, 329). Most Americans have seen John Wayne movies, which depict America's role in the world as ethical and righteous. These images are part of our culture and continue to affect the way we see ourselves on the global stage. Although they overlook the incredible damage US foreign policy decisions have exacted from the poor for decades, they do have a factual basis in history. The United States did play critical roles in the two world wars. During World Wars I and II, close to 1.4 million US servicemen were killed, wounded, or missing in action (Center for Defense Information 1997, 35). That's a lot of Gold Star mothers and a lot of collective sacrifice that still reverberates through the generations.

Further losses in Vietnam, the Gulf and Iraq wars, and other conflicts around the world reinforce the image of America's global role in the minds of the public. The United States spent nearly $13.4 trillion between 1948 and 1991 opposing the Soviets in the Cold War (Center for Defense Information 1997, 24). Little of this benefited the global poor, who were far too frequently caught in the cross fire. Nevertheless, Eastern Europeans and many others gained political freedoms after the fall of the Soviet Union. For decades, western Europeans benefited considerably from the rather expensive blanket of US military security (Zakaria 2003, 67).

In 1994, I worked briefly with an elderly Dutch surgeon then en route to western Kenya. One evening over dinner, he recalled how the American liberators had freed him and the rest of his countrymen from the Nazis, earning, in his words, his "eternal gratitude." Many older Europeans have similar memories. Most conquering powers through world history subjugated and looted the vanquished; the Americans, however, did not. One visiting priest told our parish of a friend who waited for days for a train back to the USSR in 1945; but none were available. The Soviets had commandeered all trains to transport the hoards of war booty confiscated from the Nazis at war's end; booty that is still on display at the Hermitage and other museums in Russia. There are no comparable museums in America as there was no similar pillaging. Economic and strategic considerations were certainly factors, yet the United States may well have been the first power in world history to pour significant funds into the immediate reconstruction of a vanquished foe.

Fifty years ago, former soldier and then US secretary of state George Marshall explained to the American public the urgent need to finance the rebuilding of a Europe destroyed by war. To do so, he argued, would be for everyone's benefit. What followed was the most ambitious development assistance plan in history. Known as the Marshall Plan, this effort pushed US levels of development assistance to all time highs. In 1947, foreign aid peaked at over 2% of gross national product (GNP), more than 18% of federal outlays (Sachs, 2005a, 217; Congressional Budget Office, 1997, xii). The privation stalking the major European powers in the immediate aftermath of the war carried the very real possibility that these countries could turn toward more fanatical elements or look east to communism for relief. Communist parties were particularly strong in both Italy and France in the late 1940s (Congressional Budget Office [CBO] 1997, 11). But history proved Marshall's vision correct. Former enemies have since become stable democracies and, not coincidentally, strong US trading partners. Winston Churchill called the Marshall Plan, "the most unsordid act in history" (Sachs 2001c).

It is likely that these memories of American beneficence continue to infuse our political worldview. If we spent the same levels now as we did then, the foreign aid budget in 2000 would have been $295 billion, nearly 30 times more than the $9.9 billion we actually spent that year. Most Americans assume that we have maintained funding levels larger than that of the Marshall Plan. Though Americans want to cut those perceived levels back, they present clear wishes to maintain funding levels many times the current amounts. Yet, the reality and the perception couldn't be further apart. Far from our Marshall Plan legacy as the world's benefactor, US official development assistance (ODA) (foreign aid) has plummeted since the 1960s. In 1962, the United States donated $18.5 billion (in 2001 dollars), which comprised 0.58% of GDP and 3.06% of the federal budget outlay. By 2001, that had plummeted to $10.7 billion, which comprised just 0.11% of the GDP and 0.52% of the federal budgetary outlay (Shapiro 2000).

Despite such trends, signs are emanating from the Bush administration that Washington is again interested in aid. US foreign aid reached its nadir in 1997, when total foreign aid was just over $7 billion (OECD 2002, 208). In 1998, the 21 member countries of the OECD, including the United States, increased their average aid spending by 9%, but the per percent gross national income (GNI) increased only slightly from 0.22% to 0.23%, since national income greatly increased ("Measuring Up for Aid" 2000). Since then US aid spending continued to rise steadily—though slowly—until March 2002. It was then that President Bush announced at the UN Conference on Development in Monterrey, Mexico, that he would increase US foreign aid spending by $5 billion per year, though much of this increase would not take effect until 2006 ("What the President

Giveth" 2002). This surprising pledge would increase US foreign aid to $17 billion by 2006, the largest increase in 45 years (Radelet 2003, 13). Much of this increase would come through a new Millennium Challenge Account (MCA) through which $5 billion per year in new funds would flow to those countries that demonstrated the capacity to use aid dollars well. However, this amount would still leave the United States next to the bottom of the Development Assistance Committee (DAC), at 0.17% of GNI if fully funded (12).

In sum, Americans want to do the right thing but seem constrained by their ignorance of foreign affairs and the mythical beliefs in what their government is actually doing. Very real concerns regarding the overall efficacy of foreign aid do not seem to restrain the desire of typical Americans to want to help those in need. There have been numerous efforts to better inform the US public on foreign aid expenditures, yet such attempts are repeatedly drowned out by the steady drumbeat of popular American culture. The fact that the US government is increasing its foreign aid budget, temporarily at least, begs the question, does foreign aid work? The answer is not a simple one, yet one of enormous consequence for the poor. Before answering, we need to first define development and characterize the key players involved.

Development

Development is the process through which wealthier countries seek to raise the quality of life for those in poorer countries. This usually involves the transfer of funds, materials, technologies, and expertise through well-established channels in the "foreign aid" industry, which spent roughly $50 to $60 billion per year until substantial increases followed the Monterrey conference in 2002. Foreign aid can be defined as the net transfers of financial or in-kind assistance from one country to another, either directly or through multilateral channels (Tisch and Wallace 1994, 161).[2] Although foreign aid draws the attention and occasionally the wrath of the populace in both rich and poor countries, we need to recognize that foreign aid and development are not synonymous. Development involves far more than mere resource transfers.

No one definition can fully account for the changing paradigms that have dominated development theory through the years. However, authors Tisch and Wallace offer this cogent summary,

> Development involves improvements in food production, health services, education facilities, transportation and communication infrastructure, and markets for all of these goods and services . . . advances in industrial manufacturing capacity, . . . [and] improved human skills to manage modern economies. . . . Different kinds of development are important for different countries, which have different natural and human resource bases and different social and political structures. . . . However, human beings do have similar needs and wants, so that

the overall characteristics of development are generally recognized. These include high income levels, high literacy and numeracy rates, low infant mortality, long life expectancy, a clean environment, and political freedom (1994, 17).

There are many other explanations of development that are equally broad and equally illuminating, incorporating gender and ethnic equality in addition to the standard fare just listed.[3] Further, many schools of development thought have come and gone through the years, each promising recipients that it would solve the problems in ways others could not.[4] In fairness to all the actors on the development stage, we should recognize just how difficult it is for nations to "develop." Even sound, well-planned efforts collapse under the weight of a thousand intractable problems. Further, it has been more than 200 years since the United States gained independence and began to develop, while many African countries have had less than 50 years. Many developing nations emerged from the yoke of colonialism only to watch power transfer to even more oppressive host nationals. Developing a nation, per se, is hard.

> *Even strong leadership has difficulty making lasting changes when no money is available to fund the essential functions of the state.*

One of the most important components in the process of development is the leadership of the state itself. The aid industry receives at least some of its bad press because it works with cash-strapped governments in the world's poorest countries. For many governments, problems stem chiefly from the basic constraints of poverty. Even strong leadership has difficulty making lasting changes when no money is available to fund the essential functions of the state. Further, even if all aid were well targeted, it would not be enough to overcome many of the problematic features of many poor countries: incompetence, graft, entrenched elites, ethnic divides, historical underdevelopment, fiscal mismanagement, climate, geography, and disease.

Even enlightened leaders face huge short-term problems in reforming economies and political and civic institutions. Political forces often make the cost of long-term benefits too high for a populace focused on the short term (Klitgaard 1990, 148). Those who do try to make badly needed political and economic reforms face huge obstacles. As former World Bank economist Robert Klitgaard writes, "The harsh conditions of underdevelopment encourage tropical gangsters of every variety—government, business, and international aid giver" (12). Leaders in developing countries also face the enormous power differentials that make their concerns secondary to those of more powerful nations, particularly the United States. When offered assistance by multilateral agencies or the wealthy nations that control them, they simply can't refuse—even when such "help" proves disastrous.

We should also recognize an inherent bias in the concept of development. To be "developed," as the terminology implies, is good; to be "underdeveloped," is bad. Therefore, anyone who seeks to "develop" the less fortunate of the world must be doing good work. On such a premise stands the gargantuan aid industry, well beyond reproach given the sanctity of its mission. A more disappointing return on the world's $1 trillion investment in development would be hard to conceive. Yet, any time a group seeks to impose its views on those less fortunate, there is a strong likelihood that nothing good will follow. That is as true in inner cities of industrialized countries as it is in the poorest and most isolated parts of the developing world. This tragically fatal flaw has been an unfortunate, if not dominant, characteristic of development to date. Only recently have more enlightened views begun to prevail.

Historically, some of the negative outcomes in the history of development stem from the reliance on rising GNP as the standard measuring stick for development success. Since the early 1950s, it was thought that a country was "developing" if its GNP was improving. However, although rising GNP remains an extremely important measure of progress, it tells only part of the story. Consider the following characterization of GNP from Robert Kennedy on the first day of his presidential campaign in 1968,

> Our gross national product—if we should judge America by that—counts air pollution and cigarette advertising, and ambulances to clear our highways of carnage. It counts special locks for our doors and the jails for those who break them. It counts the destruction of our redwoods and the loss of our natural wonder in chaotic sprawl. It counts napalm and the cost of a nuclear warhead, and armored cars for police who fight riots in our streets. . . . Yet the gross national product does not allow for the health of our children, the quality of their education, or the joy of their play. It does not include the beauty of our poetry or the strength of our marriages; the intelligence of our public debate or the integrity of our public officials. It measures neither our wit nor our courage; neither our wisdom nor our learning; neither our compassion nor our devotion to our country; it measures everything, in short, except that which makes life worthwhile . . . (Caufield 1996, 221).

As Robert Kennedy so eloquently described, GNP alone is a poor measure of the quality of life. It is an equally poor measure of development. A rising GNP may hide increasingly concentrated wealth among the elite, as has happened in many countries, for example, Brazil. "Development" in such cases exacerbates class differences by distributing scarce funds even more disproportionately to those at the top, while the poor's fate, as ever, worsens. Although rising incomes and expanding middle classes are of great importance, we need to view development in terms more inclusive than GNP alone. The UN's human development index (HDI) serves that purpose as well as any other measure.

The Human Development Reports, prepared annually by the United Nations Development Program (UNDP), are widely used by both those who drive policy from the largest aid agencies such as the World Bank and USAID as well as by the grassroots organizations that increasingly hold the former accountable. Such a measuring stick has created a common language that the world can use to see just how far poor countries and poor strata within all countries are advancing or falling behind. At their core, the Human Development Reports reflect a progressive development philosophy in which "enhancing human capabilities" predominates. Such language reflects the most promising and dominant voice of the modern era of development, that of Nobel Prize-winning economist Amartya Sen.

In his seminal text, *Development as Freedom*, Sen writes that in its ideal, development involves the expansion of the real freedoms that people enjoy. This entails a wide array of distinct but mutually reinforcing objectives: political freedoms in the form of free speech and democratic elections, social opportunities through education and health care, and economic freedoms through the chance to participate in trade and production (Sen 1999, 11). Sen terms such freedoms the "basic building blocks" of development. Attention should thus be focused, in his view, on expanding "the 'capabilities' of persons to lead the lives they value—and have reason to value" (18). The success of a society, he argues, should be judged not by the growth of its GNP or its accumulation of physical and human capital but by the degree to which the members of the society attain such freedoms that give life value.

Sen calls for the removal of the "unfreedoms" that restrict the agency of the majority of the world's people. Sen describes unfreedoms this way, "poverty as well as tyranny, poor economic opportunities as well as systematic social deprivation, neglect of public facilities as well as intolerance or overactivity of repressive states" (Sen 1999, 3). To this list he adds illiteracy, gender discrimination, hunger, and all the other restrictions that keep people from pursuing the lives they choose. As such, the process of development in its idealized—though not historical—form, as articulated by Sen, can be seen as simply the progressive steps of overcoming these unfreedoms.

Sen's view of development involves individual and collective transformation such that those who live in poor countries have the opportunity to change their own lives based on that which they most value. And that which they most value may differ from that which the lead development actors seek to impose on them. "With adequate social opportunities, individuals can effectively shape their own destiny and help each other," writes Sen. "They need not be seen primarily as passive recipients of cunning development programs" (1999, 11). The same principles apply to marginalized groups in rich countries (21).

By acquiring the freedom to express their views, people may force government to steer additional resources toward basic health care and education.

Sen also argues that the freedoms as stated are not only the chief goal of development but serve as its most effective means—freedoms of one type greatly help to advance freedoms of other types. By acquiring the freedom to express their views, people may force government to steer additional resources toward basic health care and education. Political freedoms allow people to determine who should govern and on what principles. As we saw in Chapter 2, societies that invest in health care and education for their people enjoy enhanced productivity from their workforce and better economic growth. These countries break out of the shackles of poverty far sooner than countries in which economic benefits are more concentrated.

The view of "development as freedom" represents a substantial step forward for the world community. UN Secretary-General Kofi Annan described Sen's thinking as having "revolutionized the theory and practice of development" (Sen 1999). Others have bestowed equally lavish and deserved praise. However, this relatively new vision articulated by Sen, the UN, and others represents progress more in theory than practice. Development work on the ground is far messier, strewn with casualties through a long history of greed, hypocrisy, corruption, conflicting motivations, strategic overrides, and the exigencies of concentrated wealth and power. The ultimate gap of the modern development era exists between the vision of Sen and the lived experiences of the poor, those who are most directly affected by the business of development.

Foreign Aid: The Players and Terms

Players, History, and Scope

Development dates back a mere 60 years to the conferences that created the World Bank and IMF in 1944 and the UN in 1945. Because many countries support and direct all three bodies, aid rendered through them or through regional development banks is termed *multilateral aid*. By contrast, direct donations between states, coordinated by oversight programs such as USAID, are termed *bilateral aid*.

For more than a half-century, developed countries have tried to help poorer countries of the world "develop" through these aid channels. Along the way there have been some successes, eg, South Korea, Taiwan, and Costa Rica. However, there have been many more failures, including most of sub-Saharan Africa, in large part due to the overriding strategic objectives of donors and a long history of very low levels of aid. These failures, combined with a long history of subjugation of the poor, unethical lending practices, and draining of natural resources, have triggered doubts about the basic motivations of aid, which some have termed "the last refuge of Western colonialism" (Maren 1997).

The measures of aid are as complex as they are multiple and account for much of the confusion that characterizes aid discussions in the media. Through such confusion, the general public remains largely unaware of where most of the money goes, and politicians on both sides stake claims that are rarely checked. To clarify, let's first look at some terms. Multilateral aid and bilateral aid together comprise ODA, which is state sponsored and paid for mostly through taxes in donor countries. To qualify as ODA, funds must go only to countries considered "developing" by widely agreed on standards.[5] Second, funds must be administered "with promotion of economic development and welfare as its main objective" (OECD 2002, 294). By definition, this excludes all forms of military aid (Congressional Budget Office 1997, 4). Third, funds must be "concessional," meaning at least 25% must be in the form of a grant (Randel et al 2002, 259). ODA can be thought of as money that flows from taxpayers in wealthy countries, through intermediaries like USAID, the UN, and the World Bank, to recipients in poor countries. It is the standard measure of aid and most closely approximates the type of assistance advocated by Sen and others.

Official aid (OA) comprises resource flows to "countries in transition," not considered developing. Such countries include Russia and the "newly independent states" of Eastern Europe (former satellite countries of the USSR), Israel, Korea, United Arab Emirates, Qatar, Libya, Kuwait, and several others (OECD 2002, 300). These countries are better off than those that receive ODA. Some of these countries, eg, Iraq, Russia, Israel, and Ukraine, are top recipients of US aid, largely for political and strategic reasons (121).

The net sum of ODA and OA, plus resource flows that do not have sufficient concessional amounts to qualify as ODA, is called *official development finance* (ODF). This last category includes many World Bank and IMF debt-refinancing schemes (discussed shortly) that would not qualify as concessional.

Quantifying aid and tracking its disbursements get very few people excited. However, by following the channels through which aid money flows and reviewing the end result, we can discern its true motivations and value. We can also figure out just how concerned we should be about the aid's impact on the health of the poor. As such, following are the breakdowns of official aid for 2002: Countries spent $62.7 billion on ODF, which includes all nonmilitary, state-supported aid. Most of this, $59.1 billion, was ODA, or traditional "foreign aid," of which $40.7 billion was bilateral and $18.4 billion was multilateral. OA to transitional countries was $7.7 billion, and other official development finance (not ODA or OA) was –$4.1 billion (flows in the opposite direction) (OECD 2004, 134).

Aid flows tend to follow the political and strategic priorities of the donors, not the recipients.

From these resource flows, we see just how important the role is for individual states. Most traditional "foreign aid" comes through direct, bilateral aid; that does not include the multibillion dollar military aid that is not counted in any of the above measures. Clearly, the power structures in Washington, London, Bonn, and Paris have enormous sway over where and how aid dollars are spent. These same centers of power also hold enormous sway over multilateral aid flows, as discussed in the next chapter. An important principle of foreign aid is this: Aid flows tend to follow the political and strategic priorities of the donors, not the recipients. By its very design, foreign aid historically has benefited the rich countries first, the recipient countries second. If we consider aid from the standpoint of the wealthy countries' interests, we can better understand some seemingly bizarre aid allocations.

Other monetary flows from rich to developing countries come from a wide variety of sources, none of them "official," and hence not included in the previous list. To get a sense of the size of these revenue flows, consider the following summary of US "private" contributions to developing countries in 2000: from foundations ($1.5 billion), universities ($1.3 billion), corporations ($2.8 billion), private voluntary organizations ($6.6 billion), religious congregations ($3.4 billion), and individual remittances, ie, sending money "home" to family members in other countries ($18.0 billion) (OECD 2002, 27). Taken together this "private assistance totaled $33.6 billion in 2000, far outstripping the $9.9 billion the United States spent on ODA that year. These represent huge flows and are often cited as evidence of our generosity. However, similar types of private flows—though less in quantity— come from all rich countries. Further, it is a stretch to claim that $18 billion in hard-earned dollars—often from low-paying jobs—sent back "home" by immigrants to the United States should be included in the "US private assistance" tally, yet USAID did just that in a 2002 report (OCED 2002, 27).

A Brief History of Bilateral Aid Flows

As the scale of aid increased during the 1950s, so did the accompanying confusion in recipient countries. It became clear that a coordinating body was needed. Meeting in Paris on December 14, 1960, the OECD, the coordinating body of the wealthy donor community, established a specialized committee to oversee foreign aid, which it called the Development Assistance Committee (DAC). As of 2005, the DAC included 22 member countries plus the Commission of the European Communities (OECD 2004, 2). The DAC publishes annual profiles of member countries' aid performance and offers a forum through which bilateral donors can review the efficacy of aid.[6] The United States played a key role in creating the DAC in 1960-1961 and has served as its chair ever since.

In 1969, the DAC recommended each member state contribute 0.7% of its GNP to ODA; this followed a 1960 UN General Assembly motion. Only five countries —Denmark, Norway, Sweden, the Netherlands, and Luxembourg—have achieved this target in recent years. (OECD 2004, 74).[7] Scandinavian countries tend to fund the poorest countries, standing apart from the rest of the developed world. Six more countries—the United

Kingdom, France, Spain, Ireland, Belgium, and Finland—have promised to join the somewhat exclusive 0.7% club by 2015 (Sachs 2005b, 87). Average aid disbursements remain low at just 0.25% of GNP ($69.03 billion) in 2003, down from 0.37% just 20 years earlier (OECD 2004, 72; Randel et al 2002, 149).

One reason for declining aid levels was the end of the Cold War, when many poor countries lost their strategic relevance. Per-person aid in the world's poorest countries fell by 40% from the 1980s to the end of the 1990s (Randel et al 2002, 152), and overall ODA from the rich OECD countries declined from 0.3% of GNP to 0.2% of GNP during the 1990s (Sachs, 2005a,213). By the year 2000, the 48 "least developed countries" according to UN rankings, received less than a third of global aid (151). These are the countries where 15% of the children don't live to their fifth birthday. In 1997, *The Economist* noted that aid to Africa in all forms was "dropping like a stone" (Kim et al 2000, 52), despite decades of stagnation and an AIDS crisis ravaging the continent (Randel et al 2002, 151). Aid per person fell from $32 in 1980 to $22 in 2001 (Sachs 2005a, 82). For many years, the wealthiest nations appeared quite reluctant to help the poorest nations; only recently has the tide begun to turn, though only slightly.

When we shift to sector allocation, ie, where funds are spent, we find an equally disturbing history. Of the aid that does flow, precious little gets to the sectors where it might make the greatest impact. In 2000, only 1.5% of bilateral commitments went to basic education and 2% to basic health (Randel et al 2002, 149). Total bilateral flows for health from 1997 to 1999 averaged just $2.5 billion per year, which is just 0.01% of donor GNP, or one penny for every $100 earned (Sachs 2001b, 93). A UN commission charged with mapping a response to the annual death toll from AIDS, malaria, and tuberculosis called for additional health expenditures of $22 billion per year by 2007 and $31 billion by 2015, amounts unlikely to come any time soon (National Public Radio, 2003a; Sachs 2001b, 11). Buttressing their call for increased aid, the commission wrote, "The AIDS pandemic will destroy African economic development unless controlled" (Sachs 2001b, 113). Because the cash-strapped governments in sub-Saharan Africa spend, on average, a mere $3 to $10 per person per year on health, they are unable to provide even basic health care, which costs $30 per person per year, let alone cover the additional costs of AIDS, malaria, and tuberculosis (UNDP, 2005, 79). Without considerable increases in aid for health care, the "perfect storm" of epidemic disease and extreme poverty will continue to ravage the continent; several of the MDGs will not be achieved.

The UN's calls for increased funding come at a time when global wealth has reached unprecedented levels. In 1961, per capita income in donor countries was $13,298, while per capita aid given was $71. By 2000, per capita income had risen to $29,769, while per capita aid given had fallen to $66 (Randel et al 2002, 145). Looked at in another way, the average aid given by OECD countries per percent of GNI is now one third lower than it was in the 1980s, and one-half the level of the 1960s (UNDP 2005, 84). With such a backdrop, even the relatively strong increases in aid levels since the Monterrey conference in 2002 represent feeble attempts to climb up from the lowest ODA levels since the DAC began. In December 2004, *The Boston Globe* reported that the Bush administration cited "budget pressures" as the reason it cut overseas food programs for the poor; however, the administration had previously cut taxes on the wealthiest Americans—$80 billion to the top 1 percent (those earning over $337,000 per year) in 2004 alone ("Reneging on Food Aid" 2004). Rising wealth has not been accompanied by rising generosity.

Aid from the rich countries has followed a complex mix of donor rationales that are strategic, economic, and historic—all of which hinder aid's efficacy. Many European countries carry a burden of guilt and use aid as a salve to make up for crimes committed during the colonial era. One Cambridge University student wrote, "We took the rubber from Malaya, the tea from India, raw materials from all over the world and gave almost nothing in return" (Hancock 1989, 7). To better understand the rationale and efficacy of aid, it is best to view aid patterns in the world's most influential country, the United States.

The United States' Role: History and Motivations

For 40 years after the end of World War II, the United States was the world's leading aid donor. Until 1968, the United States regularly accounted for more than half of the world's ODA, and as recently as 1986 its share was still more than 25% (OECD, 1996, 95). US foreign aid then declined steadily to the low levels of the late 1990s before increasing again. For the United States as for most other countries, the motives for aid generally fall into three categories: humanitarian, strategic, and economic.

Humanitarian Aid   The United States' involvement in development dates back to Harry Truman's 1949 inaugural address, in which he called for a "worldwide effort for the achievement of peace, plenty and freedom" (Hancock 1989, 69). Truman summoned the better angels of our nature, and through his address, many Americans heard for the first time about global poverty. "More than half the people in the world are living in conditions approaching misery," he said. "Their economic life is primitive and stagnant." Fresh on the heels of impressive military victories in World War II, Americans were ready to take on new challenges.

The United States emerged from World War II as a dominant global power. Through its large contributions to European reconstruction; its overwhelming influence at the World Bank, IMF, and UN; and its global economic dominance, the United States carved out a role in the early post-war years as the leader of international development, a role it has not ceded since. The US government can legitimately proclaim itself the world leader in responding to natural disasters and other humanitarian emergencies. A USAID report boasted that the US government spent $1.6 billion in official humanitarian aid in 2000, three to four times more than any other country.[8] By 2004 that amount had increased to $2.5 billion (Congressional Research Service, 2004, 6). These are the relief shipments that we read about in the wake of hurricanes in the Caribbean, tsunamis in the Indian Ocean, and civil wars in Africa. Most efforts are effective, saving countless lives.

I witnessed this aid in action in Honduras in the wake of Hurricane Mitch in December 1999. The US Army Corps of Engineers rebuilt roads and villages, supported collapsing houses, and provided immediate relief, earning widespread thanks from the poor people who were its beneficiaries. Many locals had never seen anything like the US military and humanitarian response in the storm's immediate aftermath. These forms of relief comprise some of the United States' best use of aid and engender goodwill wherever employed.

Unfortunately, in the aftermath of disasters, the rich world—with the United States in the lead—is better at making promises than keeping them. The aid for a particular disaster typically lasts only as long as the media keeps the public's attention focused on it. In the years before enormous tsunamis in the Indian Ocean killed over 300,000 people and captured the world's attention in December 2004, natural disasters in Honduras (1999) and Iran (2003) had claimed center stage ("Rapid Health Response" 2005, 61; UNDP 2005, 1). Hurricane Mitch in 1999 was the past century's worst disaster in the Western Hemisphere, killing over 9,000 and costing over $9 billion. The international community pledged $9 billion in relief, but most of that money never arrived; half of what did came in the form of loans (Thompson and Faith, 2005). The US Congress set a two-year deadline on long-term rebuilding plans, subverting pledges for long-term reconstruction. Similarly, after an earthquake with a magnitude of 6.9 killed over 40,000 people and destroyed the ancient Iranian city of Bam in December 2003, the international community pledged $1 billion to rebuild it, and then delivered just $17 million (Thompson and Faith, 2005). Hopefully, the world will better honor its pledges to the survivors of the December 2004 tsunamis.

Nevertheless, most US aid does not flow to the victims of natural disasters or follow the humanitarian direction that the US population wants. In a well-documented though tragic history, the humanitarian sentiment that launched the US role into development quickly fell to a distant third in the list of priorities. Strategic and economic concerns predominated virtually from the beginning.

Although widely touted as the humanitarian and benevolent act that it was, the Marshall Plan also served strategic and economic objectives. Between 1946 and 1952, more than 80% of US foreign aid went to Europe, most through the Marshall Plan (CBO 1997, 10). The United States needed the British, Europeans, and Japanese as strategic allies in the fight against communism. And what good would the booming war economy be if the United States had no trading partners to purchase its goods? Despite heart-warming rhetoric and some genuine efforts to alleviate global poverty, the money trail has consistently led back to US strategic and economic interests—interests that often overlap.

> *Although widely touted as the humanitarian and benevolent act that it was, the Marshall Plan also served strategic and economic objectives.*

Strategic Aid   President Kennedy bluntly summed up the priority of American aid in 1961, "Foreign aid is a method by which the United States maintains a position of influence and control around the world and sustains a good many countries which would definitely collapse or pass into the communist bloc" (Hancock 1989, 71). JFK then signed the Foreign Assistance Act of 1961, which established USAID, whose chief mission was to administer development assistance programs in countries deemed politically important to the United States (CBO 1997, 11). In the 1950s and 1960s, the bulk of US foreign aid flowed to the battlegrounds of the Cold War, particularly South Korea, Taiwan, and South Vietnam. From 1953 to 1975, that region received half of all US bilateral aid (10). As a hedge against communism, the United States increased its aid budgets to a high of 0.6% of GNP under the Johnson administration, a level it has never attained since (Easterly 2002, 33).

Following the fall of the USSR in 1991, it became painfully clear just how much of a façade Soviet leadership had projected—the USSR had been little more than a middle-income country with nuclear weapons. But there were very real fears from the 1950s that the economic machinery of communism was superior to that of capitalism, with world dominance hanging in the balance (Easterly 2002, 32). As the "other" global superpower, the United States sought to counter Soviet aggression, both real and perceived, by "buying" the support of third world dictators, no matter how corrupt. For decades, the best way to secure dollars from Washington was to befriend Moscow—and everyone knew it.

In the mid 1970s, priorities shifted again, this time to the Middle East. Following the 1979 Camp David Peace Accords, Israel and Egypt became two of the largest recipients of US aid and military assistance as a payoff for peace, a pattern that has persisted ever since. Since 1979, the Middle East has received more than half of US bilateral aid (CBO 1997, 10). From the US government's perspective, it helps to have a stable democracy in the Middle East, home to the world's largest oil reserves. Even though funding Egypt is problematic, it may enhance stability. As author Fareed Zakaria pointed out, the people in several countries in the region—and Egypt in particular—are far more extreme than their despotic and dysfunctional governments (Zakaria 2003, 119). Support of any of the area's regimes is hazardous, as US experience in Iran and Iraq has shown.

Other world regions have received US aid when their strategic importance warranted it. The Horn of Africa became a huge US aid recipient during the height of regional Cold War tensions in the late 1970s and early 1980s (Maren 1997, 1, 92). In Somalia, US food shipments flooded area markets, ruining the livelihoods of areas farmers. Up to two thirds of shipments in some areas were stolen and then sold on the black market to purchase arms, furthering the conflict and creating more refugees. Former Somali minister of the interior, Abdirahman Osman Raghe, said, "Food aid . . . had turned Somalia from a self-sufficient exporter of food to an aid-dependent 'kleptocracy'" (169). Author Michael Maren concluded from his experiences working for USAID, "Somalia added a whole new dimension to my view of the aid business. My experience there made me see that aid could be worse than incompetent and inadvertently destructive. It could be positively evil" (12).

The 2005 DAC report lists Egypt, Iraq, Israel, Pakistan, Jordan, and Afghanistan among the top 10 recipients of US ODA/OA, reflecting US strategic and political interests in the Gulf region.

Other countries have also suffered from infusions of US foreign aid. El Salvador, Nicaragua, Costa Rica, and Guatemala received substantial US aid when perceived communist threats and real threats to US business interests surfaced in the 1970s and 1980s (Chomsky 1993, 29). Much of this infusion armed authoritarian regimes that brutally repressed the poorest members of Latin American societies.[9] Saudi Arabia has long received substantial US aid in return for maintaining peace with Israel and keeping oil prices down. That US "infidel" solders are stationed on Saudi soil is ironic given the extreme conservatism of the Wahhabis in the Saudi leadership; it also provided a key motivation for the attacks of September 11 (Unger, 2004, 278). The 2005 DAC report lists Egypt, Iraq, Israel, Pakistan, Jordan, and Afghanistan among the top 10 recipients of US ODA/OA, reflecting US strategic and political interests in the Gulf region (OECD 2005, 104). And these aid tallies exclude foreign military aid expenditures, which run into the billions.

The terrorist attacks of September 11, 2001 triggered the most dramatic changes in US foreign aid in 40 years. In September 2002, President Bush released his Administration's National Security Strategy that established global development—for the first time—as the "third pillar" of U.S. national security, along with defense and diplomacy.[8]

The administration and members of Congress concluded that weak states such as Afghanistan were ideal breeding grounds for terrorists, so assistance to the front-line states in the "war on terrorism" rose substantially President Bush's 2004 budget included $657 million for Afghanistan,

$460 million for Jordan, $395 million for Pakistan, $255 million for Turkey, $136 million for Indonesia, and $87 million for the Philippines (Radelet 2003, 15).

Reconstruction programs in Iraq and Afghanistan together cost more than all other aid programs combined in 2004 (Congressional Research Service 2004, 2). However, most of the costs for Iraq's occupation and reconstruction are not included in traditional "foreign aid" tallies by the DAC. The DAC listed ODA (Iraq is a lower middle-income country) to Iraq in 2003 (the most recent compilation to date) as just $775 million, even though the United States has spent an average of $60 billion per year in the first two years of the war (Sachs 2005a, 307). Though unstated in its report, the DAC may well only include some of the costs because the United States first invaded Iraq, toppled its government, and acted primarily because of intelligence claiming that Saddam Hussein had weapons of mass destruction, weapons that have never been found. The DAC only includes aid dollars designed to promote development, not military expenditures, which comprise a large percent of the current total of US spending in Iraq. By contrast, the US government does include Iraq reconstruction costs in its foreign aid tallies, though it lists Iraq reconstruction costs separately ($18.4 billion in FY 2004 alone), as the high costs involved obscure other aid trends (Congressional Research Service 2004, 2,12). The Bush administration requested $49.1 billion for combat operations in Iraq and Afghanistan in 2006, funds not included in its $441.6 billion request for the department of defense (Center for Arms Control and Proliferation 2005). Total cost for the Iraq war from the invasion in March 2003 through September 2005, according to one estimate, were nearly $200 billion (The National Priorities Project 2005). Ironically enough, in its first two years, the Iraq War cost roughly the same amount ($120 billion) as that needed for the United States to reach 0.7% of GNP in foreign aid spending (Sachs 2005a, 307).

Strategic considerations of foreign aid through the years help to explain why thugs like Mobutu Sese Seko of Zaire, Saddam Hussein of Iraq, Daniel Arap Moi of Kenya, Ferdinand Marcos of the Philippines, Shah Reza Pahlavi of Iran, and the Duvaliers of Haiti amassed personal fortunes. The US government and its allies have turned a blind eye to even the worst human rights' abuses as long as strategic and economic objectives were met. In some cases, US aid has directly armed and trained the military forces that have carried out some of the worst atrocities of the modern era, particularly in Latin America in the 1970s and 1980s. Lars Schoultz of the University of North Carolina found a direct correlation between US foreign aid and human rights abuses. He concluded that US aid "has tended to flow to Latin American governments which torture their citizens . . . to the hemisphere's relatively egregious violators of fundamental human rights" (Chomsky 1993, 120). Although one might argue that aid tends to go to the poorest and hence most unstable governments where such repression naturally flourishes, humanitarian concerns clearly have lost out to overriding political and economic concerns.

Another category of aid, military assistance, is traditionally left out of "foreign aid" tallies, yet has been for years one of the largest categories in US aid disbursements. For example, in 2004, the United States gave nearly $4.6 billion to Israel and Egypt through the Foreign Military Financing (FMF) Program, through which the Department of Defense provides grants and loans allowing foreign governments to purchase US-manufactured military equipment (Congressional Research Service 2004, 7). This money comes right back to the United States, providing yet another means through which foreign aid creates US jobs, supports the US economy, and promotes US strategic interests. Military assistance in 2004 comprised $4.8 billion, or 23% of US foreign aid as calculated by the US government (Congressional Research Service 2004, 29).

Economic Aid   Author Edward Herman found that US aid flows tended to correlate best with improved investment climates, where organized labor and vocal opposition are quite often anathemas (Chomsky 1993, 120). The experience of Mexico's maquiladora workers makes this abundantly clear. These workers are paid little, forced to work in harsh and dangerous conditions, and are routinely fired for attempting to unionize (Kim et al 2000, 260). It is no surprise that the destruction of the free press and the killing of union leaders, organized peasants, and "agitators" like El Salvadoran Archbishop Oscar Romero have been commonplace in countries that receive large amounts of US developmental and military aid. In the words of Schoultz, state terror is required "to destroy permanently a perceived threat to the existing structure of socioeconomic privilege by eliminating the political participation of the numerical majority" (Chomsky 1993, 30). Similar forces were at work in the United States more than a century ago, as the robber barons similarly exploited workers and opposed unions.

US economic considerations are most clearly on display in Latin America and through our directives at the World Bank and IMF, which are covered in Chapter 5. Aid often helps businesses or multinational corporations to establish footholds on foreign soil, where they soon demand protection. US business interests in Central America have long been associated with US military interventions. In 1954, the United States invaded Guatemala to prevent the Guatemalan government from taking over land owned by US-based United Fruit Company (Kim et al 2000, 474). Ties between the upper echelons of US government and United Fruit were far from unusual, and plans to redistribute land to peasants reeked of communism, often the pretext for US intervention in Latin America (Farmer 1994a, 238).

Haiti presents an even more blatant example of US aggression backing powerful business interests. The US Navy sent warships to Haitian waters no fewer than 26 times between 1849–1915 "to protect the lives and property of American citizens" (Farmer 1994a, 89). Under such formidable military protection, US firms subsequently acquired 266,000 acres of Haitian land, displacing roughly 50,000 peasants. A New York financial tabloid announced in 1926 that the Haitian worker was far cheaper than contemporaries in Panama, such that, "Haiti offers a marvelous opportunity for American investment" (94). In recent years, US global domination has increased considerably, though it now assumes more covert forms.

Author John Perkins wrote about the inner workings of the international "corporatocracy," described as the new ruling elite in governments, banks, and corporations in his 2004 eye-opening book, *Confessions of an Economic Hit Man.* Perkins job as an economist to a large US international consulting firm was to "encourage world leaders to become part of a vast network that promotes US commercial interests" (Perkins 2004, xi). As a self-described "economic hit man" (EHM), he created the optimistic financial projections that would justify huge World Bank and Regional Development Bank loans to developing countries. The leaders of these countries would then hire US companies like Bechtel, Halliburton, and Brown & Root to conduct massive construction and engineering projects, enriching these companies while simultaneously ensnaring the countries in enormous debt. This debt would make them beholden to US' interests, whether for military bases, UN votes, or oil or other natural resources. Most of the money would never leave the United States, simply transferred from banking offices in Washington to engineering offices in New York, Houston, or San Francisco. Perkins writes, "The larger the loan the better. The fact that the debt burden placed on a country would deprive its poorest citizens of health, education, and other social services for decades to come was not taken into consideration" (2004, 16). According to Perkins, when the EHM's failed, CIA operatives could always step in and orchestrate coups, as they did in Guatemala, Panama, Ecuador and Iran, among others, when US corporate interests were threatened.

Aid also promotes the business interests of the United States and other wealthy countries through a phenomenon know as "tied aid." By definition, tied aid is "foreign assistance that is linked to the purchase of exports from the country extending the assistance" (Kim et al 2000, 51). As a rule, most assistance comes with strings attached. According to the Congressional Research Service, 87% of US military aid financing, over 90% of food assistance, and 81% of bilateral developmental assistance overall was used to purchase US products or services in recent years (2005, 19). Given the cozy relationships that business elites have with those in power, it follows that businesses in donor countries often receive a large share of the business of aid. Author Graham Hancock offers the following blunt and largely accurate assertion, "Here is a rule of thumb that you can safely apply wherever you may wander in the third world: if a project is funded by foreigners it will typically also be designed by foreigners and implemented by foreigners using foreign equipment procured in foreign markets" (Hancock 1989, 155).

It makes sense to some that rich nations like the United States require that their foreign aid dollars purchase goods and services that they produce. Yet this practice creates enormous problems for those in the recipient countries. Tied aid reduces the overall value of the aid by roughly 25 to 40%, because recipients are forced to buy imports that are not competitively priced (Woods 2005). The UN estimates that tied aid costs developing countries $5 to $7 billion annually, or enough to fund universal primary education; sub-Saharan Africa alone loses $1.6 to $2.3 billion annually (UNDP 2005,103). President Bush's global AIDS initiative (PEPFAR) has required poor nations to purchase US-made brand name anti-retrovirals (ARVs) at up to 50 times the cost of local, generic versions, which are just as effective (Deen 2004; Sontag 2004). The flood of these US-manufactured ARVs into poor communities has crippled local generic-producing companies, driving up the price of these medicines overall, and ultimately, costing lives. Tied aid also robs poor countries of decisions about how to allocate the aid they receive, further promotes the interests of the donors over those of the recipients, and deprives local engineers, builders, carpenters, and other craftsmen important sources of work. Because of these problems, four countries, Norway, Denmark, the Netherlands, and the United Kingdom, have untied over 90% of their aid, contributing to the overall decrease in percentage of "officially" tied aid in recent years (OECD 2002, 245). However, the practice of "unofficially" tying aid remains common.

Colleagues in the Belize government have shared their experiences with aid, which reflects aid practices everywhere (Kim et al 2000, 51). Much of the aid rendered to Belize comes in the form of specific projects, most often funded through bilateral and multilateral donors. To obtain funding, countries must compete with experienced firms based in donor countries. Requests for proposals (RFPs) demand accounting and business expertise that is often lacking in developing countries. Instead, North American and European firms with such expertise sell it—usually to northern friends—for considerable profit. Without the money to properly fine-tune such proposals or to establish links to large experienced firms, the local Belizean contractors, engineers, and business people are outmatched at the start. If you factor in political connections between those at the highest levels of the aid industry and their friends in northern firms, the deal is complete. The likelihood that regional industry will share in the business success remains exceedingly small. Because the RFPs are open to everyone, it is not technically tied aid—though the dollars flow decidedly north.

Aid may also become the vehicle for not so subtle payoffs to political "friends." One US Congressmen sent millions of poplars to Nepal via refrigerated airfreight as a payoff to friends in the tree seedling business; all the trees died shortly after planting (Tisch and Wallace 1994, 61). There are thousands of stories of aid lining the pockets of elites on both sides of the donor equation. It is ultimately the poor–the alleged beneficiaries of aid–who lose the most.

A Clear Picture of United States' Aid

Perhaps the best way to understand where US aid is going is to take a single year of aid and break it down into its components. The Congressional Research Service (CRS) did just that in 2004, offering the best glimpse into the complex workings of aid. That year, US aid totaled almost $21 billion including military aid, but not including the $18.4 billion costs of Iraq reconstruction. Of the 2004 total, $6.2 billion (30%) went for bilateral development assistance, or traditional foreign aid; $5.4 billion (26%) for five major programs that meet specific US economic, political or security concerns; $4.8 billion (23%) for military aid; $2.6 billion (12%) for traditional humanitarian aid; and $1.7 billion (8%) for multilateral assistance, eg, the UN and World Bank. Recent initiatives like PEPFAR and the MCA have the potential to dramatically increase funding to poor countries, though only if fully funded. The US government provided some form of foreign assistance to over 150 countries in 2004, yet most of the top recipients were those deemed politically and strategically important to the United States: Iraq ($18.4 billion), Israel ($2.6 billion), Egypt ($1.8 billion), Afghanistan ($1.7 billion), and Columbia ($0.6 billion). Columbia's funding is largely for counter-narcotics initiatives.

For a more detailed analysis of where US aid dollars flow, we need to go back to 2003, the most recent year for which complete DAC information is now available. That year, the US gave $16.3 billion in net ODA (0.15% of GNI), not including military aid, which would have added another $6 billion through Foreign Military Financing (OECD 2005, 104; US Department of State 2005). Of this $16.3 billion, $1.7 billion went to multilateral organizations like the World Bank, leaving $14.6 for bilateral aid. Yet very little of this last amount actually helped poor countries develop; most funds flowed toward strategic aid. The Economic Support Fund, through which we support our strategic allies like Israel and Egypt, received $4.8 billion. (Iraq received $2.2 billion in 2003 through the "Iraq Relief and Reconstruction Fund" [IRRF] was accounted for separately [US Department of State 2005].) Countries deemed important to US strategic interests, such as Iraq, Israel, Egypt, Afghanistan, and Columbia received nearly half of all US bilateral assistance in 2003, even though most are middle-income countries (Sachs, 2005b, 81).

After support for "strategic" allies is subtracted from US foreign aid totals, only $6.1 billion of 2003 totals remains to fund development in poor countries. Of this, $2 billion was allocated to emergency assistance or food aid. Of the remainder, $1.3 billion came in the form of "debt forgiveness" grants, through which the US government forgave old debts, most of which had been long since paid back. Most of the remaining $2.8 billion in 2003 bilateral aid went toward "technical cooperation," mostly consultants from US government agencies or NGOs that provide expertise to developing countries, and keep most aid decisions in Washington. No wonder "foreign aid" has failed to reverse poverty in the world's poorest countries—that was never the intention.

For those who have long decried the "trillions" of aid dollars the US government has "wasted" on developing countries, the case of sub-Saharan Africa is particularly instructive. Popular mythology holds that this region is awash in US foreign aid, yet too corrupt or incompetent to make use of any of it; but the facts belie the myths. In 2003, the US gave $4.5 billion to sub-Saharan Africa in net bilateral ODA, excluding South Africa, and a few other middle-income countries (Sachs, 2005b, 83). $1.5 billion went to emergency aid, $0.3 billion for non-emergency food aid, $1.3 billion for debt forgiveness, and $1.4 billion for technical assistance, ie, US-based consultants. This left only $118 million for African-directed efforts and US in-country operations, just 18 cents for each of the 650 million people in the world's poorest region. According to economist Jeffrey Sachs, "The next time US officials visit Africa and wonder aloud where the 'trillions and trillions' of dollars went, they should be reminded of how small those trillions actually are" (Sachs, 2005b, 83).

In 2004, US aid totals to sub-Saharan Africa did rise, mainly because of AIDS funding to Ethiopia, Uganda, and Kenya through PEPFAR. Yet against the backdrop of a near $200 billion war in Iraq, the world community, led by British Prime Minister Tony Blair, called for increased funding to Africa during the G-8 summit of world leaders in Gleneagles, Scotland in July 2005. Mr Blair stated that providing hope for Africa's millions comprised "the fundamental moral challenge of our generation" ("Africa at the Summit" 2005). During the summit, global leaders reiterated earlier promises to increase aid to Africa by 2010 to $50 billion, roughly double what it now receives ("Good, But Not Great" 2005). Speaking for many, the NGO ActionAid decried the "yawning gulf between expectations raised and policy promised delivered" ("Good But Not Great" 2005). George W. Bush also pledged to double US aid to Africa, though over 90% of the money pledged had previously been committed, mostly through PEPFAR and the MCA (Bryden 2005). Even though Tony Blair and the summit organizers could claim tangible progress on aid to the world's poorest continent, many viewed the doubling of aid to Africa by 2010 as "too little, too late," continuing longstanding traditions of providing little aid to those most in need ("Good But Not Great" 2005).

The Reality of Aid Project, a nongovernmental watchdog group, found that in the year 2000, just 19% of US aid went to the poorest countries where 60% of the global population lives with average incomes less than $2 per day. Further, less than 2% of US bilateral aid went to basic education, 3.5% to basic health, and 1% to water and sanitation (Randel et al 2002, 246). Such expenditures clearly clash with the desires of the American people and with domestic spending priorities. In a 1997 report titled *America's Vital Interest in Global Health*, the Institute of Medicine noted that the United States spent $900 billion on domestic health care, while spending just $1 billion internationally on health, primarily on child survival and AIDS, a ratio of 900:1. This international spending comprised just 0.01% of GNP (Institute of Medicine 1997, 20). The report's authors strongly advocated additional spending on international health.

It is worth reflecting briefly on the larger picture. The United States clearly prefers to spend money on its military than on development, despite the elevation of the latter to one of the three pillars of national security. The US military budget is projected to rise to $442 billion in 2006, with at least $50 billion more needed to fund ongoing operations in Iraq and Afghanistan (Center for Arms Control and Proliferation, 2005). US spending on the Pentagon outstripped US spending on foreign aid by a factor of *30* in 2004 (Sachs, 2005a, 329). Recent budget deficits (projected at $521 billion for FY 2005) may force Congress to cut funding for important new initiatives like the MCA and PEPFAR, further cutting aid to the poorest countries. Until recently, the United States spent more on narcotics control ($213 million) than it did on aid to any country in sub-Saharan Africa (OECD 2002, 121). One nuclear powered, stealth Virginia attack submarine, the world's most advanced, cost $2.3 billion, more than the entire US foreign aid budget for humanitarian aid in 2002 (Center for Defense Information 2002, 36; Congressional Budget Office 1997, 63). Tomahawk cruise missiles, which list for $1.7 million apiece, were fired with abandon during the opening salvos of the Iraq War (Sivard 1996, 39). Each missile fired required more resources than the United States individually allocated to all but three countries in 2000 (OECD 2002, 276). The US population spent $8 billion on cosmetics in 1997, more than the total US ODA budget that year of $7.1 billion. In 2000, Americans and Europeans spent more on pet food ($17 billion) than they spent on total aid to sub-Saharan Africa ($12.7 billion). Europeans annually spend six times more on alcohol and cigarettes ($155 billion) than they spend on their total foreign aid, which was $25.3 billion in 2000. The world spends $400 billion annually on narcotics, a sum that, until recently, required world foreign aid budgets seven to eight years to reach (OECD 2002, 248; UNDP 1998, 37).

The Future of US Foreign Aid

The US history of foreign aid has seen its peaks in the Marshall Plan years to its nadir in the late 1990s. But several recent initiatives will increase US foreign aid spending significantly. President Bush's $15 billion initiative to fight AIDS in Africa and the Caribbean, called PEPFAR (the President's Emergency

Plan for AIDS Relief), would add $3 billion per year if fully funded. The largest increases would come through the afore-mentioned millennium challenge account (MCA).[10] This account involves a new approach to foreign aid in which only those countries that rule justly, invest in the health and education of their people, and encourage economic and trade freedoms will receive US MCA dollars. These aid disbursements will be closely monitored and only those able to show that they have used the dollars well will be eligible for additional funds. The MCA will comprise a separate group in the State Department and will command a full $5 billion per year starting in 2006. The combination of PEPFAR and the MCA would bring US foreign assistance to early 1990s levels, at $17 billion per year by 2006 if fully funded by Congress. Although the total increase in US foreign aid will raise US totals to a mere 0.17% of GDP—second from the bottom in the OECD—such an increase will be welcomed by the global community (Radelet 2003, 12).

However, Congress may never fully fund the MCA or PEPFAR given the enormous budget deficits of recent years. After years of declining deficits in the 1990s, deficits exploded again under George W. Bush following the terrorist attacks of September 2001, the Iraq war, and large tax cuts. The devastating Hurricane Katrina in August 2005 further increased the deficits significantly. By mid 2005, only two countries, Honduras and Madagascar, had together received a total of $323 million in MCA funding, drawing wide condemnation ("A Timely Departure" 2005). In 2005 Congress authorized only $1.5 billion of the administration request for $2.5 billion for the MCA (UNDP, 2005, 87). PEPFAR is also unlikely to receive full funding; only $2.4 billion was disbursed in 2004 (Sachs 2005b, 84).

The United States has long projected its military and economic might around the world. The Bush administration rightly added the MCA and AIDS funding as a way to project US soft power, the so-called third pillar of US national security.[8] It has become increasingly clear that many around the world resent the United States' concentrated wealth and resources, as well as its repeating pattern of reneging on promises made. Generosity with other countries will enhance our national security as well as bring our foreign aid more in line with the desires of the general public.

The Host Factor

In his book *Tropical Gangsters*, World Bank economist Robert Klitgaard described his two-year effort to help the government of Equatorial Guinea realign its economy to increase exports and improve income. His is a tale of government corruption and incompetence, tribal favoritism, brutal repression, and apathy and indifference among well-paid aid workers. Many who have worked in poor countries find that Klitgaard's story reflects their own experiences. Like many African countries, Equatorial Guinea suffered horribly under the brutal regime of dictator Francisco Macias Nguema, who murdered or forced into exile one quarter to one third of the population during the late 1960s and 1970s (Klitgaard 1990, 20). Following his ouster, other military dictators retained power through favors granted to powerful constituents. One Equatorial Guinean summarized, "In Africa, first comes the family, then the clan, then the province, then the region, and finally the country" (255). Under such a system, it is little wonder that those appointed to positions of power often have a poor understanding of how to run a coun-try, particularly one overwhelmed by harsh poverty. It is also predictable that any money coming into the country will quickly find its way into the hands of those in and around power. Power and money attract—the former greatly enhances the ability of the chosen few to hold onto the latter.

Poor economic policy, incom-petent administration, and corruption within recipient governments have limited the success of various aid initia-tives through the years.

Klitgaard's story raises a key element in the story of aid that is itself political fodder, often ignored by the far left while touted as solely responsi-ble by the far right. Although donors have erred and admit it, recipient governments rarely if ever admit mistakes. We will focus on governance in a subsequent chapter; though it is impossible to understand the limits of development without briefly reviewing the role of the host government. Poor economic policy, incompetent administration, and corruption within recipient governments have limited the success of various aid initiatives through the years.

The 1997 CBO study concluded its review of foreign aid: "The useful-ness of development assistance varies with the quality of a country's governance and the economic policies it pursues" (CBO 1997, 31). For example, it compared the development efforts of four pairs of countries "matched" by region and initial GNP per capita. South Korea and the Philippines had roughly similar GNPs per capita in 1960 ($800 and $911, respectively) (40). Over the next 30 years, they diverged, with a GNP per capita of $9,790 for South Korea and $2,893 for the Philippines. In addition to much higher income levels, South Korea had higher literacy rates, higher daily calorie consumption rates, and lower infant mortality rates. While South Korea pursued a successful development path through a series of authoritarian regimes and then a more democratic system in 1987, the Philippines suffered under the rule of Ferdinand Marcos from 1966 to 1986. South Korea received substantial aid flows in the 1950s and 1960s but little since, while the Philippines continued to receive large amounts of aid (OECD 2002, 250). In 2000, the Philippines came in 12th on the US ODA disbursement list (276).

One might conclude that being a recipient of US aid has a deleterious effect on recipient countries. In fact, the CBO contends that foreign aid actu-ally hurt the Philippines' development by reinforcing Marcos' "economic mismanagement and corruption" (CBO 1997, 50). However, examples from other countries show the important roles host governments can play. Costa Rica and Honduras both received considerable aid flows from the 1970s to 1990s. Honduras devoted large amounts to its military budget (20% to 30% during the 1980s); Costa Rica, with no army since 1948, directed its resources to health care and education. While Honduras remains poor, Costa Rica is now included in the UN's "high human development" group (UNDP 2005, 219).

A more precise conclusion drawn by the CBO is no doubt correct. "Essentially," the report's authors conclude, "foreign aid given to developing countries reinforces what is there. If a country has good government and economic policies, the result is likely to be more good government and economic policies. If a country has a highly corrupt political system and has pursued counterproductive economic policies, the result is usually more of the same." Such is the motivation for the MCA. Although the aid industry has many obvious failings, we need always remember that aid is multifactorial process, with governance one of the most important.

The Economist adds, "If relief is not carefully aimed at countries with a genuine commitment to sound economic management, it will be wasted" ("How to Make Aid Work" 1999). History provides many examples to support that conclusion. Poor countries that receive large amounts of aid do no better than those that receive little, and numerous studies have failed to show a link between aid and faster growth ("How to Make Aid Work" 1999). Many advocate targeting aid only to countries that have the sound economic policies that can actually make aid work. Others, like Jeffrey Sachs, have called for donors to direct large resources to basic health and education in all countries, key sectors that have been largely ignored to date. Both approaches share in calling for increased levels of spending with increased accountability. Such aid strategies would eliminate many of the critical reviews of aid, like this one.

Conclusions

It is no surprise that global poverty has not disappeared despite the billions of bilateral aid dollars spent to date. Similarly, it is no surprise when the people who have to live under the yoke of aid-supported tyrants quite vociferously denounce the United States and its foreign policy (Zakaria 2003, 155). In discussions on aid, we should always remember that aid primarily seeks to meet the political, economic, and strategic objectives of the donors, not the recipients. Despite recent increases in funding levels for AIDS, overall aid, and aid specifically for Africa, most aid will remain largely ineffective unless donor priorities radically change.

In recent years, the World Bank and IMF have assumed increasingly important roles in development, surpassing that of the UN (Randel et al

2002, 152). This should come as no surprise. The rich countries hold far greater sway in the World Bank and IMF, where it's "one dollar one vote," than in the UN General Assembly, where it's "one country one vote" (Sachs, 2005a, 287). The United States has the largest share of votes in the IMF and World Bank and exerts considerable influence in both institutions. In 1993, the *Lancet* noted that the torch for international leadership in health had passed from the WHO to the World Bank, a finding of enormous importance given all that has transpired ("World Bank's Cure" 1993). Unfortunately, according to Jeffrey Sachs, "the IMF and World Bank simply cannot do their jobs without much closer cooperation with the UN agencies" (2005a, 287). The Bank and IMF have made considerable mistakes in their leadership roles in global health.

In the next chapter, we look at the high priests of development—the World Bank and, to a far lesser degree, the IMF. More than any other institutions, these two international financial institutions have guided development since the beginning. Although many countries disburse their bilateral foreign aid to the middle-income countries within their spheres of influence, the World Bank operates chiefly in the poorest countries. As such, the intentions of taxpayers in the United States and other Western democracies to a large extent depend on the best and brightest macroeconomists and development experts who walk their hallowed halls. Just how much blame for the failures of development should be laid at the feet of these two goliaths is a matter worth reviewing.

Endnotes

1. In 2000, the same polling group found that the public then thought the percent of the federal budget spent on foreign aid was closer to 20% (Kull 2001). For more information see online comments at www.foreignpolicy.com/issue_SeptOct_2001/kullnotes.html#3.
2. Tisch and Wallace's specific definition is "financial or in-kind assistance provided by one country to another" (1994).
3. In 1994, the UN's Human Development Report summarized development as follows:

   In the final analysis, sustainable human development is pro-people, pro-jobs and pro-nature. It gives the highest priority to poverty reduction, productive employment, social integration and environmental regeneration. It brings human numbers into balance with the coping capacities of societies and the carrying capacities of nature. It accelerates economic growth and translates it into improvements in human lives, without destroying the natural capital needed to protect the opportunities of future generations. It also recognizes that not much can be achieved without a dramatic improvement in the status of women and the opening of all economic opportunities to women. And sustainable human development empowers people—enabling them to design and participate in the processes and events that shape their lives (UNDP 1994, 4).

   In its review of the effectiveness of foreign aid in 1997, the Congressional Budget Office defined development as "a long-term trend of growth in GNP per capita, rising education levels, improving health conditions, low to moderate population growth, sustainable use of natural resources and the environment, and secure access to adequate amounts of food" (CBO 1997, 3). It added in that truly developing countries were industrializing their economies and including larger percentages of their populations in the economic growth. As such, by current measures of the UN, the US Congressional Budget Office and others, countries with rising GNPs alone may not be developing.

4. "Sectoral development" (large projects) and "integrated rural development projects" (still larger, more integrated projects) dominated early development theory well into the 1970s. Costly and often unsuccessful, these approaches saddled many poor governments with huge debts that still require repayments. "Basic needs" approaches, which emphasized building capacity from the bottom up, gave way to "sustainable development" approaches, which recognized the need to enhance internal capacities for development from within a country. Finally, following widely held doubts of development efficacy and the debt crisis of the early 1980s, the donor community—as always lead by the World Bank and IMF—saw a need to restructure entire economies through "structural adjustment" and its various stepchildren that have dominated development aid ever since (Tisch and Wallace 1994, 41).

5. For specific definitions, see any of the Development Assistance Committee Journal of Development Co-Operation Reports of the OECD.

6. For more information, see the OECD web site at www.oecd.org.

7. Saudi Arabia was the most generous country in 2002, though not a member of the OECD.

8. Information from *Foreign Aid in the National Interest*, available at the US Agency for International Development web site at www.usaid.gov/fani.

9. For the most disturbing history of US involvement in "third world" countries, see the following texts by noted scholar Noam Chomsky: *Understanding Power* (The New Press, 2002), *World Orders Old and New* (Columbia University Press, 1994), and *Year 501: The Conquest Continues* (South End Press, 1993). The British publication, *The Guardian,* had the following to say about this author's work: "Chomsky ranks with Marx, Shakespeare, and the Bible as one of the ten most quoted sources in the humanities." For a brief introduction to his thought and presentation style, I suggest his brief text, *What Uncle Sam Really Wants* (Odonian Press, 1989).

10. For a complete overview of the millennium challenge account, see Steven Radelet's *Challenging Foreign Aid: A Policymaker's Guide to the Millennium Challenge Account* (Institute for International Economics, 2003).

Chapter 5

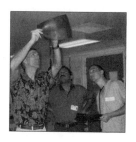

Development and Foreign Aid: Perceptions and Realities of Our Beneficence, Part II Multilateral Aid

The third world war has already started. It is a silent war. Not, for that reason, any less sinister. This war is tearing down Brazil, Latin America, and practically all the Third World. Instead of soldiers dying, there are children. It is a war over the Third World debt.

—Luis Inácio Lula da Silva, President of Brazil

When people find out what's been going on, you're going to see people out in the streets saying, 'My God, did you read this information? Why are our dollars being used to fund this kind of destruction?'

—US Senator Robert Kasten

The world's primary multilateral donor organizations are the United Nations (UN), the World Bank, and the International Monetary Fund (IMF). In this chapter, we look at the latter two, with a particular focus on the World Bank. The most influential and respected organization in the world donor community, the World Bank has also become a lightning rod for criticisms in recent decades—with much of it earned. We review several World Bank projects and then follow the steps by which many of the world's poorest countries sank deeply into debt through unrestrained World Bank lending, which nearly caused the collapse of the global monetary system in the 1980s debt crisis. The poorest citizens within these countries have since paid back some of this debt through World Bank–IMF-sponsored structural adjustment programs, in which services to the poor were cut, dramatically worsening their health and longevity. We then review the people who work in the aid organizations and aid's overall efficacy to answer the questions, why has bilateral and multilateral aid failed? And how can we help some nascent but promising attempts to reform aid and make it into a true ally of the poor?

Origins: The World Bank and the International Monetary Fund

The Economist summed up World Bank/IMF interactions with government officials from poor countries as follows, "Pointy-headed bureaucrats from Washington jet into yet another poor country and demand a slew of economic returns in return for aid. The government is overwhelmed by the numerous conditions, resents the imposition of politically unpopular reforms by outsiders, and implements them half-heartedly. The aid is ineffective and poverty continues" ("Old Battle" 2000). Such is the reality of the world's most important aid organizations—the World Bank and the IMF—over the past half century. To understand development, we must understand these two organizations, starting at their inception.

Although history and politics both played lead roles in causing World War II, there is little doubt that the economic crises of the interwar period were primarily responsible.[1] The Roaring Twenties had unleashed a period of wild, unregulated speculation in global stock markets that led directly to the crash of 1929. Because the world economy had become so interwoven, shock waves generated by economic calamities in one country forcefully struck others, worsening the crisis. All around the world in the 1930s, banks failed, factories stood idle, and tens of millions walked the streets in search of nonexistent jobs (Driscoll 1998, 3). The international systems of trade and finance had imploded, paralyzing the global economy. Between 1929 and 1932, the value of international trade fell by 63% and prices of goods fell by almost half (4). The seeds of discontent were sown everywhere and the world soon entered a war in which more than 50 million people would die.

During the war, the Allied Powers began to look for solutions that would prevent a return of a similar economic collapse in the future. Less than one month after D-Day in June 1944, delegates from 44 Allied countries gathered at the Mount Washington Hotel near Bretton Woods, New Hampshire, to fashion the institutions that would regulate the new, postwar economy. In 1941, Boston-born Harry Dexter White had posed a two-pronged plan that included a "'stabilization fund' that could keep world exchange rates in equilibrium" and a "'bank for reconstruction and development' to invest in war-damaged and poor countries" (Caufield 1996, 40). The famous British economist John Maynard Keynes had simultaneously developed a similar model. By conference's end, White, Keynes, and the other delegates had drafted plans for three global organizations with separate but mutually reinforcing functions: the World Bank, the IMF, and a third organization to regulate global trade. However, delegates could not agree on this last component, so they proposed an interim arrangement for trade liberalization called the General Agreement on Tariffs and Trade (GATT), which 23 countries signed in 1947 (Kim et al 2000, 19). It took nearly a half century before this third arm finally materialized in the form of the World Trade Organization, which replaced GATT in 1995 (see Chapter 6).

The International Monetary Fund

The first piece of the plan, the IMF, also known as the Fund, was to become the central institution of the international monetary system, charged with overseeing the health of the world's economy. According to its articles of agreement, the IMF advises countries on sound economic policy, promotes the expansion and balanced growth of international trade, maintains orderly currency exchange among its members, and keeps a "fund" to provide members with liquid resources to overcome balance of payment problems.[2] Countries pay membership fees or quotas to the IMF based on the size of their economies. As such, the IMF is like a credit union in which its member countries, which includes most of the world, may access funds in times of need.

The IMF has come to be known in popular terms as the "firefighter" in the global economy, so called because it puts out the economic fires that could lead to larger regional or even global destabilization.

It is in this last mode that the IMF has most frequently garnered world headlines. For example, following the 1997–1998 Asian financial crisis, the IMF loaned South Korea $21 billion to bolster its economy.[2] In August 2002, Brazil received the IMF's largest loan ever–$30 billion ("Brazilians Find Political Cost" 2002). Argentina, Mexico, and Russia are other recent recipients ("Doubts Inside" 2002). The IMF has come to be known in popular terms as the "firefighter" in the global economy, so called because it puts out the economic fires that could lead to larger regional or even global destabilization. Because voting in the IMF is determined by the percent contribution of its members, the world's most powerful economies run the show. It is therefore not surprising that its policies primarily serve the wealthy nations that control it, making the IMF a favorite target for criticism ("Doubts Inside" 2002).

The World Bank

The second piece of White's and Keynes' ambitious plan was a "world bank" that would reconstruct countries devastated by World War II and "develop" the poorest countries. While the IMF had the more somber task of ordering the world's finances, the World Bank would play a more humanitarian role, spreading peace and prosperity. However, it became clear early on that the World Bank would also serve other interests. With the creation of the World Bank, the era of foreign aid had begun and the industrialized, capitalist countries soon faced off against the socialist-communist countries for dominance over the third world (Kim et al 2000, 47). In addition, foreign aid would help America grow and the World Bank would become aid's champion. Eugene Black, the World Bank's third president, traveled around the United States in the 1950s drumming up public support for foreign aid, dominated then as now by the World Bank. From its earliest days, the World Bank gained a reputation for placing the interests of its New York financial supporters ahead of its clients in developing countries (Caufield 1996, 52). Richard Nixon later added his own brutally frank perspective on foreign aid, "Let us remember that the main purpose of aid is not to help other nations but to help ourselves" (Hancock 1989, 71).

> *The World Bank helps poor countries "develop" by providing their governments low-interest, long-term repayable loans.*

The first branch of the World Bank was called the International Bank for Reconstruction and Development, or IBRD. As the name implies, its founders envisioned two purposes though the IBRD played only a minor role in European reconstruction, which was largely completed through the US Marshall Plan (Rich 1994, 6).[3] The World Bank subsequently focused its efforts on development, spending more than a third of a trillion dollars between 1946 and 1996 (Caufield 1996, 1). A World Bank publication says, "The World Bank has one central purpose: to promote economic and social progress in developing countries by helping to raise productivity so that their people may live a better and fuller life" (Driscoll 1994, 2). More exactly, the World Bank helps poor countries "develop" by providing their governments low-interest, long-term repayable loans. During its early years, most World Bank loans went for infrastructure projects such as roads, dams, ports, and electric grids—the same kinds of projects that had previously helped Europe and America become global powers. Over the past 20 years, the World Bank has become less project oriented, partnering with the IMF to "restructure" developing economies toward export-oriented growth, such that recipient countries join the global economy. Although rational, both approaches have met with mixed results.

Member countries govern the World Bank by votes proportional to their relative economic strength. Initially, the United States controlled 35% of the vote and has held the largest percentage of votes ever since. Other industrial powers such as France, the United Kingdom, Japan, and Germany have long held the majority of power, effectively rendering control to G-8 countries. The Group of 8 countries (G-8) is comprised of the world's largest economies (United States, United Kingdom, France, Germany, Italy, Canada, and Japan) plus Russia.[4] Despite British preference for a World Bank/IMF location in the US financial capital of New York City, the US government prevailed, establishing the World Bank and IMF in two imposing structures on either side of 19th Street in Washington, DC, just a few short blocks from the White House and the Department of Treasury.

Such beginnings bore ominous markings, particularly to the British who saw the World Bank's founding as "little more than schemes of the United States to gain control of world trade" (Caufield 1996, 47). Still others saw the new World Bank/IMF as an "economic straightjacket" that the world powers could apply at will to the rest of the world. Such sentiments echoed through the press decades later. The *Washington Post* opined in a 1981 editorial, "successive American presidents have found the World Bank and the International Monetary Fund extremely useful. Both, with their international staffs, can set enforceable conditions for aid without threatening the infringement of national sovereignty or national pride" (205). Congress passed the Bretton Woods Agreements Act and President Truman signed it into law on July 31, 1945.

Although the US share of votes has since decreased to 20% of the total, it remains the World Bank's largest shareholder, chooses its leader, and maintains the sole veto over amendments to its articles of agreement. When the United States alone opposed a $48 million World Bank loan to rehabilitate the Polish coal industry, it failed (197). Similarly, after Egypt's President Nassar recognized the communist Chinese government in 1956, the United States and United Kingdom blocked a World Bank loan for construction of Egypt's Aswan High Dam, which the Soviets built ("Damming Evidence" 2003). When Chileans elected Salvador Allende in 1970, the Nixon administration sent out the word to "make the [Chilean] economy scream." World Bank officials complied and did not extend any loans to Chile until a few months after Allende was assassinated in 1974. Such patterns have long persisted.

The High Priests of Development   The World Bank Group is comprised of five separate entities.[5] Two of them, the International Bank for Reconstruction and Development (IBRD) and the International Development Association (IDA), comprise the overwhelming majority of lending and together are called the World Bank. These entities are technically considered to be specialized agencies of the UN, along with the IMF; however, their relationship to the UN system is tenuous at best. The budgets of the IMF and the

World Bank are listed separately from other UN agencies and each has its own funding sources.

The IBRD was the first to be founded in 1945 and has since lent more than $380 billion—$11 billion in 2004 alone (World Bank Group 2004a). It raises almost all of its money by selling its AAA-rated bonds (the most secure with the lowest risk of default) on the world financial markets, registering a profit every year since 1948.[6] As the World Bank's lending progressed, however, it became clear that most of the world's poorest countries could not afford the interest payments on IBRD loans. The IDA followed in 1960 to fill the gap, providing interest-free loans to the poorest countries.[7] As such, IDA loans are the best available. These loans, known as credits, include 10-year grace periods and reach maturity after 20, 35, or 40 years.[8] The IDA has lent $135 billion since 1960, $9 billion in 2004 alone (World Bank Group 2004a). The IDA derives most of its revenues from donor governments, which convene every three years to replenish the funds.

> *A culture of secrecy infuses the World Bank—accountability, transparency, and responsiveness are not traits for which the World Bank is known.*

Both the IBRD and IDA rely on a much larger funding source when making their loans—the taxpayers of wealthy nations. Wealthy member countries hand over certain funds and pledge the rest. Consequently, both the IDA and IDRB have immediate resources available and much larger funding "pledges," known as "callable" capital, that they can call in if things go awry. The amount actually given to the World Bank may be as little as one tenth of that pledged (Hancock 1989, 52). Because the World Bank has the backing of taxpayers from wealthy countries, it can make high-risk loans. If several large recipient countries were to suddenly and simultaneously default on their loans, these same taxpayers would foot the bill. This would seem to make the World Bank more accountable to the citizens of these respective countries for its activities. However, a culture of secrecy infuses the World Bank—accountability, transparency, and responsiveness are not traits for which the World Bank is known. During a visit in 1996, I found the tight security and sterile environs more reminiscent of a military base than a taxpayer-funded vendor of goodwill. More openness would befit an organization of such global importance.

Regardless of how one defines development, one has to recognize the World Bank as its undisputed leader. Yale international economics professor Gustav Ranis wrote, "Other lenders, public and private, may carp, resent, at times criticize, and occasionally even deviate from World Bank positions . . . but there is little question that the World Bank dominates the [development] scene in virtually every dimension" (Caufield 1996, 2). The World Bank owes its intimidating presence to its size (10,000 professional staff), wealth of experience, and level of lending ($20.1 billion in 2004) (World Bank Group 2004a). The World Bank's professional staff is among the world's best, drawn from the best schools and paid the highest salaries. When the World Bank provides economic prescriptions, poor recipient countries are rarely in a position to refuse.

Projects   The World Bank has a long history of large-scale development projects in poor countries, including a number of dams.[9] World Bank planners like dams because they can produce cheap power for industry, provide irrigation for larger-scale farming, and control flooding during monsoon seasons. They no doubt took their motivations from the experience of the industrialized world, which is covered by big dams. The United States has 6,600 dams, Japan has 2,700. Emerging countries like China (22,000 dams) and India (4300 dams) have both shown an appetite for them, with good reason. China's Yangtze River has killed millions over a long history of periodic flooding ("Damming Evidence" 2003), and India faces critical water shortages in the future. With 17% of the world's population and only 4% of its fresh water, India is seriously exploring a $120 billion proposition to increase its freshwater supply by linking all of its rivers. Further, hydropower provides one fifth of the world's power and has to date prevented consumption of some 22 billion tons of oil. There is one more compelling reason to construct a dam, as noted in *The Economist*: "No politician can resist the prestige linked to a big dam" ("Damming Evidence" 2003).

For decades, the World Bank funded construction of hundreds of dams, though at a price. World Bank water advisor John Briscoe said that lending for big dams accounts for just 10% of the World Bank's expenditures now but a full 95% of its headaches ("Damming Evidence" 2003). The problem list associated with dams is long. They have flooded miles of receding tropical rain forests, which then emit greenhouse gases as they decompose. The benefits of irrigation zones are often outweighed by the loss of fertile lands that become submerged. Dam failures kill thousands of people, erode soil and therefore crop yields, and eventually fill up with mud, limiting their usefulness. Further, their cost overruns tend to be high and their power output is frequently overstated. Most important, they displace the poor subsistence farmers who typically inhabit the areas targeted for submersion. Relocation schemes have traditionally been lacking and many of these poor, powerless people end up far worse off.

One of the World Bank's most notorious projects involved damming one of India's most sacred rivers, the Narmada. The Narmada Valley Development Project promised to be the Indian equivalent of the Tennessee Valley Authority, bringing drinking water to 30 million people and irrigating 4.8 million acres of farmland (Danaher 1994; Mehta 1994, 117). A long series of dams was planned, with the Sardar Sarovar Dam at 4,000 feet across and 45 stories high as the centerpiece (Caufield 1996, 8). However, as construction got underway, authorities began to forcibly displace hundreds of thousands of poor residents, just as they had for most of India's other large construction projects. From Independence in 1947 through the mid 1990s, dam projects displaced roughly 11 million Indians (11). Typically these indigenous people were forced from their lands into the slums of the nearest large cities. Even by the World Bank's own admissions, World Bank-funded projects pushed millions into destitution.

However, Sardar Sarovar came at a time of growing civil society, environmental, and nongovernmental organization (NGO) activism as well as activity by the increasingly vocal indigenous sector. These groups coalesced to bring increasing pressure on both the World Bank and the Indian government. A 1985 independent assessment found that resettlement plans were lacking, environmental impact studies had not been done, and the benefits of the project were overestimated. According to *The Economist*, "The Bank's own India department altered a study criticizing the resettlement, to hide the problems from the Bank's directors" (A Flood of Fiascos" 1997). Following wave after wave of protests, the World Bank canceled the loan in 1993 and the Indian Supreme Court halted construction of Sardar Sarovar in 1995. It was completed only after a long series of court rulings ("Damming Evidence" 2003).

After investing billions for dam building with mixed results, the World Bank became skittish about further dam involvement. India's Sardar Sarovar proved a public relations disaster, while the cost of China's Three Gorges' dam has risen to $22 billion and counting ("The Great Flood" 2003). Many see such massive dams as the last of their kind, and World Bank lending for dams fell from $1 billion annually in the early 1990s to less than $100 million in 2002 ("Damming Evidence" 2003).

Yet, not all of the worst World Bank projects have been dams. The Brazilian Northwest Region Integrated Development Program, or Polonoroeste, proved one of the worst debacles in World Bank history (Danaher 1994, 112). At the World Bank's behest, the government of Brazil encouraged colonization of 150,000 square miles of rainforest—widespread environmental destruction and genocide of the indigenous peoples followed. The Roman Catholic Church estimated that by decade's end, 85% of the region's native people had died through violence or newly introduced disease, a tragic replay of events 500 years earlier (Caufield 1996, 174). Tens of thousands of colonists following the call to develop the region ended up destitute and hungry.

The Polonoroeste project became a clear example of failed development, prompting hearings before Congress. World Bank President Barber Conable admitted that the World Bank had indeed "stumbled" while misreading "the human institutional and physical realities of the jungle and the frontier" (Hancock 1989, 139). Despite a long list of similar debacles, World Bank-funded construction projects will continue to receive funding, in part because they create substantial profit for those involved. One Indian official had the following to say about a failed dam project, "This project is meant only for the rich people to collect money from abroad and to put it in their pockets. The bigger the project they don't execute, the more money goes into their pockets. That is the politics" (Caufield 1996, 16). There is something inherently sinister about a project that knowingly diverts scarce resources from the poor to the rich within a society. The World Bank-funded Ukai irrigation project, located in Gujarat, India, just south of Sardar Sarovar, illustrates just how this happens.

The Ukai Dam displaced 70,000 people, mostly subsistence farmers in the region. With irrigation, the surrounding land became suitable for cash crops for export, such as wheat and sugar cane. The value of the land increased, as did the cost of farm supplies to maintain it and the taxes to keep it. Poor farmers were forced to sell their land to wealthier farmers, and vast sugar plantations came to dominate the area. In time, the small farmers became "migrant slaves," sleeping in the streets while laboring for large landowners. Some of these same people had been landowners themselves, sending their children to Baroda University. After the dam, they found themselves living with their children in Baroda's slums (Caufield 1996, 21).

The "Fog" of Development   In 1968, the World Bank received an infusion of the best and brightest from the Kennedy and Johnson administrations when Robert McNamara assumed the helm. As the chief architect of the Vietnam War, the brilliant, confident, and imposing former secretary of defense found a challenge equal to his ambition. Only decades later did he plead a *mea culpa* in the Oscar-winning documentary, *The Fog of War* (2004). The World Bank had the potential to eradicate poverty. To do so, McNamara argued, it simply had to think bigger and lend more. His style of top-down control left little room for opposing views and his clear lending targets left little time for project accountability. If countries could develop the right infrastructure, McNamara argued, they could outgrow their need for aid. Despite some ominous signs, the pressure to lend increased.

By the time McNamara took over the World Bank, third-world countries were already feeling the effects of the project-directed borrowing. By 1965, half of the export sales from poor countries was going right back to rich countries in the form of debt service payments. By 1969, South Asia had used 40% of its loans to pay debt interest alone; Latin America, 87% (Caufield 1996, 89). H. L. Mencken once said, "For any given problem, there is a solution that is simple, direct, and wrong." As third-world countries slid deeper into debt, that solution was, naturally, more lending.

During McNamara's reign (1968–1981), the World Bank dramatically increased its lending from $953 million in 1968 to $12.4 billion in 1981 (Danaher 1994, 9), totaling a staggering $77 billion worth of loans during the period. Those at the receiving end knew that careers depended on loans being made. One officer put it this way, "If you're a loan officer and you go down to Brazil and say, 'You know, if you don't fulfill these conditions you may not get the loan.' They'll say, 'That's fine buddy'—or whatever the Brazilian equivalent of buddy is—'you can just take the next plane back to Washington because we know you're going to make that loan to us. Otherwise you're out of a job'" (Caufield 1996, 102). Forty percent of all IBRD loans came through during the last two months of the fiscal year, prompting one World Bank officer to complain, "We're like a Soviet factory. The push is to maximize lending. . . . In May and June the pressures to lend are enormous and a lot of people spend sleepless nights wondering how they can unload projects."

This push to lend obscured the very real problems the lending was creating. Very few projects received any real scrutiny, and impact studies on how they affected the poor were lacking. Even earlier large-scale projects had received little review after completion. Not a single one of the 21 large-scale projects during World Bank President Eugene Black's tenure (1949–1963) were studied—and most caused more harm than good (Caufield 1996, 87). Mistakes therefore were simply replicated in subsequent projects. It was not until 1992, after almost 50 years and $140 billion of lending, that World Bank President Lewis T. Preston instructed Willi Wapenhans to critically review its work.

Wapenhans' report concluded that more than one third of the World Bank's 1,800 projects in 113 countries that were active in 1991 were "unsatisfactory," a World Bank euphemism for failure (Danaher 1994, 137). The report found that World Bank staff designed programs in accordance with World Bank policies while eschewing the wishes of borrowers and local people. The borrowers that were interviewed agreed that World Bank staff were driven more by pressure to lend than successful project outcome. Further, the report added, "The methodology for project performance rating is deficient; it lacks objective criteria and transparency. . . . The projects are too complex and often do not make allowances for the weak institutional structures in the developing country" (Danaher 1994, 139). In short, the report found "major problems" with World Bank projects.

The World Bank responded to threats of US Congressional hearings by creating the Operations Evaluations Department (OED) in 1970. Between 1974 and 1993, the OED audited more than 4000 World Bank operations and, like Wapenhans, found that more than one third of the projects were unsatisfactory. Since 1989, fewer than one third of the projects have been rated both satisfactory and sustainable (Caufield 1996, 254).

One problem frequently attributed to the World Bank is its near universal application of similar prescriptions to widely differing circumstances in different countries. The *New York Times* described the World Bank's structural adjustment policies as analogous to "an emergency room doctor who gives every patient an appendectomy regardless of the symptoms" (Altman 2002, 1). Such criticisms are widely repeated, particularly by civil society organizations working most closely with those affected. As economist Jeffrey

Sachs has said, "What might be important in one place may be irrelevant in another place. Differential diagnosis is critical. You have to be open to the wide range of things that can go wrong in the world" (Barrett 2002, 45).

In 2000, the World Commission on Dams published *Dams and Development*, a comprehensive report that reviewed the history of dam building in the developing world and posed recommendations for the future (The World Commission on Dams 2001). The report's authors concluded that the old way of forging ahead with large development projects would no longer suffice and that indigenous groups, local governments, and civil society groups had to be part of a planning process that itself was grounded in human rights (United Nations Development Program [UNDP] 2002, 109). Dams and other large development schemes can become an important source of economic development in poor countries; however, such schemes will only work if they are designed transparently, fairly, and with the involvement of those most affected. To the World Bank's credit, it dedicates far greater resources now to law and governance (25%), health (15%), and education (8%) than it ever has in its history ("A Regime Changes" 2005).

The Roots of the Debt Crisis

For years prior to the early 1960s, private banks had been reluctant to lend money to third world countries. Many poor governments had proven to be un-creditworthy and the risk of default was high. However, as the World Bank emerged in both size and stature, with its armies of well-trained economists making ever-larger loans to poor governments, private banks gained confidence and began to resume their lending, albeit tentatively. However, before the banks could jump in fully, they had to get past the US government's restrictions on foreign lending.

The dollar had long been the currency of international trade, and the US government had used its control over dollars to impose its will on those it disagreed with—most often by freezing assets held in US banks. For rival governments, this presented a real problem. Following its ascension to power in 1949, the Chinese Communist party began to transfer its US-held dollars to a Paris bank that agreed to maintain the deposits in US dollars. Russia soon followed suit, though both countries kept these transactions secret, fearing US and French government crackdowns. With time, however, more joined in; by 1960 the phenomenon of "Eurodollars" (US dollars held in banks outside the United States) was booming. To avoid tough US laws that restricted foreign lending, US banks jumped in, opening branches all over Europe (Caufield 1996, 126). From 1960 to 1972, the number of US banks with branches abroad increased from 8 to 107, and more followed the lucrative practice of lending to the third world.

Poor countries desperately sought money, and with the assurance of the World Bank, private banks were all too happy to provide such lucrative loans. In 1977, the nine largest US banks derived half their earnings from these loans, despite holding only 8% of their assets there (Caufield 1996, 128). The countries' poor credit risk justified—at least to the lending banks—high interest rates and administrative fees. The banks used these profits to compete for the wealth of Middle Eastern clients, which flowed like gold crude into the Eurodollar market following the oil price increases of the early 1970s. This process triggered what some have called "a virtual orgy of lending," in which private bank lending drastically increased the debt of third world countries (Kim et al 2000, 21), from $100 billion in 1972 to more than $600 billion in 1981 (Caufield 1996, 134). Poor countries had to take out additional loans and "reschedule" the old ones, all with hefty administrative fees added in. One banker described a "nearly insolvent developing country" in this way, "That country is a cash cow for us. We hope they never repay" (139).

It is unlikely that banks would have lent such large sums to developing countries without the tacit understanding that the Bretton Woods Institutions would bail them out should any country default. After all, the IMF was charged with protecting the international financial system and the World Bank was the most knowledgeable organization working in the developing world. The IMF simply could not allow defaults on billions of dollars of debt that might destabilize the banking systems of large donor countries. The World Bank, on the other hand, far from sending out warnings of an impending crisis, stepped up its lending and encouraged private banks to follow suit, which they did. From 1977 to 1982, loans to developing countries tripled (Caufield 1996, 136). Unfortunately for poor countries, more and more of this borrowing was used to pay interest on existing debt. By 1978, 25% of money borrowed by Third World countries went for interest payments on the debt. By 1982, Latin America was spending all its billions in annual loans on debt payments (137).

Still worse, most of these loans paid for massive, failed projects or were siphoned off by the elites in power. Author Patricia Adams has termed the resultant debt "odious," citing historical precedent for wiping out debts incurred illegitimately (Danaher 1994, 35). Philippine President Ferdinand Marcos had racked up a total of $26 billion in national debt by the time he was overthrown in 1986. Much of this went for elaborate development projects that padded his ego, though a substantial total, at least $10 billion, disappeared into foreign banks to finance his and his wife Imelda's extravagant lifestyle (Hancock 1989, 175). While Philippinos languished in some of the worst poverty in Southeast Asia during the 1970s, the Marcoses acquired an art collection valued at $100 million and luxury residencies in New York, Hawaii, and Paris.

From 1965 until 1997, Mobutu Sese Seko ruled Zaire (now the Democratic Republic of the Congo), one of the world's poorest countries. The country had accumulated a foreign debt of $5 billion by 1992, yet

Mobutu became one of the world's richest men, with an estimated fortune of $4 billion, much of that from World Bank loans (Caufield 1996, 132; Hancock 1989, 139). Haiti, too, has long been one of the world's poorest countries. From 1957 to 1986 it suffered under the Duvalier kleptocracy, during which an estimated 63% of government funds were misappropriated. Two days after the IMF deposited a $22 million loan into the national treasury, Fund officials found that $20 million of it was withdrawn for Jean-Claude ("Baby-Doc") Duvalier's personal use (Hancock 1989, 179). Other infamous kleptocrats include Kenya's Daniel Arap Moi, Liberia's Samuel Doe, Somalia's Siad Barre, the Argentine junta, and Chile's Auguste Pinochet, to name a few.[10]

> *Wealthy elites in poor countries had developed ways to grab incoming dollars and send them abroad for safekeeping, a phenomenon known as "capital flight."*

Although these celebrated crooks garnered the headlines and corruption became the favored reason why four decades of development policies had failed so miserably, collectively they accounted for just a small amount of the cash diversions. The real problem was that wealthy elites in poor countries had developed ways to grab incoming dollars and send them abroad for safekeeping, a phenomenon known as "capital flight." While dollars from private banks, bilateral donors, and the Bretton Woods Institutions poured into developing countries during the 1970s and 1980s, roughly equal dollar amounts left those countries, destined for private bank accounts and various investment schemes in the United States and Europe. The World Bank estimated that from 1976 to 1984, Latin America's debt increase roughly equaled the region's capital flight (Caufield 1996, 132). Morgan Guaranty Trust Company studied the problem and concluded, "This was no coincidence," estimating that from 1983 to 1985, 70% of borrowings by Latin America's 10 largest countries had financed capital flight. This prompted one US Federal Reserve Board member to say, "The problem is not that Latin Americans don't have assets. They do. The problem is, they're all in Miami" (133).

Yet the problem stretched far beyond the Americas. In 1985, capital flight from 18 developing countries totaled $198 billion, with enormous repercussions for the poor in each. Another firm found that from 1976 to 1986, capital flight from specific developing countries was as follows: Mexico, $56 billion; Argentina, $26 billion; Brazil, $10 billion; India, $10 billion; Indonesia, $5 billion; Nigeria, $10 billion; Philippines, $9 billion (Hancock 1989, 182). Through this process, money from the banks and development institutions of the North passed through the hands of ruling elites—and their well-connected friends—in the South and then came right back up North. One consultant summed up the exercise as, "cooperation among the world's powerful for exploitation of the world's weak" (Caufield 1996, 133).

Clearly a crisis was looming, yet one that would not harm the elites on either side of the equation. The first warning sounded when Zaire stopped making payments on its $700 million debt to private banks in June 1976 (Caufield 1996, 135). Following failed negotiations, banks wrote off their loans to Zaire. A few months later, Peru loomed on the brink of defaulting on its $4.4 billion foreign debt. Following the World Bank's failed attempt to stabilize the Peruvian economy through currency devaluation, tax increases, and government spending decreases, the IMF stepped in with a $200 million loan in exchange for the Peruvian government's agreeing to its harsh economic reforms. Similar crises soon followed in Turkey (1978), Iran (1979), and Poland (1981).

Other forces caused growing debt burdens to explode to unsustainable levels. In 1979, the Organization of the Petroleum Exporting Countries (OPEC) hiked oil prices for a second time, causing an increase in the costs of producing goods everywhere. Overnight, third world economies saw their import prices rise while export prices stayed the same or declined. For the poorest countries, trade deficits increased, from $45 billion in 1979 to $90 billion just two years later (Hancock 1989, 60). However, it was not just the poor countries that felt the impact of this "second oil shock"; rich countries felt it, too. In the late 1970s and early 1980s, US Federal Reserve Chairman Paul Volcker increased interest rates to keep inflation at bay. Because most foreign loans were held in US dollars, their cost suddenly went up–a lot. A global recession in the early 1980s meant people everywhere were buying fewer goods, including those imported from poor countries. Consequently, those in poor countries had smaller markets to export to, and export earnings decreased still further. This combination of increased import prices, rapidly increasing interest rates and debt burdens, and decreased export earnings dealt a deathblow to poor countries, which soon found they could no longer service their rising debts.

The first backlash of these cumulative events was the reversal of net financial flows from northern banks to southern governments, which had totaled $20 billion per year during the 1970s. However, between 1983 and 1989, more than $242 billion flowed from the South to the North–at enormous cost to the poor (Watkins, 1995, 174).

Then, on August 13, 1982, the Mexican finance minister informed the US government that Mexico would be unable to repay the $81 billion it owed its foreign creditors. The debt crisis had officially begun. At the time, Mexico owed US-based Citibank $3.3 billion and served as the repository for 80% of the assets of the Bank of Tokyo (Caufield 1996, 138). Many other large banks had considerable assets tied up in Mexico and other Latin American countries. In the luxury suites of the world's largest banks, near panic ensued as the threat of a global domino effect loomed. Argentina and Brazil soon followed with similar threats of default. If Mexico, Brazil, Venezuela, Argentina, and Chile defaulted on even half of their loans, the six largest US banks would go bankrupt. And such massive bank failures, eerily reminiscent of the 1930s, could potentially cause the global financial system to collapse. The very disaster that had spawned the IMF and World Bank suddenly loomed as a very real possibility, ironically, due to the policies and practices of these two institutions.

Structural Adjustment Programs

The world's leading economic powers faced the greatest international financial crisis since the years prior to World War II. What can at best be termed irresponsible lending produced the real possibility that private citizens would lose large sums of money to governments unable to repay their loans. The elites who ran these governments also shared a considerable amount of blame for the crisis, having borrowed irresponsibly and badly mismanaged their economies. In earlier times, countries went to war to protect their citizen's assets from default by foreign powers. This time, however, the world's wealthy countries sent in the IMF instead of troops.

The IMF bailed out Mexico with an emergency loan that required Mexico to maintain payments on its debt and drastically cut back on government spending. In the process, the IMF essentially restructured the Mexican economy. The IMF also coaxed private banks in wealthy countries to extend additional loans to Mexico by allowing them to charge high rescheduling fees, which of course they did. But the IMF alone could not accommodate all of the outstanding debt; it needed help from its sister organization just across 19th Street. Concerned that loan defaults would hurt its bond rating as well as its reputation as the global development leader, the World Bank came up with huge, rapidly deployable loans that would help countries with their balance-of-payment problems. Overnight, the World Bank evolved from an institution that dispersed million-dollar loans for projects to one that dispersed billion-dollar loans for debt repayment. The World Bank and IMF began to work more closely together.

The brain trusts of both institutions recognized that developing countries could benefit from their armies of economists and development experts. As such, these new loans would proceed only if the developing countries adhered to the recommendations on how they should "restructure" their economies. Consequently, they became far more than just loans. They were emergency funds with long strings attached, financial Trojan horses that released their minions under cover of darkness to assault national sovereignty. The World Bank and IMF essentially told poor countries—in no position to refuse—that they would "readjust" the very "structure" of their economies according to World Bank- and IMF-approved neoliberal lines. As such, these loans became known as "structural adjustment" loans. The responsibility for running the economies of most poor countries quietly shifted from local capitals to Washington.

On the surface, it was not inherently wrong for the world's most acclaimed group of development experts to help poor countries realign their economies. After all, the governments did need the help—their policy decisions had contributed to the crisis and the World Bank's staff was the world's best and brightest. However, the pressure to lend from the World Bank, private banks, and other bilateral and multilateral lenders had been largely responsible for the crisis, and the "restructuring" of poor economies has been an outright disaster for the poor. The motivations behind the imposed economic advice remain questionable and, quite expectedly, reflect the beliefs of those in power at the time. In the early 1980s, the newly elected administrations of Reagan, Thatcher, and Kohl shared an economic philosophy that largely blamed problems in poor and rich countries on the interference of the state. Reagan had famously said, "The best government is the least government." The private sector, this theory held, would create wealth and the chief role of governments was to get out of the way so the market could work its magic. This "neoliberalism" or "Washington consensus," as it was more broadly known, has been the dominant development paradigm since the 1980s. The adjustment loans that embodied this paradigm included three essential components: privatization, liberalization, and deregulation (Kim et al 2000, 22). The IMF and World Bank implemented these remedies as a form of "shock therapy" to the economies of poor countries.

Draconian cuts in government spending often mean devastating reductions in services on which the poor rely heavily—health, education, and food subsidies.

Privatization meant that state-controlled firms or services, including health care and education, were sold off or taken over by NGOs or for-profit firms that often added user fees. While a boon to industry, privatization can prove disastrous to health and education in developing countries. The World Bank itself has shown that once user fees are imposed, people use fewer services. For example, following imposition of $30 to $80 fees for tuberculosis drugs in China, 1 to 1.5 million cases went untreated, producing an additional 10 million infections. According to the *Lancet*, "many of the 3 million Chinese who died of tuberculosis during the 1980s could have been saved" ("World Bank's Cure" 1993, 63). *Liberalization* referred to the reduction of barriers to free trade and investment, essentially opening up poor economies to the world's free markets, despite the fact that the wealthy economies of the world had developed under strong protectionist policies. Even the Asian tigers, the models of development success, had only gradually reduced the protections governing their fledgling industries (Zakaria 2003, 55). *Deregulation* meant that the state had significantly less power to regulate capital, labor, and goods and services.

During the 1980s, structural adjustment loans dominated the development scene. Eighteen Latin American countries received 107 World Bank–IMF-sponsored programs. By 1991, 75 countries, 30 in Africa alone, had received similar loans totaling $41 billion (Kim et al 2000, 23). These policies have translated into a literal assault on the poor. Countries often have to devalue their currencies, which decreases the amount a given shilingi or peso can buy. This makes imports more expensive (and therefore less desirable) and exports less expensive (favoring export-mediated growth). It also means that available money suddenly purchases less—the poor become even poorer. Draconian cuts in government spending often mean devastating reductions in services on which the poor rely heavily—health, education, and food subsidies. Tax increases and increased costs for state-run staples such as water and electricity add to the poor man's burden. Elimination of labor protections often leads to union busting and the imposition of harsh conditions that the poor can neither control nor contest.

To the creditor nations, however, structural adjustment has been a remarkable success—the loans are being repaid (Kim et al 2000, 11). Between 1983 and 1989, poor countries paid $242 billion more to their creditors than they received in new loans, while net transfers paralleled this shift. In 1981 a net $43 billion flowed to poor nations, while in 1989 a net $33 billion flowed from them. Still, the debt stock for poor countries continued to grow, from $616 billion in 1980 to an incredible $2.2 trillion in 1997. While a considerable amount of this debt remains private, much has been transferred to official aid agencies. By 1997, sub-Saharan Africa owed $179.2 billion, of which 74% was official. By contrast, in Latin America and the Caribbean, less than one third was official debt. The bottom line is that northern banks, investors, and official aid agencies have all benefited from the reversal of monetary flows.

On the other hand, those paying the price are the same as they have always been—the poor. Following the mistakes and miscalculations, the boondoggles in the jungle, the siphoned fortunes and backroom dealings, the outrageously irresponsible lending and borrowing that nearly sank the global financial system, the ones to bear the brunt of it all are those with the least ability to protest against it. Consider the following:

- As of June 2005, Nigeria spends $1.7 billion per year on debt service payments, an amount that is five times larger than it spends on education, and 13 times larger than it spends on health (Kar and Watkins 2005). Naturally, those most reliant on public education and health are the poor.
- During Peru's two structural adjustment programs from 1977 to 1985, unemployment soared while per-capita income fell by 20%. By 1985 a worker's paycheck was worth less than half of what it had been worth a decade earlier. Meanwhile, government expenditures on health care and education decreased; food and fuel subsidies per family were eliminated; and childhood malnutrition increased by more than 60% (Hancock 1989, 62).

- Despite being one of the world's poorest countries, Niger spends more on debt service than it does on health and education combined. This reflects broader trends in Africa; during the late 1990s governments transferred four times more to their northern creditors than they spent on health and education (Kim et al 2000, 25).
- In Mexico, adjustment intensified poverty and widened disparities in wealth between those at the top and those at the bottom (Caufield 1996, 153). In January 1994, simmering tensions over inequality exploded when a band of poor rebels captured six towns in the southern state of Chiapas;. more than 150 died in the subsequent fighting with Mexican government forces. *The Economist* concluded, "Mexico's Zapatista rebellion is not the only recent sign, merely the fiercest, that ordinary Latin Americans want more of the cake" (154).
- In the Congo, the United Nations Children's Fund (UNICEF) found that malnutrition and stunting among poor children rose, while the percent of low birth-weight babies almost doubled following structural adjustment. Similar nutritional deficiencies followed rising poverty in the wake of adjustment in Cote d'Ivoire (Kim et al 2000, 113).
- In a number of heavily indebted countries, rising child mortality rates have reversed decades of progress. Child mortality rates have risen in Zimbabwe, Zambia, Nicaragua, Chile, and Jamaica, in part due to cutbacks on basic health care and vaccinations.

In retrospect, it is clear just how detrimental structural adjustment has been and still is under its new terms. In 1989, UNICEF concluded that half a million children had died in the previous year due to the adjustment-mediated reversal of progress in the developing world (Caufield 1996, 162). Further, during the 1980s, average incomes in Africa and a number of Latin American countries decreased 10% to 25%, while per capita spending on health and education decreased by 25% and 50%, respectively, in the world's 37 poorest countries. UNICEF concluded the following about structural adjustment and the lending frenzy that had preceded it, "It is hardly too brutal an oversimplification to say that the rich got the loans and the poor got the debts. . . . The fact so much of today's staggering debt was irresponsibly lent and irresponsibly borrowed would matter less if the consequences of such folly were falling on its perpetrators" (162).

Protests and Violence

During the 1980s, poor people aligned with groups from civil society and nongovernmental organizations to form a global activist network. These activists were able to present firsthand evidence in the form of photographs and testimony that, for the first time, gave the World Bank pause. As one staff member recalled, "It's a lot easier to argue endlessly about policy approaches to energy conservation in the abstract than to find that someone's just returned from Indonesia and has photographs of what you just finished saying couldn't possibly be happening" (Caufield 1996, 168).

Activists prompted two days of hearings before Congress in 1983, the first of 20 such hearings on the social and environmental impact of World Bank projects. Following extensive revelations, conservative US Senator Robert Kasten said, "When people find out what's been going on, you're going to see people out in the streets saying, 'My God, did you read this information? Why are our dollars being used to fund this kind of destruction?'" (Caufield 1996, 172). The World Bank responded by admitting past mistakes but informed the Congress and the general public that it had changed its ways. Such professions have continued ever since. In a 2002 *New York Times* interview, World Bank President James Wolfensohn responded to a question about the World Bank's quite vocal critics, "Reform takes time in an organization with a 57 year history," he said. "But I wouldn't underestimate how much change has already taken place at the bank. Some of our critics seem to be stuck somewhere in the bank of the 1980s" (Altman 2002, 1). Because much of the restructured debt burden came from the 1980s, it has proven a difficult decade to forget.

By the year 2000, protests against the policies of structural adjustment had been going on for 20 years, led by the civil society organizations 50 Years is Enough and Jubilee 2000. Although some adjustment is necessary for poor countries, the central objections stem from the draconian nature of the adjustments prescribed (Altman 2002, 1). Clare Short, Britain's popular former secretary of state for international development, said, "A lot of structural adjustment was right, but was too brutally implemented" (1). Most see the adjustments as inconsistent with poverty reduction. According to Bread for the World, "[Structural adjustment policies] are perceived as undermining government subsidies and social safety nets; and as privileging export industries over domestic production, the private sector over the public sector, large farmers over small farmers, foreign debt servicing over domestic citizen needs, and economic growth over employment generation" (Grusky 2000). Between 1976 and 1992, 146 protests and demonstrations against structural adjustment policies occurred in 39 countries (Grusky 2000), while national protests in Poland, Jordan, Bolivia, and Zimbabwe and in the cities of Caracas, Buenos Aires, and Bucharest have involved tens of thousands taking to the streets in well-coordinated campaigns (Caufield 1996, 161).

At times, enraged citizens have taken more violent courses of action. One of the bloodiest riots occurred in 1984 in the Dominican Republic. Following implementation of an IMF-World Bank adjustment plan, the price of food doubled and that of medicine quadrupled. In the ensuing riots, 112 people died and 500 were wounded (Jubilee 2000a). Riots broke out in Caracas, Venezuela, in 1989 after an adjustment program caused wages to collapse to less than half their value nine years earlier while prices skyrocketed. Estimates of the number of dead caused by the riots range from 300 to 1,500 (Jubilee 2000a).

In Africa, rising debt and the considerable destabilization produced by adjustment contributed to rising violence and war (Kim et al 2000, 91). The Hutu genocide of thousands of Tutsis and Hutu members of opposition parties in Rwanda in 1994 stemmed in large part from the economic distress brought on by adjustment (103). The plane crash that killed the presidents of Rwanda and Burundi in April 1994 provided the pretext for a military coup that produced "the fastest, most efficient killing spree of the twentieth century" in which 800,000 Tutsi and "politically moderate" Hutu were killed in just 100 days (Power 2003, 334). Authors Schoepf, Schoepf, and Millen concluded,

> The extreme violence did not erupt unforeseeably, out of irrational "ethnic hatreds." It was the culmination of a long history of economic deterioration and political conflict, every stage of which Rwanda had been observed by representatives of international financial institutions—some of whom mandated the very processes and policies that led to the bloodshed (Kim et al 2000, 106).

Debt Relief

In 1996, the World Bank and IMF developed the $12.5 billion Heavily Indebted Poor Countries (HIPC) Initiative,[11] in which they and bilateral donors began to reduce the debt burdens of the poorest countries to "sustainable" levels (Jubilee 2000b). Such sustainable levels were defined in 1996 as a debt stock of no more than 200% to 250% of a country's exports. To qualify for the HIPC program, countries need to demonstrate good governance and economic management according to World Bank/IMF criteria. Once accepted, (the so-called Decision Point) the countries prepare Poverty Reduction Strategy Papers (PRSPs) that introduce reforms designed to reduce poverty.[11] Once countries fully implement the PRSP's to the satisfaction of World Bank/IMF oversight committees, they reach the Completion Point, in which they receive the full amount of debt cancellation previously committed. This does not include the entire debt, but merely the amount that the World Bank/IMF views as "sustainable," ie, that amount—often contested—with which the country can continue to function economically. The International Financial Institutions (IFIs) had never previously written off debt, but took such an extraordinary step in response to the pressures brought by global activists, including some unlikely allies. Convinced that the $12.5 billion HIPC Initiative fell far short of what was needed, Pope John Paul II, Bono of U2 fame, the Dalai Lama, economist Jeffrey Sachs, and others joined the Jubilee 2000 coalition to call for further debt reductions (Easterly 2002, 123). The world's 42 most heavily indebted countries had a debt stock of more than $141 billion at the time.[12]

In 1999, the G8 leaders pledged at their meeting in Cologne, Germany, that they would increase the amount of debt relief to $29.3 billion, equally divided between bilateral and multilateral donors, and redefine "sustainable" debt as 150% of a country's exports (World Bank Group 1999a). Given Organization for Economic Cooperation and Development (OECD) financial assets at the time of $53 trillion, the net value of debt held by poor countries represented 0.13% of their holdings, a small amount by any measure. By 2004, nearly $34 billion of debt had been cancelled, another $18 billion of debt relief had been pledged, and $89 billion of debt remained in the HIPCs.[12] Because the HIPC Initiative debt relief targets those countries with "sound economic management," less of the funds are wasted ("How to Make Aid Work" 1999). The Cologne Initiative sped up the timetable for qualifications and repayments. Consequently, some of that relief has already made an impact. With money saved from debt relief, Uganda doubled its school enrollments while Mozambique saved the equivalent of twice its health budget ("Can Debt Relief" 2000).

However, not everyone agrees that even the 1999 HIPC Initiative goes far enough. Oxfam has criticized the response as far too little, serving more to restructure debt burdens so poor countries can continue paying to their wealthy creditors. Oxfam, Jubilee 2000, the Reality of Aid Project, and 50 Years is Enough have called for an outright cancellation of all third world debt. One of the stronger arguments for debt cancellation is that the principle of the debts has already been paid back, in some cases many times over.[10] Further, large amounts of the loaned money went directly back north to the hordes of well-connected consultants, contractors, construction companies, and experts who built the different projects.[10] Debates about the adequacy of the HIPC Initiative continue apace, while the poorest people continue to struggle under the weight of their countries' oppressive debts.

Meeting in Gleneagles, Scotland in July 2005, members of the G-8 agreed to an outright cancellation of the debts of the poorest 18 countries in the HIPC initiative, most of which are in Africa. This amounts to roughly $1 billion per year, totaling $40 billion. To its credit, the US government had favored debt cancellation and carried the day. Most countries carry debt, though wealthy countries can sustain enormous debt burdens with relatively little harm to their economies. For perspective, according to the Central Intelligence Agency, the US debt to foreign creditors in 2001 was $1.4 trillion—the world debt in 2004 was $12.7 trillion (Central Intelligence Agency 2005). Yet the US debt was a mere 13% of its GDP of $10.4 trillion, a burden that has failed to slow US economic growth significantly. (*The Economist*, 2005, 26, 40) By contrast, in many developing countries, debt burdens are many times the GDP, strangling any potential growth, and contributing to the poverty traps that constrict so many. In 2000–2002, the following countries had these respective foreign debt burdens as a percentage of their GDPs: Liberia 526%, Guinea-Bissau 354%, Sierra Leone 201%, Congo 178%, Zambia 177%, and Burundi 174%. Given their small economies and high debt burdens, it is not surprising that so many pay significantly more to their creditors than to the health and education needs of their poorest citizens.

A "New" World Bank

In 1999, the World Bank and IMF together evolved the structural adjustment programs into more inclusive "Poverty Reduction Strategy Papers (PRSPs)" that require World Bank and IMF officials to involve host governments, members of civil society, and those most impacted by programs, such as indigenous groups. Instead of Washington-based designs, programs must now be "owned" by host governments. Through PRSPs, the World Bank and IMF encourage governments to target a few broad parameters such as reduced infant mortality or better school enrollment. In fact, the PRSPs must line up with the UN's millennium development goals (MDGs). If such policies do foster a broader consensus on the part of bilateral and multilateral donors, aid could become more effective ("Old Battle" 2000). Aid is generally at its greatest efficacy when it supports reasonable policies undertaken by equally reasonable governments.

The World Bank's web site offers an impressive array of facts showing how the "changing World Bank" has responded to its critics and sharpened its focus. Comparing the World Bank of 1996 with the World Bank of 2003, it notes that it has improved in a number of areas. Among them, "client-owned PRSPs" have gone from 0 to 25 fully implemented and another 50 nearly so; anticorruption and governance work has increased from "few" to more than 95 countries; increased involvement of civil society in projects has increased from less than 50% to more than 70%; debt relief increased from 0 to more than $50 billion in 34 countries; and community-driven pieces in projects, ie those conceived at the local level, increased from $700 million to $2 billion (World Bank Group 2004b).

Whether this most recent version of the World Bank's outward rhetoric is real or yet another glossy veneer remains to be seen. The World Bank and development institutions in general have gone through a number of fads over the years, each with equally limited results. Even the *Economist* has questioned whether this most recent change is merely "window dressing" ("Old Battle" 2000). The World Bank's critics, however, are even more skeptical.[13] Senior policy analyst Soren Ambrose of *50 Years is Enough* found the change from SAPs to PRSPs "Orwellian," noting "It was as if they chose precisely what structural adjustment doesn't do, and renamed it for those qualities."[10] He adds, "A PRSP would attract the requested funding only if it pledged adherence to the same macroeconomic principles that the IMF had always insisted on in [earlier] programs." Further, despite rhetoric to the contrary, the public and members of civil society groups continue to have limited input into the process, as evidenced by a 2003 PRSP in Sri Lanka.[13]

In June 2003, the World Bank commissioned a survey of 2,600 opinion leaders in 48 countries. To the World Bank's dismay, many still found the World Bank "too bureaucratic and arrogant," while remaining "too much at the beck and call of its largest shareholder, the United States" (Willard 2003).

In addition, those responding from Latin America, the Middle East, and North Africa felt that World Bank-mandated economic reforms generally "do more harm than good." However, not all the news was bad. Many respondents found the World Bank "positive and improving" in their countries and had been "more useful, relevant, transparent, responsive, and better at communication." Respondents also felt the World Bank had improved its performance in poverty reduction, health, education, environment, governance, and economic growth.

Whether such trends represent real change at the World Bank remains to be seen. Despite some promising rhetoric emanating from the World Bank, it is difficult to look ahead optimistically. The same forces that have always dominated the World Bank and IMF continue: they remain closely aligned with US and OECD interests; their well-paid consultants, contractors, and middlemen remain eager to capitalize on available financing for World Bank-funded initiatives; and their only real incentive for change remains a small but vocal group of activists. Although the two phases of HIPC have come as welcome, and hard fought, they are far from enough given that many sub-Saharan countries still pay more in debt payments than for health and education for their people.

In sum, the World Bank and IMF have served chiefly the interests of the powerful at the expense of the poor for more than 50 years. During that time, the rhetoric that emanated from the World Bank in particular has been lofty, even inspirational at times, though blatantly hollow in the face of what has transpired on the ground. The gaps between rich and poor have widened in much of the world, despite the billions of dollars that have flowed through aid channels for more than half a century. In the end, the IFIs have served primarily to funnel funds from poor taxpayers in rich countries to wealthy elites in poor countries; the poor have gained little (Caufield 1996, 338).

The People of Aid

The people who carry out the business of aid largely determine whether aid projects succeed or fail. As such, it is worth briefly reviewing their motivations. Naturally, for both bilateral and multilateral donors, these people are in an ideal position to first take care of themselves and their own interests. That is as true in the United States as it is elsewhere. Author Graham Hancock calls this the "triumph of the intermediaries," and the logic makes perfect sense. If a World Bank staffer travels abroad, he or she most likely stays at the best hotel around and meets with the ruling elite of the developing country. There is a certain destructive irony involved. As former (UN) Food and Agriculture Organization staffer Raymond Lloyd said, there is a "paradox of working for the poor and underprivileged from a position of wealth and power" (Hancock 1989, 87). The World Bank staffer makes the loan, buttressing a career, while the ruling elite secures money that can then be turned around to buy votes, as in Kenya, or be put into pet projects that will appeal to the ruling and moneyed classes, as in any number of power or dam schemes. That the poor end up far worse off is tragic, even criminal, though obvious and expected when human nature is factored in.

Further, although operatives on both sides of the equation do extremely well financially, the principal players concerned, the poor in the developing countries and the taxpayers in the wealthy ones, are largely kept on the outside. Despite recent rhetoric to the contrary, the poor are still rarely consulted and taxpayers and virtually anyone else seeking information from the World Bank and other multilaterals are kept safely at arm's length (Danaher 1994, 159). (By contrast, USAID and some other bilateral donor agencies are quite open.) As such, unsupervised and largely unaccountable middlemen shape the fates of millions. According to Hancock, the process of development thus becomes, "nothing more than a transaction between bureaucrats and autocrats—a deal that gets done, in the name of others, by intermediaries and brokers" (1989, 67).

Social events for one annual World Bank-IMF board of governors meeting cost more than $10 million, a sum that Hancock suggests might have been more appropriately spent preventing 47 million children from going blind by providing them with vitamin A supplements.

One doesn't have to look far to discover why those at the World Bank might be unfamiliar with poverty and hence oblivious to program decisions that worsen the lives of the poor. Much of its staff still resides in Washington, DC, where they enjoy high, tax-free salaries and generous benefits packages (Danaher 1994, 152). The World Bank's administrative budget reached $1.4 billion in 2000 (World Bank Group 1999b)—employee retreats alone cost millions (Danaher 1994). Social events for one annual World Bank-IMF board of governors meeting cost more than $10 million, a sum that Hancock suggests might have been more appropriately spent preventing 47 million children from going blind by providing them with vitamin A supplements (Hancock 1989, 38). Hancock adds, "Pomp and ceremony of just about every kind, gourmet dinners, and five-star hotels are integral components of the day-to-day existence of those employed by international organizations to solve the problems of global poverty" (40). It is little wonder that poverty reduction has been more rhetoric than reality.

According to World Bank insider Michael Irwin, cozy relationships with those of similarly elite status in poor countries serve to isolate World Bank operatives from the poor who define the World Bank's mission (Danaher 1994, 152). When living abroad, Irwin recalls, "the World Bank representative always seemed to have the best house in town." Since most interactions are with local elites, staffers tend to be "out of touch" with the poor and the realities of their lives. Further, a tendency to stress academic credentials has resulted in fewer staff with hands-on experiences in the field. And because few ever leave, what experience there is tends to fade. As such, according to author Catherine Caufield, "many Bank officials have spent their professional lives telling people in countries where they have never lived how to do things they themselves have never done" (214).

However, in fairness to those who work for bilateral and multilateral agencies, we must recognize that the individuals who comprise their staffs are typically well intentioned but must fulfill political and strategic agendas not of their own making. Following a text filled with well-documented, blistering attacks on the Bretton Woods organizations, Kim and colleagues wrote in 2000, "Most men and women working for the World Bank, the IMF, and international development organizations are committed to reducing human suffering and enabling the majority of people to lead more satisfying lives" (2000, 388). It is their "collective decisions and institutional policies" that far too often prove devastating to the poor. As neo-conservative architect Paul Wolfowitz assumed the World Bank helm on June 1, 2005, he took over an organization burdened by a checkered past, hemmed in by protests at each new meeting, but still retaining the ability—perhaps more than any other organization—to truly affect change for the global poor ("A Regime Changes" 2005).

I recall walking down the halls of USAID offices in Alexandria, Virginia, in 1994 and noticing the carvings, batiks, and exotic tribal masks that adorned virtually every office wall. I learned then that many of these USAID workers had formerly been Peace Corps volunteers, hardly a group known for greed, materialism, or "anti-poor" views. In the United States, former Peace Corps workers not infrequently receive USAID jobs as repayment for service rendered abroad. Similar arrangements characterize Britain's Volunteer Services Organization (VSO) and other bilateral agencies. We can only understand the massive failings of such good people by viewing the motivations of the organizations that employ them.

Understanding the Failure of Aid

From the last two chapters, it is clear that the hopes and expectations of the American public are quite distant from the reality of day-to-day development work. We may want to do well in the world through both the bilateral and multilateral agencies that render aid for us. However, the forces aligned against this possibility are simply overwhelming, while the public focuses on other matters it deems more pressing. If aid were as important to the average US voter as, say, Medicare, its reform would be immediate and its impact far different. But it is not; aid remains in the shadows of public inter-est, distorted by politicians, and its effects buried in a few select journals or in the back pages of newspapers.

For the average health worker interested in serving in poor countries, aid poses a great irony. We all want to see more resources and expertise flow to the poor. Yet, it is clear that we have not yet seen the ideal means of doing this. When US Senator Jesse Helms, for many years no friend to the global poor, refers to aid as money that has gone down "foreign rat holes," it pains those who really care about such matters to admit he has a point.

We are left with the following rather disquieting question: after nearly six decades of developmental assistance, why are there still so many poor people? More specifically, have the large development institutions achieved what they originally set out to do, and if not why? It is not as straightforward a question as the preceding may lead one to think. The reality is that some development programs have worked well while many others have gone awry. We are left with the uncomfortable conclusion that aid is both good and bad. My own conclusion is that historically aid has done more harm than good, but given its promise, I would not advocate for its termination, nor for that of any of its key players. I would rather see an engaged and informed citizenry exert enough political pressures to reform the aid business. The Bush administration's Millennial Challenge Account represents real progress in the form and amount of aid, but we will not know the efficacy of this approach until several years after its full deployment in 2006. For now, let's review why aid has largely failed thus far.

1. **True "foreign aid" has not worked well chiefly because it has not been tried since the Marshall Plan.** Although rich countries have spent 1 trillion dollars on "aid" through the years, most of it has served their political and strategic interests, not the interests of those trapped by poverty. Recall from the last chapter where US aid dollars actually go; many other rich country donors follow suit. After subtracting the aid given to political and strategic allies (who are mostly middle-income countries), humanitarian emergencies, debt forgiveness, and "technical cooperation," ie, experts from rich countries, there is very little left to help poor countries help themselves. This so-called "transformational aid" holds the greatest potential to effect lasting change, but remains largely ignored. One can only hope that the rich world will combine recent initiatives like GAVI, the Global Fund, the MCA, and to a lesser extent PEPFAR, with substantial increases in both the quantity and quality of aid to the poorest countries.

2. **Poverty exerts its own constraints on development.** Those countries caught in "poverty traps" face a daunting array of obstacles, including overpopulation, high disease burdens, poor infrastructure, low levels of literacy, distance from navigable rivers for trade, adverse geography, crushing debt burdens, and extreme poverty itself. These governments simply lack the resources to help their citizens out of poverty. When the paltry amounts of aid are factored in, it should be

of no surprise to see how few countries have been able to escape the shackles of poverty.

3. **Development is difficult and complex work.** Risk for failure is high even under ideal circumstances. The UN counts less than one third of the world's countries as "highly developed," while including such dubious entries as Croatia, Latvia, and Kuwait (UNDP 2003, 237). Although aid has certainly had its share of problems, it is wrong to lay the failure of poor countries to develop solely at the feet of aid. The reality is far more complex and multifactorial.

4. **The overall amount of aid remains small.** In a world economy of $31.5 trillion, a mere $50 or even $80 billion per year cannot possibly be expected to radically effect change. Aid comprises just a small amount of most recipient countries budgets, typically 2% to 3% of their GNP, though considerably higher in some countries in sub-Saharan Africa (CBO 1997, xiv). These amounts can't possibly be expected to overcome the problems with which host governments must contend. To effect radical change, aid budgets will have to scale up significantly, as prescribed by the MDGs. If rich countries would simply honor promises already made, there would be enough to meet the MDG goals and millions more would be lifted out of poverty. Rising income levels in rich countries provide more than enough funds to cover the MDGs; the money is not lacking, only the will.

5. **Historically, the quality of aid has been poor.** Most bilateral aid has come through specific programs run by donor countries, with little coordination with other donors or even host nationals. As a result, duplication of efforts is common, and government employees in poor countries are forced to fill out mountains of paperwork from multiple donor agencies. Because recipient countries must follow specific program designs from a variety of donors, they often have little input into the programs in their own countries. Wild fluctuations in the levels of aid from year to year also make it impossible for governments to implement long-term strategies. Tied aid also considerably reduces aid quality and redirects aid dollars away from people and firms in poor countries that desperately need the work.

6. **What goes into developing countries generally supports what is already there.** Anyone who has dealt with bureaucrats in poor countries understands this completely. At least some of the blame for the failure of aid has to lie with host governments and their collective histories of poor economic policies, entrenched elites, graft and incompetence. As such, newer aid program designs that make further aid contingent on current performance are more likely to have greater success in the long run. The Global Fund and the MCA both

share this design feature. Also, aid that is targeted at specific, basic requirements of the state such as health care and education is more likely to help countries develop in the long run.

7. **Many of the "intermediaries" involved in the business of aid follow incentives to first improve their own lot and only secondarily improve the lot of the poor.** Those who play ineffective, self-enriching intermediary roles will continue to do so in whatever form aid takes, even in the best-designed systems. There are simply not enough counterincentives or police available to change such practices.

A Future for Aid?

Based on the preceding, we are forced to conclude that our collective decision to leave "development" to others in the bilateral and multilateral aid communities is pure folly. It simply hasn't worked well thus far, and without a concerted effort by an engaged citizenry, little will change. However, recent campaigns to increase the quality and quantity of aid, including the Millennium Development Goals, and the Make Poverty History Campaign prior to the July 2005 G-8 meetings in Gleneagles, Scotland offer hope. Health providers can voice their concerns to government—particularly the US government, with its dominant global influence. Or they can join any number of civil society organizations, or act directly through any of the NGOs listed in the sequel to this book, *A Practical Guide to Global Health Service.*

Although many have advocated for an end to aid, including many in poor countries, the answer is not to end aid, but to reform it. The US government's Millennium Challenge Account, the Global Fund, and the Global Alliance for Vaccines Initiative (GAVI) all offer better operating paradigms. In each of these initiatives, future fund allocations are based on performance, encouraging better use. Waste, corruption, and some of the worst abuses of the past should be markedly reduced. It will be impossible for any aid organization to overcome the entrenched minions who thrive on the business of aid, yet more of the billions involved may actually help the poor. Countries with governments that are too corrupt or ineffective to receive money from the MCA, GAVI, or the Global Fund will still receive help through bilateral donors such as USAID. Because most poor countries are now aligned with the MDGs, it should be easier to target aid to have the greatest impact.

In the final analysis of aid, we must recognize that the opportunity of our time is truly historic. It is unfortunate that the history of aid is littered with so many failures that many see it as little more than wasted money. Yet, for the first time in history, the rich world has both the money and the knowledge to end extreme poverty and dramatically improve the ill health that has plagued the poor since antiquity. The evolving story of aid does not have to read like the dark chapters that have been written over the past 40 years. Current world leaders have taken positive, though decidedly tentative steps toward changing the fundamental nature of aid, from strategic and self-serving to humanitarian and transformational. Yet it is up to each of us, particularly those in the health professions, to exert a collective influence on our leaders to do what true ethics demands. Aid can and should be of better quality and far greater quantity. Much more of it should be directed to improving health. Instead of comprising yet another cross that the poor must bear, aid could become one of several key components, like fair trade and economic growth, that helps those in poor countries improve their lives.

Endnotes

1. In this chapter, I use a large number of sources to tell the story of how bank lending drove the debt crisis and the structural adjustment programs that followed. However, the chief source was Catherine Caufield's *Masters of Illusion: The World Bank and the Poverty of Nations* (Henry Holt, 1996), which is by far the best source on the subject.
2. For more information see the International Monetary Fund web site at www.imf.org/external/pubs/ft/exrp/what.htm.
3. The World Bank did extend loans to France, the Netherlands, Denmark, and Luxembourg totaling $497 million. However, the timely infusion of $41.3 billion by 1953 in grants and concessional loans (soft loans, well below commercial rates) made by the US government's Marshall Plan rebuilt Europe.
4. The G-6 originated in the aftermath of the 1973 oil crisis and subsequent global recession. Canada joined at the behest of President Ford, forming the G-7 in 1975. Russia became an informal member in 1991. Despite its ranking as the world's sixth largest economy, China is not a part of the G-8. However, it did participate at the G-8 meetings in Gleneagles, Scotland in 2005, and may well have greater involvement in time.
5. The World Bank Group includes the International Bank for Reconstruction and Development (IBRD) and the International Development Association (IDA), the International Finance Corporation (IFC), the Multilateral Investment Guarantee Agency (MIGA), and the International Centre for Settlement of Investment Disputes (ICSID).
6. According to the World Bank web site, it raises funds on the open markets, and then lends to middle income and higher-income developing countries, that benefit by receiving loans at interest rates far less than they could get from commercial banks. Countries also benefit from a grace period of 3 to 5 years before principle repayment begins and at 25 to 30 years, a longer term to repay the loan than would be available from private banks. For more information see the World Bank web site at http://web.worldbank.org/WBSITE/EXTERNAL/EXTABOUTUS/0,contentMDK: 20040580~menuPK:34588~pagePK:34542~piPK:36600~theSitePK:29708,00.html.
7. The International Development Association considers the "poorest countries" those with annual per capita income of less than $875 in 2002 dollars.
8. The World Bank attaches a "service charge" of 0.75% to dispersed balances, roughly $7.5 million for every $1 billion dispersed.
9. Among the better book sources are Catherine Caufield's *Masters of Illusion, The World Bank and the Poverty of Nations* (Henry Holt, 1996), Graham Hancock's *Lords of Poverty* (Atlantic Monthly Press, 1989), Kim et al's *Dying for Growth* (Common Courage Press, 2000), Kevin Danaher et al's *50 Years is Enough: The Case Against the*

World Bank and the International Monetary Fund (South End Press, 1994), and William Easterly's *The Elusive Quest for Growth* (MIT Press, 2002).

10. For more information, see Soren Ambrose's "Responding to 'Mainstream' Attitudes on the IMF and World Bank" on the 50 Years is Enough web site at www.50years.org.
11. Information from the World Bank web site at www.worldbank.org/hipc/about/hipcbr.htm.
12. Information from the Jubilee Research web site at www.jubileeplus.org.
13. Dr Edward O'Neil, Stacy McDougal (staff member from 50 Years is Enough web site), personal communication, 2003.

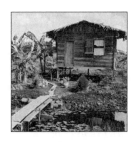

Chapter 6

Forces of Disparity I: Private Financial Flows, Trade, Multinational Corporations, and Inequality

There should exist among the citizens neither extreme poverty nor again excessive wealth, for both are productive of great evil.

—Plato

Them that's got shall get, them that's not shall lose So the Bible says, and it still is news Momma may have, Poppa may have But God bless the child who's got his own, who's got his own.

—Arthur Herzog, Jr and Billie Holiday

In the next three chapters, we review many of the forces of disparity that keep the lives of the poor unchanged: global financial flows, trade, inequality, history, racism, governance, militarism, population growth, sexism, geography, infectious diseases, and AIDS. In this chapter, we look at the financial forces that foster an unequal and unsustainable world economic order. Increasingly volatile global financial flows have destabilized entire economies and cast millions into poverty. Trade barriers and subsidies place insurmountable barriers in the path of poor farmers and workers, making fair competition in the global marketplace a distant dream. The ruthless practices of some multinational corporations (MNCs), reminiscent of century-old practices of the developed world, have spawned riots and enslaved millions in the satanic mills of free enterprise zones. Finally, inequality itself may well be our greatest plague, holding sway over those in power, shortening the lives of those at the bottom, and numbing those of us in the privileged world to the dire needs of the rest of humanity. Each of these forces expands the steep gradients of wealth both within and between countries that exacerbate poverty and the poor health it causes.

Global Financial Flows

In the last two chapters, we saw how widely divergent our perceptions are from the reality of how we help others. Yet foreign aid pales in both size and impact when viewed in the larger context of global trade and finance. According to the United Nations (UN), "The concept of development cooperation (foreign aid) should be broadened to include all flows, not just aid—especially trade, investment, technology and labour flows. Greater attention should be paid to the freer movement of non-aid flows, as these are more decisive for the future growth of the developing countries than aid flows" (United Nations Development Program [UNDP] 1994, 5). To fully understand why so many countries fail to escape from the grip of poverty, we need to track global financial flows in their entirety.

Regional Wealth

The first order of business is to characterize the framework. According to *The Economist*, the total amount of goods and services produced in the world in 2002 (global gross domestic products [GDP]) was $32.3 trillion (*The Economist* 2005, 27). Of this, the industrialized economies produced $25.8 trillion, while just seven countries, the G7, (US, UK, France, Germany, Italy, Canada, and Japan) produced $21.2 trillion—global financial resources are extremely concentrated. It is not surprising that huge disparities in health follow these general financial trends.

When viewed by country, these indices are equally telling (*The Economist* 2005, 25). US GDP in 2002 was $10.4 trillion, nearly one third (32%) of total global output. Japan came in second at $4.0 trillion, while the only other countries with more than $1 trillion in output were Germany ($2.0 trillion), the United Kingdom ($1.6 trillion), France ($1.4 trillion), China ($1.3 trillion), and Italy ($1.2 trillion). US economic predominance eclipses even that of the European Union 15 (UN15) at $8.6 trillion.

By comparison, the entire continent of Africa produced only $430 billion in 2002, just 1.3% of global economic output and less than $\frac{1}{23}$ that of the

United States. Latin American countries produced $1.8 trillion, Eastern European countries produced $970 billion, and Middle Eastern countries produced $860 billion. Given the concentrations of people in these areas, it is easy to understand how available resources are stretched. It also follows that areas with poor infrastructure, unstable locales, and low economic output attract little foreign investment, a finding of enormous consequence.

Financial Flows

Global financial flows fall into two broad categories: official aid flows, including all the bilateral and multilateral aid flows just covered, and private flows, which include all individual, foundation, university, and nongovernmental organization (NGO) flows; bank lending; stock and bond investment flows; and export credits—defined as loans for trade extended either by the states, multilateral donors, or individuals. Money in both the official and private sectors flows both ways. As illustrated during the debt crisis, flows can rapidly reverse with net transfers going *from* poor *to* rich countries, hardly ideal for the poor.

Although the net total of official aid flows has remained in the $60 to $90 billion per year range for the past decade, private financial flows between rich and poor countries have exploded in recent years, reaching a high of $273.1 billion in 1996 (Organization for Economic Co-Operation and Development [OCED] 2004, 134). Following the Asian financial crisis of 1997–1998, private flows fell off (Wider 2002) but still accounted for $149.2 billion in 2001, well over twice the amount of official aid that year (OECD 2004, 134).

All types of private financial flows have increased dramatically in recent years. Foreign currency trading increased from $10 to $20 billion per day in 1973 to $1.5 trillion per day in 1998, while regional stock markets soared (Kim et al 2000, 11, 39). As recently as 1990, financial flows from public sources like the World Bank and UN were considerably larger than those from private sources. Following the capital revolution in the 1990s, however, the flows have changed dramatically. By 1996, private flows comprised more than 85% of the total amount of funds entering developing countries (Anderson 1998). Of the many types of private financial flows between rich and poor countries, the two most important are foreign direct investment (FDI) and portfolio investment.

Foreign Direct Investment   Foreign direct investment involves any foreign holding of a firm or other enterprise in a country other than the home country of the company involved, eg, Euro Disney. In the past, FDI occurred chiefly between industrialized countries, though in recent years ever-increasing amounts of FDI have flowed to select developing countries.

From 1990 to 1996, FDI in the developing world increased from 15% to 40% of all FDI totals, even as the amount of foreign aid fell (DeMartino 1998). In the 1970s and 1980s, foreign investment flows to developing countries comprised only $11 billion per year; by 1999, it had reached $188 billion, more than three times that of official aid flows (US Agency for International Development [USAID] 2003, 14). The main sources of funds for poor countries quietly shifted from foreign aid to MNCs and private investors—a decidedly mixed blessing.

Only those countries with the requisite conditions of strong governance, little corruption, stable rule of law, open trade relations, and transparent regulations attract FDI (USAID 2003, 14). World Bank economist William Easterly showed that during the 1990s, countries around the world flooded the United States with investment dollars equal to $371 for each US citizen for each year of the decade. By comparison, global investment flows into India were equal to a mere four cents per person (Easterly 2002, 58). The investment incentives in India were simply not there, although that has changed recently with the explosion of technology in southern cities like Bangalore (Friedman, 2005, 11). Home to more than 1 billion people, China has grown explosively in recent years, in part due to its ability to attract FDI. In 2004, China attracted $54.9 billion in FDI, far more than any other developing country. ("Wrong Way Round" 2005) In the 1990s, China cut its extreme poverty nearly in half (OECD 2004, 55), during which time a number of health indices, quite expectedly, have improved. The multinational companies behind FDI import much-needed foreign capital, technologies, marketing and management skills, and, of course, jobs—all of which are much needed by the poor.

However, FDI shares a problem with portfolio flows—both are extremely concentrated in countries that can turn around money for profit (Congressional Budget Office [CBO] 1997, 17).[1] According to the OECD, most private investments remain attracted to "the most dynamic countries and sectors of the developing world" (OECD 1996, 57). That excludes, almost by definition, the countries and sectors that are most in need. Upper middle-income countries (UMICs) such as Argentina, Brazil, Korea, Malaysia, Mexico, and Venezuela, still termed "developing," received more than 70% of the growth in private flows between 1990 and 1995 (63). China alone received nearly a fifth of all FDI in 1999 (USAID 2003, 14). By contrast, flows to the world's poorest region, sub-Saharan Africa, are miniscule (Kim et al 2000, 52).[2] Almost all of the external flows going there come through aid.

Portfolio Investment Perhaps the most salient feature of the modern global economy is how freely money can move across borders. The sector benefiting most from this change is known as portfolio investment (PI), which includes the pension funds, 401(k) plans, and individual retirement accounts (IRAs) that comprise retirement nest eggs for the US and European middle class. In 1987, portfolio investment flows into developing countries totaled $800 million. By 1996, they had soared to $45.7 billion (Grabel 1998). Until the 1990s, governments and banks closely regulated the flow of money. Following the debt crisis, however, many developing countries were forced by World Bank and International Monetary Fund (IMF) structural adjustment programs to open up their stock markets to foreign investors and to deregulate their financial markets, prompting huge surges in investment dollars (Anderson 1998). A revolution in communications allowed traders to move more than $2 trillion a day of this so-called hot money freely in and out of developing countries, capitalizing on opportunities for quick profit (Mander and Goldsmith 1996, 361).

When investors rapidly pour billions of dollars in and out of a poor country, they can destabilize entire economies. Rapid withdrawals force banks and individuals to dump currency holdings, which may force governments to devalue the currency. This triggers further investor withdrawals, and the crisis deepens. With no foreign capital available, governments cannot meet their foreign debt obligations and soon the IMF arrives on the scene to put out the fire.

A number of financial crises in the 1990s started when unregulated, massive capital investments entered and then exited unstable countries. During the Asian economic crisis of 1997, panicked investors pulled capital from Indonesian investments, collapsing the economy and triggering a rise in unemployment, inflation, poverty, and childhood malnutrition. Other economic crises that directly followed similar flows include those in Mexico and Latin America in 1994 and 1995, Asia in 1997, and Russia in 1998 (Kim et al 2000, 38). Each proved particularly devastating to those at the bottom of the economic ladder in each country. Authors John Gershman and Alec Irwin remind us of the costs of this "economic casino." "The manipulation of money," they wrote, "even in its 'hottest' and most disembodied forms, has consequences for real human bodies: for the health and indeed the very survival of vulnerable individuals, families and communities" (41). The vulnerability of the poor to such fluctuations and the shocks that come from these money flows is a key, though tragic, characteristic of the emerging global economy (38). This free capital flow might be viewed as another form of aid, unfettered by the concerns of governments or individuals and solely benefiting those of us in the privileged position to send capital in search of profit at the outset.

Trade

"Free" Trade

On November 29, 1999, more than 50,000 trade unionists, environmentalists, and activists descended on the World Trade Organization (WTO) meeting in Seattle, Washington. During an internationally televised struggle that involved tear gas, rubber bullets, and large-scale property destruction, the protesters succeeded in shutting down the WTO talks, signifying one of the most effective and best-organized protests in recent years ("The Non-Governmental Order" 1999). An expert from a progressive think tank in Washington, DC, called it "a kick in the groin of the ruling class" (Dolan 2003).

Although the media focused on the property destruction and the antics of some of the more extreme elements, many of the more substantive issues were buried under the piles of trash that covered Seattle's streets. For most observers, the reason for such a large outpouring was either jobs or the environment and little more. Lost in the ruckus were complex histories of trade imbalances and the ever-widening gap between rich and poor. In short, there was a lot underlying the protest. To understand what happened in Seattle is to understand why trade, MNCs, and international financial flows mean so much to the global poor. For them, all that we have seen in the realm of foreign aid amounts to mere window dressing when compared to that which strong trade can provide.

Trade and MNCs both comprise a paradox at the heart of the debate on how to best cure the world's extremes of poverty. The two are so closely intertwined that it is nearly impossible to discuss one without the other.

Trade has helped lift millions to higher living standards; however, the current system fails many more.

Roughly two thirds of all world trade now occurs within companies, and the foreign sales of the largest MNCs comprise a full one fourth of world trade (Oxfam 2002a, 8). Given such enormous economic power, MNCs and world trade clearly hold enormous potential to lift millions out of poverty. Oxfam noted succinctly, "History makes a mockery of the claim that trade cannot work for the poor" (8). Columbia University Professor of International Economics Jagdish Bhagwati calls trade "the poor's best hope" (Bhagwati 2002). Yet, therein lies the paradox. Trade has helped lift millions to higher living standards; however, the current system fails many more. In short, the most promising global solution for poverty reduction has been co-opted by the same concentrations of wealth and power that have turned trade into yet one more cross the poor must bear.

No nation has ever successfully developed without trade. Since the 1970s, Japan, Korea, Taiwan, and China have lifted 300 million people out of poverty, chiefly through trade (Rosenberg 2002). Economic growth in recent years for China (> 8% per year) and India (> 6% per year) has been among the highest in the world (Sachs, 2005a, 18).[3] Following this growth have come great advances for many of their people, particularly China. Success stories such as the East Asian tigers and Chile, which have all demonstrated considerable economic growth in recent years prove that trade can serve as one of the most powerful engines of growth (Watkins 1995, 115).

Economist Jeffrey Sachs showed that between 1970 and 1989, countries more inclined toward trade, called "open" economies, grew at an average rate of 4.5% while those with relatively "closed" economies grew only at 0.7%. The World Bank similarly found that countries with strong outward orientation had far greater "economic performance" than more inward-oriented economies "in almost all respects" (CBO 1997, 26).

"Free trade" has an intuitive appeal, one that is more than substantiated by success stories throughout the developed world. If only it were that simple, the Seattle protesters could have stayed home. But reality is far more complex, and the history of trade much darker. As Oxfam summarized, "The problem is not that international trade is inherently opposed to the needs and interests of the poor, but that the rules that govern it are rigged in favor of the rich" (Oxfam 2002a, 5).

The Mechanics of Trade

The history of trade follows that of larger world orders. Following years of exploiting their former colonies, rich countries ordered trade to their own advantage and have maintained unequal orders ever since. Although they no longer extract minerals, oil, and timber with the barrel of a gun, they now use tariffs, subsidies, and import quotas. One order of exploitation has given way to a subtler but equally lethal version.

Subsidies   On September 10, 2003, a middle-aged South Korean farmer named Lee Kyoung Hae climbed to the top of a police barricade as 10,000 people protested rich country subsidies at the WTO meetings in Cancun, Mexico (Vidal 2003). After waving a banner that read "WTO Kills Farmers," Mr Lee plunged a knife into his chest and died later in a nearby hospital, even as "peasants, unions and students from more than 30 countries" fought pitched battles with police. Lee's final act of desperation dramatically illustrated the frustration born by small farmers from developing countries, many of whom can no longer compete against farmers in rich countries whose subsidized products are sold on world markets at far lower prices. According to the United Nations Development Program (UNDP), industrialized countries spent $353 billion protecting their agriculture in 1998 through subsidies (Randel et al 2002, 5). That single expenditure, one of many in the murky waters of trade protectionism, comprises a full seven times the amount of foreign aid rendered during the same year (OECD 2000, 172).[4] By September 2003, that amount remained above $300 billion, prompting considerable angst when the subject became a focus of trade talks at the WTO Summit in Cancun, Mexico (Becker 2003a). Poor farmers rightly complain that they cannot compete with US and European subsidized exports. More than three quarters of the world's poor live in rural areas, depending largely on agriculture for their basic survival ("The Cancun Challenge" 2003). Oxfam aptly likened the international trading system to a hurdle race in which "the weakest athletes face the highest hurdles" (Oxfam 2002a, 10). Former US Secretary of Labor Robert Reich said simply, "We ought to be ashamed" (National Public Radio 2003b).

As trade barriers fall around the world at the behest of the WTO, World Bank, and IMF, subsidies become that much more important. Because farmers in the United States and European Union can produce crops for export at substantially less cost due to heavy subsidies, they overproduce and then "dump" these cheap exports on poor countries where they drive prices lower, often destroying local markets. Mexican corn suffered such a fate after cheap US imports flooded local markets following the North American Free Trade Agreement (NAFTA) (Rosenberg 2002, 33). Before NAFTA, corn covered a full 60% of Mexican farmland. Once Mexico agreed to open its borders to heavily subsidized corn from north of the border, farmers could not compete. They abandoned their farms in droves, often migrating to cities or the *maquiladora* sector along the border. US corn, after subsidization, sells at 20% less overseas than it costs to produce. Combined with advanced technology that helps to cut costs and boost production, US corn now comprises one half of the world's stock.

In May 2002, President Bush signed a $248.6 billion farm bill (The Farm Security and Rural Investment Act of 2002) that provides large subsidies for eight crops: corn, wheat, cotton, soybeans, rice, barley, oats, and sorghum, further inflaming the ministers who assembled at the WTO talks in Cancun. Former UNDP President Mark Malloch Brown estimates that US farm subsidies costs developing countries $50 billion per year in lost agricultural exports, while the World Bank former president James Wolfensohn said, "these subsidies are crippling Africa's chance to export its way out of poverty" (Mittal 2002). The $248.6 billion bill increased US taxpayer spending over its 1996 predecessor bill by more than 80%. Food First Codirector Anuradha Mittal aptly noted that the eight commodities affected by the bill's "agribusiness welfare" are grown in the "bread-basket states, which also happen to be swing states" for presidential elections (Mittal 2002). Further, the bill's provisions provide a huge boon to large agribusiness giants like ADM and Cargill. These giants lobby US government, WTO, World Bank, and IMF representatives to force open foreign markets, then flood them with low-cost, heavily subsidized produce. Then the forces of industry and politics await the next bill six years later, when they exert their enormous influence again. While activists protest in Seattle and Cancun and poor farmers drown in the flood of cheap commodity imports from the world's wealthiest nations, business goes on as usual in the unseemly world of international trade.

Ian Goldin, the World Bank's vice president for external affairs said, "Reducing these subsidies and removing agricultural trade barriers is one of the most important things that rich countries can do for millions of people to escape poverty all over the world. . . . It's not an exaggeration to say that rich countries' agricultural policies lead to starvation" (Becker 2003a). The most obvious fix would be to reduce or abandon such subsidies, yet this underestimates both how entrenched these subsidies are and how formidable the power blocs that keep them in place are. US farmers receive 20% of their income from government subsidies, while their European counterparts receive 35%. Both groups have powerful lobbies. Farm subsidies in the United States comprise a "huge corporate-welfare program," in which 70% of payments go to the largest 10% of producers (Rosenberg 2002, 33, 50). From these flows comes the political influence of such conglomerates as Archer Daniels Midland Company, which, like its other large agribusiness rivals, buys influence on both sides of the aisle in Congress.

US political history, like that of Europe, is riddled with the influence of moneyed interest groups. One percent of US wool producers receive a $100 million mohair subsidy as the result of intense lobbyist pressures (Zakaria 2003, 173). A 1954 congressional determination that mohair, a type of wool from Angora goats, was a "strategic commodity" because it was used to make military uniforms offers the lobbyists an absurd means to hold onto the money. Even though Dacron replaced wool in military uniforms decades ago, the wool lobby has maintained the mohair subsidy ever since. US cotton growers have fared even better. Just 25,000 cotton growers with an average net worth of $800,000 receive $4 billion in annual government subsidies while producing just $3 billion worth of cotton (Zakaria 2003, 173). Poor cotton farmers in the least developed countries are simply unable to compete.

Tariffs and Nontariff Trade Barriers   Although subsidies comprise the largest trade barriers, they are far from the only ones in play. When poor countries export to rich countries, they face tariff barriers of $100 billion, more than twice as much annually as foreign aid expenditures in recent years (Oxfam 2002a, 5). In the European Union, agricultural tariffs average 20% and those in the United States are roughly 12%. Some specific products face even stiffer tariffs. For example, rice imports to Japan face tariffs of 1000% ("The Cancun Challenge" 2003). The very produce that creates work for the majority of the world's poor faces the stiffest import tariffs from the world's wealthiest countries. One can only wonder at the logic that sends $50 to $80 billion of aid to developing countries but then takes more than $450 billion back through subsidies and tariffs.

The New York Times noted the irony of the situation in a September 2003 article on the WTO talks in Cancun, "Africans find this double attack of subsidies and tariffs especially maddening since they have been told they should trade their way out of poverty, not look for foreign aid" (Becker 2003a). One agricultural expert from Sierra Leone said, "For Africa, it's a major problem. . . . People can't better themselves if they can't feed themselves, and farmers are being driven off their land" (Becker 2003a). Such frustrations are one reason why protesters, joined by thousands of poor Mexican farmers and laborers, protested the WTO talks at Cancun ("Poor, Rich Face Off" 2003). Their frustration is easily understood—they should have an advantage in agriculture due to cheap labor and sizable arable lands. Instead, they continue to lose, largely because of the subsidies and artificial trade barriers the wealthy countries use to maintain their stranglehold on commodities.

Although agricultural subsidies and tariffs rightly cause the most vocal clamor abroad, some specific aspects of tariff design exacerbate the problems. When poor countries export manufactured goods to developed countries, they face tariffs that are four times higher than those imposed on rich countries, sometimes more (Oxfam 2002a, 5). For example, the United States imposes tariffs of 14% on imports from Bangladesh but only 1% on imports from France ("The Cancun Challenge" 2003). Further, wealthy countries tend to erect the highest tariff barriers against the products that poor countries most often manufacture, such as textiles and footwear.

However, not all trade barriers are imposed by rich nations on poor ones. One of the few ways for poor countries to help themselves is by reducing the tariffs they impose on each other's manufactured goods. Trade between developing countries is rising twice as fast as overall global trade, now accounting for 11% of all trade. At present, tariffs that poor countries impose on each other are many times higher than those imposed on them by developed countries. Overall, tariffs imposed by rich country average 3% while those imposed by poor country average 13% (Bhagwati 2002). In the United States, the average tariff on industrialized goods from poor countries is 4%, those imposed by Brazil and India are 14% and 30%, respectively ("The Cancun Challenge" 2003). This is a sticking point to rich countries, which see these tariffs in the more advanced developing countries as being problematic. Professor Jagdish Bhagwati claimed that "trade barriers of the poor countries against one another are more significant restraints on their own development than those imposed by rich countries" (Bhagwati 2002). Naturally, this view excludes subsidies and several nontariff barriers.

Many other nontariff barriers further restrict trade and inflict still more damage on the global poor. Many countries impose quotas through which other countries can only export a limited amount of a given product. Other nontariff barriers include nebulous factors that often follow "health and safety regulations," referred to as "thinly veiled disguises for restricting imports" (Sider 1997, 150). For example, France once required imported VCRs from Japan to clear customs in the tiny southern town of Poitiers, hundreds of miles from any port. Immigration officials then laboriously followed customs regulations to the letter, producing the desired effect—the monthly total imported VCRs dropped from 64,000 to 10,000 (150). Barriers against poor countries lacking the funds and political muscle of an industrialized country suffer even more.

Friends in the Belize government have told me of barriers that Central American farmers routinely face.[5] As tariffs fall under WTO agreements, the United States and European Union (EU) simply design lists of restrictions that Belizean and other exporters have to meet. For example, oranges must be orange (not their real color), soaked in a certain disinfectant, have a certain weight, and on and on. The United States can then legally exclude the crop in full compliance with WTO articles. Smaller nations without much power have little recourse against US and EU giants. As power increasingly shifts from the UN to the WTO, avenues for recourse diminish further.

The Export-Import Bank helps US businesses abroad, acting as yet another subsidy in a relentless drive to crush business opposition in developing countries as well as rich countries.

Among US government plans to foster its business interests abroad is the Export-Import Bank, which "promotes US exports by offering insurance guarantees and loans to US companies operating or selling abroad, including in developing countries" (CBO 1997, 62). The Export-Import Bank helps US businesses abroad, acting as yet another subsidy in a relentless drive to crush business opposition in developing countries as well as rich countries. Another subsidy falls under Public Law (P.L.) 480, Title I, which finances US agriculture exports through low-interest loans. Like the Export-Import Bank, this can be loosely viewed as another subsidy, this time for US agriculture.

Some trade policies immediately contradict rationale for foreign aid. The US government gave aid to encourage the government of Bangladesh to pursue labor-intensive clothing manufacturing for export. Following a successful policy, assisted by aid, with a resultant boom in clothing exports, the United States subsequently restricted Bangladeshi apparel exports to the United States and has maintained such restrictions ever since (1986) (CBO 1997, 35). Thus the United States imposed import quotas on the very industry it had helped expand through its foreign aid. Does this make any sense?

Such actions make it easy to understand why many people in poor countries mock rich country rhetoric of a "global village." The reality of trade policies more accurately fits a "divided village," replete with those in the rich countries maintaining concentrations of extreme wealth through policies of their own design.

The Birth of Industry   In addition to tariffs against manufactured products, which serve to restrain industry in poor countries, other forces can crush nascent industries before they reach maturity. New industries in any country find it difficult to compete against older, more established rivals whose experience, technologies, production methods, and marketing savvy make them intimidating foes to those in poor countries. Nascent industries need protection, in the form of tariffs and other barriers, to keep foreign rivals' identical products from sinking the industry at its outset. In turning back the clock, we find that the United States and Germany used tariff barriers to fiercely protect their nascent industries from the predations of the more developed Great Britain, the first nation to industrialize (CBO 1997, 25). France and Japan also grew to their present state behind protectionist trade barriers (Rosenberg 2002, 30).

Similarly, the Asian tigers rose through a gradual removal of industry protections, guided by a strong hand of state, which ensured that the right amount of tariffs were in place long enough to allow industry to develop. A period of protection that is too brief may cause an industry to fail by premature exposure to rivals. However, if protections continue for too long, industries lose their incentive to more efficiently and competitively produce. As the saying goes, markets punish insularity. This is the reason why the former Soviet Union and the Soviet bloc countries stayed viable for as long as they did and then failed on the open market. The state controlled their industries, by definition, and without the impetus from global competitors, they churned out Trabants. Scores of state-owned industries imploded after the fall of communism.

As reviewed in Chapter 5, the World Bank, IMF, and WTO press countries to privatize, liberalize, remove trade barriers, and deregulate in a process that reorients their economic policies toward export-oriented growth. While a gradual opening of the economies worked for China, Singapore, Chile, Taiwan, Hong Kong, and others, similar prescriptions don't work everywhere. China opened its economy up to trade when its industries could compete globally. The same is not true, however, for Haiti, which finds itself simultaneously at the top of the IMF's index of trade openness and near the bottom of the UN's human development index (Rosenberg 2002, 31; UNDP 2002, 155). According to Oxfam, "Many of the industrial policies that facilitated successful integration into world markets in East Asia are now either restricted or prohibited by WTO rules. . . . By requiring countries at very different levels of economic development to apply the same rules, the WTO system is out of touch with the challenges that confront poor countries" (Oxfam 2002a, 16).

The Structures of Trade

For 50 years, the Global Agreement on Tariffs and Trade (GATT) Treaty structured global trade. Rich countries largely ignored it, creating the current global trade imbalances (Watkins 1995, 117). In 1994, delegates to Uruguay negotiated the terms for the nascent WTO, in what is called the Uruguay Round. This was the first of many highly publicized talks in which ministers of trade from a growing number of countries voiced concerns over global trade. After the disruptions in Seattle in 1999, talks resumed in Doha,

Qatar, in 2001, during which little changed. Fearing a complete breakdown of further talks in Cancun, Mexico, in 2003, several industrialized countries made a few modest agreements prior to the meetings, including provision of greater freedom for developing countries to replicate life-saving drugs and hints at liberalizing agricultural trade ("The Cancun Challenge" 2003). However, the talks in Cancun also ended in failure, amidst massive protests and a refusal by the rich countries to discuss subsidies ("Raising the Barricades" 2003).

However, the WTO may well represent the poor's best hope for the future. *The Economist* had this to say about globalization, "far from being the greatest cause of poverty, is its only feasible cure" ("Globalization and Its Critics" 2001). And the WTO should jumpstart the engines of globalization. Likewise, lest we return to the chaos that led directly to World War II, there must be an overarching structure in place to regulate trade, and the WTO remains the best hope. A World Bank analysis suggested that an achievable round of trade barrier reduction in the Doha Round could boost global trade by $290 to $520 billion annually, with more than half of these gains going to poor countries (The Cancun Challenge 2003). If accomplished, an additional 144 million people could escape poverty.

That said, those who rioted in the streets in Seattle and attempted to scale fences in Cancun have a considerable arsenal of arguments to make against the WTO. First, a *1984* atmosphere of "four legs good, two legs better" permeates what was supposed to be a much more egalitarian body. According to *New York Times* writer Tina Rosenberg, the WTO has become "an unbalanced institution largely controlled by the United States and the nations of Europe, and especially the agribusiness, pharmaceutical and financial-services industries in these countries" (2002, 30). As the forces of globalization continue to spread throughout the world, it is the rich countries and their concentrated business elites who have gained most from it. The WTO and its GATT predecessor have done little thus far to curb their power. The residual subsidies, tariffs, and other nontariff barriers supply ample evidence that the WTO has not succeeded in equaling the global playing field.

Most power imbalances at the WTO reflect larger economic imbalances in the world. Powerful voices resonate within its halls, just as they do at the World Bank and IMF. To simply maintain a WTO delegation in Geneva costs about $2 million per year, well out of the reach of many poor countries (National Public Radio 2003b). Thirty member countries have no Geneva delegate because of this cost barrier. One delegate from Jamaica commented, "If you're not there, your concerns are not heard." Thus, as so many have alleged, policy at the WTO largely reflects the wishes of the wealthy industrialized countries. Poor countries are, once again, marginalized.

Reflecting such power imbalances, the TRIPS Agreement, or trade-related aspects of intellectual property rights, regulates international copyright, trademarks, and patent laws, allowing rich countries to impose trade sanctions on the predominantly poor countries that violate it (UNDP 1999, 67). TRIPS dealt a body blow to the poor countries unable to afford medicines to treat AIDS. Since 1996, Brazil cut AIDS deaths in half, primarily by manufacturing its own knockoff antiretrovirals and distributing them free ("The Right Fix?" 2003). Naturally, US pharmaceutical representatives and the US trade representatives who (are well paid to) represent their interests at the WTO grumbled about such matters but finally agreed to limited generic copies for more widespread use in poor countries (Becker 2003b). The political pressures from Cancun proved too much even for the well-financed pharmaceutical industry. Many other trade agreements involve such conflicting arguments, most favor the rich countries and their powerful lobbies.

The Global Structures of Trade and the Commodities Disaster: Oxfam's Story of Coffee in 2002

Most of the world's coffee comes from small, family-owned farms in tropical and subtropical regions. Among these regions are some of the world's poorest countries: Uganda; Kenya; Ethiopia; Tanzania; Burundi; Rwanda; Honduras; Nicaragua; Guatemala; the Chiapas, Veracruz, and Oaxaca regions of Mexico; as well as poor, rural regions of Brazil and Vietnam (Oxfam 2002b). For many of these areas, coffee is a staple product upon which the health of the economy depends. For generations, many poor subsistence farmers, now numbering 25 million, have made their living by trading coffee beans. As such, they are dependent on fair trade and fair prices for their produce. They are also extremely vulnerable to shocks in the commodities markets.

The International Coffee Agreement, which had regulated both the supply and minimum price for coffee globally, ended in 1989. US opposition, buoyed by major US-based industry giants, played a major role in scuttling the agreement. What followed was a rapid decline in the price of coffee, exacerbated by increased supply from Brazil and Vietnam, a decrease in global coffee consumption, and lack of any clear regulating body to ensure price flooring. Such a business environment quite logically favored large companies over small farmers. By the end of 2001, farmers received the lowest price for their coffee beans in 100 years, earning them roughly 25% of their level in 1960. "Coffee is a waste of time from a strictly economic point of view," said one, since it earns less than the cost of its production. Accompanying the falling prices for coffee are the inevitable declines in health, education, and life expectancy. In coffee-producing regions, malnutrition, illiteracy, and poor health have all risen dramatically as farmers increasingly are unable to cover the basic needs of their families.

continued

South American farmers unapologetically report turning former coffee fields into dangerous but profitable coca fields.

While 25 million coffee-dependent poor farmers and their families struggle to survive, the largest companies attain record profits. Greatly benefiting from the more business-friendly climate, the four largest coffee roasters—Kraft, Nestle, Proctor & Gamble, and Sara Lee—all have annual sales of more than $1 billion. Reflecting wider trends, Sara Lee's profit margin is 17% while Nestle earned 26% on its instant coffee, both considered very high by industry standards. The same coffee that pays poor Ugandan farmers just 14 cents per kilogram, sells for $26.40 per kilogram on supermarket shelves in the United Kingdom, a markup of 7000%. As Oxfam so aptly summarized, "companies' booming business is being paid for by some of the poorest people in the world."

As this story so clearly illustrates, capitalism per se does not necessarily create the extreme privations and inequalities in our world. Rather, it is often the failed systems—fueled by political influence of MNCs—coupled with greed and a callous disregard for the working poor that causes misery on such a wide scale. The larger institutions involved, including the WTO, World Bank, and IMF, have met obligations to their wealthiest supporters while abandoning the poor. In the face of such disparities, it is useless to talk about aid or charity. What is needed is basic restructuring, fairness, and corporate accountability. At the least, consumers can look for the Fair Trade label on many products.[6]

Multinational Corporations

MNCs have attained prominence in both rich and poor countries through their size, economic importance, and political influence. Proponents and critics alike have legitimate arguments. *The Economist* has argued that MNCs should be seen largely "as a powerful force for good" ("The World's View of Multinationals" 2000). Multinational firms create jobs, spread technologies, and bring much-needed sources of wealth generation to developing countries. In both rich and poor countries, the multinationals typically pay better than domestic firms and create jobs faster. In many developing countries where unemployment rates commonly run from 10% to 40%, jobs at multinational firms are highly prized (Glain 2003; *The Economist* 2003, 55). Long lines rapidly form at the hint of new job openings—even under working conditions that many in rich countries would find deplorable. Such conditions have drawn fire from the watchdog civil society organizations that monitor MNC activities abroad. To this the MNCs have replied that they set guidelines for dealing with environmental safety and sexual harassment in countries "where no such words exist in the local tongue" ("The World's View of Multinationals" 2000). *The Economist* concluded, "Big, border-crossing companies are now many people's favorite devils. Yet they actually do more good than harm, both to the third world and the first" (2000). Economist Jeffrey Sachs agrees, pointing out that all poor countries that have developed successfully have passed through these "first stages of industrialization." Further, despite the dire work conditions, most workers describe the opportunity to work in such jobs as the "greatest opportunity" they could ever have imagined (Sachs, 2005a, 12).

MNCs have funded the research and development of a number of medical and technological breakthroughs over the past century and then facilitated their diffusion throughout the world (Kim et al 2000, 177). In 1997 the UN estimated that 70% of the international royalties on technology involve payments between parent firms and their foreign affiliates, reflecting the important role multinational firms play in disseminating technologies globally ("Worldbeater, Inc" 1997). MNCs also bring in badly needed foreign currency and provide host governments with needed sources of tax revenues—even though far too many poor governments contract Faustian bargains just to lure them.

Size and Power

Although many of the issues surrounding large MNCs are controversial, what is indisputable is their dominance in the world. In 1995, multinational firms created $7 trillion in sales through foreign affiliates, a sum greater than the world's total exports ("Worldbeater, Inc" 1997). As such, multinationals constitute one of the "main conduits" through which globalization occurs. Their sheer size has become a source of consternation for rich and poor countries. In Ireland, foreign firms supply half the country's jobs and two thirds of its output ("The World's View of Multinationals" 2000). The largest MNCs dwarf the economic output of most of the world's countries. Each of the world's 15 largest MNCs has gross revenues greater than the GDP of 120 countries (Kim et al 2000, 181). In fact, of the world's 100 largest economies, half are corporations (UNDP 1997, 92). A UN ranking of "country or corporation" ranked by GDP or total sales at first seems surreal. General Motors, with sales of $168.8 billion, would have placed 24th among 174 countries ranked in such a fashion in 1997 (UNDP 1999, 180). Following GM comes Thailand, Norway, the Ford Motor Company, Mitsui & Company, Saudi Arabia, Mitsubishi, Poland, Itochu, and South Africa (32). Further, the total revenues of the top 200 corporations totals $7.1 trillion, while the poorest four fifths of humanity, or 4.5 billion people, earned only $3.9 trillion (Kim et al 2000, 181).

Corporations of such magnitude generate trepidations throughout the world. While the United States and other industrialized countries fret over what Ross Perot once termed the "giant sucking sound" of jobs moving south—many courtesy of large MNCs that find better "operating conditions" elsewhere—those in the poor countries have a different set of concerns. These companies are of sufficient size and power to force poor countries to crush unions, foul the environment, and concentrate wealth in the hands of an elite and connected few while the most vulnerable sectors suffer. What is frustrating to most, however, is that MNCs could significantly improve the lives of the poor at little cost. Although many companies do improve upon the dismal labor conditions they find when they arrive in developing countries, they are still responsible for the deplorable conditions that they continue to propagate.

During a visit to Belize in March 2003, I sat in on a memorable conversation on such issues between a physician in our service programs, Dr John O'Brien, and Mr Austin Flores, a former high school principal, political activist, and cultural guardian of the Garifuna people. Mr Flores now runs a small inn along a run-down section of town with dirt streets and ample dogs. Often unshaven, chain-smoking, and occasionally sipping an evening rum, his outward appearance belies the fiery intellect and wealth of experience that lie beneath. Although he was friendly with the political elites who established a free Belize at the time of its independence from Great Britain in 1981, Mr Flores knows poverty and has worked much of his life to bring a better life to those in the communities around him.

At one point during a long conversation, Dr O'Brien posed the following question to Mr Flores, "OK, so the large multinational companies bring in jobs, foreign currency, and pay comparatively higher wages. In fact, people line up around the block if a new Nike factory opens up. Sure, people still earn peanuts and live horribly while the company pockets billions. But, what to do you say to the executives at Nike who provide the classic argument, 'Nike is helping these people by providing them jobs. If we weren't there, they would have no jobs at all. Even if they only make $1.98 per day, they are better off.'"

Mr Flores took a drag on his cigarette and responded with characteristic fire, pointing a bony finger as if to discipline an unruly student. "To the executives at Nike, I would say this, 'You sir, are taking advantage of my poverty.' True, people are better off working for little than not working at all. But, what they are doing is immoral. Look at Enron. Look at these executives who make millions while laying off thousands of workers. It's the same here." He compared his own experiences with the local man who looks after the tourists. They come in with their wealth and leave him with none of it, often scorning him in the process. He may smile and accept their various insults. "But," Mr Flores adds, "he is angry. He knows he is getting merely a pittance."

What Mr Flores refers to is not an inherent immorality of capitalism per se. Rather, it is the degree to which those in positions of great power routinely choose to ignore—even exacerbate—that which they could so readily change. Transnational corporations have great opportunities to improve the lives of the workers under their employ. Even small wage hikes can allow locals, many of whom are women and girls, to afford adequate food, education, and health care, as well as provide for young children. Given the comparative differences in salaries between rich and poor countries, such wage increases would hardly affect the bottom line. The failure of these large corporations to act reflects far more concerning undercurrents of greed, opportunism, and disengagement. The corporate responsibility so often touted in ads represents little more than imaginative advertising.

> *Transnational corporations have great opportunities to improve the lives of the workers under their employ.*

Concerns of labor unions, activists, environmentalists, and the poor are frequently drowned out until egregious corporate behaviors prompt protests and confrontations. Such was the case with Enron's $3 billion Dabhol power project in India, where Enron officials were accused of bribing Indian officials and tolerating police brutality to quell protests to get it built ("Generation Gaps" 2001; "Enron, and on" 2001). In Bolivia, hundreds of workers went on strike opposing construction of the Aguas del Tunari water corporation project; only the imposition of martial law slowed the protests, during which one protester was killed. Such cases only heighten an already suspicious general public's concerns about corporate behaviors. The many corporate scandals of 2002 through 2004—typified by Enron—reinforced unflattering stereotypes. Such concerns surfaced earlier in the 1999 Millennial Survey in which 57,000 people in 60 countries expressed "widespread suspicion and scorn" over corporate behaviors (UNDP 2002, 68).

Fueling the tension is the fact that corporations and states have different missions. The state is ultimately responsible for safeguarding the lives of its weakest members, while the corporations must generate income to meet their shareholders' expectations. Those pursuing profit rarely list the welfare of the poor among their main concerns—understandably, doing so would not help them to meet their objectives. It is this fundamental difference between corporations and states that causes such consternation among those concerned with the welfare of the global poor, particularly in light of the growth of many corporations in size and wealth.

Before coming to a premature conclusion about the role of MNCs, however, we must recall just who it is we are talking about when we talk about "foreign governments." Far too often we think of foreign regimes as virtual replacements for the United States with which we are so familiar—with all of its strengths and weaknesses. Consider Iraq under Saddam Hussein, with 300,000 bodies found in mass graves in the first few months following the fall of Baghdad. Or, how about Kenya? If given the choice between the government of Kenya or the board of General Motors, I would choose the board—profit-driven competence trumps incompetence and corruption.

The point is this: Foreign nationals intruding on foreign regimes, while certainly in violation of principles of sovereignty, is not always a bad thing. In an ideal world, poor governments stand up for their poor citizenry against the deplorable demands of invading multinationals. And such cases do exist. But there are far too many other cases, as in much of sub-Saharan Africa, where government structures are too weak or incompetent to adequately care for their own people.

Political Influence

MNCs have long wielded enormous political clout, occasionally determining the fates of governments. Britain's East India Trading Company leveraged its 1690 foothold in India to become a military and administrative arm of the British government, which ruled for the next two centuries (Wolf 1982, 239). Modern day influence comes more covertly through the WTO-, World Bank-, and IMF-sponsored trade and development policies (Kim et al 2000, 182). In the process, host governments have surrendered power to corporations following the standard prescriptions of privatization, deregulation, and trade liberalization, creating the ideal conditions for MNCs. Through such power imbalances, states have lost the ability to regulate foreign industries within their borders. Through similar mechanisms, MNCs influence policies of the United States and other OECD countries that may adversely affect small farmers thousands of miles away. In one study of three US trade advisory committees, only 2 of 111 members represented trade unions, none represented consumers, and the remaining members represented corporate interests (UNDP 2002, 68). Whose interests will be best served under such structures?

Other political influences are more overt, as evidenced by MNC political power in the United States. The world's largest agricultural commodities firm, US-based Archer Daniels Midland Company, contributed millions to the Democratic and Republican parties in the 1990s alone, purchasing $3 billion in corporate welfare in the process (Kim et al 2000, 227). Through extensive lobbying on Capitol Hill, corporations obtain grants, tax deductions, loopholes, and publicly funded research and development contracts worth more than $100 billion per year (231).

Corporations have sufficient resources to essentially drown out any competing voices in the political process. During the 2000 US elections, corporations gave $1.2 billion in political contributions, 14 times that contributed by labor unions and 16 times that of other interest groups. Similar trends exist elsewhere. In India, businesses provided 80% of the financing for the major parties in the 1996 elections (UNDP 2002, 68). Although the US government's positions on environmental issues such as the Kyoto Protocol are widely viewed with incredulity, well-financed business lobbies such as the US Global Climate Coalition repeatedly steer the debate outcome in their favor. Finances determine the outcome, regardless of the amount and quality of the science opposed.

Labor Relations, Environmental Destruction, and Worker Health

The best place to view the labor, environmental, and health impacts of MNCs is in the export processing zones that have sprouted up all over the world. Poor countries set aside areas where cheap labor and relaxed environmental, labor, and health standards would attract MNCs (Kim et al 2000, 188). First established in the 1970s, these zones have mushroomed to cover 50 countries and 2 million workers, primarily single women between the ages 18 and 25. Well-publicized zones in Mexico, China, Vietnam, Nigeria, Bangladesh, and scores of other developing countries account for an increasing percentage of global trade. During a 1996 visit to a factory in Wushi, Jiang Su Province in China, I asked a factory supervisor what happened to workers who were injured on the job. Did they have any insurance? Through the interpreter, it became clear that he had not understood my question—there were no such safeguards. If someone is injured, they are replaced.

Mexico's *maquiladora* workers provide evidence of the dangers of allowing MNCs the opportunity to police themselves. Starting in 1965, Mexico created an export-processing zone along the US border and lured US corporations by allowing them to bring in parts and materials duty-free, while paying export taxes only on the value added. US MNCs built scores of plants and employed thousands of low-wage workers, known as *maquiladoras*. The plants afforded corporations the opportunity to employ cheap labor while maintaining low transportation costs in shipping to the United States, a decided advantage over similar sectors in Asia. Following the passage of NAFTA in 1994, the sector exploded. By 1997, the area had become a chief driver of Mexico's economy, soon accounting for 45% of all of Mexico's exports, supplanting other sectors in the process (Kim et al 2000, 265). By 1998, 4,050 plants employed nearly 1 million workers. One Oxfam worker described the *maquiladora* zone as "a facsimile of hell on earth," while the American Medical Association called it, "a virtual cesspool and breeding ground for infectious disease" (Watkins 1995, 123). While such export processing zones are a necessary step out of poverty for many developing nations, one wonders at the ethics of the corporations that maintain such conditions; only pressure from consumers in rich countries seems to alter their behaviors.

The *maquiladora* workers have not fared well under the system that mandates overtime and seven-day work weeks, pays poverty-level wages, busts unions, and causes environmental devastation and poor health (Kim et al 2000, 261). Given intense competition for low-wage labor, large firms often coerce governments to oppose unions. "What we won't permit," one Mexican labor minister said, "are the unions who chase away the sources of employment" (267). Consequently, the overwhelming majority of *maquiladora* workers are not unionized. Those who attempt to organize routinely lose their jobs and become blacklisted. When Sony's *maquiladora* firm increased the workweek from 40 hours to 48 hours in 1994, workers attempted to organize and fight the new demands. The effort failed and many workers, 80% to 90% of whom were female, were subsequently brought up on criminal charges or fired (268). Similar abuses occurred routinely in the United States during its early period of industrialization more than 100 years earlier, until unions evolved to catalyze protective legislation.

From an environmental perspective, the *maquiladora* sector, roughly the size of France, is one of the most "contaminated regions in the Americas," according to author Joel Brenner (Kim et al 2000, 276). Industries dump waste directly into the tributaries of the Rio Grande, and from just a half million Nuevo Laredo residents, 25 million gallons of raw waste flow into the Rio Grande every day, making the river unsafe for 25 miles downstream. Ninety-one percent of well water samples in the area tested positive for fecal coliform bacteria, a sure sign of unsafe drinking water (279). In addition, pesticides banned in the United States, including DDT and heptachlor, turned up in residents' blood and urine samples and measurable levels of arsenic, lead, and other toxins exceeded allowable US limits.

Such environmental degradation invariably leads to health problems, as do poverty-level wages and overcrowding in the squatter settlements that spring up around these industrial sectors. The *maquiladora* sectors and other export processing zones throughout the world are, in effect, disease traps. When malnourished, impoverished people crowd together in unsanitary conditions, microbes flourish. Occurrences of tuberculosis and hepatitis A are at least two times higher in the *maquiladora* sector than across the border in the United States (Kim et al 2000, 280). Mexican cities in the *maquiladora* sectors had six times the infant mortality rates of their US counterparts. Rates of congenital abnormalities and various cancers are higher than elsewhere in Mexico and much higher than in the United States. Industrial accidents are also far more common; not surprisingly, so is depression.

According to Oxfam, MNCs globally are "failing the poor." Through "poverty-level wages and severe forms of exploitation," they maximize profit at the expense of human dignity (Oxfam 2002a, 176). Salary levels are far often too low for workers (most of whom are women) to provide adequate nutrition for themselves and their families. Nor do they provide health care, education, or adequate shelter.

Workers in Guatemala and El Salvador describe being beaten and sexually harassed and others complain of the "sheer exhaustion" that follows routine 12-hour shifts combined with 8-hour overtime shifts mandated two to three times per week (Kim et al 2000, 188). These factory workers sleep together on cardboard boxes on the floor before the process starts over again. Workers in many *maquiladora* factories face required pregnancy testing and summary firing if found positive. Globally, the International Confederation of International Trade Unions reported 299 documented murders of trade unionists in 1998, 4,210 cases of trade-union harassment, and 2,330 arrests or detentions of workers in union activities (190).

The Infant Formula Industry

Western-style advertising causes its share of damage in poor countries by enticing the poor to spend what little they have on products they don't need. Cosmetics, soft drinks, and tobacco chew up a disproportionate share of the budgets of those who cannot afford basic nutrition, education, and health care. The two worst marketing and advertising campaigns involve infant formula and tobacco, which together kill millions annually. The infant formula industry pressures poor mothers to replace breast milk with industry products, despite a mountain of evidence that breast-feeding is superior (Werner and Sanders 1997, 89). In poor countries, bottle-feeding is particularly lethal because mothers often dilute the formula to save money and use contaminated water to mix the formula—water that frequently transmits lethal diarrheal illness. In addition, formula lacks the protective antibodies found in breast milk that these often malnourished infants need to survive. This combination of factors conspires to kill 1.5 million formula-fed infants annually (UNDP 1998, 63). Two successive studies, one by the WHO and the other from the Philippines found, respectively, that that bottle-fed infants were 25 times more likely to die of diarrhea than breast-fed infants, and that bottle-fed infants were 40 times more likely to die than breast-fed infants of all causes (Werner and Sanders 1997, 89). In 1939, Dr Cicely Williams said, "If your lives were as embittered as mine is, by seeing day after day this massacre of innocents by unsuitable feeding, then I believe you would feel as I do that misguided propaganda on infant feeding should be punished as the most criminal form of sedition and that those deaths should be regarded as murder" (Kim et al 2000, 205).

Experts have long known the risks of using infant formula in poor countries, though such knowledge failed to slow market expansion by industry giants such as American Home Products, Abbott, Bristol-Meyers, and industry leader Nestle, which controls between 35% and 50% of the market. Aggressive marketing tactics, eg, handing out free formula samples in hospital wards, distributing misleading product literature, and providing free samples through doctors and medical students, give the impression of broad support from the medical profession, leading to widely increased usage. One 1986 study from five developing countries showed that 40% of mothers surveyed used infant formula (Werner and Sanders 1997, 91).

Following growing outrage over millions of deaths related to bottle-feeding, the WHO's governing body, the World Health Assembly, adopted the International Code of Marketing of Breast Milk Substitutes in 1981 (Kim et al 2000, 206). This code required corporations, governments, and health workers to encourage breast-feeding and protect mothers from the pressure to use breast milk substitutes. More specifically, the code states that corporations should not provide formula samples to mothers or health care personnel; should not provide information to health professionals that "implies or creates the belief that bottle feeding is equivalent or superior to breast feeding"; and should provide no inducements to health workers (Taylor 1998, 1117). The United States was the only government to oppose the measure, citing the potential damaging effect the code might have on US business interests (Werner and Sanders 1997, 92). One can almost hear the sound of industry lobbyists dialing their cell phones in the halls of Congress. It was not until 1996 that all 191 WHO member countries, including the United States, affirmed their support for the code.

Nestle first attracted the indignation of global activists in 1977, when consumers, religious groups, and academics launched the first boycott against Nestle products (1977–1984) (Kim et al 2000, 206). Although this boycott contributed to the creation of the WHO code four years later, it by no means ended the aggressive sales tactics. In 1988, a watchdog group accused Nestle of promoting its infant formula to health facilities in developing country through "posters, advertisements, free and low cost supplements, bribes, competitions and sales representatives" (Werner and Sanders 1997, 92). The boycott was reinstated that same year. Also in 1988, UNICEF found that many transnational corporations continued to violate the code in Bangladesh, Poland, South Africa, and Thailand, publishing its findings in the *British Medical Journal (BMJ)* (Taylor 1998, 1117). In this study, it was found that 8% to 50% of health facilities had received free formula samples and 18% of health workers had received "gifts" from companies. A 2003 *BMJ* study that monitored compliance in West Africa showed significant violations, with Nestle still in the lead (Aguayo et al 2003, 127).

Selling formula with full knowledge that millions of infants will die as a result must rank as one of the most egregious crimes against humanity.

Selling formula with full knowledge that millions of infants will die as a result must rank as one of the most egregious crimes against humanity. While it is convenient to call the practice merely a by-product of "progress," this falls short of the reality of what has and continues to transpire. We have reached a point in time when knowledge is readily available and those in positions of power must be held accountable. So little of this type of news fills our newspapers, a testament to the power of the multinationals that use their power to buy influence and suppress dissent. Even well-documented studies proving how deadly the practice of bottle-feeding is in poor communities are not enough to reel in the arrogance of power. More public attention and more political pressures are warranted.

The Tobacco Industry

Since 1950, more than 70,000 articles have shown that smoking causes premature death and disability (World Health Organization [WHO] 1999, 65). In the developed world, smoking caused 62 million deaths between 1950 and 2000 and now causes 4 million deaths annually (66). As former WHO director general Gro Harlem Brundtland said, "Tobacco is the only product that, when used as intended, will kill one half of its consumers" (Oxfam 2002a, 202). Such details seem to have escaped those in powerful positions in the multibillion-dollar tobacco industry. To the contrary, industry executives have refuted any causal relationship between cigarettes and illness for decades. Through well-financed marketing and legal campaigns, the tobacco industry created doubt about the potential harm of its products. Following the first "Big Tobacco" trial in Minnesota in 1994, however, literally millions of pages of previously confidential internal documents taken from the major tobacco companies revealed just how extensive the cover-up, deceptions, and lies had been (Hurt et al 1998, 1173).

In addition to the obvious harm their products caused, something else troubled tobacco executives. For decades executives argued that smokers had a "right" to smoke and that millions chose to light up because they liked the taste of the product. However, cigarettes do serve one other purpose—they provide the drug nicotine. Tobacco insiders acknowledged its addictive properties as early as 1963. Fears that the larger public would realize this fact plagued industry lawyers and executives for years. A public relations executive for "Big Tobacco" wrote in 1980 that legal advisers had cautioned, "the entire matter of addiction is the most potent weapon a prosecuting attorney can have in a lung cancer/cigarette case. We can't defend continued smoking as 'free choice' if the person was 'addicted'" (Hurt et al 1998, 1173).

It is clear both to those who design cigarettes and those who treat the resultant illnesses that nicotine is powerfully addictive. Most health professionals have seen the patient in the intensive care unit wheel out to have a cigarette right after his or her "breathing tube" is removed. I have treated emphysema patients who sustained extensive facial burns after lighting cigarettes while wearing their portable oxygen—ironically delivering the oxygen their blackened lungs could no longer supply. According to some studies, nicotine is as addictive as cocaine and heroin (Centers for Disease Control and Prevention 1988, 4). A 1979 report of the US Surgeon General called nicotine addiction "the prototypical substance-abuse dependency." Those in the tobacco industry call cigarettes, simply, "a delivery device for nicotine" (60 Minutes 1996). The records from the Minnesota trial make clear that tobacco companies have known for decades that nicotine is addictive, despite repeated denials to the contrary (Hurt et al 1998, 1173).

In April 1994 testimony to Congress, which was investigating claims of massive deceit and cover-up by the tobacco industry, the chief executive officers (CEOs) of the US largest tobacco companies, including RJ Reynolds, Phillip Morris, US Tobacco, American Tobacco Company, and Brown & Williamson, testified, "Nicotine is not addictive."[7] They were lying, as a mountain of evidence subsequently proved during the discovery phase of the lawsuits in several states (Hurt et al 1998, 1173). In *JAMA* in 1995, Dr Stanton Glantz published a series of articles describing the content of information forwarded to him from an insider at two tobacco companies. During a *60 Minutes* interview, Dr Glantz described what he had learned from these files, "They told me that thirty years ago, Brown & Williamson and British American Tobacco, its parent, knew nicotine was an addictive drug and they knew smoking caused cancer and other diseases" (60 Minutes 1996).

Whistle-blower Dr Jeffrey Wigand, later the subject of the movie *The Insider*, ran the research and development division of the third largest tobacco company in the United States, Brown & Williamson, until 1993 when his guilty conscience won out. It was then that he turned states witness against the tobacco industry. In a *60 Minutes* interview in 1996, Wigand said, "I felt an obligation to tell the truth. There were things I saw. There were things I learned. There were things I observed that I felt that needed to be told" (60 Minutes 1996). Called "the most sophisticated source who has ever come forward from the tobacco industry," Wigand became the target of legal intimidation, a multimillion dollar smear campaign sponsored by Brown & Williamson, and numerous death threats (Brenner 1996). One afternoon, a voice on the phone said to Wigand, "Leave tobacco alone or else you'll find your kids hurt. They're pretty girls now" (60 Minutes 1996). Dr Wigand provided the expert testimony the government needed to win settlements against the tobacco industry. He also testified that tobacco companies knew about the health risks of their product but countered such charges with their own fabricated evidence.

It is clear that Big Tobacco committed one of the most egregious acts in US corporate history. The attorney general of Mississippi, Michael Moore, said,

> This industry, in my opinion, is an industry [that] has perpetrated the biggest fraud on the American public in history. They have lied to the American public for years and years. They have killed millions and millions of people and made a profit on it. . . . I'm used to dealing with cocaine dealers and crack dealers and I have never seen damage done like the tobacco company has done. There's no comparison (60 Minutes 1996).

In 1998, Big Tobacco settled a lawsuit with the attorneys general of 46 states for $206 billion in the Master Settlement Agreement, the largest settlement in US history (Centers for Disease Control and Prevention 1999e, 986). Despite overwhelming evidence, the defendants still denied any wrongdoing. Six years later, they were still advertising their product to young people, in defiance of the terms of the agreement (King and Siegel 2001, 504; Woolner 2004, 42).

From a purely economic perspective, the motivations of those who work for the tobacco industry are clear. Tobacco is a $300 billion per year industry with an estimated $20 billion per year in profits (WHO 1999, 65). Given global consumption of 6 trillion cigarettes annually, the industry will not simply go away. Following costly litigation and steadily declining sales in the United States and other developed countries, tobacco companies simply took their wares overseas, where rudimentary and poorly funded public health departments were unable to inform an unsuspecting public of the impending danger.

While cigarette sales in the United States fell between 1970 and 1990, sales in poor countries rose 64%; China alone saw a 260% increase over the same period (Kim et al 2000, 208). Such trends reflect huge demographic shifts in the murderous path of cigarettes. The WHO estimates that 4 million people die each year from causes related to tobacco use, with more than half of these deaths occurring in industrialized countries (WHO 1999, 65). By 2020, more than 10 million globally will die each year from tobacco-related causes, with more than 70% of deaths occurring in developing countries. By 2020, smoking will cause roughly one of every three deaths worldwide, up from one of every six in 1990. These trends indicate that tobacco will cause 150 million deaths in the first quarter of the 21st century and 300 million deaths in the second quarter (65).

Despite laudable attempts to control tobacco's spread, eg, the WHO's "Tobacco Free Initiative," the reality is that no developing country has the resources to combat the well-funded and experienced marketing machinery of Big Tobacco. The growing toll from cigarettes is one of the most important public health challenges facing the world community.

As in other stories in this text, the forces aligned against the poor are simply overwhelming. The combination of a strong profit motive, enormous financial resources to deceive on a massive scale, and minimal legal and governmental obstacles makes both the infant formula and tobacco stories understandable—despite the enormous death toll exacted by each. Unfortunately, these two industries are not alone in their destructive practices—the arms industry has a similarly ignoble history, as do others (Kim et al 2000, 177). Where checks on corporate power are lacking, only greater corporate morality and continued vigilance by the UN and civil society will rein in the worst abuses.

Inequality

The Super Rich

In a tony London restaurant in November 1997, three businessmen enjoyed a rather costly dinner, prompting the *Boston Globe* to ask the following question in a subsequent headline, "What's the tip on $22,000? Ask Table for 3" ("What's the Tip" 1997, A27). The meal of lobster mousses and salmon papillotte, beef fillets and navarin of lamb was certainly costly, but the bulk of the expense came from the $21,700 wine bill. The group found the $8,348 bottle of 1985 Romanee Conti "a bit young," so they gave it to the waitstaff. No one seemed to mind the extravagant spending; La Gavroche is an exclusive restaurant accustomed to high dinner bills. And this dinner bill was far from the record.

That honor came six years later, when a group of six celebrating a business deal racked up a bill of $62,679 in another London restaurant. *Guinness World Records* described the dinner as "the most expensive meal per capita ever" (Lawless 2002). The businessmen, all from Barclay's Bank, ordered four bottles of wine totaling $60,500 with cigarettes and tax adding another $2,179. Given the size of the liquor bill, the restaurant threw in the meal for free. One of the businessmen, Dayananda Kumar, was quoted in London's *Evening Standard* as saying, "To be honest, I'm not that bothered about it . . . I went climbing on Everest, I've just come back from Kilimanjaro, and I'm off to the North Pole soon. It's no real problem." Yet Kumar was troubled by one subsequent inconvenience, "The biggest problem that has arisen from this is that nobody in the City is prepared to eat in restaurants any more after big deals. It's too risky."

"Trophy mansions" and mega-yachts defined success in the Roaring '90s, while entertainers and athletes routinely earn millions. Concentrated wealth is far from unusual—ours is a world defined by the extremes of poverty and wealth and always has been. The Bible warns about the dangers of wealth, while the pyramids stand as permanent reminders that the few have always commanded the resources of the many. In 1998, the UN offered the following from its widely quoted Human Development Report (UNDP 1998, 30):

- The world's three richest people in 1998 had assets exceeding the combined GDP of the 48 least developed countries.
- The 15 richest people have assets that exceed the total GDP of sub-Saharan Africa.
- The 225 richest people have a combined wealth of more than $1 trillion, equal to the annual income of nearly half the world's people.
- Just 4% of the assets of these 225 people could cover basic health care, basic education, reproductive health care, adequate food, safe water, and sanitation for all of the world's people.

In America such concentrations of wealth represent the surface of much deeper and more disturbing trends. The *Christian Science Monitor* reported that between 1992 and 1995, the wealthiest $\frac{1}{2}$% of US households (500,000) gained $1.6 trillion in assets, or "enough new wealth to write a check for the entire US budget deficit . . . cover the annual economic output of Italy . . . and then buy any company traded on the New York Stock Exchange—General Electric for example" (Collins et al 1999, 15). Since the 1970s, the top 1% has doubled its share of national wealth while others have stagnated or declined (5). It seems that we have entered a second Gilded Age in which those with the most have increased their share of the pie for more than a quarter century while everyone else has lost their share. One author noted, "Put simply and bluntly, the great American middle class has become a non-participant in the American dream" (2). *Boston Globe* columnist Derrick Jackson noted in 1999 that the last time wealth was so concentrated in the United States was in 1929, just before the stock market crash (1999, A21). President George W. Bush's tax cuts have only exacerbated the problem, with 53% of the cuts going to people with incomes in the top 10% over the first 15 years of the cuts, which began in 2001. The top 0.1% of income earners in the United States earned $3 million in 2002, over two and one half times what they earned in 1980, making them the group with the most rapidly rising incomes (Jackson 1999, A21).

Such income gaps have been no more readily apparent than in the stunning rise in executive pay in the United States. In 1980, CEOs made 45 times more than production and nonsupervisory workers. By 1990, they made 96 times more and, by 2000, they made an incredible 458 times more (Overholser 2001, C7). In fact, CEO pay increased by 571% during the decade of the 1990s, which the NGO United for a Fair Economy appropriately termed the "decade of greed" (Anderson et al 2001, 2). Even staunch business supporter *The Wall Street Journal* called CEO pay "out of control." According to *Business Week*, average annual CEO pay for the largest 365 US companies averaged $13.1 million in 2000 (4).

Some of the individual payments defy belief. In 2001, Apple's CEO Steve Jobs received an $872 million options grant, the largest ever, according to *Fortune* magazine. Other CEOs raked in multimillion dollar salaries as a matter of course. In 2000, Citigroup's Sandy Weill received $151 million, General Electric's Jack Welch received $125 million, and Oracle's Larry Ellison received $92 million (Colvin 2001). In April 2002, the *New York Times* ran a special report on executive pay, reviewing the cash, stock options, and other forms of compensation paid to CEOs of 200 large US-based companies in 2001 ("Executive Pay" 2002). The average total compensation was $15.5 million for the year and the average "total value of equity" or stock value in the respective companies came in considerably higher at $386.1 million. No wonder the number of billionaires keeps rising steadily.[8] In 2005, *Forbes* reported that there were 691 billionaires in the world, worth some $2.2 trillion, or slightly more than the GDP of Germany (Kroll and Goldman 2003).

The Bad and the Good of the Wealthy Diaspora

It is unclear just how many of the fortunes that are accumulating for the few are justifiably earned. Most US companies saw profits decline during 2001, a year of terrorist attacks and recession, yet only half of their CEOs saw their pay decline as well. Some CEOs made out handsomely, eg, the CEO of Cisco Systems, John T. Chambers, made $154 million while the company lost $1 billion (Leonhardt 2002). As Global Crossing hurtled toward bankruptcy, CEO Gary Winnick cashed in $735 million of company stock (Eisenberg 2002, 48). As University of Texas professor James K. Galbraith said, "It is a runaway and wildly corrupt system in which executives have come to form their own reference group. Their pay doesn't depend on performance of their companies, but on the pay of other executives" (Krasner and Lewis 2002).

In September 2002, *Fortune* reported new levels of avarice on what it termed "the greedy bunch." Following a review of the years 1999 through 2002, the authors concluded that executives and directors of 1,035 of America's worst-performing companies sold off $66 billion of stock holdings while their companies' share prices dropped 75% or more. The authors noted, "The not-so-dirty secret of the crash is that even as investors were losing 70%, 90%, even in some cases all of their holdings, top officials of many of the companies that have crashed the hardest were getting immensely, extraordinarily, obscenely wealthy" (Gimein 2002). Such glimpses into the world of executive excesses proved to be a harbinger of even worse depravities. The Enron debacle may well be, as author Robert Bryce says, "the most egregious example of executive piracy in American corporate history" (2002, 7). Yet it was hardly the only corporation to fall from grace. Seemingly for months on end in 2002 and 2003, one corporate scandal after another rocked the business world. Employees of Tyco, Adelphia, World Com, Freddie Mac, and several other companies watched their CEOs paraded before the national media in handcuffs. Even Martha Stewart was convicted of insider trading in selling off shares of IMClone stock ("Courtroom Tales" 2004). She emerged from prison in March 2005 newly added to the list of the world's billionaires. (Kroll and Goodman 2005) She was one of the rare ones to be caught cheating, an all-too-common practice among the moneyed elite. Just look how far in advance shares fall in advance of bad corporate news.

Even though millions have lost pensions due to the aftershocks of corporate scandal and the resultant plummeting of the stock market, only a few of those guilty of the worst offenses—until recently—have done jail time. *New York Times* columnist Kurt Eichenwald posed the irony this way, "How is it that someone is more likely to go to jail for robbing a liquor store than for defrauding the equivalent of the population of a mid-sized city?" (2002). But history proves him right. Although the Savings and Loan scandal cost US taxpayers $153 billion, only a handful of executives served short-term jail sentences. In the 1980s and 1990s, E.F. Hutton, National Medical Enterprises, and Prudential Securities all committed fraud or outright theft and no executives ever served jail time. After Columbia/HCA pleaded guilty to defrauding government health programs in the worst health care scandal in US history, they paid only fines. Archer Daniels Midland Company executives received just two years of prison time, later increased to three, for "stealing millions from their own customers" (Eichenwald 2002).

In a response to the spate of recent fraud cases, the US Department of Justice (DOJ) created a task force in 2002 to tackle corporate fraud ("The Case Against the Prosecution" 2004). It soon increased the number of convictions from 50 per year before 2002 to 250 after 2002. At the DOJ's prodding, the US Sentencing Commission raised penalties for corporate fraud twice in 2003. Although such convictions appear to satisfy the calls for blood from a battered public and an irate Congress, the real reforms have remained elusive. Executive pay remains ridiculously high and the "looting" of Tyco and Adelphia are far from an uncommon practice in corporate America.

Other fortunes are also questionable. Recall that the heads of several poor countries joined the billionaires' club at the expense of their countrymen. In the business world, Philip Morris' Hamish Maxwell earned more than $15 million selling cigarettes, a product linked to 3 million global deaths per year (Collins 1999). Toys "R" Us CEO Nolan Archibald raked in more than $64 million in 1992, mostly from Chinese laborers who work 20-hour shifts for 20 cents per hour. Certainly only a small percentage of corporate executives are thieves. Most are honest and hard working. Some, like Malden Mills CEO Aaron Feuerstein, are exceptional. Feuerstein kept all 3,000 of his employees on the payroll with full benefits for several months following a devastating fire in December 1995, citing an obligation to his workers and to the communities of Lawrence and Methuen in Massachusetts. His convictions cost him $25 million but earned him the love and respect of his workers. Similarly, CEO Thomas J. White has been the financial engine behind the Boston-based NGO Partners In Health since its founding in 1987. The organization leaders have dubbed him their "patron saint," and it is clear that their trajectory would have been quite different without him. Many of the NGOs that comprise the database in *A Practical Guide to Global Health Service* (AMA 2006) depend on the goodwill and philanthropy of those in corporate power, Omni Med included. Finally, the names of wealthy individuals from

Wealth affords those who have come to it, by whatever means, the opportunity to do either great good or great malice in the world.

the first Gilded Age and today now front the foundations that lend considerable support to the sector most effectively engaged in the developing world, including Kellogg, Rockefeller, Ford, Pew, Carnegie-Mellon, Soros, and Gates.

It may well be impossible to properly dissect the good from the bad within the wealthy diaspora. For every Jeffrey Skillings (Enron), there is an Aaron Feuerstein; for every Dennis Kozlowski (Tyco), a Tom White. It is not the wealth that is so inherently dangerous, because so many have put wealth to good use. Rather, the wealth affords those who have come to it, by whatever means, the opportunity to do either great good or great malice in the world. The central challenge remains how one handles such responsibility.

Other countries have seen some of the fraud, though less of the inequity, compared to their US counterparts. Parmalat, Italy's largest dairy company, collapsed amid one of the largest frauds in corporate history ("Milking Lessons" 2003). Yet, the ratio of the average CEO's pay to that of the average worker's pay in the United States in 1998 was 419:1, that ratio in Japan was 20:1, and in the United Kingdom was 35:1. A study by the nonprofit groups Institute for Policy Studies and United for a Fair Economy found that CEOs of seven large foreign corporations made between 4% and 27% of the amounts made by average US CEOs (Anderson et al 2001, 4). And while the pay for US CEOs shot up 571% during the 1990s, the pay for Japanese CEOs rose little (Anderson et al 2001, 3). Many countries consider the common US nine-figure pay packages obscene.

A World Divided

All of the previous examples serve merely as a window into the enormous inequalities that characterize our world. In 1992, the UN first showed that the richest one fifth of the world's people earn 82.7% of the income while the poorest one-fifth earn just 1.4%, a differential of nearly 60. The richest fifth also accounts for 86% of global consumption, including 87% of cars, 74% of telephones, 58% of energy, 65% of electricity, and 46% of meat (UNDP 1998, 50). The bottom fifth, by contrast consume less than 10% of each of these respective commodities.

The UN reported that between the 1950s and the 1990s, of 77 countries with 82% of the world's people, inequality rose in 45 countries and fell in 16 (UNDP 2001, 17). By 1993, the richest 1% of the world's people earned as much income as the poorest 57% (19). Also according to the UN, the income gap between the fifth of the world's people living in the richest countries and that of the fifth living in the world's poorest countries had steadily risen from 30 to 1 in 1960, to 60 to 1 in 1990, to 82 to 1 by 1995 (UNDP 1999, 3; UNDP 1998, 29). The trends are clear. By the late 1990s, the world's wealthiest fifth had 86% of global GDP, 82% of world export markets, and 68% of FDI, while the bottom fifth had just 1% in each of these respective categories (UNDP 1999, 3).

So What? Why Inequality Matters

Why does it matter if there is concentrated wealth? Conventional wisdom holds that rich people, through their spending, create jobs, pay more taxes, and drive the economy. Further, the concentrations of wealth don't make people poor, other factors do. Economist Jeffrey Sachs said, "My own analysis doesn't suggest that the reason that poor people are poor is that rich people are rich. I think rich people are rich because they developed technology successfully to address a lot of challenges and because they were lucky enough not to have some of the ecological barriers that the poor have" (Barrett 2002). History proves this correct. Until 1800, there was little economic growth anywhere and people in all countries were equally poor. It was only through the explosive economic growth that followed the Industrial Revolution in Europe and the United States in the 17th century that vast disparities in wealth between nations began to emerge. According to Sachs, "Today's vast income inequalities illuminate two centuries of highly uneven patterns of economic growth" (Sachs, 2005a, 29). *The Economist* has concurred with this view for years, adding that blaming global poverty on the rich is counterproductive at best ("A Question of Justice" 2004).

Yet, there are significant reasons for concerns over the inequality in the world, both between and within nations. Beyond the lethality of basic deprivations, there is the destructive nature of class differentials, operating both in wealthy and poor nations alike. Recall the striking correlation between British class distinctions and resultant life expectancies; as income inequalities rise, so do the resultant gaps in life expectancy., More unequal societies tend to have worse general indices. As Richard Wilkinson wrote, "It is now clear that the scale of income differences in a society is one of the most powerful determinants of health standards in different countries" (Farmer 1994b, 15).

Another important concept of inequality is the effect it has on growth in developing countries. As we saw in Chapter 2, when economic growth is combined with "pro-poor" strategies, more people benefit. Countries that more broadly share the benefits of growth tend to grow faster. By contrast, when the benefits of economic growth are concentrated in the hands of the elite few, the poor often gain little, if at all. In fact, uneven growth strategies serve as one of the greatest deterrents to poverty reduction. Far too often, overly aggressive growth strategies produce dramatic worsening for the poor, as occurred in the IMF-World Bank–sponsored structural adjustment programs discussed in Chapter 5. These strategies have the additional effect of slowing down overall economic growth, a further consequence of short-sighted policies.

Dr James Gilligan has shown how the relative inequality between rich and poor increases violence in societies. He wrote, "Relative poverty—poverty for some groups coexisting with wealth for others—is much more effective in stimulating shame, and hence violence, than is a level of poverty that is higher in absolute terms but is universally shared" (Gilligan 1996, 239). Shame, in Gilligan's view, is the major contributor to violence, both domestic and international. De Tocqueville noted how revolutions occurred not when things worsened but precisely when things improved slightly for the poor, an insight long since corroborated by others (289). Such was the case with the French Revolution and the US Civil Rights Movement in the 1960s. The US National Commission on the Causes and Prevention of Violence concluded, "a rapid increase in human expectations followed by obvious failure to meet those expectations has been and continues to be a prescription for violence. Disappointment has manifested itself not only in riots . . . but may also be reflected in the increasing levels of violent crime" (289).

Such feelings of frustration stem from the advertising machinery that drives global consumerism and broadens class differentials through cultures of acquisition. While in Kenya for three months in 1994, I listened only to one radio station that was comparatively commercial free. After returning home, I recall the barrage of radio, television, and print media telling me the things that I had to have, the things I needed. We who live within "the beast" rarely notice its profound hold over us—yet it controls us. The average American watches 21,000 commercials per year (Sider 1997, 145); global spending on advertisement is conservatively estimated at $435 billion (UNDP 1998, 7). US schoolchildren now spend nearly as much time watching television as they do in school (64). The industry would not spend such amounts if there was no clear outcome. Yet, surveys have shown that what comprises the "American dream" has consistently risen through the decades. Many more survey respondents in 1991 rated the need for such amenities as a "vacation home," "swimming pool," and "job that pays more" as required for "the good life" than did respondents in 1975 (61). We strongly believe that we need more "stuff" to lead better, happier lives.

Another form of violence catalyzed by inequality comes in the familiar form of terrorism. Following the September 11, 2001, attacks, broad consensus emerged among both the US Administration and Congress that significant and effective foreign aid was both morally justified and an important ingredient of US national security (OECD 2004, 30). Although the Al Quada operatives who attacked New York City and Washington, DC, were mostly middle class, educated men from middle-income countries with little disparities (Saudi Arabia, Egypt, and the United Arab Emirates) (Zakaria 2003, 136), the fact remains that the hotbeds for recruiting terrorists—Afghanistan, Pakistan, and Sudan—are mired in poverty. According to Oxfam, following these attacks, the governments of many industrialized countries "acknowlededged the threat to collective security posed by poverty and inequality" (Oxfam 2002a, 29).

Economist Jeffrey Sachs, among others, has repeatedly written on the importance of the United States addressing global poverty as a way to limit our inclusion in foreign conflicts (Sachs 2001c). Oxfam termed such engagement "enlightened self-interest," adding, "The anger, despair, and social tensions that accompany vast inequalities in wealth and opportunity will not respect national borders. The instability that they will generate threatens us all" (2002, 7). Recall the CIA study mentioned in this book's introduction that found that every time the United States became enmeshed in a foreign conflict over the period studied, rising indicators of poverty had previously led to failed states and war.

Perhaps one of the most pernicious effects of concentrated wealth is its impact on power in societies, even democratic ones. When societies are widely split between an entrenched elite few and a vast poor majority, quite expectedly, the elite exploit their considerable advantages while the majority suffers. The ultra wealthy often have little need for the safety nets government provides such as social security, basic education, and health care. When there is no middle class to hold governments accountable, the wealthy in power tend to cut services and enrich themselves, as happened in Kenya under Daniel Arap Moi and many others previously cited.

Yet, the damage is not limited to dictatorships or sham democracies. The US government has been under siege by well-funded special interest groups for years. According to author Fareed Zakaria, "lobbyists have become Washington's greatest growth industry" (2003, 173). Lobbyists, representing concentrated wealth and influence, have become the dominant players in Congress. Subsidies for cotton, mohair, and other maritime and agricultural products persist only because lobbyists—and the powerful interests who finance them—wish it so (173). Former representative Dan Rostenkowski recalled watching members of Congress looking over at lobbyists to see how to vote on the lobbyists' pet projects. If a member failed to vote as expected, the lobbyists immediately began to work the phones, generating intense political pressure from the well-oiled machinery that was fully capable of changing the outcome. Numerous attempts to eliminate some of the "corporate welfare" in Congress, both by Republican and Democratic presidents, have failed miserably. Newt Gingrich trimmed a mere $1.5 billion from government subsidies after targeting $15 billion during the "Republican Revolution of 1994" (175). The power of vested interest groups was simply too strong.

No matter which side one took in the 1993–1994 debate on the Clinton administration's attempt to reform health care, it was clear that the ultimate winners were the lobbyists. According to the Center for Public Integrity, the debate was "the most heavily lobbied legislative event in recent US history . . . hundreds of special interests cumulatively spent in excess of $100 million to influence the outcome" (Skocpol 1996, 141). Among them, the Health Insurance Association of America (HIAA), which spent $15 million. Of course, the attempt was defeated, costing Clinton dearly in the mid-term elections and helping to launch Gingrich's Republican Revolution of 1994.

In modern US elections, money controls both the issues and the winners and losers of elections. As elsewhere, money equals power and power decides which issues carry the day—certainly not a healthy situation for the poor. Because most US campaign contributions come from the wealthiest 1% of the people, it is not surprising that the rich have far more sway over elected officials than do the poor (Sider 1997, 144). It is equally unsurprising that legislation passed on such issues as subsidies, tax structure, and the estate tax tend to reflect the preferences of the wealthy. It becomes increasingly difficult for politicians to bite the wealthy hand that feeds when political parties can no longer provide cover, the political process is completely out in the open, and elections so greatly depend on fund-raising. It is hard to call such a system truly democratic—the respective parties have been marginalized into near irrelevance, replaced by money. The candidate who is able to raise enough money can move up in the polls and raise more money. It is in this way that modern elections are won.

Nearly half of the incoming freshmen congressmen in the 2002 election were millionaires (Salant 2002, A23). Further, many had significant financial holdings in pharmaceutical and oil industries, posing clear conflicts of interest. According to Gary Ruskin, director of the Congressional Accountability Project, "Only richer people tend to win office. It's those very same people who tend to hold lots of stock. They tend to have conflicts of interest in respect to their voting" (A23). According to the Center for Responsive Politics, 75% of the US Senate races and more than 95% of the US House races in 2002 went to the candidate who spent the most money.[9] Similar patterns hold for statewide elections. Candidates, parties, and issues groups spent more than $1 billion during 2002 political campaigns, much of it on television ads (Lewis 2004, 5). New York City Mayor Michael Bloomberg is worth more than $4 billion, so spending "millions" to win the New York City mayoral elections was not much of a sacrifice for him ("The Forbes 400" 2001). Arnold Schwarzenegger claimed a salary of $29 million before winning the California gubernatorial race in 2003. Italy's richest man, Silvio Berlusconi, became its prime minister (Kuttner 2001, C7).

A relatively new wrinkle has furthered the importance of money in politics. In 1978 Howard Jarvis coordinated California's Proposition 13 and launched the era of the referendum. Posed to place democracy directly with the voters and away from powerful lobbyists, the effect has been exactly the opposite. Increasingly, wealthy individuals are the ones who sponsor ballot issues ranging from immigration to education, taxes to health care. In California, the number of ballot initiatives increased from 181 in the 1970s to 378 in 2000 (Zakaria 2003, 187). In 1996 such ballot initiatives cost $141 million—one-third more than the total spending by candidates for the state legislature. George Soros, Amway cofounder Richard DeVos, Microsoft cofounder Paul Allen, and venture capitalist Timothy Draper have all sponsored referenda to push favorite agenda forward (197). Such political misadventures short-circuit the deliberative processes that are so essential to the proper working of democratic systems. More directly, they caused the near total loss of control of the budget in California. Due largely to the restrictions of various referenda, 85% of the California state budget, which at $1.3 trillion GNP represents the world's fifth largest economy, is outside the control of either the legislature or the governor.

A more subtle cost of income inequality arises when certain wealthy individuals with a heightened sense of self-importance travel abroad. During my travels in East Africa, the Caribbean, and elsewhere, I have noticed the common phenomenon of American tourists treating native peoples poorly or in a patronizing fashion that speaks volumes about underlying beliefs. Those beliefs are rarely voiced but essentially can be expressed as follows: "I have wealth, and therefore I am better than you. You should serve me." We have all seen such behaviors at home and abroad. It is a key attitude that has earned us the "Ugly American" moniker. It plays here in the United States as well, as "entitlement." I have encountered it a thousand times while treating patients in the emergency department. Columnist Robert Kuttner writes, "We are back to a kind of unitary society in which there is one yardstick of influence and achievement, and it is financial" (2001, C7). In my opinion, this sense of entitlement is one of the most insidious and destructive forces gnawing at the very fiber of American culture.

The images that now flood our television screens and newspapers serve more as a backdrop to the day-to-day activities of our lives than any impending apocalypse— as it so often is for the poor so depicted.

Inequality also drives both the AIDS and tuberculosis epidemics. When we fail or only partially treat HIV and tuberculosis, millions of patients then serve as incubators for further resistant strains. Because poverty has always been the most virulent cofactor in these epidemics, reducing inequality can be seen as the only rational response to containing them, as well as the other epidemics that will no doubt follow.

The final point about inequality is perhaps the most troubling. The longer such extreme wealth gradients exist, the greater our danger of intransigent, blind complacency about these gradients. Perhaps it is already too late. Long ago we acquiesced to extreme suffering and premature mortality in poor countries. The images that now flood our television screens and newspapers serve more as a backdrop to the day-to-day activities of our lives than any impending apocalypse—as it so often is for the poor so depicted. As John Kenneth Galbraith wrote 40 years after publication of his text *The Affluent Society*, "The fortunate individuals and fortunate countries enjoy their well-being without the burden of conscience, without a troublesome sense of responsibility" (UNDP 1998, 42). Further, they tend to ignore the poor or, worse, blame them for their poverty. Their poverty is somehow inevitable and quite likely deserved. It is this moral certitude that spells the most troubling challenge of inequality.

The response of many of the wealthy is to recede behind walls that separate them from the less well-off. The ultrarich in São Paulo, Brazil, found a way to overcome a rash of rising crime and overpopulation—helicopter travel (Faiola 2002, A14). Instead of wrestling with urban blight and poverty, the rich of São Paulo wall themselves off in heavily guarded compounds and travel to and from work via the safety of a helicopter. Helicopter companies take off an average of 100 times per hour in a city that boasts 240 helipads, compared to just 10 in New York City.

Of the devastating effects of wealth gradients in the world, Paul Farmer writes, "In a very real way, inequality itself constitutes our modern plague" (1994b, 15). Given the clear pathology it produces in both rich and poor countries alike, the violence and disease it fosters, the imbalanced power it provides to political elites, the cultural dominance it confers, and the inexorable drive it exerts in pulling a sheet over our collective consciences, there is little doubt that Farmer is correct. Inequality is the deadliest of plagues and one that we dare not ignore.

Endnotes

1. Other countries include Indonesia (a low-income country [LIC]), Thailand (a low middle-income country [LMIC]), and Argentina and Indonesia (middle-income countries [UMIC]).
2. Sub-Saharan Africa received just 1% of all free financial flows between 1989 and 1993.
3. Figures are listed for the years 1990–2000.
4. OECD official development assistance in 1998 totaled $51.8 billion.
5. Dr Edward O'Neil, Ambassador Fred Martinez (Belizean Ambassador to Guatemala and former Belizean Ambassador to Mexico), personal communication, 2003.
6. A number of organizations work to develop fair pricing policies in global commodities markets. For example, see the Make Trade Fair web site at www.maketradefair.com/en/index.htm and the Fair Trade Certified web site at www.fairtradecertified.org.
7. Information from Congressional testimony on April 14,1994. For more information, see www.jeffreywigand.com/insider/7ceos.html.
8. The number of billionaires has fallen from 538 in 2001 to 497 in 2002, although the long-term trends are clearly in the opposite direction. For more information, see the *Forbes* web site at www.forbes.com.
9. Information from the *Washington Post*, as quoted in *The Week*, November 22, 2002, pg. 16.

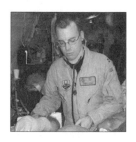

Chapter 7

Forces of Disparity II: History, Racism, Governance, and Militarism

*Until the lions have their historians, tales
of hunting will always glorify the hunter.*

—African proverb

*Mother, mother, there's too many of you crying
Brother, brother, brother, there's far
too many of you dying
You know we've got to find a way
To bring some love in here today
Father, father, we don't need to escalate
You see, war is not the answer, for only love
   can conquer hate
You know we've got to find a way
To bring some understanding here today*

—"What's Going On" by Marvin Gaye

*In this chapter, we view some of the most important forces shaping current
world orders: history, governance, racism, and militarism. By reviewing
history, we can better understand how certain world regions, such as sub-
Saharan Africa, or certain peoples, such as indigenous peoples everywhere,*

have remained mired in poverty for generations. The historically powerful forces of racism and intolerance explain in large part why so many have remained in poverty for so long. As we have seen, governance is one of the most important forces in determining whether a people will remain largely impoverished, as in much of Africa, or begin to emerge from poverty, as in China and to a lesser degree India. Poor governance explains the lack of development in other regions, eg, the Middle East, while military expenditures propagate cycles of violence and absorb spending that should go to health, education, and much needed infrastructure development.

History

History, more than any other factor, has shaped current world orders. When we seek to understand why poverty predominates in certain regions of the world, we search blindly if we do not start with history. Through its lingering effects, history is very much alive, though largely forgotten by and invisible to those in rich countries who benefit most from its alteration.

The first step in understanding how history affects poverty is to recognize the biased version that each of us learned during our formative years. Most of us learned how the early American colonists fought wars with "Indian savages" to establish a new country, most of which was uninhabited. Estimates of small native populations in an empty continent justified white conquest. This "shining city upon a hill," as Massachusetts governor John Winthrop called early America, was to serve as a moral beacon for the world, and those who spread our nation westward followed a certain "manifest destiny" in which white Europeans were both compelled and destined to succeed. Similar biases characterize European and world history. As the expression goes, history is written by the winners—it is little wonder that our views of premodern history are so partial and inaccurate.

Such views contradict history as it actually occurred. When Europeans arrived in the New World in the 15th century, they found a continent populated by Inca, Maya, Chibcha, Aztec, Cree, Blackfoot, Apache, Sioux, Hopi, and countless others who had evolved complex civilizations through long histories of their own. The invading Europeans called these diverse peoples "Indians," whose immediate fate included genocide, disease, and marginalization for the few who survived the initial onslaught. According to current estimates, at the time of the first European arrivals, there were roughly 20 million people in what is now the United States, with millions more inhabiting Central and South America and the islands of the Caribbean. The genocide that followed is often been painted over with the brush of "moral destiny," erasing the histories of those who were here already.

A second casualty to the mythology of history is that of the interconnected nature of things. There is no "American" history in isolation, just as there is no European, Asian, or African history in isolation. Rather, Europe and then the United States developed directly from the conquest and subjugation of those in the New World, Asia, and Africa, with riches from the latter supplying wealth and hence power to the former—the histories of each quite inseparable. In short, there is but one history—a tangled, interdependent, and ongoing world history in which the dominant powers of the day compete for raw materials and cheap labor. In the process, the dominant powers erase the histories of the conquered while enshrouding their own histories in mythology.

Like those in other cultures, Americans hold ethnocentric views that elevate our current and historic roles in the world. As such, we run the risk of dismissing the views of history that run counter to our own. Nevertheless, in fairness to earlier American generations, the United States does have a lot to be proud of in its history. America has played significant roles in the fall of Imperial Germany, the Axis Powers, and the Soviet Union, at a cost of hundreds of thousands of US lives and trillions of US dollars. America has served as the flagship for liberal democracy and capitalism, both of which now dominate the world order. Given history's succession of empires: Greek, Roman, Ottoman, Spanish, Portuguese, French, and British, the United States has been the most benevolent and enlightened. With some justification, according to our worldview, we are indeed the shining city upon the hill.

> *There is but one history—a tangled, interdependent, and ongoing world history in which the dominant powers of the day compete for raw materials and cheap labor.*

Yet it is important to accommodate some complexity if we are to appreciate fully the US role in the world. America plays both positive roles and, simultaneously, self-serving and destructive roles. Unlike the view from the US heartland, quite a different view prevails in reservations in the southwestern United States, the barrios in Guatemala City, and the slums in Port au Prince, Haiti. In these places, the view is of a superpower wielding its influence to maintain elite power structures that repeatedly punish the poor. Similar sentiments reverberate through the Middle East, Southeast Asia, and much of Africa, where the United States has used its dominance to protect its interest in oil, raw materials, and cheap labor, often by supporting regimes that favor an elite aristocratic class at the expense of the poor. In addition, US support for many corrupt and repressive dictators during the Cold War caused strong anti-US sentiments to take root in a number of regions.

These are the views from the other side of history, and it is hard for many in the United States to accept it. When I first heard anti-American attacks while working in Tanzania in 1987, I had not previously lived outside the United States and was stunned by the degree to which people from other countries resented US foreign policy. An American physician/nun who ran the hospital I was working at said, "Our country does some awful things in the world." She was right. It is a view that most Americans encounter when traveling, assuming they travel with eyes and minds open. Yet many resist such views, preferring the sanitized view of the world they get from their local news. It is with great reluctance that most Americans accept, according to Paul Farmer, "the ugly realities about the role of our government in the Third World" (1994b, 53).

When people from the United States travel together, there is the danger of "cocooning," ie, staying among themselves so that the more disturbing ideas, sights, and sounds can be properly sanitized through collective, subconscious filters. This tactic serves to maintain the most comfortable of illusions for all concerned. However, to open ourselves we must reread history accurately. Given the inculcation that occurs from the earliest television viewing in the United States, that is a sizable obstacle to overcome. Our news, like our popular movies, is partial and limited in scope. Just ask any visitor to the United States or listen to the BBC World Service for comparison views. We view the world through lenses designed and manufactured in the United States and appropriately tinted for an American audience. Yet this view creates havoc for many developing countries. Consequently, part of our charge when traveling abroad is to reinterpret history, with eyes and minds open, particularly to the versions of history that are written by the poor.

History's force is readily apparent when one arrives in Belize or Guyana, just as it is in other parts of the Caribbean and Latin America. Throughout the Americas, these questions arise: why are there so many poor black people?, why are the "Indians," as the indigenous peoples are often called, invariably at the bottom of the pecking order, always with the worst jobs and most likely to suffer from the most brutal attacks by government forces? In Belize, the indigenous Maya, like natives everywhere, were displaced by the conquistadors and forced into the most uninhabitable lands. Those descendents who were not killed outright by weapons or germs either intermarried to form the Mestisos, who now dominate in politics and business, or survived in small bands in remote rural areas. The Garifuna, descendents of runaway African slaves, occupied a lower tier of society and, as in the United States, still bear the markings of a group facing widespread discrimination. These people were kidnapped from their homeland and sold into slavery, and still they fight to keep their native traditions. The memory of history still shapes modern elections and fuels the disparities that persist to this day. In Guyana, political parties split clearly along racial lines, Indian and Black; and national elections scheduled for early in 2006 will likely fuel another explosive round of ethnic violence.

Dr Jared Diamond, who won the Pulitzer Prize for his 1999 book *Guns, Germs, and Steel,* clearly and convincingly explains the fates of human societies over the past 13,000 years. When we seek to understand the force of history that is still active in our world, Diamond offers an important starting point. He writes,

> The history of interactions among disparate peoples is what shaped the modern world through conquest, epidemics, and genocide. Those collisions created rever- berations that have still not died down after many centuries, and that are actively continuing in some of the world's most troubled areas today. For example, much of Africa is still struggling with its legacies from recent colonialism. In other regions—including much of Central America, Mexico, Peru, New Caledonia, the former Soviet Union, and parts of Indonesia—civil unrest or guerilla warfare pits still-numerous indigenous populations against governments dominated by descen- dants of invading conquerors (Diamond 1999, 16).

The Force of History

World history centers on the theme of one race or one group conquering another. This stems from our ancestral roots as competing bands of hunter- gatherers, which evolved into larger groups that conquered others. The spread of Europeans throughout the Americas, the Bantu throughout Africa, and the ancestral Chinese throughout Southeast Asia all shows how groups of similar race, ethnicity, or religion subjugate other groups that are seen in some way as "other" (Diamond 1999). Groups of peoples have always com- peted for limited resources, though the outcomes depend less on their genetic makeup than on their surrounding environs. Author Jared Diamond offers this succinct view, "History followed different courses for different peoples because of differences in peoples' environments, not because of bio- logical differences among peoples themselves" (25). According to Diamond, the most important reasons why certain peoples prevailed are: available plants, available animals for domestication, the germs that came with those animals, the geography that made transmission of these advances possible, and the abilities of the different civilizations to incorporate these advances.

The most successful early civilizations sprang up around 8500 B.C. in the Fertile Crescent, the area roughly encompassing some or all of modern Jordan, Israel, Iraq, Iran, Syria, and Turkey (Diamond 1999, 98). Along with areas now comprising Mexico, the Andes, parts of China, and Africa's Sahel zone in the north, these areas hosted the species and climates most con- ducive to agriculture. The Fertile Crescent produced most of the world's "founder crops," ie, those that initiated agriculture—wheat, barley, peas, lentils, chickpeas, and flax. Native also to the Fertile Crescent were four of the world's most important domesticated big mammals: goats, sheep, pigs, and cows (159). Thirteen of these large mammalian species have been domesticated in Eurasia vs none in sub-Saharan Africa and just one (llamas) in the Americas. Most large mammals in the Americas were hunted to extinction by 11,000 B.C., and all of the efforts to domesticate the large mammals indigenous to sub-Saharan Africa failed. The combination of edible plants, hospitable climate, and domesticable large mammals conferred a huge evolutionary advantage to the peoples in the Fertile Crescent and then Eurasia. Yet the close relationships to these animals came at a price.

Humans and individual animal species have their own set of host-specific microbial pathogens, most of which remain confined to their hosts. Occasionally, however, certain pathogens jump species, causing human epidemics with devastating consequences. Recent examples include AIDS, severe acute respiratory syndrome (SARS), Lyme disease, Lassa fever, and Bolivian hemorrhagic fever.[1] Some epidemics inexplicably die out with time; others infect humans in perpetuity, as happened with some of the first microbes that jumped from animals to humans. From cattle, came measles, tuberculosis, and smallpox; from pigs came influenza and pertussis; from birds came malaria (Diamond 1999, 195). Populations that had long exposure to domesticated animals developed protective immunity. Those without long exposure suffered the fate of the nonimmune everywhere—death on a massive scale.

An accident of geography conferred an additional advantage to the peoples of Europe and Asia (Eurasia) (Diamond 1999, 176). The land mass that stretches from the Atlantic coast of Ireland to the Pacific coast of Japan is 8,000 miles long, the longest west–east continuous distance on earth. The diverse regions within this land mass share a similar climate—mild, moist winters that favor edible crops and the animals that feed upon them, as in the Fertile Crescent. By contrast, the primary axis of the Americas is north–south, with markedly differing climates and a host of geographic barriers. Crops and animals cannot be widely shared. Similarly, the Saharan Desert cuts off sub-Saharan Africa from Eurasia, with a tropical climate throughout most of its interior that is markedly different from that of Eurasia. The net result of this geography is that crops and animals (along with the microbes they shared) in the world's most fertile region spread west to Europe and east to China and the Far East. The Americas and Australia remained isolated by water and sub-Saharan Africa by desert and climate.

In the regions favorable to growing edible crops and domesticating animals, populations swelled. Food surpluses afforded populations the opportunity to diversify. Some were freed to invent useful things for agriculture or war, others could become the first politicians, soldiers, and craftsmen. Language, writing, metallurgy, and societal structure developed in societies that first perfected their agrarian base and spread along the axes, favoring broad exchanges of ideas and burgeoning technologies—chiefly within Eurasia. When these more advanced peoples clashed with those still trapped in prior modes of existence such as the hunter–gatherers, as they inevitably did, the more advanced peoples won, taking the conquered as slaves or annihilating them outright. It is no accident of history that the three dominant monotheistic religions all arose in or near the Fertile Crescent.

A visitor to Europe, the Middle East, or China any time after 8500 B.C. well into the 15th century would have predicted that Europe would be the least likely region to forge ahead to global dominance (Diamond 1999, 409). Until 1450, technologies flowed from China and the Fertile Crescent into Europe. Until global power began to shift over the 16th and 17th centuries, the Muslims of the Middle East viewed Europe as "an outer darkness of barbarism and unbelief from which there was nothing to learn and little even to be imported, except slaves and raw materials" (Lewis 2002, 4). So, why did the peoples of the Middle East and China not dominate as the Europeans did?

The native Chinese did proliferate through Southeast Asia, but not much further. In addition, China has always been subjected to central rule, which served to stifle political and technological innovations. The oft-warring kingdoms of Western Europe, by contrast, had to fully adapt to advances in agriculture, war, communication, and other realms or perish. Advancements in science, politics, weaponry, and language were quickly adapted and widely disseminated. European climate and geography favored crops and animals that could sustain large populations. By contrast, the Middle East, which was once covered by forests and the world leader in food production, committed "ecological suicide." The low rainfall of the region could not sustain the swelling human populations. Plants and trees died off and large areas became desert. Curious relics like Petra (present-day Jordan) offer glimpses into a fertile past; the last forests around Petra were felled prior to World War I (Diamond 1999, 410). Only huge stores of oil have prevented the region from collapsing into sub-Saharan–like levels of poverty.

It is clear that surrounding flora and fauna, geographic position of regions, a people's relative immunity to a multitude of microbes, lines of communication, and freedoms to adapt to changing times have shaped history and established current world orders. The ethnic differences of the various peoples involved have had no bearing. A host of peoples separated through time have repeatedly shown that groups with identical genetic make-ups will flourish or fail in direct proportion to the surrounding environment. As civilizations grew and flourished in disparate world regions, they evolved the technologies that brought them into direct conflict. As Europeans piloted ships to the New World in the 15th century, the Incas and Aztecs ruled over empires with stone tools, completely unaware of the approaching doom. The resultant clashes were of epic proportions, shaping our modern world.

The Great Dying: European Invasion of the Americas

While the great civilizations around the Fertile Crescent spread east and west, the Maya, Inca, Aztec, Navajo, and other native civilizations experienced their own, though considerably slower, rise in the Americas. When Columbus first landed in the densely populated Caribbean islands in 1492, he initiated history's most important collision between civilizations. People who had developed separately over thousands of years suddenly came together, with devastating consequences for the natives of the New World. On November 16, 1532, in one of history's most pivotal moments, a Spanish conquistador named Francisco Pizarro led an army of 168 soldiers against 80,000 Incans in the Peruvian highland town of Cajamarca. Pizarro prevailed (Diamond 1999, 67). The Spaniards' horses, guns, armor, and steel weapons frightened the Indians into a panic, allowing Pizarro to capture the Incan emperor Atahuallpa and paralyzing those not initially slaughtered. Not a single Spaniard died on that day, while at least 7,000 Indians fell. Because the Indians lacked writing and communicated poorly, distant tribes never heard of the Spaniard's advance, and the episode replayed all over the New World. By contrast, Pizarro's exploits spread quickly through a literate Spanish world. It was not the genetic superiority of the Spanish that allowed them to prevail, it was their advanced weaponry, immunity to Old World germs, and ability to communicate through writing that determined the outcome. Although most New World natives died from exposure to previously unseen microbes, the World Health Organization (WHO) estimates that 10 million died at the hands of the European invaders (World Health Organization [WHO] 2002a, 218).

Bartolome de Las Casas was one of the first to describe, in graphic detail, the brutality the conquerors inflicted on the indigenous peoples of the Americas. A contemporary of Cortez, Pizarro, and Velasquez, Las Casas was a priest who witnessed—and opposed—countless acts of brutality. He returned to Spain and published *The Devastation of the Indies* in 1592, which soon triggered a "storm of controversy that persists to the present day" (de las Casas 1965). It is hard to understand such brutality against people widely described as peaceful. Columbus was hailed as a god when he first encountered the peoples of the "Indies," the modern day Caribbean. "People began to come to the beach, as naked as their mothers bore them," he had said. "They are friendly and well-dispositioned people who bare no arms except for small spears. I know that they are a people who can be made free and converted to our Holy Faith more by love than by force" (Donovan 1974, 13).

Yet, they were met with anything but love—the conquistadors viewed the natives as subhuman, in part because they had not been mentioned in the Bible. As de Las Casas wrote,

> And the Christians, with their horses and swords and pikes began to carry out massacres and strange cruelties against them. They attacked the towns and spared neither the children nor the aged nor pregnant women nor women in childbed, not only stabbing them and dismembering them but cutting them to pieces as if dealing with sheep in the slaughter house. They laid bets as to who, with one stroke of the sword, could split a man in two or could cut off his head or spill out his entrails with a single stroke of the pike. They took infants from their mothers' breasts, snatching them by the legs and pitching them headfirst against the crags or snatched them by the arms and threw them into the rivers,

roaring with laughter and saying as the babies fell into the water, 'Boil there, you offspring of the devil!' Other infants they put to the sword along with their mothers and anyone else who happened to be nearby. They made low wide gallows on which the hanged victim's feet almost touched the ground, stringing up their victims in lots of thirteen, in memory of Our Redeemer and His twelve Apostles, then set burning wood at their feet and thus burned them alive (1965, 33).

Although such cruelty strikes us now as incomprehensible, remember that Hutus hacked 800,000 Tutsi and moderate Hutus to death in Rwanda in 1994 with machetes and that Serbs committed atrocities against Muslims in Srebrenica in the heart of Europe just one year later (Maass 1996). The human capacity for good and evil has not changed and we have not advanced as much as we might like to think.

In addition to their advanced technologies, the invading Spaniards carried with them the microbes against which none of the indigenous peoples of the New World had immunity. Smallpox, measles, influenza, typhus, diphtheria, malaria, mumps, pertussis, plague, tuberculosis, and yellow fever claimed many more lives than genocide. One smallpox epidemic killed more than half the Aztecs. Mesoamerica's population (Central America, Mexico, and the southwestern United States) decreased from 25 million before Europeans arrived to 1.6 million by 1650 (Wolf 1982, 133). Some estimate that number of people killed in the New World is as high as 100 million (Ubelaker 1999, 14). According to current best estimates, 95% of the New World population succumbed to the invading armies and microbes (Diamond 1999, 210). Those who survived either intermarried with the conquerors or remained sequestered in the most uninhabitable locations and continue to bear the worst forms of oppression at the hands of their conqueror's descendents.

European Invasion of Africa and the Slave Trade

The European conquest of the Americas proceeded swiftly; most indigenous peoples were gone by the 16th century. Similar scenarios played out in other world regions, with Eurasian germs decimating native peoples in the Pacific Islands, Australia, and Southern Africa. It took nearly 400 years longer to subjugate Africa, however, primarily because of its own host of deadly pathogens, eg, malaria, yellow fever, and sleeping sickness. These microbes earned Africa the moniker, "the white man's grave."

Nevertheless, the Europeans persisted, and the story of the Africa's subjugation is well known. England, France, Portugal, Belgium, Germany, and Spain competed for the spoils in what author Joseph Conrad once called, "the vilest scramble for loot that has ever disfigured the history of human conscience" (Harden 1990, 28). Slaves, ivory, rubber, and land upon which to grow export crops prompted the "Great Powers" to annihilate or subjugate all of Africa's peoples.

Belgium's King Leopold II's raping of the Belgian Congo in the late 19th century stands with history's worst crimes against humanity (Hochschild 1998). Belgium's occupying army routinely tortured, mutilated, and killed their African captives in their drive for ivory and rubber. Through a combination of murder, starvation, introduction of new diseases, and a plummeting birth rate (due to the capture and elimination of young Africans), Leopold's armies decimated the Congo population by an estimated 10 million between 1880 and 1920 (225). Few outside the Congo knew the extent of the brutality and killing until the early 1900s (185). Yet the brutality and inhumanity was enough to inspire the first humanitarian rights movement of the 20th century, ultimately stopping the killing.

Following centuries of incursions into Africa, 14 competing colonial powers convened in October 1884 at the Conference of the Great Powers in Berlin, where delegates began carving Africa up into European-dominated "spheres of influence," arbitrarily separating people long associated by language and culture (Lamb 1987, 103). Not one African was present at the conference. Author Adam Hochschild wrote, "The Berlin Conference was the ultimate expression of an age whose newfound enthusiasm for democracy had clear limits, and slaughtered game had no vote" (1998, 84). When five centuries of European domination ultimately came to an end in Djibouti in June 1977, the arbitrary lines had become permanent, contributing to continuing chaos and disorder (Lamb 1987, 134).

Some have argued that European colonialism afforded the former colonies an advantage over those never colonized, such as Liberia and Ethiopia (Lamb 1987, 137). According to this view, the Europeans ultimately abolished slavery; improved the standard of living; developed natural resources; introduced Christianity, public health, education, and the rule of law; and paved the way for democracy.

Such a view, however, again revises history in favor of the "winners." During their long reign, Europeans did little to establish the institutions necessary for development. Instead, they governed as if colonialism would last forever. As David Lamb writes, "The Europeans built artificial foundations for Africa's fledgling nations, and when the tide changed, they crumbled like sand castles. Only one aspect of colonialism was strong enough to survive the transition to independence—economic enslavement" (1987, 137). The corrupt, greedy, and incompetent practice of colonial governance served as a blueprint for native African governments for decades after independence. Governance in much of sub-Saharan Africa still follows a colonial-based model through which those in power access the largest share of the available wealth, whether through diamonds, oil, minerals, or other natural resources. Now, as then, holding office simply shores up the interests of a powerful elite class, replacing colonial governors with African despots and ultimately prolonging the institution of colonialism in another form.

President Kwame Nkrumah, Ghana's first president following its liberation from the United Kingdom in 1957, offered the following testimony to the lingering effects of colonialism,

> [The colonial powers] were all rapacious; they all subserved the needs of the subject lands to their own demands; they all circumscribed human rights and liberties; they all repressed and despoiled, degraded and oppressed. They took our lands, our lives, our resources and our dignity. Without exception, they left us nothing but our resentment. . . . It was when they had gone and we were faced with the stark realities—as in Ghana on the morrow of our independence—that the destitution of the land after long years of colonial rule was brought sharply home to us (Hancock 1989, 71).

Ghana was the first African country to emerge from the yoke of colonialism, with successive waves following throughout the 1960s. By 1977, it was all over, though such recent emergence has given the countries little time to right themselves following centuries of oppression. Yet colonialism was not the worst burden the Europeans cast down on Africa. That burden was slavery.

Slavery

Slavery dates back to our earliest recorded history and has occurred in most societies throughout time. Muslims kept European slaves during the first millennium, and Native Americans, Africans, and Asians enslaved foes captured in battle. As the competing European powers acquired raw materials and new lands for cultivation of export crops in the New World, they increasingly turned to Africans for their supply of labor. From 1451 to 1600, more than a quarter of a million slaves went to Europe and the Americas. During the 17th century, slave exports increased to 1,341,000, primarily in response to the rise of sugar cane plantations in the Caribbean islands (Wolf 1982, 195). In the 18th century, the slave trade reached its peak—more than 6 million people made the Middle Passage to the New World. Despite Britain's abolition of slavery in 1807, more than 2 million additional slaves were transported from Africa in the 19th century, many to sugar plantations in Cuba. Although no one knows the actual number of slaves taken from Africa, estimates of 10 to 15 million are common, with some as high as 50 million (Lamb 1987, 146). The WHO estimates that more than 6 million died during capture and transport over four centuries (WHO 2002a, 18).

Slavery produced one of the major population shifts in history. Millions of people were uprooted from their homes, cut off from their families and tribes, and sent to other countries to work under bondage for the rest of their lives—as did their progeny. These African slaves replaced the indigenous populations of the Caribbean and the Americas, which were wiped out by the European invaders. And the descendents of these captive peoples constitute the lower classes of many of today's societies, their ongoing marginalization a legacy of a sordid history. In addition to displacing millions of people, slavery inflicted a psychological burden on Africans that persists today. Unlike their New World contemporaries, the black Africans surrendered without a struggle. In the words of author David Lamb, "The first seeds of uncertainty and inferiority Africa still feels in its dealings with the outside world had been planted" (1987, 150).

When European invaders came to the New World, they traded for gold and silver in the south, beaver pelts in the north. In Africa, they traded for people. Upon their arrival, they found that slavery, an integral part of most societies, was widespread throughout the continent. People could become slaves through the settling of debts (known as pawnship), through the judicial process, or through capture in war. The widespread practice of trading in humans naturally lent itself to other forms of commerce. Europeans arrived in West African ports with iron, copper, hardware, cloth, spirits, tobacco, and firearms. As local chiefdoms acquired guns and additional soldiers, they embarked on slave raids to further trade with the Europeans. As a result, slavery became the central commerce of West Africa, causing the rise of polities and the collapse of kingdoms, such as that of the Kongo. Europeans rarely staged slave raids themselves. Instead, Africans were responsible for capture, maintenance, and overland transport, while the Europeans covered the overseas transportation, "seasoning" (breaking), and distribution (Wolf 1982, 229).

Contrary to common belief, Africans were not primitive savages "brought to the light of day" by their European captors. Rather, they came from established, complex societies with preexisting trade routes upon which the slave trade was grafted. Some African states, such as the Asante and Oyo, emerged as a result, while others such as the LoDagaa, Tallensi, and Kokomba, were pushed into fringe areas and marginalized. The trade triggered the proliferation of entrepreneurial bands that pushed ever eastward seeking more lucrative slaving grounds. In its wake, slavery re-ordered the political economy of Africa. The impact of slavery was not limited to the African victims, slavers, and tradesmen: By supplying a labor force to the New World, slavery wielded a sizable impact on the growth of port cities and nation-states in Europe. England, France, Spain, and Portugal reaped enormous profits from their American colonies, which in turn triggered periods of rapid economic growth. This trans-Atlantic trade, fueled by slave labor, provided the capital for the British Industrial Revolution that followed in the 19th century (Wolf 1982, 199).

Slavery comprises one of the major forces shaping human history and the current world order.

It is clear that slavery comprises one of the major forces shaping human history and the current world order. In addition to accelerating the development of European powers and New World economies, slavery changed the population makeup of most of the Western Hemisphere (Farmer 1994a, 62). It raised port cities from Liverpool to Lisbon and altered the dynamics of power in Africa, Europe, and the New World. Ultimately, slavery was about the sacrifice of human lives in a relentless drive for wealth and power. It set in motion forces that have long since polarized societies everywhere, helped to fuel a civil war in the United States, and set back the continent of Africa for generations. Its reverberations still affect us all.

Unfortunately, slavery is still widely practiced in a number of countries. In the context of a 20-year-old civil war in Sudan, government-backed militia routinely take slaves from the civilian Dinka population in the southern part of the country ("Slavery and Slave" 2005; "Slavery Returns" 1998). Because the Dinka are predominantly Christian or animist and the government-backed "raiders" are Muslim, several Christian groups have organized pilgrimages to the Sudan to purchase the slaves' freedom. Christian Solidarity International estimates that Arabs own "tens of thousands" of black slaves in northern Sudan (Slavery Returns" 1998). Far from limited to war-torn Sudan, slavery continues in Ghana, Mauritania, Benin, Brazil, Bangladesh, India, Nepal, Thailand, and a number of other countries. London-based Anti-Slavery International (ASI) estimates that there are at least 27 million people worldwide in bondage (Jacobs 1996).

Racism and Intolerance

History provides the background to better understand one of our most prevalent and destructive forces—racism and intolerance. Whether discussing the redlining of blacks in US cities, the assaults on Turks in West Germany, or the genocide of Muslims in Srebrenica, racism remains a potent force in our world. Jonathan Mann, a pioneer of the modern human rights movement, wrote,

> Discrimination against ethnic, religious, and racial minorities, as well as on account of gender, political opinion, or immigration status, compromises or threatens the health and well-being and, all too often, the very lives of millions. In its most extreme forms, prejudice or the devaluation of human beings because they are classified as "other" has led to apartheid, ethnic cleansing, and genocide. Discriminatory practices threaten physical and mental health and result in the denial of access to care, inappropriate therapies, or inferior care (Mann et al 1999, 1).

Its impact on health is clear. From the victims of genocide to the significantly and consistently lowered life expectancies of blacks and indigenous peoples, there are clear correlates regarding race, health, and longevity, as there have been through history. The constancy, universality, and, at times, invisibility of racism and intolerance make it an ongoing threat and one that functions most often by stealth. The universality of racism and intolerance makes it one of the most important forces, albeit one secluded in a darker side of our nature.

By racism and intolerance, I mean the exclusion or outright persecution of any group viewed by the dominant group as "other." That characteristic of "other" can take the form of race, faith, nationality, ethnicity, sexual orientation, or a host of other characteristics endemic to a specific time or place, eg, the Tutsis in Rwanda in 1994. Once this "force" is brought to light, we must recognize it as one of the most powerful forces coursing through world history. It is, and always has been, a part of us, passing through the generations like a structural component of our genes. At selected times through history, it has reared up to dominate a time and place, though seemingly less often now than in our ignoble past. It remains a constant presence, infusing modern structures that favor one group over another, existing in such a veiled manner that it evades detection by most, particularly those who stand to gain the most from its employment.

Although most of us consider ourselves pure in conscience, we are still subjected to the "recordings" all around us, that series of conversations, Hollywood-generated stereotypes, and popular myths that instill lingering questions in our subconscious about any group of people that we might define as "other." We best remember that this force is in each of us and the right constellation of factors can bring it forth with a deadly vengeance, resulting in riots, war, and genocide. One of the most frightening aspects of the Holocaust and other genocides is the fact that some of the worst individuals involved are depicted as "ordinary" men. Every war has its monsters, but it is the cruelty of the men on the line that is most alarming. Such is the "banality of evil" (Maas 1996, 37). In a host of stories from Rwanda, Bosnia, and Nazi Germany, the "man next door" turned into a ravenous killer.

A simple question can demonstrate the presence of "recordings" within most of us. Why are the aborigines of Australia less developed than the whites that rule the country? Consider your answer briefly before reading on. Many well-educated people would probably answer that the aborigines are simple, primitive people, genetically inferior in some way to the whites who came in and developed Australia (Diamond 1999, 18). The reality, however, is far different. Australian aborigines developed more slowly because their surrounding environment offered few advantages and effectively cut them off from the progress attained by the outside world. They are as intelligent and capable as the whites that rule the country and quickly master industrial technologies when given the chance. However, most people still default to the racist explanation, accepting it without thinking. Despite our progress and our protestations to the contrary, racist views—often unexamined—still infect most of us.

Genocide and War

Historically, when the force of racism flares into riots, war, and genocide, some common elements have been seen at widely disparate times and places. Frequently, there is underlying social tension, eg, poverty, unemployment, large influxes of immigrants, or a demographic spike in the number of young men. The ensuing civil unrest prompts people to look for scapegoats, always an easier option than deciphering complex underlying causes. Often there are triggers, such as the Rodney King trial verdict in California or the plane crash in Rwanda that killed the presidents of Burundi and Rwanda. Often there are depraved leaders, such as Hitler, Milosevic, or Hussein. Author Peter Maass rightly concludes, "the capacity for self-destruction exists in every society, and its eruption into war depends not on the will of God but on the acts of men, especially their leaders" (1996, 207). When leaders tap into underlying tensions and incite the masses through nationalistic and inflammatory rhetoric, the results are often disastrous, as history has too often shown.

The Holocaust remains the standard against which all acts of racial and religious persecution will forever be compared.

The most familiar modern example is that of the Nazi rise to power amidst the economic, social, and political turmoil of the 1920s and 1930s. Hitler and his nascent Nazi party exploited the indignation felt by the German people regarding the humiliating terms of the Treaty of Versailles. They tapped into old European anti-Semitism and advocated Volk, the idea of the superiority of German culture that warranted a "racially pure" Germany. The Holocaust remains the standard against which all acts of racial and religious persecution will forever be compared. In his drive to "purify" the Aryan race, Hitler "exterminated" 6 million Jews along with 5 million Poles, Roma, political opponents, and others (Power 2002, 90). The number and nature of the atrocities committed still strain the boundaries of our comprehension. Earlier genocides, such as those in the New World and Africa during European conquest, occurred before the advent of the newsreel and will forever be afforded less attention due to the vagaries of the numbers killed.

Health providers should recall that physicians, many among the most prominent in Germany at the time, committed some of the worst individual acts of the Holocaust. Thousands of captive Jews, Poles, Russians, and Gypsies died from experiments in freezing; high-altitude exposure; sterilization; mustard gas exposure; incendiary device exposure; infection with malaria, yellow fever, smallpox, typhus, and cholera; various bone, muscle, and nerve resections and transplantations; and other horrors (Mann et al 1999, 292). During the Nuremberg Doctor's Trial in December 1946, chief prosecutor Telford Taylor reminded the court, "The wrongs which we seek to condemn and punish have been so calculated, so malignant, and so devastating, that civilization cannot tolerate their being ignored because it cannot survive their being repeated" (285). Yet, subsequent massacres in Phnom Pen, Srebrenica, and Kigali belie the statement's promise and reveal a darker constancy to our nature.

Turkey's "slaughter" of 1 million Armenians in 1915 evolved through the Turks attempt, like that of the Third Reich, "to achieve 'nothing more or less than the annihilation of a whole people'" (Power 2002, 9). Iraq's Saddam Hussein killed 100,000 Kurds in 1987 and –1988 alone, many through poison gas. Columnist Hazem Saghiya estimated that Saddam killed 1–1.5 million, a total rivaling that of Cambodia's Pol Pot (Unger 2004, 81).

In the former Yugoslavia, strongman Tito's death in 1980 opened the gates for war a decade later, as formerly autonomous provinces suddenly emerged from the yoke of communism. While leaders fanned the flames of nationalism and ethnic hatred, 200,000 Bosnians were killed between 1992 and 1995. The West, following patterns established in the genocides that predated it, largely stood by silently watching for more than three years (Maass 1996, 207). It is possible that these "tribal rivalries and century-old hatreds" may have ignited on their own. Yet, provocateurs like Serb leader Slobodan Milosevic made war inevitable where more thoughtful leaders might have prevented or at least contained it (204). While on trial in The Hague for crimes against humanity, including genocide, in 2002, Milosevic listened as his accusers charged him with creating "rivers of blood" while "bent on creating an ethnically pure Greater Serbia" (Simons 2002).

In 1994, the Hutu-dominated government of Rwanda armed 20,000 to 30,000 unemployed men and taught them to "kill Tutsi 'cockroaches' without mercy" (Kim et al 2000, 106). In just 100 days, 800,000 died. Far from being a problem "over there," for those inclined to think in such terms, racism remains a problem everywhere. Its explosive potential can flare at any time, given the right combination of circumstances and misdirected leadership.

US Aspects of Racism

The large-scale horrors of war attract considerable and much warranted attention. However, it is the structural components of racism that create the most damaging effects, particularly from the health perspective. Racism seldom acts alone, and although poverty is the engine that generates the bulk of the worst health indices, a disproportionate share of the American poor is comprised of people of color. There are certainly other forms of racism in the United States and other countries. However, the American black–white rifts are the most pointed, the most discussed, and the most valuable for understanding the consequences of institutionalized racism. The United States has a clear and well-documented history on race matters, from slavery to civil rights. It also, uniquely, has a long history of studying health indices by racial and ethnic categories. By contrast, many other countries have neither tracked racial disparities nor begun their own civil rights struggles. One can only assume that problems similar to those encountered in the United States are even worse. There is a lot to learn from the US experience, so I will continue that focus here.

Many have openly questioned arguments that cite race as a factor in health or resource disparities. Many also view the United States as a "color-blind" society that has dealt with its race problems and must now simply move forward. However, such arguments underestimate the legacy of history. *Something* is going on that consistently causes blacks in the United States—and other minority groups in other countries—to die younger, live in poorer areas, and have higher levels of unemployment, violence, incarceration, and poor health (Prothrow-Stith 1991, 11). Consider the following evidence:

- According to *Morbidity and Mortality Weekly Report*, life expectancy for blacks in the United States has been consistently less than that of whites since it was first tracked the early 1900s. In 1998, blacks lived an average of six years less than whites, with heart disease, cancer, and homicide contributing most to the differential (Centers for Disease Control and Prevention [CDC] 2001, 780).
- In 1990, the average life expectancy for black men in our nation's capital was 58 years vs 72 years nationally for white men. As such, a black man in Washington, DC, in 1990 could expect a shorter life than the average person living in India, Pakistan, Nicaragua, Zimbabwe, and many other poor countries (Kim et al 2000, 427).
- In the United States, seven out of eight ghetto residents in urban areas in 1990 were minorities, mostly African-Americans (Wilson 1996, 51).
- As elsewhere, the AIDS epidemic in the United States has exploded in the poorest communities, comprised mostly by people of color. In the 1980s AIDS struck black women 11 times more frequently than white women (Farmer et al 1996, 21). Similarly, in 1994 alone, US black and Latino women had AIDS rates 16 and 7 times that of white women, respectively (62).
- When Hurricane Katrina decimated New Orleans in August 2005, it focused an international spotlight on America's urban underbelly. Those who fled prior to the hurricane were largely white and afflu-ent; those left behind were poor and black. Prior to Katrina, 28% of people in New Orleans lived in poverty (twice the national average); of these, 84% were black (DeParle 2005). In 2004, there were 264 murders in New Orleans (population 500,000), compared with 572 murders in New York City (population 8 million) (Herbert 2005).

The previous data clearly demonstrate marked differences in life expectancy and violence in black and Hispanic communities in the United States, placing human development indices for poorer communities at levels similar to those for some of the world's poorest countries (Sider 1997, 178). An oft-cited study found that black men living in Harlem in the late 1980s were less likely to reach the age of 65 than men living in Bangladesh, one of the world's poorest countries (McCord and Freeman 1990, 173). The same study reported that blacks and Hispanics in New York under age 65 had mortality rates twice as high as whites. The authors concluded that the main source of the excess deaths in the minority groups were "vicious poverty and inadequate access to basic health care. . . ." (173). How shocking a picture to paint for the average American. Walk a few blocks to Harlem from Manhattan or to Roxbury from downtown Boston and life expectancies plummet, homicide surges, and hopelessness descends like a coastal fog.

From a health perspective, racial and ethnic disparities exist in the availability, provision, and outcome of health care for black, Hispanic, and other minority groups. A large number of studies have shown that black Americans receive significantly less medical care than their white counterparts. The most compelling data comes from cardiovascular care, which takes on increased importance when recalling that heart disease contributes more than any other to white–black disparities in life expectancy. In relation to their white counterparts, black patients are less likely to receive cardiac catheterization (Chen et al 2001, 1443), coronary reperfusion therapy (Canto et al 2000, 1094), or bypass surgery (Peterson et al 1994) following an acute myocardial infarction (heart attack). Management of virtually all aspects of heart attacks in blacks is inferior to that of whites (Vaccarino et al 2005, 671). Blacks are also less likely to undergo renal transplantation (Alexander and Sehgal 1998, 1148); receive appropriate treatment and analgesia for cancer, which is also more commonly found at later stages in black patients (Smedley et al 2001, 43); undergo fewer diagnostic and therapeutic procedures for cerebrovascular disease (46); receive antiretroviral therapy for HIV; or receive prophylactic therapies to prevent the opportunistic infections that define AIDS, despite a significantly increased risk for both. They are also more likely to receive their asthma or diabetes care in emergency rooms instead of primary care offices, with poorer long-term management as a result (Smedley et al 2001, 50), and they are less likely to receive expensive surgical procedures (Jha et al 2005, 683). Recent studies show that most of these disparities remain unchanged (Lurie 2005, 727).

Alarmed by such data, the US Congress requested in 1999 that the Institute of Medicine (IOM) study the reasons for the persistent health disparities between white and nonwhite populations. The commission subsequently reviewed more than 600 studies published over a 10-year period, summarizing the most relevant 100 in one of the most comprehensive reports ever written on the subject (Smedley et al 2001). The commission's findings were clear, "Racial and ethnic minority patients are found to receive a lower quality and intensity of healthcare and diagnostic services across a wide range of procedures and disease areas" (61). It further found that the racial and ethnic disparities were attenuated but remained, after controlling for socio-demographic characteristics, insurance status, and clinical factors. The committee found the disparities "unacceptable" because they were frequently associated with worse outcomes. They concluded, "many sources— including health systems, healthcare providers, patients, and utilization managers—may contribute to racial and ethnic disparities in health care" (17). They added that providers also contributed to the problem through "bias, stereotyping, prejudice, and clinical uncertainty." It is a problem with a long history but no imminent solutions.

Providers have found similar difficulty finding solutions to another epidemic that lowers both life expectancies and hope in black communities: violence. In communities where job prospects are dim, "children are raised without fathers and social institutions are in disarray" and violence soars (Prothrow-Stith 1991, 17). Contrary to popular beliefs, more than 90% of the victims of black violence are other blacks (Gilligan 1996, 197). Dr James Gilligan, a professor at Harvard Medical School and the former medical director for Bridgewater State Hospital for the Criminally Insane, spent a lifetime working with the most hardened criminals, roughly half of them black. In his book *Violence: Our Deadly Epidemic and Its Causes*, he writes, "You cannot work for one day with the violent people who fill our prisons and mental hospitals for the criminally insane without being forcibly and constantly reminded of the extreme poverty and discrimination that characterize their lives" (Gilligan 1996, 191). In addition to the historic and economic factors, Gilligan sees a deeper psychological root to much of the violence, which stems from "the endless circle of shame, humiliation, and the implied unacceptability of one's own person" that many American blacks experience (203).

This "implied unacceptability" is best described by the United States' most celebrated advocate of nonviolent approaches to racial healing. Dr Martin Luther King Jr's legacy may have taken some public hits (Boyd 2002, A19), but he remains a timeless voice in the quest for a just and tolerant world. While in jail for "parading without a permit" in 1963, King responded to a group of clergy calling for him and others to "wait" for a better time to hold protest marches. In his famed response, *Letter from a Birmingham Jail*, King summarized the oppression of "Negroes" of the time and spoke eloquently to the ills that characterize overt racism everywhere:

> I guess it is easy for those who have never felt the stinging darts of segregation to say, "Wait." But when you have seen vicious mobs lynch your mothers and fathers at will and drown your sisters and brothers at whim; when you have seen hate-filled policemen curse, kick, brutalize and even kill your black brothers and

sisters with impunity; when you see the vast majority of your twenty million Negro brothers smothering in an airtight cage of poverty in the midst of an afflu-ent society . . . when you are harried by day and haunted by night by the fact that you are a Negro, living constantly at tip-toe stance, never quite knowing what to expect next, and are plagued with inner fears and outer resentments; when you go on forever fighting a degenerating sense of "nobodiness" then you will under-stand why we find it difficult to wait. . . .[2]

King's description of racism represents a period from which the United States has certainly evolved, in no small way from his own work. Yet human nature evolves slowly. It is easy to take the next logical step and see how those same racial and ethnic biases quietly become "institutionalized" in the legal, economic, and political structures of society. The predictable result is the marginalization of certain groups, borne out by differential group indices in virtually all countries.

Like King, contemporary commentators such as Cornel West push the discussion toward an analysis of the deeper effects of such marginalization. "*Nihilism*," West writes, defined as "the lived experience of coping with a life of horrifying meaninglessness, hopelessness, and (most important) lovelessness," grips black communities throughout the United States (West 1994, 22). This is the force we should most fear, when large numbers of marginalized people develop a "numbing detachment from others and a self-destructive disposition toward the world" (23). Such is part of the backdrop to the murder rates in US urban ghettoes, reflected in the "gangsta" music emanating from them. The reflective and healing prayer of Marvin Gaye's "What's Going On?" has been replaced by what Rev Eugene Rivers has called the "justifiable anger" that courses through much of hip-hop and rap. Such music similarly reflects disillusionment with the hopeful rhetoric of the 1960s civil rights leaders, and an angry rejection of what has become a hard and permanent reality.

So how do we answer the fundamental question, "What's going on?" Is it pure racism that accounts for so much of the misery detailed here, as many liberals claim, or is there some group moral or character deficiency, as the conservatives claim? Extreme polar viewpoints dominate the public dis-course in their respective responses, and both have their limitations. Liberals tend to dismiss culturally destructive behaviors and attitudes from ghetto residents, and conservatives tend to see group deficiencies of character or intelligence as popularized in *The Bell Curve* (Wilson 1996, xciii). Both viewpoints inform practitioners and help shape some of the unconscious bias that the IOM study warned of. This "bias" may also shape attitudes that become land mines when transported to different cultures in other coun-tries. As such, it is worth exploring a little further.

William Julius Wilson, one of America's most prominent sociologists, argues that many factors are responsible for the misery of urban blacks, but chief among them is the "disappearance of work, and the consequences of that disappearance for both social and cultural life" of inner-city ghetto residents (Wilson 1996, xix). Rising levels of unemployment have pushed segregated urban ghettos in the United States into ever-worsening crisis. Of crucial importance, however, is how such large numbers of black and Hispanic people became concentrated in urban ghettoes in the first place.

Recall that most Africans first came to the United States as captive slaves from West Africa during the 17th through 19th centuries. Following emancipation in the aftermath of the Civil War, many blacks moved to burgeoning, though segregated, cities to pursue work. Similar agrarian to urban population shifts occurred in other countries during this period as part of the Industrial Revolution, with similar concentrations of poor people resulting.[3] Though now freed men, blacks were not viewed as equals by their white counterparts—they moved into segregated areas that slowly evolved into modern ghettos. The current residents did not make voluntary decisions to stay in what have become concentrated centers of poverty, drugs, and violence. Their options remained limited. According to Wilson, these urban ghettos were "the product of systemic racial practices such as restrictive covenants, redlining by banks and insurance companies, zoning, panic peddling by real estate agents, and the creation of massive public housing projects in low-income areas" (Wilson 1996, 23). People became trapped in the same areas their ancestors were forced into generations earlier. Even conservative republican President George W. Bush acknowledged this ignoble history after Hurricane Katrina revealed to the world that the urban underclass in the American south was largely black. In a nationally televised address from New Orleans, the president said, "As all of us saw on television, there's also some deep, resistant poverty in this region [the Gulf] as well. That poverty has roots in a history of racial discrimination, which cut off generations from the opportunity of America" (The White House 2005).

Thus, the legacy of slavery and racial segregation in the United States has been the concentration of predominantly black and Latino individuals in ever-increasing "ghetto poverty areas," creating "chocolate cities and vanilla suburbs" (West 1994, 9). Although these locations afforded work opportunities in earlier times, they also made their residents vulnerable to the inevitable industrial shifts that characterized much of the 20th century. When industries left the cities for the suburbs or for foreign, cheaper labor markets in the 1970s and after, urban minorities were stranded and unemployment rates soared. Fewer role models were employed to model work-friendly behaviors like punctuality, dependability, good attitude, and customer-friendly interpersonal skills. Instead, destructive behaviors predominated, prompting both white and black employers to avoid hiring those from certain residential areas (Wilson 1996, 111). Racist practices continue in the form of glass ceilings, continued redlining, less opportunity for high-quality education, political voice, and life advancement. Despite the rise of a thriving black middle class, many more millions remain trapped by the poverty, violence, crime, drugs, and hopelessness of their urban ghetto prisons. The net result: poor health, higher infant mortality, and lowered life expectancies. Both the legacy and active components of racism translate into very real differences in the health of people. Limiting care by removing public health measures, doctors, and hospitals would have a comparable effect.

Global Aspects of Racism

Turning our gaze internationally, we see that patterns similar to those in the United States exist in virtually all countries studied. Certain groups occupy the bottom rungs of most societies, to an extent that cannot be explained by chance alone. As is the case around the world, those who occupy a community's bottom economic rungs have the worst health. Since 1990, the United Nation's (UN) human development reports have "disaggregated" countries to reveal hidden disparities by region, race, ethnicity, and gender. The reports reveal a consistently worse quality of life for those of the nondominant ethnic, religious, or racial groups within a country or region. Indigenous people, in particular, tend to fare the worst. People of darker skin color or those from nondominant tribes or ethnic backgrounds frequently occupy the next lowest rungs.

According to the UN, indigenous people remain poorer than most other groups "in almost all societies where they are to be found. . . . In developing countries, the poorest regions are those with the most indigenous people" (United Nations Development Programme [UNDP] 1997, 43). This represents the logical, though tragic, consequence of historical forces in which invading groups conquered, mostly destroyed, and then marginalized indigenous groups. Australian aboriginals earn only half as much income as non-aboriginals. In Guatemala, only 40% of indigenous people are literate and half of their "earnings shortfall" is estimated to come from discrimination (43). In my travels in Guatemala, Brazil, Belize, Guyana, and the United States, the indigenous people always appear to be the worst off. As in the United States, they are forced onto the most arid lands and have the highest levels of unemployment, the least education, and the least hope for the future. It is a universally heart-breaking phenomenon.

During a Kellogg Fellowship visit to Brazil in 1995, our group visited several indigenous tribes and observed their poverty, their hopelessness, and their dwindling numbers. We subsequently visited the Brazilian Parliament, where a Native American woman from our group named Deborah Harry stood up and, with tears streaming down her face, asked one of the Brazilian senators, "Can you please tell me . . . how we can stop this ongoing genocide from wiping out my people?" Based on population surveys, time is running out for indigenous people everywhere.

According to the *Boston Globe*, since the 1980s, a "silent rebellion" in the form of multiple suicides has swept through many of Brazil's indigenous tribes peoples (Christie 1995, 21). Facing increasingly dismal life prospects, at least 236 of the Guarani Indians in the Mato Grosso region of Brazil killed themselves between 1982 and 1995—many of them children (21). Five million Indians in the territory have been decimated through genocide, disease, and poverty, reducing their population to a mere 23,000. The phenomenon of suicide continues in 2005 throughout Latin and North American tribes (Forero 2004). One villager in Bororo, where "the squalor surpasses many city slums," said, "We don't have food, we don't have water, and we don't have medicine" (Christie 1995, 21). In an analysis reminiscent of the plight of their US counterparts (Sahagun 1997), the *Boston Globe* reports, "Experts agree that the Guarani are suffering a spiritual crisis brought by the loss of their traditional lands and lifestyles, the proximity of modern cities and the grinding poverty in which most of them live" (Christie 1995, 21).

Similar trends occur in other countries. In Mexico, indigenous people have poverty rates of 81% vs 18% among nonindigenous people (UNDP 1996, 31). Like indigenous people everywhere, those in Mexico have, according to the UN, "less access to social services and basic infrastructure, leading to lower literacy rates, higher infant mortality, and a higher incidence of poverty" (32).

Although indigenous people face the very real threat of extinction in a number of countries, by far the worst of any group, other groups also face widespread discrimination. Globally, people of African descent tend to reflect the US experience, though with considerably worse living standards and far less progress in acquiring their civil rights. Roughly 8 million Africans were forcibly transported to Brazil between 1540 and 1850, then subsequently turned out after emancipation to become "vagrants, homeless, jobless, penniless" (Rocha 2000). A 1999 report by the Minority Rights Group found that black and mixed race Brazilians have less schooling, higher infant mortality rates, higher unemployment, and receive less pay for the same work as their white counterparts (Rocha 2000). Not surprisingly, the BBC reports "racism exists here" and Brazil is "only just starting to recognize it may have a problem with race equality."[4]

South Africa was long seen as an international pariah for its apartheid policies, abandoned only after a concerted global push. The legacy of its long history of racial segregation is a country still divided, one wealthy and white, the other poor and black. The health indices clearly reflect the difference. If the two populations were separately indexed in the UN's Human Development Report, white South Africans would come in at 24, and black South Africans would come in at 123 (Sider 1997). Two South African provinces tell a story of a vast divide between the races. The province of North Transvaal is 90% black and would rank just ahead of Myanmar at the human development index (HDI) of 133. Contrast this with the province of Western Cape, with a black population of only 17%, where the HDI rank would be 61, next to Belarus. The per capita income of Western Cape

is $6,000 while that of North Transvaal is only $1190.00, a difference
of a factor of 5 (UNDP 1996, 32). Health follows wealth, and wealth flows
preferably to the dominant groups.

In the Western Hemisphere, Haiti constitutes an example of the lingering and destructive effects of discrimination (Farmer 1994a). Haiti's isolation, marginalization, and impoverishment all stem from its origins as a slave
colony. The slave revolt of 1803 defeated the French occupying force, establishing the second oldest democracy in the New World while simultaneously
sending shivers down the spines of the slave-holding powers in Europe and
the Americas. As a consequence of their hard-fought freedom, Haiti's former
slaves embarked on a long road of backbreaking poverty, largely rooted in
international trade imbalances, colonial governance practices, and environmental destruction. Nearly 200 years later, Haiti remains the poorest country
in the Western Hemisphere, with an HDI that places it firmly in the midst of
the sub-Saharan Africa diaspora. Life expectancy at birth is 52.6 years, the
lowest in the Western Hemisphere. Less than half its people are literate;
newborns have a 32% chance of not surviving until age 40; and its infant
mortality rate (IMR) is 81 per 1,000 (vs 7 per 1,000 in the United States). Of
interest to health providers is the fact that there are only 8 physicians per
every 100,000 people in Haiti, while there are nearly 300 physicians per
100,000 people in the United States (UNDP 2002, 149).

Other forms of racism and intolerance reflect regional variances yet still
serve the needs of those in power. Kenya's president Daniel Arap Moi
"inflamed ethnic divisions" to keep his grip on power for 24 years ("The
View from the Slums" 2002). During his long tenure, which ended in
January 2003 due to constitutional requirements, Moi pitted Kenya's many
tribes against each other, in a time-tested strategy that worked to spur
Kenya's 30 million to vote along tribal lines, thus maintaining Moi's KANU
party in power—and in money. The ethnic tensions and occasional killings
also served to distract attention from the corruption and incompetence that
ruined the country during his watch ("The View from the Slums" 2002).
Members of his own tribe, the Kalenjin, were free to grab land from the
indigenous Ogiek, who have made the forest their home for centuries. *The
Economist* concludes, "In Kenya, it is politically correct to burn forests and
evict indigenous people." Moi's tactics were far from unique among African
strongmen.

The AIDS epidemic brings into relief racism and intolerance on a number of levels. The paranoia, blame, and discrimination that have emanated
from this epidemic have served as a barometer of intolerance in the modern
world. Various groups have felt the backlash, including homosexuals,
Haitians, Africans, intravenous drug users, and the poor. Prostitutes have
been rounded up and summarily executed in Burma, and homosexuals have
been beaten and killed in the United States. This epidemic is the worst in

human history, with profound implications for human rights. We will explore it in depth in Chapter 9.

In summary, it is clear that through history the force of racism has worked on the international stage to elevate certain dominant groups over others; at times producing genocide, though most commonly inflicting damage more furtively through structural violence. The reallocation of the often scant resources this entails has direct implications for the health of those who receive less, in the form of lowered life expectancies, higher infant mortalities, and reduced access to potentially life-saving health care. Rather than stemming from the character deficiencies of any particular group, sources of disparity originate in the complex interplay of the economic, political, health, and social structures of a given society, themselves tracing origins to foreign conquest, slavery, and segregation.

> *Rather than stemming from the character deficiencies of any particular group, sources of disparity originate in the complex interplay of the economic, political, health, and social structures of a given society.*

Part of the solution to the problem is to first recognize it, realize its impact, and then openly discuss it across lines of race, faith, gender, and other differences. That conversation is already occurring in many formats in the United States, including clinical ones (Srinivasan 2001, 1474). It is only fitting to conclude this section by recalling the words of one familiar with the problems engendered by racism.

Martin Luther King Jr won the 1964 Nobel Peace Prize in recognition of his lifetime contribution to nonviolent racial healing. In his *Letter from a Birmingham Jail*, he wrote, "Injustice anywhere is a threat to justice everywhere. We are caught in an inescapable network of mutuality, tied in a single garment of destiny."[2] He dedicated his life to combating the forces of racism and intolerance, following the examples of Jesus Christ and Mahatma Gandhi. In so doing, he helped to raise the debates on race and economic justice to a higher plane, summoning the better angels within us all. By the time of his death in 1968, the Civil Rights Movement had begun to pass him by, responding to more radical elements. King's writings and speeches, however, remain as beacons directing us all toward a better, more inclusive world. He had evolved his civil rights positions from voting rights to economic justice, challenging the more covert structures, still in force, that had institutionalized racism. In an eerily prophetic speech delivered on the rainy night of April 3, 1968, he told his followers that he'd been to the mountain, looked over, and seen the Promised Land. "I may not get there with you," he said. "But I want you to know tonight, that we, as a people, will get to the Promised Land."[2]

The next day he was shot and killed while standing on the balcony of the Lorraine Hotel in Memphis, Tennessee. Although his death has become a part of American history familiar to every school child, few recall the events that brought King to Memphis in the first place. He had answered a call for help from 1,300 of the city's mostly black sanitation, sewer, and road workers in their strike for safer working conditions and decent pay. In a proclamation that echoes from those Memphis streets to the abundant slums of our current world, the sanitation workers carried signs that read simply, "I am a man" (Jordan 1998).

Governance

Governments largely determine the fates of their people. From our review of development and foreign aid, the importance of governance should be abundantly clear—no amount of aid can overcome incompetent governance. Governments that spend too much on the military (Idi Amin's Uganda, Saddam Hussein's Iraq) or on the leaders (Marcos's Philippines) or that mismanage their economies (Mexico, Equatorial Guinea) strangle development, punishing their most vulnerable citizens. Recall Amartya Sen's vision for development in which all people attain the right and ability to live the lives they value. We must recognize that this can only happen when governments foster it.

A broad array of factors account for good governance, not all of which reside with the leadership (Congressional Budget Office [CBO] 1997, xiii). Those in the best position to state what factors are important in governance are those who have seen so much of their aid dollars squandered by a lack thereof—the large donor countries. When officials from the Bush administration designed the millennium challenge account (MCA), they decided to fund only strong, stable governments that would use the funds well (Radelet 2003, 19). According to the MCA, some of the more important factors contributing to good governance include *stability, ruling justly and wisely, sound economic management, and political openness.*

Stability

Countries that have political and social stability tend to develop more rapidly than those plagued by instability and disorder. Seven of the 10 countries with the lowest HDIs in 2002 had recently fought civil wars (UNDP 2002, 16). Political stability is a given for those who live in the West, but not so for most of the world's people. Coups, social upheavals, and civil wars are commonplace in much of sub-Saharan Africa and Central Asia. In addition to the enormous loss of life that such upheavals cost, countries embroiled in struggle do not grow economically. Too often the key institutions important for development are lost, and no foreigners send investment dollars to war zones (CBO 1997, 21). During Mozambique's 16-year civil war, more than 40% of the health centers and schools were destroyed, as were its industries—postwar production decreased by 60% to 80% (UNDP 2002, 16).

Ruling Justly and Wisely

Although a favorite target of the Right and a common scapegoat for all the ills of the third world, corruption is not the dominant factor most suspect. Most countries remain poor for the host of reasons detailed here. Nevertheless, in countries where it is endemic, corruption hinders economic growth and causes damage at every level. Transparency International, a nonprofit group, has long ranked the most corrupt governments; in 2004 it published a corruption "all-star" list of rulers over the past 20 years (Transparency International 2004). Among them, Indonesian President Mohamed Suharto, who stole $15 to $35 billion between 1967 and 1998; the Philippine President Ferdinand Marcos who stole $5 to $10 billion from 1972 to 1986; and the former ruler of Zaire Mobuto Sese Seko, who stole $5 billion from 1965 to 1997. Less successful thieves included Nigeria's Sani Abacha ($2 to $5 billion), Serbia/Yugoslavia's Slobodan Milsevic ($1 billion), and Haiti's Jean-Claude Duvalier ($300 to $800 million).[5] A tragic part of this pattern is the depth of poverty most of these men ruled over. Gross Domestic Product (GDP) per capita in Zaire was just $99 in 2001, that of Haiti was $460, and Nigeria just $319 (Transparency International 2004).

Unfortunately, corruption at the top is not the sole problem. It is the graft that spreads through an entire system that is so cancerous. When landing at Nairobi's Wilson International Airport in 1994, I brought an envelope stuffed with wrinkled $1 bills. When an airport baggage handler told me that my bag of medical supplies would require "customs review," an obvious pretext for extorting money, the envelope quickly improved my fortunes. My supplies and I were very soon on our way; customs, it seemed, was happy. Seven years earlier in Tanzania, I learned not to bite into the rice. Since rice was sold by weight, farmers and everyone else involved in the transaction added small rocks to increase their take. The end product was heavier and hence more valuable, though no friend to molars. Although corruption is prominent in sub-Saharan Africa, it is by no means limited to that continent. Stories from Moscow in the early 1990s invoked memories of Al Capone's Chicago in the 1920s. Only four of the most corrupt countries in Transparency International's 2003 corruption perception index were in sub-Saharan Africa. According to that survey, the 10 most corrupt countries in the world were, in order, Bangladesh, Nigeria, Haiti, Paraguay, Myanmar, Tajikistan, Georgia, Cameroon, Azerbaijan, and Angola (Transparency International 2003). Kenya was 11th, Russia 47th. Further, those who tend to blame all of Africa's problems on corruption should note that African countries are no more corrupt than other countries with the same income level (Sachs 2005a, 312).

To fully comprehend the corrosive quality of graft, imagine every transaction in life requiring a bribe. Commerce as we know it virtually stops. When a fuse blew out on my refrigerator when I was in Tanzania in 1987, it was not sufficient to bribe the regional parts distributor for a replacement. The local police, government regulators, and a series of other "officials" all found ways to get a piece of the action for what they saw as a valuable commodity. In the end, it would have been cheaper to buy a new refrigerator. This culture of graft extends to every aspect of life, and the poorer one is, the more one faces it. Street children living in the mean streets of Nairobi's Kibera slum talk about the brutality of local police, "All they do is take bribes and beat people" (Harding 2002). Police were responsible for more than 90% of Kenya's fatal shootings in 2001 ("Nairobbery" 2000). Graft extends through all levels of some developing countries, destroying any sense of trust and civility. It also strongly dissuades foreign businesses from investing in a country and kills economic growth. Studies have shown that corruption and economic growth are inversely related (Easterly 2002, 241).

Graft extends through all levels of some developing countries, destroying any sense of trust and civility.

Beyond the problems of corruption, poor countries must also spend what little revenue they have wisely. Irresponsible spending and mismanagement leaves precious little for basic services. Unfortunately, a number of countries still spend more on their military than they spend on education or health care for their citizens (Sivard 1996, 44). Honduras spent between 20% to 30% of its budget on the military during the 1980s, relying heavily on aid for support (CBO 1997, 39). A number of African and Middle Eastern rulers have built lavish palaces while letting their people starve. In democracies, civil society organizations and a freestanding media call attention to such abuses and mobilize the citizenry, making such abuses far less common.

Governments have to create the infrastructure for a just and fair society by securing property rights, guaranteeing the validity of contracts, and maintaining fair and strong judicial systems. Imagine spending a lifetime building up a business only to have someone else steal it from you, then glower as their connected friends beat you in a rigged court system. This is commonplace in countries with weak legal systems, such as Kenya.

Governments must also provide the infrastructure within which people and businesses can flourish. Education fosters economic growth, best proven by East Asian countries that invested heavily in education and now reap the benefits (CBO 1997, 22). Expenditures in health and education spread the wealth of economic growth more evenly throughout a population. Roads, ports, communications systems, water, and sewer are all important for development, and invariably come through governments.

Sound Economic Management

Governments also hold the chief responsibility for creating a stable environment for business, which in turn drives the economy. Yet a host of problems plague businesses of all kinds in developing countries.

Thriving black markets undermine economies by acting like a tax on exports (Easterly 2002, 221). Because US dollars can serve as a hedge against deflation of local currencies, they are worth more and people will pay higher than official rates to exchange for them. When in Tanzania in 1987, people in the street offered significantly higher rates for my US dollars than I could find in any bank. Such exchanges seemed like a harmless way to extend my student budget, but the consequences were and remain far-reaching and damaging. Consider the poor farmer who is forced to purchases supplies in the local economy at black market rates but must sell his produce through government-regulated exporters at government-fixed rates. He must pay an artificially higher rate for his needs in local currency but receives a low rate in return for his goods, which are traded in US dollars. In effect, the artificially high price in his home (black) market punishes him, as it does all who sells their wares abroad. Such circumstances strongly hinder export-oriented economic growth and contribute to the stagnation of a number of poor countries—black market premiums caused Ghana's cocoa market collapse in the 1980s (222). Those visiting poor countries can help spur local economies by shunning local black markets.

As discussed previously, trade policies are of great importance to development. Countries that adopt export-oriented trade policies are far more likely to have sustained economic growth than those who keep their economies closed by restricting imports through high tariffs and nontariff barriers. Export-oriented growth fueled the rise of the Asian tigers while China, India, and Israel all showed markedly increased economic growth in the 1980s after their economies became more market oriented (Zakaria 2003, 53). Sachs and Warner found that between 1970 and 1989, poor countries with closed economies grew at 0.7% per year while those with open, export-oriented economies grew at an average of 4.5% per year (CBO 1997, 26).

Additionally, when countries respond to budget shortfalls by printing more money, the value of money falls, triggering inflation. This has been a common problem for a diverse group of countries during the last 30 years. Argentina, Bolivia, Brazil, the Dominican Republic, Ghana, Jamaica, Mexico, Peru, and Zambia, among others, all had two-year periods when inflation averaged more than 40% per year (Easterly 2002, 219). An inflation rate of 40% means that 1 dollar is worth only 60 cents in a year and 36 cents in two years. People have no incentive to save, and foreigners have little reason to invest. Countries cannot grow economically with such inflationary pressures.

The End of History? Liberalism and the Emergence of Democracy

In 1992, the noted scholar Francis Fukuyama presented a forceful argument that history had ended (Fukuyama 1992). Following centuries of governance failures that included monarchism, totalitarianism, socialism,

and communism, liberal democracy had emerged as the ideal means to preserve the rights, dignity, and freedom of man. No other form of governance
has been able to provide what democracy has. Even Islamic theocracy holds
an appeal for a diminishing few. The "last man," Fukuyama said, was a liberal democrat—history was over.

Recent history has provided considerable support to Fukuyama's claim.
Two hundred years after the French Revolution and the ratification of the
US Constitution, the Soviet Union collapsed, signaling the end of the Cold
War and victory for the great experiment with democracy (Fukuyama 1992,
25). In the aftermath of the collapse, democracies sprouted up all over
Eastern Europe and even in Russia in 1991. These events followed years of
upheaval throughout world capitals. Authoritarian governments fell during
the 1970s and 1980s in southern Europe (Portugal, Greece, and Spain) and
Latin America (Peru, Argentina, Uruguay, Brazil, and Chile), and during the
1980s and early 1990s in the Philippines, South Korea, Nicaragua, and
South Africa (13). The emergence of liberal democracies, accompanied by
economic liberalism, has become, according to Fukuyama, "the most
remarkable macropolitical phenomenon of the last four hundred years" (48).

For a given country, the mode of governance is of enormous importance
for both development and poverty eradication. Although some dictators have
bestowed better living conditions and improved economic performance, the
opposite is more commonly true. Lord Acton's dictum applies: power tends
to corrupt, and absolute power corrupts absolutely. As such, governments
headed by monarchs, dictators, or military coup leaders tend to fail and corruption reigns supreme. Modern history has clearly shown how fragile such
leadership is. World War I ended the rule of many European monarchies, and
World War II disposed of the fascists (Zakaria 2003, 86). Systems that incorporate checks on power have worked better over time. The Roman standard,
dividing power among the executive, judicial, and legislative branches, has
enshrined checks against arbitrary power. From Uganda, Kenya, Iraq,
Cambodia, and a host of other modern tragedies, we can see how important
these checks on power are. In governance, democracy—along with civil society and the free press—offers the most effective checks on power.

Yet there is far more to what makes the United States' and other Western
governments strong than democracy alone. Recall that democracy simply
means that individuals have a right to choose their government through free
and fair multiparty elections. This choice has not always produced better
societies—the Nazis won Germany's democratic elections by a large margin
in 1933. However, as author Fareed Zakaria wrote in his brilliant book, *The
Future of Freedom: A Liberal Democracy at Home and Abroad* (Norton
Press, 2003), the real strength of American governance is not the freedoms
that come from its democracy but the individual protections enshrined in
the Bill of Rights. We are in fact less democratic than any other democracy
in the world today, given the restrictions our constitution places on the will

of the majority. Our strength resides in the power of our "constitutional liberalism," defined as the individual "inalienable" rights that are guaranteed by our constitution. These rights are protected from intervention by any force, including the state, church, or society. Our Bill of Rights establishes individual protections that exist despite what the majority thinks. This places human rights within the rule of law—even the state cannot override them.

Democracy and constitutional liberalism may be at odds, as in the example of the Jim Crow laws. The majority in the South would have maintained segregation if asked to vote on it—integration came through other means. President Truman integrated the armed forces through executive fiat, while school desegregation came through a Supreme Court ruling. More democratically, the Civil Rights Act of 1964 came through an act of Congress (Fukuyama 1992, 17). For a long time after the founding of the republic, electoral choice resided only in the hands of rich, white men. Women, blacks, and poor whites were excluded—hardly our modern idea of a participatory democracy. Not until the eve of the Civil War could all white men vote. Blacks acquired that right in 1870, though not for another 96 years in the South. Women only gained suffrage in 1920.

For all of its limitations and flaws, however, democracy has become the world's dominant form of government. According to the UN, 81 countries have taken "significant steps towards democracy" since 1980; 140 of 200 countries in 2002 held multiparty elections, a greater number than at any time in history (UNDP 2002, 1). During this span, civilian-run regimes replaced military ones in 33 countries. This recent "third wave" of democratization has produced only the most recent change in a long succession of countries' ascension toward democracy. In 1790, there were only three: the United States, France, and Switzerland (Fukuyama 1992, 48).

Although we in the United States think of democracy as a static system, it is not. It is a concept that continues to evolve over time in theory and in practice. In a historic address before the US Congress in 1990, Vaclav Havel, the newly elected president of Czechoslovakia, said, "Democracy in the full sense of the word will always be no more than an idea; one may approach it as one would a horizon, in ways that may be better or worse, but it can never be fully attained" (Noviny 1995, 41). As a philosopher, playwright, and political activist, Havel had spent a lifetime fighting the communists, and admiring the political freedoms of the West from afar, for a long time from prison. Those under the yoke of communism had a greater appreciation for the beauty of American democracy than those who have known no other form of governance. Havel acknowledged the debt the world owed the United States for forging ahead with such a grand experiment and "inspiring" the world. However, Havel also reminded the Congress that the United States had a 200-year head start over most of the world's democracies. Many countries, including those in Africa, Latin America, and Eastern Europe, were wrestling with the inevitable problems that accompany this trend. Just as the United States had grappled with a host of difficulties, even fought a bloody civil war, all emerging democracies require time to build stable democracies and liberal societies.

Accompanying the surge of democracy has been the spread of economic liberalism. Following Japan's stunning rise to economic prominence following World War II, many other countries in East Asia industrialized, opened up their economies, and joined the global capitalist economic system (Fukuyama 1992, 41). The resultant "East Asian miracle" was not lost on China or other states with central control of their economies, chiefly those in Latin America. The former USSR had also come to recognize that its economic policies could not compete with the West. Gorbachov's perestroika and glasnost inadvertently opened the doors to political freedoms from which the Soviet Union and bloc countries could never retreat. Their fall became inevitable, particularly when these freedoms were combined with falling oil revenues and rising external debt (Sachs 2005a, 132). China's leadership had closely observed the events leading up to the collapse, slowly opening up its economy while holding tightly to power, most clearly shown in Tiananmen Square in 1989. As incomes in China rise, individual liberties inevitably follow. Rich countries invariably find democracy.

As those in China will likely see over the next generation, democracies give people the opportunity to shape their lives according to what they value. Democracies avail the citizenry a means of voicing concerns that is unavailable to those under authoritarian regimes. Repressed frustration and anger always find a vent, often in the form of bloody revolutions that overthrow dictatorships. Although riots and strikes are far more common in democracies—as are changes in government, they do not slow economic growth as they do in dictatorships, which are also more prone to war (UNDP 2002, 57).

Democracy also protects people from catastrophes such as famines. Amartya Sen has argued that although famines may kill millions of poor people, they rarely reach the rulers. In fact, he argues, famines are entirely avoidable if governments have the incentive to act (Sen 1993, 43). Democratic countries with freestanding presses rarely experience famines, primarily because democratically elected rulers have to be more responsive to the concerns of their constituencies. India has experienced no famine since it won its independence from the British in 1947. By contrast, famines have long characterized those living under colonial or authoritarian rule. While under British rule, Ireland's famine of 1846 to 1850 killed 1 million people, transformed Irish society, and spawned millions of émigrés to the United States and Canada. Soviet leader Joseph Stalin tried to break Ukrainian resistance by imposing policies that caused a famine that killed 5 to 10 million Ukrains between 1923 and 1933.[6] Chairman Mao's disastrous Great Leap Forward, launched in 1958, caused the worst famine in human history, killing 30 million Chinese. The previous worst famine had also occurred in China, killing

10 million in 1870 (Kristof and Wudunn 1995, 66). Recent history has shown us famines in Biafra and Bangladesh in the 1970s, Ethiopia in the 1980s, Somalia and North Korea in the 1990s, and Iraq, Mozambique, North Korea, Sudan, and Angola in the 2000s (Fackler 2002). None of these countries are blessed with democratic leadership.

Democracies are also better at informing the public about health issues such as the benefits of limiting family size, the benefits of breast feeding, and the dangers of unprotected sex (UNDP 2002, 58). In democracies, people enjoy a better quality of life through participation in the decisions that affect their lives. Despite problems of entrenched elites and the influence of special interests, it is still easier for the poor to voice their concerns and lobby for the funding to broaden their political and economic opportunities (3).

> *There is no evidence to support the idea that robust economic growth only happens in democracies.*

What is the best system of governance for sustained economic growth, itself the best source of poverty eradication and development? One would think democracy. All but two of the world's richest countries have the most democratic regimes, and 42 of the 48 countries with high human development ratings are democracies (UNDP 2002, 56). However, there is no evidence to support the idea that robust economic growth only happens in democracies. Several dictatorships have led their countries to strong growth. Strong regimes, the argument goes, can more easily spurn interest groups. The broad inclusiveness of democracy, on the other hand, requires more equitable sharing, helping the future more than the present. Dictatorships have registered some of the best growth (South Korea and China) and some of the worst (Uganda and Iraq). Democratic countries avoid the extremes, tending to cluster around the middle. It is clear, however, that as countries gain wealth, they are more likely to become and remain democratic.

Democracy and Capitalism

Capitalism has become the dominant economic system in the world, largely paving the way for democracy and serving as the most important force shaping our world order. As Fareed Zakaria writes, "Nothing has shaped the modern world more powerfully than capitalism, destroying as it has the millennia-old patterns of economic, social, and political life" (Zakaria 2003, 45). In societies that protected property rights, such as England, a new class of wealthy and powerful men emerged. Because they benefited from the individual liberties and market conditions that were essential to the success of capitalism, they lobbied for the reforms that caused these characteristics to multiply. As Zakaria said, "No bourgeoisie, no democracy" (47).

The ties between capitalism and democracy remain strong. The single most important factor in determining whether a country will sustain its democratic impulses is its per capita GDP. Prezeworski and Limongi calculated the odds of a country sustaining a democracy for a given GDP per capita income level (Zakaria 2003, 69). When national GDP per capita was under $1,500, the regime had a life expectancy of 8 years; between $1,500 and $3,000, it lasted 18 years. Once over $6,000, the odds of the regime failing were 1 in 500. None have ever failed with income levels above $9,000, with a total of 32 regimes having existed continuously for 736 years. This trend has held up through time and through markedly differing regions, from early Western Europe to postcommunist Eastern Europe.

When Church and State Aren't Separate: The Troubled Middle East

When the Roman Emperor Constantine moved the capital from Rome to Byzantium (later renamed Constantinople) near the Black Sea in AD 324, he initiated one of the most important movements in history (Zakaria 2003, 29). The bishop of Rome did not go with him, and the separation between church and state had begun. For the next 1,500 years in Europe, the church and state struggled against each other for power, and from these struggles came the origins of liberalism. Later struggles between monarchs and aristocrats, Protestants and Catholics, businesses and the state produced added pressure for individual liberties, first in England and later in the United States (31). By 1648 at the end of the wars resulting from the Reformation, the separation of church and state in wider Christendom had become complete and irrevocable. The path in the West was clear for the rise of capitalism.

By contrast, a number of predominantly Muslim countries in the Middle East have never made a similar separation. Although most of the world's Muslims, including those living in Turkey, Indonesia, Pakistan, Bangladesh, and India, live in secular societies, most Middle Eastern Muslims live in countries trending toward fundamentalism, among them, Iran, Egypt, Syria, and the Persian Gulf states. None of the 22 members of the Arab League are electoral democracies, that compared to 63% of the countries in the rest of the world (Zakaria 2003, 129). In these countries, Islam offers no separation between the law of the church and that of the state. There is only the *sharia*, the divine law that governs all aspects of life, whether civil, criminal, economic, constitutional, or spiritual. This aspect still characterizes most Islamic countries, and simultaneously restricts their development. This is to say nothing against Islam, which is a noble and worthy faith. However, just as the separation of Christianity from Western governments freed men to develop more tolerant and liberal forms of government, Islam has proven equally restrictive and intolerant. Much of the "fundamentalist" movement in Islam calls for a return to more restrictive interpretations of the Koran and, according to author Bernard Lewis, to "remove the alien and pagan laws and customs imposed by foreign imperialists and native reformers" (Lewis 2002, 105).

Reformers adhering to these beliefs currently hold significant power in Iran, the Sudan, and, to a lesser degree, in Afghanistan.

The problems stemming from such close ties between Islam and state governments are legion. The most glaring problem is the restriction of the freedoms of women, most apparent in countries under the sway of more fundamentalist elements. It is difficult to advance for societies in which half its members remain largely illiterate and subjugated. Ayatolla Khomeini spoke with anger about the "inevitable immorality" that would follow women teaching young boys. Women still cannot vote in Brunei Darussalam, Kuwait, Oman, Qatar, Saudi Arabia, or the United Arab Emirates (UNDP 2002, 3). It follows that when governments must follow 1,200-year-old laws, they will be hindered in a modern world—economically, socially, and politically. The entrepreneurs' spirit—the ability to think freely and creatively and to adapt to changing circumstances and environments—will be compromised, as will the opportunity to develop a strong, vibrant middle class upon which solid governments rely. Lewis writes that the problems of the Muslim world stem from a "lack of freedom—freedom of the mind to question and inquire and speak; freedom of the economy from corrupt and pervasive mismanagement; freedom of women from male oppression; freedom of citizens from tyranny" (Lewis 2002, 159).

Such a state serves as a striking contrast to an earlier time, when the Middle East was the center of civilization, right up until 1000–1200 AD. It was a stunning setback when Europeans outmaneuvered and outgunned Muslim opposition following the Ottomans. Somewhere around 1200–1400 A.D. power shifted to the West, and it has never returned to an increasingly dysfunctional Muslim world.

Beyond the restrictions imposed by religion, the region faces a huge array of other problems, largely due to its governments. The region has degenerated into impoverishment, backwardness, and repression. Far from its enlightened past, it is now the home to "flag-burners, fiery mullahs, and suicide bombers" (Zakaria 2003, 127). Among them, a vast demographic bulge of young men raised on anti-Semitic and anti-US rhetoric used by their leaders to cover their own inadequacies. These young men dislike the regimes that rule them and blame the United States and Israel for supporting them. Lacking a political voice, they gravitate toward fundamentalists who offer the very thing their governments deny—an opportunity to participate (139). Because the religious community offers the one place where people can vent their frustrations, the Mosque spawned the more radical elements. It was of little surprise when US Marines in Iraq received enemy fire from within Mosques.

Further, the region did not grow economically as did those in the West, which developed the institutions required for good governance. Instead, many of the region's rulers simply dug holes in the ground, reaping unimaginable oil wealth (Saudi's King Fahd was worth $25 billion prior to his death in 2005) that afforded them the opportunity to buy off their people. As Zakaria says, "regimes that get rich through natural resources tend never to develop, modernize, or gain legitimacy." The easy money that flows from oil allows governments to avoid taxing their people and, in return, provide them with "accountability, transparency, even representation." Jeffrey Sachs and Andrew Warner looked at 97 developing countries over 20 years and found that those countries with the richest mineral, agricultural, and fuel resources were most likely to fail economically, because these resources "tend to impede the development of modern political institutions, laws, and bureaucracies" (Zakaria 2003, 74).

A lack of democracy is not the chief problem of the Middle East, it is a lack of constitutional liberalism and the institutions required to support it. Many of the region's governments have been appropriately described as "stuck in a time warp" (Zakaria 2003, 131). One can only hope that democracy and liberalism will flourish somewhere in the region, a process that seems increasingly unlikely in Iraq, given the current widespread chaos. The next best hope would be that the region's theocracies will utterly discredit themselves, as is already occurring in Iran. Ultimately, a region with economies based on a single, finite resource will have to adapt to a changing world, starting by changing its fundamental political structures. Many of these changes will be painful, and in all probability, violent. Hopefully, the region's wealthy and omnipotent leaders will start by looking within.

Africa

The best example of governments that have failed on a massive scale is in sub-Saharan Africa, which we have discussed already. Although corruption is most frequently cited as causative, Africa's poor governance stems primarily from its widespread poverty. Low incomes mean low tax receipts, leaving precious little for governments to work with. Rising incomes produce a more literate and responsible society better able to keep a watchful eye on government, and higher tax revenues provide funds for improved infrastructure, professional staff, and better communication within government. According to Jeffrey Sachs, "African governance is poor because Africa is poor" (Sachs 2005a, 312). Non-African countries with similar levels of income have similar governance. African countries do have slower economic growth than countries in other parts of the world with similar levels of income and governance, but this is primarily due to the additional burdens of African geography, disease, and poor infrastructure. Ultimately, African governments will continue to receive an inordinate share of the blame for the ongoing problems throughout the continent. Yet these problems will continue no matter who is in power as long as the continent remains trapped in poverty.

Violence and Militarism

Peace has yet to come to Flanders, one of the great battlegrounds of the First World War. Unexploded shells from World Wars I and II, even from the 19th century Napoleonic wars, still rise from the mud—either from frost upheavals or farmers' ploughs—to claim lives. As of the late 1990s, 73 Belgian soldiers and civilians comprising World War I's last active detachment still worked full-time to collect the unexploded ordinance, roughly 3,000 shells each year, almost all of which had outlived its builders. As one bomb disposal commander said, "For us, the First World War has not stopped" (Fesperman 1996). One tenth of the shells from World War I contained poison gas. As in Flanders, mines laid during conflicts in Cambodia and Afghanistan, Iraq, and Angola still kill and maim years after the hostilities have ended (Stover et al 1994, 331). Land mines still plague 82 countries and cause 15,000 to 20,000 casualties each year, often poor farmers and their families.[7]

As Flanders and countless other battlefields have shown, war is the deadliest business. July 1917 saw 250,000 British troops die capturing just a few square miles of mud around the Belgian village of Passchendaele, representing just one episode of futility brought by war. Roughly 20 million people died in World War I (Sivard 1996, 18); 50 million were lost in the Second World War ("Concerns Over WWII" 1995). Both wars were part of history's bloodiest century, in which nearly 110 million died in conflict. Millions more died in the great purges of Stalin and Mao, while famines stemming from conflict or genocide claimed another 40 million more lives (WHO 2002a, 218).

Genocide itself is a 20th century term, born in the Turkish killing of 1 million Armenians in 1915 and first uttered during the Holocaust. However, despite frequent proclamations of "Never again" by a succession of American presidents and other world leaders, the term has since surfaced recurrently to describe the large-scale killings in Cambodia, Iraq, Bosnia, and Rwanda (Power 2002, 17). The only US citizen to remain in Rwanda throughout the genocide, Carl Wilkens, commented, "we've got to recognize in each one of us, there's such a potential for good and there's such a potential for evil . . ." ("Ghosts of Rwanda" 2004). That evil has shown no signs of abating.

The 20th century saw more than 250 wars, with nearly six times as many deaths per war as occurred in the 19th century.

Conflicts became more frequent and more deadly during the latter half of the last century. The 20th century saw more than 250 wars, with nearly six times as many deaths per war as occurred in the 19th century (Sivard 1996, 7). Conflicts now occur almost exclusively within states and increasingly target civilians, who now comprise more than 90% of war-related casualties (17). Half of all civilian war casualties are children (UNDP 2002, 11). The WHO estimates that 310,000 people died from war-related injuries in 2000 alone, with more than half occurring in Africa (WHO 2002a, 217, 282). Like most other problems, wars occur far more often in poor countries than in wealthy ones. Less than 1,000 of the 310,000 deaths in 2000 occurred in high-income countries (282).

A host of forces fuel conflict, with poverty chief among them. Scarcity triggers competition between disparate groups, often with lethal consequences. In wealthy democracies, competing groups fight politically through the ballot box. In nonrepresentative states, people often resort to violence. One author found more than 50 ethnicity-based conflicts in 1993 to 1994 alone (Easterly 2002, 268). Recent conflicts in Rwanda, East Timor, Nigeria, Bosnia, Kosovo, and the Democratic Republic of the Congo all had twin economic and ethnic forces driving the violence. Other forces also trigger conflict: stark inequalities, particularly between distinct population groups; unequal access to power; unequal access to and control of natural resources, eg, diamonds in Angola, oil in Sudan, and drugs in Afghanistan; and ethnic tensions, political repression, and the ready availability of small arms (WHO 2002a, 220).

Death on a large scale is not the sole consequence of conflict. Millions become disabled from physical or psychological trauma. Rape has long served as an instrument of intimidation and demoralization in warfare in addition to spreading communicable disease. Survivors commonly suffer from life-altering psychological trauma and are often ostracized from their communities. Mutilations have become a common practice in some recent conflicts as another means of demoralizing the enemy: cutting off ears or lips during Mozambique's civil war, and severing limbs in Sierra Leone (WHO 2002a, 224). Torture has also been widespread in recent years. Amnesty International found "widespread" practice of torture in more than 70 countries in 2000, with torture-induced deaths in 80 countries (219). Many of these victims suffer from prolonged posttraumatic stress disorder, depression, and anxiety (Shrestha et al 1998, 443).

Accompanying the prodigious rise in the number of internal conflicts has been a marked increase in the number of refugees and internally displaced persons, largely in the developing world. In 1970, 2.5 million people sought refuge across borders. By 1997, that number had risen to 23 million. During the early 1990s, 20 to 30 million people were internally displaced at any given time, most fleeing conflict. Unlike refugees, those internally displaced people often suffer from malnutrition and communicable disease and remain at considerable risk of ongoing violence, stalked by those (often government forces) within their own borders. Mortality rates for refugees and internally displaced persons typically soar, at times up to 60 times higher than the norm (WHO 2002a, 225). Recall the 1.5 million Kurds who fled into the mountains from Saddam Hussein following the Gulf War in 1991 and the thousands of Rwandan refugees who fled to Goma, Zaire, from the Hutu killing squads in 1994. At highest risk are the children, who commonly die from malnutrition and diarrhea.

War also destroys the infrastructures that sustain quality of life: health care systems, schools, industries, and water and sanitation systems. Recent internal conflicts in Haiti, Mozambique, Sudan, and the Congo have produced deplorable health indices in their respective populations. In and after wars, childhood immunization and life expectancy commonly plummet, while infant mortality, maternal mortality, and communicable disease outbreaks skyrocket. Preventable illnesses like measles, tetanus, malaria, tuberculosis, and diphtheria increase, as do sexually transmitted diseases. AIDS thrives in conflict, partly because of the rapes that increasingly accompany war and partly because conflict disrupts economies, forcing more women into prostitution (WHO 2002a, 223). Infectious illnesses of all types thrive during conflict for a host of reasons. War disrupts basic services like immunizations and mosquito spraying while starvation-induced immunodeficiency and overcrowding in refugee camps makes war-torn populations far more vulnerable. Many conflicts claim more victims after the fighting stops.

The Business of War

Given the millions of deaths and disabilities that collective violence has spawned through the ages, it is no wonder that countries choose to invest in arms. As a close friend and West Point graduate Malcolm Visser often says, "There are wolves out there." The 20th century showed us a virtual parade of wolves, headed by Hitler, Hussein, Pol Pot, Stalin, Bagosora (Rwanda), and Milosevic. Virtually all countries have experienced the horrors of war, so it is no surprise how heavily armed our modern world has become. However, the imminent threat of instability and war has spurred an arms industry that has become self-perpetuating. Conflicts have grown more frequent and more deadly in part due to the global proliferation of arms.

Dwight Eisenhower famously warned of the dangers of the "military-industrial complex." Arms manufacturing in the United States and other developed countries is big business, accounting for $29 billion in annual sales. Despite the collapse of the Soviet Union, the main protagonist of the United States in the arms race, the manufacturing and export of arms has proceeded apace. As state military budgets shrank in the 1990s, arms manufacturers simply shipped their wares overseas. The five permanent members of the UN Security Council—the United States, the United Kingdom, France, China, and Russia—produced more than 70% of the world's conventional arms for export in 2002 (Stohl 2003). At the head of the pack stands the United States, by far the global leader in arms manufacturing and sales. Its 2002 sales stood at $13.3 billion, or 45% of the total of world sales. The United States is also responsible for half the arms sales to developing countries—$8.6 billion in 2002 alone—helping to destabilize entire regions and fuel deadly conflicts (Stohl 2003).

Many of these weapons eventually find their way into the hands of terrorists, rebel groups, or despotic governments that use them to intimidate and kill their own people. Governments of Afghanistan, Iraq, Liberia, Columbia, and Uganda have used US arms to commit abuses, as have terrorist groups such as al Qaeda and insurgents in Sri Lanka and the Philippines (Stohl 2003). During 1993 to 1994, US-supplied weapons were used on one or both sides of 45 of the 50 largest ethnic or territorial conflicts (Kim et al 2000, 212).

The United States exports 400,000 small arms annually. Small arms from all countries now kill half a million people a year, or roughly one person every minute (UNDP 2005, 173). In Jamaica, Kenya, Haiti, Somalia, and a host of other countries, escalating arms trafficking–almost always originating through state-sanctioned sales–have markedly increased regional violence and instability. Some of those arms, along with far more sophisticated and deadly weapons systems, increasingly boomerang back on US soldiers. Those in the military call it "blow-back," a term defined as the use of American-made weapons against American troops. In almost every conflict in which the United States has sent troops since 1989–Panama, Haiti, Somalia, Afghanistan, Iraq, and Bosnia–US forces have faced US-made weapons. In one of the world's most troubled regions, the Middle East/North Africa, the United States delivered $34.4 billion worth of arms from 1987 to 1994 alone (Sennott 1996, B1).

US Military Expenditures and Choices

The Bush administration's fiscal year 2005 military budget called for $430 billion in expenditures, not including the costs of the ongoing conflicts in Iraq and Afghanistan (Corbin and Pemberton 2004). This amount also does not include the amount of the federal debt incurred through military spending, which would add at least another $100 billion, nor does it include military retirement pay, veterans' benefits, foreign military aid, the space program, peacekeeping, and other expenditures (Center for Defense Information [CDI] 2002, 34). These additional costs brought the 2005 fiscal year defense and defense-related budget to more than $600 billion, with additional funds required for Iraq and Afghanistan.

The United States increased its military expenditures by 50% between 2000 and 2004, primarily in response to the attacks on September 11, 2001, and the subsequent war on terrorism (Corbin and Pemberton 2004). However, even though a subsequent commission found considerable weaknesses in domestic intelligence and security, most budgetary increases have gone toward traditional military expenditures. The Bush administration's 2005 budget requested seven times more for military expenditures than for domestic homeland security.

Additionally, much of the military expenditures cover conventional large-scale opposition that the United States no longer faces. According to the Center for Defense Information's Marcus Corbin, funds would be more wisely spent restructuring and retraining forces for counterterrorism and smaller-scale peace and security operations, improving flack jackets, reinforcing truck armor, and developing helicopter protection systems (Corbin and Levitsky 2003). Marines in Iraq echoed these sentiments in widely publicized comments to Secretary of Defense Donald Rumsfeld in December 2004. Corbin adds, more should be spent on shoring up our reserve to protect ourselves and prepare for future threats stemming from failed states and much less spent on the "obsolete" offensive and nuclear capabilities where we have been spending most defense dollars. On October 26, 2001, the Pentagon awarded $200 billion (the largest military contract in history) to Lockheed Martin to build the F-35 "joint-strike fighter," an aircraft that will no doubt further American and its allies' air supremacy but add little to our ability to fight insurgents in Baghdad or Kabul.

When we compare national military expenditures, the United States is by far the world leader, eclipsing all other NATO member countries combined and US enemies by a factor of 20. When strictly viewing traditional tallies of military expenditures, the United States in 2002 spent $349 billion. By contrast, six countries with historically poor relationships with the United States—Iran, North Korea, Syria, Cuba, Sudan, and Libya—spent a combined $15 billion. US allies spent a combined $257 billion, while other strategically important countries spent a combined $159 billion, including China ($51 billion), Russia ($51 billion), Saudi Arabia ($22 billion), India ($14 billion), Israel ($10), Taiwan ($8 billion), and Pakistan ($3 billion). Despite the huge imbalance, these expenditures still do not tell the entire story of US dominance. Many other countries rely on outdated and poorly maintained weaponry and lack US technology, training, and coordination. These spending disparities are reflected in the United States' vast superiority in numbers and quality of warships, helicopters, tanks, armored vehicles, and airplanes (Corbin and Levitsky 2003, 4). In short, there is no country in the world that can challenge US military supremacy in a conventional war. Present spending levels, even during current conflicts in Iraq and Afghanistan, are difficult to justify.

All governmental expenditures reflect choices made by those in power. In the United States those choices have remained surprisingly constant through time. In 2003, the US government spent $2.2 trillion, with roughly 60% spent on "mandatory" aspects such as Medicare, Medicaid, Social Security, and interest payments on the national debt and 40% on "discretionary" programs, which include everything else. In 2003, nearly half of the $860 billion available for discretionary spending ($425 billion) was spent on national defense. By contrast, all other areas received paltry amounts, including transportation ($61 billion), education ($52 billion), health ($44 billion), housing assistance ($34 billion), justice ($33 billion), environment ($29 billion), and veterans' benefits and services ($25 billion) (Corbin and Levitsky 2003, 4). Areas of government spending that give life value have often been shortchanged because inordinate amounts are spent on military expenditures. Building roads, protecting the environment, providing housing and education for the less fortunate, and enforcing the law all fall under budget-cutting axes, while far too many pork-laden military programs receive little scrutiny.

Such trends have long existed for a number of reasons, some quite valid. The United States has carried an inordinate amount of responsibility to safeguard the world for decades. Scandinavian countries that spend large percentages of GDP on foreign aid have long done so under the protective cover of the US military. Troop deployments from Asia to Europe, to the Caribbean have enhanced global security, as have US warships. Lacking a police force, shipping lanes would quickly revert to the piracy that was the norm before the British began to police them. Less principled powers such as Iraq, the former Soviet Union, Libya, or North Korea would certainly have taken advantage of a power vacuum if the United States ever scaled back its forces.

However, two essential questions remain. First, given the enormous differentials that exist between the United States and its enemies, do we need to spend as much as we do on the military, even in times of war? The short answer is no. As CDI and others have shown, we could make significant cuts while shifting portions of the existing military budget to more effectively counter the main threats to US security now, primarily terrorism and failed states such as Afghanistan.

It makes sense that the United States might make more progress by shifting funds from its enormous military budget to its development budget, helping countries become more open, democratic, and better able to provide for their citizens.

Second, are there other ways to enhance global security than through military spending? To answer this question, recall from the introduction to this book that the CIA found that in every instance of the US military becoming entangled in a foreign war from 1960 to 1994 the war had begun in a failed state (Sachs 2001a). A failed state is one characterized by war, genocide, or political overthrow and often follows three common elements: a lack of free trade, a lack of democracy, and a high infant mortality rate. In short, states that are poor, closed, and fail to listen to their people tend to fail, often precipitating US military involvement. As such, it makes sense that the United States might make more progress by shifting funds from its enormous military budget to its development budget, helping countries become more open, democratic, and better able to provide for their citizens. President Bush was right in 2002 when he made significant increases for foreign aid and more rational means of choosing aid recipients. Yet, even after the millennium challenge account is fully funded (which seems increasingly unlikely), the United States will still be the second from the bottom in donations in the OECD. We could do so much more in the world by redirecting some of our military funding toward rational aid to poor states that tend to fail. The Reality of Aid Project concluded that the United States in the 1990s spent roughly 33 times as much on its military as it spent on aid (Randel et al 2002, 155). These patterns persist today; in 2004 the United States spent 30 times more on the military

($450 billion) than on foreign aid ($15 billion) (Sachs 2005a, 329). In his book, *The Sorrows of Empire*, author Chalmers Johnson wrote, "We now station innumerably more uniformed military officers than civilian diplomats, aid workers, or environmental specialists in foreign countries— a point not lost on the lands to which they are assigned (2004, 4).

Although the nation remains divided on the rationale for the war in Iraq, some have rightly questioned whether the United States was right to mobilize world donors to give such a large amount of aid to one middle-income country, while calls from so many poor countries went unheeded (Singh 2003, 1672). The US government's investment thus far in Iraq must give those in poor countries pause. Iraq sits on the world's second largest oil reserve and is far from poor (Sachs 2003). Other countries like Rwanda, Sierra Leone, and Somalia have far lower life expectancies and higher infant mortalities than Iraq, and these countries pose ideal havens for terrorists. Yet they receive little international attention and aid. Iraq may or may not have posed a significant threat to the world, and the grand plan to establish a model democracy in the troubled Middle East certainly has merit. Yet no one country should soak up so much of the available international aid that others suffer inordinately, as is occurring now.

Given such a dichotomy between goals and actual funding, why do we still continue to spend as much as we do on the military? This gets back to our first question. Beyond the need to maintain a strong global military presence, there are other, more powerful forces at work. The industries that make the tanks, jet fighters, bombs, and missile guidance systems are multibillion-dollar firms that wield enormous clout in Washington. Department of Defense (DoD) contracts create thousands of US jobs and keep sizeable industries running strong profit margins. Naturally, some of these profits find their way to lobbyists and political campaigns. In 2002 Lockheed Martin had $17 billion of DoD contracts and contributed $8.7 million to political campaigns, while Boeing had $16.6 billion worth of DoD contracts and contributed $1.1 million to political campaigns (Corbin and Levitsky 2003, 7). Other familiar names had similarly large DoD contracts and large campaign contributions: Northrup Gruman Corporation ($8.7 billion/$4.8 million), Raytheon ($7.0 billion/$4.0 million), and General Dynamics Corporation ($7.0 billion/$5.1 million). Just as in other sectors, large industries exert significant influence over the political process, keeping their interests in the forefront of politicians' minds.

It takes a courageous politician to oppose the wealth of the defense industry. Those seeking the highest office surely know that the electorally dense states of California, Texas, and Florida receive the most lucrative military contracts (CDI 2002, 30). No presidential candidate will campaign in Florida stating he wants to cut the military. In the 2004 US presidential election, the only plausible candidate to take this position was the one with no chance of winning—Ralph Nader. Similarly, no senator or congressmen will oppose lucrative defense contracts for his or her state. The resultant job and revenue loss would spell a certain end to that political career.

Even after the end of the Cold War, the government found ways to maintain defense spending; in part because of the long-term stability that this spending has brought to the US economy (CDI 2002, 35). In 1996, Congress created the Defense Export Loan Guarantee Program, which helped finance US weapons sales to foreign governments, with a subsequent increase in US weapons market share (Kim et al 2000, 211). While "military aid" is traditionally left out of "foreign aid" tallies, it represents one of largest categories in US aid disbursements, comprising $7.1 billion in 2001 and 2002 (CDI 2002, 34), and $4.8 billion (23% of the aid budget) in 2003 (Congressional Research Service [CRS] 2004, 29). The Foreign Military Financing (FMF) Program provides grants and loans allowing foreign governments (chiefly Israel and Egypt) to purchase US-manufactured military equipment, driving the US economy (CBO 1997, 13). Manufacturers of high-tech jets, tanks, and missiles sell their wares abroad and then require government support to develop the next generation to stay one step ahead of the competition—which we just armed. The rationale strains logic. Former assistant secretary of defense Lawrence Korb said, "The brakes are off the system . . . It has become a money game: an absurd spiral in which we export arms only to develop more sophisticated ones to counter those spread out all over the world. . . . It is a frightening trend that undermines our moral authority in the New World Order. It is very hard for us to tell other people—the Russians, the Chinese, the French—not to sell arms, when we are out there peddling and fighting to control the market" (Sennott 1996, B1).

In their respective farewell addresses in 1796 and 1961, Presidents Washington and Eisenhower, each of whom knew the bitter taste of war from personal experience, warned future generations of the dangers of an expanding military. Washington warned that "overgrown military establishments" were "inauspicious to liberty," and Eisenhower of a "disastrous rise of misplaced power" of the "military-industrial complex" (Johnson 2004, 39). Both were prescient. At the time of the September 11, 2001, attacks, the United States had become a true "empire" with more than 250,000 military personnel deployed around the world in at least 725 overseas bases, often on prime real estate, valued at $118 billion (24, 156, 190). While some bases are needed, many others serve more as sources of angst for host nationals or vacation retreats for upper echelon military brass than as strategic bulwarks against America's enemies in the world. All of these bases add to the bottom line of the Pentagon, which has continued to rise.

Yet for all the hundreds of billions spent annually on our increasingly militaristic worldview, there is another side to the equation: the social side. For every submarine, missile, or nuclear warhead purchased, there are many fewer schools built, fewer babies vaccinated, fewer mothers attended by qualified midwives during childbirth. As Nobel Peace Laureate Oscar Arias

Sanchez says, "It is the greed of the arms trade that threatens our common future in a world where 900 million adults do not know how to read or write, one billion people do not have access to potable water. The arms merchants bear much of the blame for this poverty. . . . Sadly, the peace dividends seem to have escaped our grasp" (Sennott 1996, B1).

We fund our vast military at the expense of other priorities, mortgaging our collective future in the process. Roughly half of the world's countries spend more on defense than on health (Sivard 1996, 39). President Eisenhower said in April 1953, "Every gun that is made, every warship launched, every rocket fired signifies in the final sense a theft from those who hunger and are not fed, those who are cold and are not clothed. This world in arms is not spending money alone. It is spending the sweat of its laborers, the genius of its scientists and the hopes of its children" (Sidel 1988, 442).

No one would sensibly argue that we should gut the strong military that has maintained US and global security for nearly a century. Yet there is considerable room to reallocate funding, both within the United States and abroad. By shifting more current military spending toward domestic security and preparation for the small scale, intra-state conflicts that most threaten our current security, we can better prepare and safeguard our troops. By redirecting some funds from large-scale conventional military preparations toward rational and well-targeted development, we can better prevent the next conflict from occurring.

Endnotes

1. See *The Coming Plague: Newly Emerging Diseases in a World Out of Balance* by Laurie Garrett (Penguin Books, 1994) for the best summary of recent plagues, though not including SARS.
2. Excerpt from Martin Luther King, "Letter from a Birmingham Jail," available online at http://almaz.com/nobel/peace/MLK-jail.html.
3. Information from the faculty web page of Professor Gerhard Rempel at Western New England Collage at http://mars.acnet.wnec.edu/~grempel/courses/wc2/lectures/industrialrev.html.
4. Information from a BBC report from São Paulo, October 4, 2002.
5. Other notables include Peru's Alberto Fujimori ($600 million); Ukraine's Pavol Lazarenko ($114–200 million); Nicaragua's Arnoldo Aleman ($100 million); and the Philippines' Joseph Estrada ($70–80 million).
6. Information from the Info Ukes web site at http://www.infoukes.com/history/famine.
7. For more information see the International Campaign to Ban Landmines web site at http://www.icbl.org/lm/2003/findings.html.

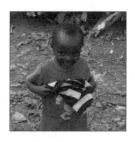

Chapter 8

Forces of Disparity III: Children, Sexism, Population, Nature, and Infectious Diseases

Without a global revolution in the sphere of human consciousness, nothing will change for the better in the sphere of our being as humans, and the catastrophe toward which this world is headed, whether it be ecological, social, demographic, or a general breakdown of civilization, will be unavoidable.

—Vaclav Havel, former Prime Minister, Czech Republic

One love, one heart
Let's get together and feel all right
Hear the children crying (One love)
Hear the children crying (One heart)
Sayin', "Give thanks and praise to the Lord
and I will feel all right."
Sayin', "Let's get together and feel all right."

—Bob Marley

Of the remaining forces that determine the fate of the world's poor, the vulnerability of children, sexism, population pressures, geography, and infectious diseases all take their toll. The world's children bear

an inordinate share of this burden and their story is highlighted here.
Women comprise the world's most discriminated against group and
shoulder the main burden of raising the world's children. When they
suffer, so do the children. Population growth is another force that
exerts its most harmful effects on the poor, who rely on larger families to
ensure against those who will inevitably be lost at young ages. Nature,
with water and sanitation control in particular, also contributes to
health and illness globally. Geography plays an underappreciated role
in fostering poverty and wealth differentials, with global concentrations
of wealth all assuming a number of similar geographic and climatic
features. Finally, the major infectious diseases of our world target
the poor with a relentless predilection. Malaria, tuberculosis, and
a host of "tropical" illnesses serve to sicken and kill millions while
slowing economic growth of entire world regions, particularly that
of sub-Saharan Africa. Given the enormity of the AIDS crisis and its
importance in determining the fate of untold millions, we focus on
this epidemic in the next chapter.

The War on Children

Perhaps the most tragic aspect of poverty is the toll it exacts from the
world's children. In the developing world, 27,000 children under the age of
five die every single day from preventable or treatable causes, such as diarrhea, acute respiratory illness, or malaria.[1] Put another way, a child under
age five dies needlessly every three seconds. More than half of these deaths
are associated with malnutrition (UNICEF 2001; Pelletier et al 1993, 1130).
Nutritionally acquired immunodeficiency syndrome (NAIDS) has stalked the
poor for centuries. With weakened immune systems from malnutrition,
children get sicker more frequently, stay sicker longer, and suffer from more
serious disease (Strickland 2000, 968). Globally, 177 million children are
malnourished, which leaves them easy targets for the microbes that thrive in
the tropical settings of many poor countries (UNICEF 2001). Fully half of
Africa's one-year-olds are not immunized against the common illnesses of
childhood: diphtheria, pertussis, tetanus, polio, and measles, leaving them
vulnerable to serious illness and death (United Nations Development
Program [UNDP] 2001, 3). Noting the dire state of child health in Africa,
David French of the World Health Organization (WHO) said, "People in
Africa don't live long enough to worry about cancer or the other diseases
that concern us in the Western world. In Africa, the big trick is to get to be
five years old" (Lamb 1987, 258).

Malnutrition in children causes a plethora of other problems, such as
muscle wasting, intellectual impairment, skin sloughing, profound weakness, and severe limitation of growth. In 1994, UNICEF (the United Nations
Children's Fund) reported that half the world's children in the least

developed countries suffered moderate to severe growth stunting, which is commonly associated with marked reductions in IQ scores (UNICEF 1998, 16; UNICEF 1997a, 98).

Delays in brain development produce irreversible damage, thus sentencing poor children, during their infancy, to significantly and permanently compromised lives.

These and other unfortunate children miss life's most critical period of brain development, 80% of which occurs during the first two years (Sider, 1997, 11). Two Brazilian studies showed conclusively that recurrent bouts of diarrhea in early childhood impairs brain function years later (Nichaus et al, 2002; Guerrant et al, 1999). UNICEF notes that "adequate nutrition, good health, clean water and a safe environment free from violence, abuse, exploitation and discrimination all contribute to how the brain grows and develops" (UNICEF 2001, 14). This constellation of factors remains simply beyond the reach of many families in poverty. A South African study showed dramatic images of cerebral "shrinkage" in brain magnetic resonance imaging (MRI) scans of 12 children ages 6 to 37 months admitted with severe malnutrition. The images were similar to the changes we see in elderly or alcoholic adults in the United States who have similar shrinkage due to atrophy—along with the cognitive deficits that track the pathology. The important "structural abnormalities" cited by this study that stemmed directly from "cerebral shrinkage" reversed once the children were fed, leaving the reader to ponder what happens to all those other severely shrunken brains lacking similar intervention (Gunston et al 1992, 1030). Delays in brain development produce irreversible damage, thus sentencing poor children, during their infancy, to significantly and permanently compromised lives.

Even in industrialized countries, extreme poverty during the first five years causes particularly harmful effects on children's "future life chances" (Aber et al 1997, 465). One study found that family income correlated better with age-five IQ than maternal education, ethnicity, or female headship; it also found a strong correlation with behavioral problems (475). Another US study showed poor children and adolescents had more vision and hearing problems, oral health problems, higher blood lead levels, and more chronic illnesses that limited their attendance in school than their wealthier counterparts (Newacheck et al 1995, 232). Nearly three fourths of homeless children in a study in New York City had insufficient or unknown immunization status (Redlener 1994, 328).

Turning back to the developing world, we find that those fortunate enough to survive into childhood and adolescence find other obstacles lying in wait. The International Labor Organization (ILO) estimates that 73 million children are employed, many in physically demanding or dangerous work (UNICEF 1997b, 26); UNICEF found that nearly a fifth of the 5- to 14-year-olds in developing countries are working (UNICEF 2004). Poverty limits choices for poor families, forcing many children to work in lieu of school. Nearly

120 million children, mostly female, are not in school and receive no formal education (UNICEF 2002).

One of the worst forms of exploitation is that of child prostitution, the profession forced upon the young girl that opened this book. The UN estimates that 1 million children are forced into prostitution every year (UNDP 1995, 7). Unlike stereotypes popularized in the US mainstream media, most commercial sex workers, especially children, are not individuals lacking the appropriate moral values–they are just poor. An author studying in the Philippines concluded that prostitution there was, "caused mainly by severe economic privation" (Farmer et al 1996, 87). In a study of prostitutes in Calcutta, half became prostitutes to escape poverty and 84% were illiterate (85). For many women, the result of this occupational "choice" is the inevitable acquisition of AIDS. The authors of *Women, Poverty, and AIDS* concluded that the majority of HIV-infected women reside in the world's poorest communities "because poverty and gender inequality act to increase women's HIV risks" (89). While tracking the Haitian AIDS epidemic, Paul Farmer noted that the price of men's and women's bodies became cheaper as Haiti became poorer (1994b, 122). Some desperate parents in poor communities are forced to sell their daughters to fraudulent "middlemen" who promise to find them work in the cities. Hundreds of thousands of girls in India, Nepal, Thailand, and other locales thus end up as slaves in the sex industry. Half of Bombay's prostitutes were recruited through trickery or abduction (Farmer et al 1996, 22). Participants in the burgeoning sex industry cause increasingly younger girls to be taken from the countryside in order to satisfy the demand for "AIDS-free" prostitutes (84).

In one final glimpse into madness, Human Rights Watch reports that some 300,000 child soldiers, most taken from extreme poverty, have been involved in 33 ongoing or recent armed conflicts throughout the world ("Slavery and Slave" 2005). *Newsweek* interviewed four child soldiers, the so-called cannon fodder of choice for the brutal civil war in Sierra Leone, for its May 2002 issue (Masland 2002). Two of the boys were age eight and nine years old when they were forcibly conscripted; one watched as his father was murdered. The four boys told stories of gang-raping women, amputating the hands of victims, drinking victims' blood, and burning victims alive. The four who were interviewed were a small fraction of the estimated 10,000 children used as combatants in the decade-long war that is now over. A few years earlier, Liberia's Charles Taylor had used 15,000 child soldiers in "small-boy units" in that country's war (Masland 2002). Such outrageous actions most often occur in the most extreme settings of poverty. In the Human Development Index of 2001, Sierra Leone ranked last out of 162 countries (UNDP 2001, 144). When last ranked in 1996, Liberia was 158 out of 174 countries, 16 from the bottom (UNDP 1996, 137).

One of the most important inputs into the developing life of a child is love. In his book *Violence: Our Deadly Epidemic and Its Causes* (Putnam

Books, 1996), James Gilligan describes the inmates in Massachusetts' Bridgewater State Prison for the most severe offenders. In the holding unit for the worst offenders, inmates cut themselves "just to know they are alive." Gilligan points out that the self-starved of love dies, emphatically making the point that the psychological well-being of our young is just as important as their physical well-being. We ignore the latter at our peril. Bridgewater's prison, like prisons around the world, fill up with those who bear the scars of abuse, neglect, discrimination, and vicious poverty. Inmates should not be freed, but we must pay attention to the circumstances that mold such individuals at the outset. Imagine the generation looming that was formed in the massacres in Rwanda or is being inexorably orphaned by the global AIDS epidemic. Without love, we are all mere shadows of what we could become and may in time pose threats to all around us.

We have seen how children bear a disproportional amount of the pain from poverty, malnutrition, and illness. Far from coddling our young as a species, as any parent would hope, humans inflict incredible suffering on our young. Children have no political voice of their own and remain particularly vulnerable to the economic and political forces that have historically turned many into victims. Recognizing these and other factors, in 1989 the United Nations adopted the Convention on the Rights of the Child (CRC), which has subsequently become the most universally accepted document in history. Of 192 countries, 191 have ratified this convention, making it enforceable law in each (UNDP 2000, 51). The lone exception remains the United States, citing articles 37 and 38, which respectively ban capital punishment and military recruiting until age 18. In this most impressive document, the UN laid out a series of 54 articles that requires countries to afford full dignity, opportunity, and freedom for all children to become fully developed adults capable of participating in the full spectrum of life in their societies.[2] This beautifully and inspirationally written document remains filled with more promise than results thus far; many countries remain too poor to meet its most basic requirements. Still, it points a way to a more promising future for the most vulnerable among us.

Sexism

The hills around Nairobi are known for the "flame trees" that bloom every spring, made famous by a well-known Elspeth Huxley novel *The Flame Trees of Thika: Memories of an African Childhood* (Penguin Classics, 2000). During one warm Sunday afternoon in April 1994, I was with a group that ventured outside the gates of Nazareth Hospital to see these trees in full bloom. While out walking, we came upon a woman who had brought several of her children to the hospital. A physician in our group had recently treated her eldest son for asthma and knew her well, so we stopped to visit. Just as she had done most every day of her life, the woman had been out working in the fields with her elderly mother. All of her children were with her–her asthmatic son was doing well–and we went inside their one-room hut. The walls were blackened from the fire in the middle of the dirt floor and there were no windows. We stayed for a short while and ate some home-grown fruit that the grandmother graciously offered–it seems to me a universal truth that the less people have, the more they are likely to give. As we were leaving, her husband came home. He tried to walk toward us and say something but had a hard time doing either. He soon fell sideways into some tall grass and then, gave up, and lay there mumbling. His drunkenness would have been funny if we hadn't just seen the sweat pouring off the females in the family. The woman smiled at us embarrassed, as people there often do. She confided to us, "*pole*"–this has happened before; we'll be fine.

Women comprise the world's most discriminated against group.

In male-dominated cultures, which comprise virtually our entire present world, it is not unusual for scenes like this to play out. I don't mean to imply that all African men are similar to the one depicted here; they're not. The kernel of inequity relayed in the story, however, represents a broader truth in Africa and the world at large. Men hold the bulk of land, political power, and wealth, while women often live under forced subjugation. For this they suffer, as do the children wholly dependent upon them.

Representing just more than half of humanity, women comprise the world's most discriminated against group. Suffering more than the effects of race, religion, nationality, ethnicity, or any other "ism" that defines someone as "other," women bear the brunt of discriminatory policies and practices throughout the world. The UN notes, "Poverty has a woman's face"; 70% of the 1.3 billion people living in poverty are women (UNDP 1995, 4). Despite long-understood connections between child survival and women's education (Commission on Macroeconomics and Health 2001, 35), women still receive considerably less education than men. Of the 900 million illiterates in the developing world, two thirds are women. Of the 130 million children with no access to primary school, 60% are girls (UNDP 1995, 4).

Similar patterns of discrimination hold for other areas, including work. A UN survey of 30 countries showed that women work longer hours in virtually all countries and carry a larger share of the total workload than men (UNDP 1995, 88). Yet, much of the work that women do is unpaid and untracked. Traditional accounting methods that track the value of the total output of goods and services generated by a nation's citizens (gross national product [GNP]) do not factor in women's contributions, such as raising a family and doing domestic work at home. Economist Amartya Sen and others have pointed out that these traditional methods grossly underestimate the "value" of women's contributions. If women's invisible contributions to the global work output were measured as other market transactions, the world output would increase by 70% (6).

In return for their hard labor, women receive a bevy of setbacks. In developing countries, 76% of men are paid for their work, but only 34% of women are paid. Women frequently work in low-paying jobs or in the informal sector, averaging only three-fourths the salary of their male counterparts (UNDP 1995, 4). They also work longer hours than men in every country surveyed. In Kenya, women work an average of 56 hours per week in their fields, 62 hours if there are cash crops involved (92). Since Kenyan men legally hold title to all of the land, a woman only has access to land if she has a living husband or son. Hence, it becomes a necessity to smile when he is incapacitated by alcohol. Kenya's land ownership policies find resonance with many other developing countries, where women lack legal control over land they farm, even when a woman is head of the household (38). Author and economist Robert Klitgaard wrote of Equatorial Guinea in West Africa, "I often had trouble deadlifting the weights the women routinely bore." He learned what most who have lived in Africa know to be true—it is the women who breathe life into the long-suffering continent:

> Men monopolize formal organizations from village councils to government ministries. Men are forces of control but also a lack of control, of dissipation. Women are the creators, the sinews of both home and economy. It is the men who are wasting Africa's money on armaments and corruption and luxuries, the women who nurture the young, grow the subsistence crops, tend the houses, and make markets work (Klitgaard 1990, 173).

Women encounter many other obstacles throughout the world. In many countries, it is much harder for a woman to open a new business. Women receive only a small percent of the available credit from formal banking institutions, eg, only 7% to 11% in Latin America and the Caribbean. It is also considerably harder for women to advance in business and government. As recently as 1995, women comprised less than 14% of administrative and managerial positions in developing countries and held only 10% of the seats in parliament and 6% of cabinet positions (UNDP 1995, 1).

Women in the formal sector, particularly domestic servants, may be obliged to supply sex as a condition of employment (Farmer et al 1996, 51). Still others may have to supplement meager wages with commercial sex work to support their families. Vulnerable social and financial positions force many women into unfavorable relationships with men who may beat them, infect them with HIV, or kill them outright. According to *The New York Times*, wife beating is an "entrenched epidemic" in sub-Saharan Africa; one in three Nigerian women report having been beaten by a male partner (LaFraniere 2005). As evidence of widespread vulnerability induced by poverty, the UN estimates that 2 million girls age 5 to 15 enter the commercial sex market annually (Griffiths 2000).

Women have been particularly vulnerable to the AIDS epidemic because so many lack the ability to control their sexual choices. Those in the middle and upper classes in the United States may fail to appreciate how coercive money and power are, particularly when the lives of one's children are at risk. Yet, the poor know all too well. Poverty and gender inequality are powerful cofactors directing HIV's murderous spread among women. In explaining why a deafening silence greeted the AIDS epidemic of women in the United States, Paul Farmer writes that the women most at risk have been previously "robbed of their voices." "In settings of entrenched elitism," he writes, "they have been poor. In settings of entrenched racism, they have been women of color. In settings of entrenched sexism, they have been, of course, women" (Farmer et al 1996, 6).

Women also receive less health care than men. When poor women deliver their babies, they face difficult odds: half a million die from complications of pregnancy and childbirth at rates 10 to 100 times higher than those in industrialized countries (UNDP 1997, 3). When an African woman delivers, she is 180 times more likely to die from complications than a woman in western Europe (UNDP 1995, 36). Further, many of those same African women likely bear scars already. An estimated 130 million women worldwide have undergone forced genital mutilations, often following accepted cultural "norms" (Griffiths 2000).

The most striking aspect of the global injustice perpetrated against women is the phenomenon of the "missing" women described by economist Amartya Sen. Globally, there are large disparities between the number of women and men. Women outnumber men by 5% in North America and Europe, where women tend to outlive men. Even impoverished sub-Saharan Africa shows a female:male ratio of 1:02. Yet, in several Asian countries, men significantly outnumber women, raising the disturbing question of what happened to the "missing" women. Sen and others have reported that in Asia there are more than 100 million fewer women than expected, including 44 million in China and 37 million in India. This data reflect sex-selective abortions or female infanticide (often through bedside drowning just after birth) prevalent in some locales, particularly in China with its "one child" policy. Higher female mortality rates also follow a "staunch anti-female bias" in these countries (UNDP 1995, 35; Sen 1993, 46). When poor parents are forced to choose, it is generally the boy who receives food, education, and health care; it is the boy who will work the farm, inherit the land, and accept a dowry.

Less has become the female standard in wealth, education, health care, land holding, inheritance, legal protection, managerial and administrative power, political voice, and employment.

In short, women face discrimination that severely restricts their life's agency from the cradle to the often-premature grave. From their murders before or immediately after birth in some parts of the world, to the less available nutrition, education, and development early in life, women of the world face significant obstacles to survival. Later, they face unfavorable unions with men through an ancient, well-established power imbalance that defines less as the "norm" for women. Less has become the female standard in wealth, education, health care, land holding, inheritance, legal protection, managerial and administrative power, political voice, and employment. Is it any wonder that women and the children who depend upon them suffer the most in a world of entrenched inequality?

Just months after my own son James was born in 1999, I stood watching a poor Mayan woman and her young child begging in a crowded market in Belize City. Picturing my own wife and son under similar circumstances gave me pause. For those of us who have been through it, there is full agreement that the love of a child is a unique force of nature in this our shared human experience. There is a universality of love that transcends boundaries of culture, race, and wealth. The love any of us feels for our children is the same as that felt by the poor, particularly poor mothers who must bury their children with alarming frequency. Perhaps, with more effort to help poor women in the poorest countries, we can make such occurrences less frequent.

Population

Population growth has been widely cited as one of the great threats to geopolitical stability, in addition to straining fragile natural resources and continuing cycles of poverty. Although alarmist rhetoric from the 1970s has diminished in intensity, there is still sufficient cause for concern. The human population is expanding, pushing poor people ever deeper into fragile ecosystems, where they encounter newly emerging pathogens such as Lassa fever, Ebola, Marburg virus, HIV, and a host of others (Garrett 1994, 13). Population pressures simultaneously force millions to live in environmentally risky areas, subject to obliteration from the next hurricane or monsoon. Population pressures strain scarce resources and the resultant environmental destruction further worsens health. Such are the concerns over the population explosion—one that has shown rapid growth for years.

According to UN estimates, the human population surpassed the 6 billion mark some time around October 12, 1999 (Crossette 1999, 1, 4). It took roughly 7 million years for humankind to reach the 1 billion mark in 1804; it then took just 123 years to reach 2 billion in 1927 (Crossette 1999, 1, 4; Diamond 1999, 36). Subsequent milestones have increasingly shortened, reaching 3 billion people in 33 years, 4 billion in 14 years, and 6 billion in just 12 years (Crossette 1999, 1, 4). The BBC reports current global population increases of 240,000 per day and 88 million per year (BBC News 1999). UN population projections peg human totals at 9.5 billion by 2050, with 8 billion in developing countries (UNDP 1998, 66) where 98% of the annual population increase now occurs (Cornelius and Cover 1997). Projections have the world's population leveling off at around 10 billion by the year 2200 if current trends hold true (Crossette 1999, 1, 4). As such, we are now in the midst of the steepest population growth phase in human history. The curve is flattening only slightly and won't sufficiently slow for another 50 to 100 years.

Those who envision nightmarish scenarios triggered by these population trajectories have always had company, starting with Thomas Malthus in 1798. Malthus thought that unchecked population growth would eventually outstrip available resources, causing persistent famine and the ultimate destruction of man.[3] His habit of making doomsday prophecies and then blaming the poor for the myriad problems ensuing from overpopulation reverberate into modern times. One can easily picture a world in which there is simply not enough food for everyone, water shortages are common, and rising population pressures push large groups of people ever closer to war or civil conflict.

The environmental effects of this population bomb hit the poor the hardest, according to the UN. "People in poverty are forced to deplete resources to survive, and this degradation of the environment further impoverishes people" (UNDP 1998, 66). Consider Haiti, for example. More than 500 million people—almost half of the world's extreme poor—live on marginal lands (66). It was primarily the poor who died by the thousands when their favellas slid into the swollen Choluteca River in Teguciagalpa and the surrounding countryside when Hurricane Mitch devastated Honduras and several other Central American countries in 1998.[4] Few mansions are built on such precarious perches; such unsafe locales are the exclusive domain of the poor throughout the world. The killer tsunamis of December 2004 also claimed predominantly poor people in Asia, though thousands of European tourists perished along with them. As population pressures force more poor people into fragile areas, future environmental disasters are likely to exact still higher tolls.

However, it is not the unsafe locales that cause the most environmental harm for poor populations. The industrialized world burns the bulk of the world's natural resources, generates most of the air and water pollution, and causes global warming through emission of greenhouse gases. Ironically, while the rich create the problems, the poor suffer most from their effects. The poor comprise the "overwhelming majority" of those who die each year from the effects of water and air pollution, lose land to desertification, and feel most acutely the brunt of the flooding, storms, and crop failures caused by global warming (UNDP 1998, 66). In 1997, the average person in the United States contributed 19.1 metric tons of carbon dioxide to the atmosphere—by far the world's largest amount—while the average person in Indonesia, Bangladesh, and Tanzania contributed 1, 0.2, and 0.1 metric tons, respectively (Cornelius and Cover 1997). It is hard to point fingers at the poor given such data, though many still do.

In addition to the environmental effects of population expansion, poverty itself is both a cause and a result of rapid population growth. Poor families respond to their dire conditions in predictable fashion—in most cases, by reproducing in sufficient numbers to insure that they and their children have a better chance at survival. A significant body of evidence shows that high annual birthrates correlate with generally poor health and low life expectancy. The poorest countries tend to have the highest population growth rates. While Western democracies have annual population growth rates of 0% to 1%, poor countries have rates of 3% to 3.5%.[5] The average woman in the United States from 2000 to 2005 had 2.0 children (average fertility); the average woman in Kenya had 5.0; in Sierra Leone, 6.5; and in Niger, 7.9 (UNDP 2005, 234). Overall, in 2000–2005, the average woman in high-income Organization for Economic Co-operation and Development (OECD) countries had 1.6 children, while the average woman in the least-developed countries had 5.0 children (235). Thus, the worse conditions are in a given country, the higher the average fertility and the more likely there will be sustained, large-scale population growth.

It is not surprising that those who are at greatest risk of losing their children tend to have more of them. Morally offensive arguments that include "weeding out" the poor or upbraiding them on their "errant ways" serve only to obscure potential solutions to the problems of overpopulation. It is better to first understand the nature of the problem and the reasons behind such trends. As in several of the areas described earlier, there are lessons that come from the experience of developed countries that warrant a look.

Population Transitions in Developed Countries

Rich countries offer two valuable lessons to the world on population control. First, fertility rates fall as average incomes rise, people can then afford food, education, and health care. Second, fertility rates fall still farther when contraceptive methods allow women to gain control over when and how many children they want to have. The family size in the United States decreased from 7.0 children in 1800 to 3.5 children in 1900. Rising prosperity, better medical care, increasing educational level and economic stability of women, falling infant mortality rates, and better contraception all contributed to declining birthrates. Following introduction of the birth control pill and intrauterine device (IUD) in the 1960s and enhanced family planning services through Medicaid in the 1970s and 1980s, fertility rates fell and stabilized to the current level of 2.0 children per family. The Centers for Disease Control and Prevention (CDC) estimates that by 1994 public family planning services were preventing an estimated 1.3 million unintended pregnancies in the United States each year, including 534,000 unintended births, 632,000 abortions, and 165,000 miscarriages (CDC 1999k, 1073). The experience of many industrialized countries is similar to that of the United States (UNDP 2002, 165).

One lasting lesson of this population slow down from the developed countries lies in what is termed the "epidemiological transition." In 1971, Abdel Omran theorized that countries transition from those with short-lived, high-birthrate populations that die from infectious disease related illnesses to those characterized by long-lived, low-birthrate populations that die from noninfectious causes such as heart disease and cancer (1971, 509). Today, the United States represents the latter while Kenya represents the former. Most countries are gradually undergoing this transition, with the late 20th century as the midpoint of a two-century transition of the world's population from Omran's first group to his later (WHO 1999, 3). Then as now, many of those premature deaths occurred in infants and children. To compensate, families traditionally had more of them. Economist Jeffrey Sachs notes the same phenomenon operating in poor countries today, citing "painfully clear" logic in which, "Poor families compensate for children's deaths by having large numbers of children . . . just to assure themselves of a high probability that at least one son (or daughter, or both) will survive till the parents' old age" (Sachs 2001b, 35). Most countries don't have social safety nets like Medicare and Social Security, so children serve as their parents' caretakers.

Jeffrey Sachs and others have shown that countries with infant mortality rates higher than 100 have average total fertility rates of 6.2 children and countries with infant mortality rates of less than 20 have total fertility rates of 1.7 children. Households whose children have a 75% chance of survival have 6 children on average, of which 4.5 survive. By contrast, households where children have a 95% chance of survival tend to have 2 children, of which 1.9 survive (Sachs 2001b, 36).

Lowering the infant mortality rate, therefore, is one of the best ways to lower population growth rates.

When more children survive, parents and governments alike can concentrate resources on fewer individuals. More education, more health care, better nutrition, and more individual attention lead to healthier kids who grow up to be more productive workers; they, in turn, help to break cycles of poverty and disease and force fertility rates ever downward. As health improves and infant mortality rates fall, population growth initially rises, then quickly falls. Parents lengthen the birth interval and have fewer children. Consequently, improving health of a population is a key factor to overall reduction of population growth. Developing countries today benefit from the diffusion and direct transfer of medical technology as well as advances in contraception and family planning to reduce fertility more directly (Omran 1971, 509).

Lowering the infant mortality rate, therefore, is one of the best ways to lower population growth rates. Yet, there are other factors that are equally important. Many studies point to the importance of the educational status of the mother in lowering fertility rates. Educated women have more economic opportunity, more control over reproductive choices, and are better able to keep themselves and their children healthy. The UN concludes that "universal access to reproductive health care, universal education, and women's empowerment" are keys to decreasing fertility rates and reducing the conditions that contribute to poverty creation (United Nations 2002a).

Poor women face other obstacles not often factored into discussions on overpopulation by the Western media. Women who lack economic and political power are often unable to refuse unwanted sexual advances by more socially powerful men. In addition to the risk of acquiring HIV and other sexually transmitted diseases (STDs), this imbalance of power contributes to the large number of unintended pregnancies each year. Poor women are often unable to delay motherhood, space births, or stop childbearing after reaching the desired family size.[6] The US National Academy of Sciences estimates that between 20% and 40% of births in developing countries are unwanted or ill-timed, jeopardizing the health of millions of women and families through increased strains on precarious resources (Tsui et al 1997). The Institute of Medicine estimated, rather conservatively, that roughly 100 to 200 million women worldwide who would like to space or limit childbirth are not using modern contraceptives (Institute of Medicine 1997, 16). An additional indication of unintended pregnancy rates is abortion. In 1987 there were 26 to 31 million legal and 10 to 22 million illegal abortions worldwide (Tsui et al 1997, 14). Given the high rates of maternal mortality in poor countries—99% of the 600,000 annual pregnancy-related deaths occur in developing countries—each subsequent pregnancy also increases the risk of death for the mother, which in turn has devastating consequences for the children (3). When a mother dies in some poor countries, the likelihood for her children who are under five to die is as high as 50% (14).

Family Planning and Medical Technology

Fortunately, not all is so bleak. Contraceptive technologies have diffused into poor countries, causing birthrates to plummet. The CDC claims that the most important reason for declining fertility rates in developing countries is contraceptive use (CDC 1999k, 1073). Through family planning programs, new contraceptive technologies, and mass educational campaigns through television, millions of women in developing countries have reduced family sizes (Robey et al 1993, 60). Overall global fertility rates fell by one-third from the 1960s through the 1980s, from an average of six to an average of four children per woman, with even more dramatic changes in some countries (24% decline in Asia and Latin America, 50% decline in Thailand) (CDC 1999k, 1073). According to *The Economist*, the "typical" East Asian woman in 1950 had six children, today she has two ("Does Population Matter" 2002). The UN reports that family planning programs are responsible for almost one third of the global declines in fertility from 1972 to 1994 (United Nations 2002a).

Family planning may be the single most important determinant in overall fertility in developing countries. *Scientific American* reports, "A country's contraceptive prevalence rate—the percentage of married women of reproductive age who use any method of contraception—largely determines its total fertility rate" (Robey et al 1993, 60). Differences in the overall use of contraceptive methods may account for as much as 90% of the country-to-country variability in fertility rates. A large survey of 300,000 women in 18 developing countries sponsored by the US Agency for International Development (USAID) showed that a 15% increase in contraceptive use resulted in the average woman having one less child during her lifetime. In Kenya, contraceptive use increased 59% between 1984 and 1989 and fertility fell 16%. Bangladesh saw fertility rates fall 21% from 1970 to 1991—from 7.0 to 5.5 children per woman. Use of contraceptives among married women of reproductive age increased from 3% to 40% during the same period; Robey and others conclude increased contraceptive use is the chief reason for the decline (1993, 60). Given such data, it would make sense for the global community to fund programs that will afford poor women better reproductive control. However, there are significant barriers, among them the influence of some conservatives in the United States.

Politics remains a significant barrier to diffusion of funds and knowledge to developing countries. USAID has sponsored family planning programs in many countries (Robey et al 1993, 60). However, conservatives in the US House and Senate have delayed promised funding for family planning efforts out of concerns over involvement in abortion services ("Playing Politics" 1999). The Bush administration withheld $34 million in UN-designated family planning funds because the UN Population Fund worked in China, even though the UN strongly opposes the forced sterilizations and forced abortions that comprise China's one-child policy. Ironically, money from the UN Population Fund, which is spent on family planning, literacy, and health care, actually decreases the number of abortions.

Further support of global family planning initiatives would serve an additional economic interest for those in poor countries. Countries with slower population growth rates have a more productive citizenry, which can help many more poor people rise out of poverty. The previously cited declining birthrates in East Asia caused a 57% increase in the working age sector of the population, increasing four times faster than the number of dependents. This alone contributed one third of the region's per capita income during the period ("Does Population Matter" 2002). In other words, more working-aged people with fewer dependents are more productive, and this propels more and more people out of poverty and ill health. Fertility declines accounted for one fifth of the economic growth in the region between 1960 and 1995 (United Nations 2002a). "Since 1970," the UN notes, "developing countries with lower fertility and slower population growth have seen higher productivity, more savings and more productive investment" (United Nations 2003).

Following a groundbreaking 1994 UN population conference in Cairo, Egypt, 179 nations ratified a comprehensive program to go beyond simply providing birth control. Policymakers instead added maternal and child health, improved education, reproductive health education and services, and women's empowerment as part of a comprehensive strategy to rein in population growth (Hartman 1999).

Malthus and others have purported the idea of controlling population growth rates by restricting the reproductive capacity of the poor. China has gone further, introducing a draconian one-child policy in the late 1970s that has served to lower that country's burgeoning population growth through restrictive fines, forced sterilizations, forced abortions, and infanticide in a policy that most find morally repulsive (Kristof and Wudunn 1995, 240). The data, however, favor more humane and less radical approaches to the problem of population expansion. Just as examples from developed countries have shown, by increasing nutritional status, health care, and educational status for the poor, fewer infants and children will die, fertility rates will fall, and more resources will be concentrated on each child. Better family planning and more available contraceptives will give poor women more reproductive control over their own lives, allowing those in poor countries to directly constrain their own population growth, even before countries undergo the transitions described by Omran and others. The medical profession can—and should—help directly by enhancing obstetric and pediatric care, providing family planning services, and providing local health providers with the knowledge and skills to afford their poor patients a real choice. We all benefit in the end.

UNICEF summarized, ". . . the responsible planning of births is one of the most effective and least expensive ways of improving the quality of life on earth—both now and in the future—and . . . one of the greatest mistakes of our times is the failure to realize that potential."[5]

Nature

December 26, 2004, will long be remembered as a day when nature turned wicked, claiming 300,000 lives following an earthquake and several tsunamis in the Indian Ocean (UNDP, 2005, 1). Such disasters force us to confront the raw power of nature, as have similar disasters before it. Earthquakes, hurricanes, cyclones, tsunamis, and droughts have each wrought their own devastation on humanity for millennia. Over the past century, droughts claimed more than 10 million lives; floods claimed nearly 7 million; wind storms, including hurricanes and cyclones, claimed nearly 2 million; and earthquakes claimed nearly 2 million. Following marked increases in global population and increased migration to dangerous areas, even moderate earthquakes, cyclones, and droughts will claim far more, predominantly poor lives (Revkin 2005).

Yet, nature does not rule over humanity chiefly through the occasional natural disaster. Illnesses from contaminated water and improperly disposed of waste claim far more lives. Similarly, the location of one's country is more important in determining one's longevity than the likelihood that one will be trapped by one of nature's upsurges. Although it is the violence of nature that makes headlines, it is the more mundane water and basic sanitation, that dictate life and death for the poor.

Water and Sanitation

In 1996, I had the opportunity to travel deep into the rain forest in Brazil to visit an indigenous tribe.[7] A group of local "Western" Brazilians nearby were celebrating a national holiday with a large party at the river's edge, drinking large quantities of alcohol and urinating in the water, gunning jet skies with engines that discharged into the river. Our group boarded several boats and traveled downstream past a factory that emptied its waste into the river. Once within the sanctity of a small indigenous village along the river, I watched a small boy walk down to the water's edge, bend over, and cup his hands to drink. "What is he doing?" I asked. Surely someone would stop him from drinking such polluted water. Through an interpreter, one of the elders replied that the young boy was doing what they all did, drinking the only source of water they had. The villagers were frequently sick and many rightly blamed the water. As was the case in industrialized countries a century ago, many of the premature deaths in poor countries today stem from the twin burdens of unsafe drinking water and poor sanitation. UNICEF reports that 2 million children die every year from a lack of access to safe water and proper sanitation (UNICEF 2002).

Clean drinking water is a highly sought after commodity for the poor. According to the WHO, more than 1 billion people in developing countries, roughly 18% of the world's population, lack access to safe drinking water (United Nations 2002b; WHO 1998, 124). The UN estimates that only 56% of the rural populations in Latin America and the Caribbean have access to safe water (UNDP 1995, 26). Of the 12.2 million childhood deaths in 1993, a quarter of them came from diarrheal illnesses and 99.6% of them occurred in poor countries (Werner and Sanders 1997, 33). The water supply functions both as cause and cure. When the water supply is contaminated by human waste, even life-saving oral rehydration solutions can prove lethal. The UN estimates that with adequate supplies of safe drinking water and sanitation, "the incidences of some illnesses and death could drop by as much as 75%" (United Nations 2002b).

In most poor countries, it is the woman's job to haul the water. Anyone who has carried water knows its oppressive weight. In rural Tanzania, where I worked as a medical student in 1987, women hauled large containers filled with water over large distances. The WHO estimates that women and girls annually spend more than 10 million person-years hauling water from wells to residencies (United Nations 2002b). That the water is safe is far from a given in many locales. Waterborne illnesses such as cholera, schistosomiasis, salmonella, dracunculiasis, and all forms of gastroenteritis are caused by common waterborne opportunistic pathogens. Other toxins haunt water and well supplies in poor communities worldwide.

In Bangladesh, some 35 million people routinely drink arsenic-contaminated water in what the WHO has called the "largest mass poisoning of a population in history" (Bearak 2002, 1). Scientists and public health officials have speculated that from 1 to 5 million people may eventually die from arsenic-related causes. Changing wells could save countless lives, but the wells are privately owned and most are unavailable to the women who fetch the water (Stephenson 2002, 1708). It would seem a painfully ironic task to explain to an arsenic-toxic Bangladeshi or an African mother with several deceased children the reasons why Americans prefer to drink "pure" bottled water (more than 6.4 billion gallons in 2003) instead of US tap water which is, by comparison, impeccably clean (International Bottled Water Association 2004).

Sanitation represents the other half of the equation, with enormous consequences for those who lack access to proper disposal of human waste. For example, more than half of Bombay's 6.7 million people live in slums, most lacking any toilet facilities. The poor suffer the indignity of having to publicly relieve themselves while packed commuter trains ramble past. It is not uncommon for some of these poor people to be killed by trains when they sprint across the tracks in search of more secluded areas for relief. Women are forced to "undergo a punishing daily self-discipline: to relieve yourself only before sunrise or after sunset" (Sengupta 2002, 3). In Bombay's Dharavi Slum, believed to be one of the world's largest, there is just one toilet for every 800 people; theoretically, one could wait for more than a week just to use the facilities (3).

In southern Belize in Central America, the poor bring buckets of their waste to the ocean's edge under the cover of darkness, prompting the descriptive term "night soil." Fecal coliform bacterial counts in the bays and rivers near urban areas have been, not surprisingly, high.[8] When massive influxes of humanity strain the local capacity for sanitation, disaster often follows. Following the genocide in Rwanda in 1994, millions of refugees fled across the border into Goma, Zaire, now the Congo (Power 2002, 334). The subsequent cholera epidemic killed between 10,000 and 20,000 people (Werner and Sanders 1997, 5). Other cholera epidemics have followed civil strife or natural disasters in Afghanistan, Brazil, Guinea, Guinea-Bissau, and Somalia (Strickland 2000, 325). Cholera, like typhus, tuberculosis, and HIV, is just one of many pathogens whose opportunities dramatically improve when humans subject large numbers of their brethren to conditions of strife and want. Cholera thrives in the water and explodes in crisis. Considerably more damage occurs due to the structural components of poor sanitation that characterize everyday life for millions.

The UN estimates that 800 million people in South Asia (UNDP 1995, 26) and an additional 1.6 billion people elsewhere lack access to even basic sanitation (UNDP 2001, 9). Further, between 90% and 95% of sewage and 70% of industrial wastes in developing countries are dumped untreated into the usable water supply (United Nations 2002b). In Nairobi's Kibera Slum, people defecate in open drainage ditches or in plastic bags subsequently thrown onto the roofs. Then the rains come. . . .

Solutions to the problem are the same as they were for those in the United States and other rich countries a century ago. However, developing countries require funding to create proper public sanitation, filter or chlorinate public drinking water, or drill wells. The UN has provided considerable funds for these tasks, though the problem remains staggering in many countries. The solution lies in the hands of governments, international agencies, nongovernmental organizations (NGOs), and individuals. Larrimer Mellon, the Gulf Oil heir who went to medical school at age 37 and built Hospital Albert Schweitzer in Deschapelles, Haiti, in 1950, trained first as a physician, then spent much of his time in Haiti digging wells for clean water, earning the affectionate nickname "watermelon" from the local villagers.[9] The point is that although medical care is always important, first things should come first. Time spent treating recurrent illness from consistent problematic sources such as contaminated drinking water prompts those involved in health care to correct the underlying problems whenever possible.

In its World Summit on Sustainable Development in Johannesburg, Republic of South Africa, in 2002, the UN highlighted the contribution that unsanitary conditions made toward poor health and called on all nations to reduce by half the number of poor people who lack sanitation by 2015 (Swarns 2002). Like other UN goals, it raises the bar for poor countries—and the rich countries who should fund them—but quite understandably offers no guarantee of change.

Geography

To a large extent, global poverty is determined by climate and location. In a study published in *Scientific American,* economist Jeffrey Sachs and colleagues showed that merely by looking at a map, one could predict a country's wealth. The world's wealthiest countries are chiefly found in temperate regions, while most of the poorest countries lie in the tropics, that region between the tropic of Cancer and the tropic of Capricorn (Sachs et al 2001d, 70). Of the world's 28 high-income countries, only Hong Kong, Singapore, and part of Taiwan lie in the tropics, comprising just 2% of the population of the high-income regions. By contrast, almost all countries that lie in temperate zones are either high-income or middle-income but burdened by a socialist or communist past. Similar disparities exist within countries as well—the richest states of Brazil lie in a temperate zone in the country's southernmost region.

Countries that lie in temperate zones have two distinct advantages over those that lie in the tropics. First, temperate climates favor agriculture. The major food grains like wheat, corn, and rice grow better in temperate and subtropical zones (Sachs 2001d, 70). While 1 hectare of land in a tropical zone typically yields 2.3 metric tons of maize, 1 hectare in a temperate zone yields 6.4 tons. Land in tropical zones suffers the twin assaults of high temperatures and torrential rains, both of which leach minerals from the soil. Tropical regions also serve as perpetual hosts to a variety of pests and infestations that destroy crops. The ever-present threat of drought is a further threat to agriculture in the tropics.

Those in tropical regions also face diseases largely unknown in temperate zones. As Sachs writes, "Winter could be considered the world's most effective public health intervention" (2001d, 70). Mosquitoes bearing malaria, dengue, and yellow fever; worms; tsetse flies; and a host of other parasites plague tropical zones, adversely affecting the health and productivity of local populations. Most of these pests do not survive in northern winters, affording a huge economic advantage to countries in those regions. It was far easier to rid the United States of malaria than it ever will be to rid a sub-Saharan African country of the same.

Naturally, countries with difficult geographic barriers, eg, the mountains of Tibet and Bhutan or the large deserts of the Sudan and Chad, face impossible obstacles. Given the environs, it is understandable though tragic that these countries face perpetual poverty.

Another important component of geography is the distance of a given country from shipping lanes, either through navigable rivers or coastline. The 18th century economist Adam Smith predicted that countries without such access would be poorer, and Sachs and colleagues proved him right. Countries that are landlocked tend to be among the poorest. Shipping freight by the sea is far cheaper than by land or air. Port cities become focal points of economic growth and gathering points for ideas and technologies, which furthers development. Countries that lack such ports suffer clear disadvantages.

When Sachs and colleagues combined the features of climate and distance from shipping lanes, they found some not unexpected results. Most global commerce occurs in temperate regions near shipping lanes, so-called temperate-near by the study authors. This temperate-near category comprises just 8.2% of the world's inhabited land area but holds 22.8% of the world's population and produces 52.9% of the world's GNP (Sachs 2001d, 70). By contrast, tropical regions that are far from shipping lanes comprise the world's poorest, with average GNP that is roughly one-third the world average.

By turning back to the map, we can predict certain characteristics of our world. We would expect that Africa, which lies primarily in the tropics and has an enormous land mass compared to its coast, would harbor extensive poverty, which it does. We would also expect that much of Central and South America, Asia, and Oceania would be poor based on their locations within the tropics, which they are. By contrast, much of western Europe, the United States, Canada, and Japan are in temperate locales with extensive coastlines and waterways. Their wealth, at least in part, reflects their geography. Where one's country sits geographically determines to a great extent how poor one will be.

Infectious Disease

The infectious diseases of our world determine our collective fates far more than we realize. Those of us in the West are far enough removed from plague, malaria, smallpox, and other scourges that we rarely think of infectious diseases. We live under the false belief that we are somehow safe from the ravages of the next plague. Despite the devastation of HIV/AIDS, multidrug-resistant tuberculosis (MDR-TB), and the potential devastation of severe acute respiratory syndrome (SARS), we go about our business unaware of the microbes that live among us and inhabit the deep recesses of tropical jungles, quietly waiting for the opportune moment to emerge.

Yet the destructive impact that microbes have had on humans through time is incalculable. In the natural order, it is microbes that are predator and we who are their prey. Fleas, ticks, rats, lice, and their various microbial freeloaders have raised and crushed civilizations, while decisively shaping history. In 1934, the noted bacteriologist and author Hans Zinsser wrote, "Swords and lances, arrows, machine guns, and even high explosives have had far less power over fates of the nations than the typhus louse, the plague flea, and the yellow-fever mosquito. Civilizations have retreated from the plasmodium of malaria, and armies have crumpled into rabbles under the onslaught of cholera, spirilla, or of dysentery and typhoid bacilli. . . . War and conquest and that herd existence which is an accompaniment of what we call civilization have merely set the stage for these more powerful agents of human tragedy" (1934, 9).

The world has strong memories of prior scourges that descended on hapless men and women without warning, destroying entire cities and redefining world orders, old and new. Our common fear of rodents stems from a distant memory of European ancestors fitfully awaiting the arrival of the Black Death from their stricken neighbors, borne through the bacterium harbored in rats. More recent plagues, such as Lyme disease, hantavirus, and HIV/AIDS, stem from human disruption of previously stable ecological systems or from the relentless human encroachment on habitats largely untouched by humans.

Author Laurie Garrett wrote one of the great books of the 1990s, *The Coming Plague*, published in 1994 (1994). In it, she meticulously documents the emergence of Ebola, Lassa fever, Marburg virus, *Legionella*, hantavirus, and HIV, among others. Following such a consistent history of microbes winning out over the best our science can offer, it seems clear that such trends will continue. Judging by our slow, pained, and markedly biased response to HIV, along with a growing tendency to relegate the struggle against microbes to a passed era, Garrett writes, "The skills needed to describe and recognize perturbations in the *Homo sapiens* microecology are disappearing with the passing of the generations, leaving humanity, lulled into a complacency born of proud discoveries and medical triumphs, unprepared for the coming plague" (1994, 12). Whether that plague comes in the form of SARS, MDR-TB, or a previously unknown virus now mutating in a distant jungle, its arrival seems inevitable.

Yet it is not the new or the exotic that inflicts the most damage on the poor on a daily basis. It is the common case of diarrhea or pneumonia and the well-established pathogens like tuberculosis, malaria, and HIV that claim the most lives. The world's poor consider these "bugs" among their chief concerns. Few of the patients I treated in Kenya or Tanzania were unfamiliar with malaria. Their recurrent bouts of drenching sweats and shaking chills were as familiar to them as the change of seasons is to many of us. Their dormant malarial parasites flared and attacked frequently, often at the most inopportune time, during an illness, surgery, or childbirth—virtually any stressor. The poor routinely lose children to treatable respiratory or diarrheal illness and watch hopelessly while family members die of tuberculosis, curable since the 1960s.

For many people in developing countries, infectious disease defines their lives. HIV has irrevocably changed the lives of the 12 million AIDS orphans in Africa, along with the extended families who now assume their care and child-rearing. Entire communities have suffered from the scourge of multidrug-resistant tuberculosis, with rare pockets receiving effective, albeit expensive, medications. Other "bugs" such as the tsetse fly, sand fleas, kissing bugs, and worms of various types all take their toll on the global poor. Their health bows inexorably to their microbial freeloaders, ever a constituent part of their bodies.

The health burden of these microbes is immeasurable. Globally, infectious diseases accounted for one quarter to one third of 1998s estimated 54 million deaths worldwide (National Intelligence Council 2000, 5). In poorer regions, the toll from infectious diseases is far higher. In many sub-Saharan African and poor Asian countries, infectious diseases contribute to roughly 45% of all deaths. According to the National Intelligence Council, an advisory body to the Central Intelligence Agency (CIA), if current trends continue, by 2020 tuberculosis and HIV/AIDS will have caused the "overwhelming majority" of deaths from infectious diseases in developing countries (5). In addition to established pathogens, newly recognized diseases continue to emerge. Since 1973, at least 30 previously unknown diseases have surfaced, including AIDS, SARS, Ebola, hepatitis C, hantavirus, Lyme disease, and *Legionella*.

The pathogens that kill the largest number of people per year include the following: HIV/AIDS, 3.1 million; tuberculosis, 2 million; malaria, 1.1 million; hepatitis B and hepatitis C (millions will die of cirrhosis or cancer), lower respiratory infections, 3.5 million, mostly children; diarrheal disease, 2.2 million, mostly children; and measles, 0.9 million, mostly children (UNAIDS 2004; National Intelligence Council 2000, 14; WHO 1999, 49). Although the last three pathogens have peaked, the first four are surging, becoming more widespread and drug-resistant (National Intelligence Council 2000, 14). A number of factors, largely borne of human behaviors, contribute to the increasing spread of these pathogens. Steadily rising population growth and increasing concentrations of poor, starving people in the world's growing urban landscapes favor the microbes. The growing numbers of refugees and internally displaced people do the same. Changing patterns of land use, such as reforestation and human encroachment on tropical rain forests, will continue to afford previously unseen microbes the opportunity to prey upon human hosts. Ever-increasing travel will ensure that pathogens arising in remote jungles or markets will quickly spread throughout the world, as SARS did in 2003. Roughly 2 million people cross borders each day and 1 million cross borders between the developing and developed world each week. Further, overuse of antibiotics by both farmers (for use in livestock) and doctors will continue to stimulate antibiotic resistance among microbes.

Contributing to the continued rise of the microbes are poor responses from the global community to problems arising in developing countries. As previously discussed, most bilateral and multilateral foreign aid serves the needs of donors. Not surprisingly, relatively few funds are used to address the basic health needs of those in the developing world. Although low- and middle-income countries spend roughly $250 billion on health care annually, the developed countries provide only $2 billion to $3 billion annually in health-related aid (National Intelligence Council 2000, 33). The sheer size of the need places health in developing countries well beyond the capacities of both the WHO and NGO communities. Recognizing the importance of health to economic development, the World Bank has shifted its lending priorities toward health, accounting for $2.5 billion in health loans for 2002 alone (34). Yet, the combined efforts of donors have fallen far short of the needs. In far too many developing countries, few people have access to even basic medical care. For example, fewer than 40% of people in Nigeria and the Democratic Republic of the Congo have access to basic medical care (27).

As mentioned in the introduction to this book, infectious diseases also threaten global political and economic stability. A number of infectious pathogens have disrupted global trade. From cyclospora stopping importation of Guatemalan raspberries to SARS halting tourist visits to Hong Kong and Toronto, Canada, infectious disease outbreaks continue to take their economic tolls. A 1994 outbreak of plague in India cost the country $2 billion, according to the WHO (National Intelligence Council 2000, 48). As the HIV/AIDS epidemic spreads, it will claim more young lives and sideline more workers in developing countries who become ill or have to take on the role of caretaker. Economies will decline, which is a longstanding lead-in to war and chaos. Given the murderous spread of HIV/AIDS throughout Africa, Asia, the Caribbean, and Eastern Europe, countries will feel the economic impact of a reduced workforce and rising medical bills. AIDS will also contribute to instability due to the relatively high rates of infection among soldiers and officers, decreasing combat readiness. In some countries, fewer soldiers are better for all; however, the deteriorating militaries may invite insurgencies and contribute to further upheaval. Additionally, fewer soldiers will be available for peacekeeping missions.

Microbes not only contribute to political and economic instability, they feed off of it. Following Idi Amin's murderous reign, Uganda saw an upsurge in virtually every conceivable pathogen. Measles, malaria, leprosy, kala-azar, and cholera, among others, thrived on the chaos (Garrett 1994, 210). In virtually every war through history, the end of hostilities fails to stem the surge of deaths caused by infectious diseases. It is not uncommon to lose more people in the aftermath of war through infectious outbreaks than through the actual war. For every violent death in Congo's war zone, there are 62 deaths attributed to non-violent, mostly infection-related causes like diarrhea, pneumonia, and "fever" (Lacey, 2005). The microbes exploit their opportunities, and few present a better opportunity for this than war and its immediate aftermath. Conflict also redirects precious resources from health infrastructures to armaments in countries that commonly cannot afford either.

Three infectious illnesses hold particular sway over those in poor countries and those at the lower end of the economic ladder in many rich countries. These three infections attracted the attention of the WHO, which in 2000 proposed a plan through which the rich countries would spend $27 billion per year to save up to 8 million lives as part of the Global Fund (Sachs 2002). Unfortunately, the Global Fund has been chronically under funded since its inception. But the three illnesses continue to exact their toll from the poor at alarming rates. These three illnesses—tuberculosis, malaria, and AIDS—comprise a disease burden that claims millions of lives annually, reverses decades of development, and holds the potential to drag entire world regions down into chaos and war. We'll start by reviewing tuberculosis and malaria.

Tuberculosis

When combined, HIV/AIDS, tuberculosis, and malaria claimed 6 million lives each year during the early 21st century, and the numbers are rising (WHO 1999, 49). HIV/AIDS, tuberculosis, and malaria all share the following characteristics: they target primarily the poor, respond to antibiotics, develop resistance to existing drugs, and remain beyond the reach of vaccines (Partners In Health 2002, i). We will review HIV/AIDS shortly, after first reviewing two ancient scourges that continue to wreak havoc on the world's poorest countries. Tuberculosis was labeled "the forgotten illness" until it "reemerged" in the rich countries after the HIV epidemic struck in the early 1980s. Notions of tuberculosis' "reemergence" struck a particularly dissonant chord among those who had been forever living under its long shadow (Farmer 1994b, 47). Malaria has received relatively little attention from the world's rich countries since its eradication from Europe and the United States in the 1950s and 1960s. Both of these infectious killers remain distant concerns for the world research community. Precious few research dollars have targeted them, despite their position atop the list of infectious disease killers. Unfortunately for their victims, neither of these disease entities proves cost effective for major research efforts given the poor state of the majority of their victims. Yet their virulence remains.

Consumption, as tuberculosis is known, has been a part of human history since at least 5,000 B.C. (Garrett 1994, 241), claiming more than 1 billion victims through the centuries (Global Alliance 2004a). In ancient times, tuberculosis affected virtually all cultures, except those in the Americas, who succumbed to it in droves after acquiring it from their European colonizers. As populations expanded everywhere and more people lived huddled together in poor housing, rates of tuberculosis increased. In 1850, Lemuel Shattuck named consumption the leading cause of US deaths, a trend that continued for decades (Institute for Health 1996, 20). As living standards and general hygiene improved in developed countries following the reforms ushered in as a response to the living conditions of the Industrial Revolution, the incidence of tuberculosis fell. However, it remained prevalent in poor countries and then surged worldwide in the 1980s following the spread of HIV. As recently as 1995, the WHO reported that there were 8 million new cases and 3 million deaths, with 95% of all cases and 98% of all deaths occurring in developing countries (WHO 2004a). As poverty rates fell throughout the developing world, the death rate from tuberculosis had fallen to 2 million by 2002, though more than one third of the world's population remained infected. Such a high incidence is not surprising given tuberculosis' ease of transmission. Someone with tuberculosis who is coughing infects an average of 10 to 15 people per year, earning tuberculosis the moniker of, "Ebola with wings." From 2000 to 2020, 1 billion people will become newly infected, 200 million will become sick, and 35 million will die from tuberculosis, unless current efforts at detection and treatment are strengthened (WHO 2002b).

Tuberculosis has killed so many for so long, not because of its biological or clinical characteristics, but because of the social patterns of its prey, generally those at the bottom of unequal societies and in the poorest countries. Such trends reveal a long-standing "pernicious synergy" between poverty and tuberculosis, confirmed by the literature (Farmer 1994b, 201). English death registries from the 1830s showed that the likelihood of dying from tuberculosis increased with decreasing socioeconomic status (Institute for Health 1996, 2). In the United States and other developed countries, tuberculosis continues to preferentially attack the poor, along with minorities, alcoholics, drug injectors, and the homeless. In one 1996 study, tuberculosis attack rates among New York City welfare recipients who "abused drugs and alcohol" were 70 times the national average and 4 times higher than those found in developing countries (Friedman et al 1996, 828).

More than 90% of people infected with tuberculosis will simply wall off the bacillus in the lung and live unaffected for decades or for life. Yet, in the unfortunate 10% who are less able to fight the bacillus due to malnutrition (from poverty) or immunodeficiency (from AIDS and/or malnutrition), tuberculosis attacks relentlessly. Hence, its high attack and fatality rates in developing countries. To see an acute case of tuberculosis is to see infectious illness at its most inexorable. The afflicted cough relentlessly, long beyond that which it appears their frail bodies can stand; their coughs often produce blood. In time they evolve a depleted, emaciated countenance that is not unlike that of an end-stage AIDS patient—often the two illnesses coincide. It is little wonder that tuberculosis is likely the most common opportunistic infection found in HIV/AIDS patients. In many countries, a sudden spike in tuberculosis cases heralded the arrival of HIV. Until overtaken by HIV/AIDS in the early 2000s, tuberculosis had been the leading infectious disease killer. Tuberculosis and AIDS share another unfortunate characteristic for the afflicted—both have long fostered discrimination and blame.

Prior to Koch's discovery of the tubercle bacillus in 1873, some thought tuberculosis was an inherited condition, with proclivities among some racial groups. US blacks in particular attracted theories of tuberculosis susceptibility due to their "deficient brain capacity" or belief in "superstition" that produced a "menace to whites" (Institute for Health 1996, 21). Such explanations were cited as rationale for keeping white and black youths segregated.

Modern equivalents hold that the poor are "noncompliant" or somehow "unfit" to receive appropriate treatment when the real obstacles are money, distance from care, and increasing drug resistance. Often such reprimands come from their health providers (Farmer 1994b, 184). And although poverty largely determines who becomes sick once infected, a poor health infrastructure largely determines who among the sick will receive appropriate care. Writing on tuberculosis' dubious status in the late 1990s, Paul Farmer wrote, "Tuberculosis is thus two things at once: a completely curable disease and the leading cause of young adult deaths in much of the world" (185). As such, tuberculosis has joined the ranks of those illnesses for which effective therapies only serve to further exacerbate disparities in health—the rich are cured while the poor are left to suffer the natural course of the illness, often resulting in death. Most tuberculosis deaths continue to occur in settings of abject poverty with "abysmal tuberculosis services" (212). It is not surprising that no new drug breakthroughs have been developed in more than 30 years. Although tuberculosis would seem an ideal investment vehicle for pharmaceutical companies given its global prevalence, only 5% of those currently infected can pay for treatment (Global Alliance 2004b).

Because tuberculosis is a slow-growing bacillus, it takes months of effective drug treatment to eradicate it. When people take only part of their full therapy course, they foster drug resistance. As such, it is important that health workers observe patients taking every pill, a practice called directly observed treatment, short-course, or DOTS. This labor-intensive therapy has worked well in both rich and poor countries, including some of the poorest locales (Mitnick et al 2003, 119). The WHO initiated the first global DOTS campaign in 1991. Other campaigns have since cured millions, with new countries adding DOTS campaigns each year. Like all other infectious agents, tuberculosis bacilli have evolved multidrug-resistant strains, contributing to the lethality of the disease. Such strains are labeled MDR-TB and they have contributed to a surging worldwide epidemic that is raging through Eastern Europe, Asia, Africa, and South America (Espinal et al 2001, 1294). A green-light committee from the WHO, in partnership with Médecins Sans Frontières (MSF), Partners In Health, and other NGOs, was able to bring down the cost of second-line agents essential to treating MDR-TB. Two physicians intimately involved in this process were Jim Yong Kim and Paul Farmer, profiled in Chapter 13. Halving the tuberculosis prevalence and deaths rates by 2015 is included among the UN's Millennium Development Goals, though attaining this goal is unlikely without significantly more money. The battle against MDR-TB continues and the epidemic serves as a harbinger of things to come, as more and more microbes acquire resistance to the best efforts of scientists. Perhaps tuberculosis' greatest lesson is how an infectious threat long ignored by the rich countries will ultimately ensnare them as well.

Malaria

Malaria has long afflicted tropical and subtropical regions around the world. During the first half of the 20th century, malaria claimed 2 million lives per year, mostly in Asia and the Pacific tropics (WHO 1999, 50). Following the discovery of DDT and the founding of the WHO, anti-malarial campaigns became widespread, with some modicum of success. Malaria was once rampant in the United States and western Europe. As recently as the 1850s, malaria was considered the most important disease in the United States, killing thousands in seasonal outbreaks and afflicting 1 million soldiers during the Civil War (Farmer 1994b, 40). As recently as the 1920s, malaria continued to infect 1 million people in the US South annually. Drainage of swamps, netting, agriculture development, improved housing, mosquito repellents, and eradication campaigns that followed the invention of DDT in 1939 all stemmed from large-scale reductions in poverty–the United States was free of malaria by the mid-1960s. Europe and other developed countries had similar success. In Sri Lanka, malaria cases plummeted from 1 million cases per year to just 20 cases in 1963 (WHO 1999, 53). In recent years, Hong Kong, Singapore, and even China have had great success rolling back malaria through spraying, prevention through treated nets, and strong treatment programs. China now has roughly 100 malaria-related deaths per year vs the hundreds of thousands of cases per year during the early 20th century.

As with HIV and tuberculosis, malaria preys on the poor preferentially, and those countries that host the malaria protozoa are among the world's poorest. Malaria causes nearly 250 times as many deaths in the world's poorest countries as in the richest countries. Poor countries have been unable to mount successful public health ventures, and their people simply have had to bear the scourge of the protozoa. Because of its effects on workers, students, and tourism, malaria is a major contributor to economic stagnation so common in afflicted countries. In its dual role as both a cause of and result from poverty, malaria is a key component of underdevelopment and any strategies to reverse it (WHO 1999, 51).

More than 90% of all global malarial deaths occur in sub-Saharan Africa, a region that sees malaria cause one fifth of all childhood deaths.

As with HIV and several other life-shortening infectious diseases, the prime center for malaria infection and death remains sub-Saharan Africa. The toll this one disease takes on Africans annually is staggering. Nearly three fourths of Africa's population lives in highly endemic areas; 270 million cases occur annually, with almost 1 million deaths (WHO 1999, 55). In fact, more than 90% of all global malarial deaths occur in sub-Saharan Africa, a region that sees malaria cause one fifth of all childhood deaths. The death toll from malaria rose in the 1980s just as it was falling elsewhere.

In part, this stemmed from the difficulty of achieving adequate vector (mosquito) control, as was achieved elsewhere—it is beyond the means of many African governments. It also stems from the fact that the prime form of malaria in Africa is *Plasmodium falciparum*, by far the most deadly strain and one that has evolved resistance to the affordable and effective drug chloroquine in recent years. Armed conflict and refugee movements that have plagued Africa for decades have contributed to the increase burden of malaria since the 1980s (53).

In addition to its enormous health burden, malaria inflicts a substantial economic burden, particularly for those countries with *P. falciparum*. The economies of Spain, Greece, Italy, and Portugal soared in the 1940s and 1950s following marked reductions in the number of malaria cases. Rolling back that one disease galvanized these economies through tourism and foreign direct investment (Commission on Macroeconomics and Health 2001, 38). By contrast, malaria alone costs Africa between 1% and 2% of its GDP per year (National Intelligence Council 2000, 46). Estimates for specific countries are higher—2% to 6% per year in Kenya and 1% to 5% per year in Nigeria (WHO 1999, 51). Such estimates stem largely from the loss of productivity due to sickness and premature mortality. Yet, malaria slows economic growth through indirect means as well. Students miss school due to illness and are less attentive. Additionally, foreign investment, tourism, and trade opportunities are lost due to malaria infestation. Malaria also serves as a significant drain on already strained health systems in affected countries. In Africa, between 20% and 40% of outpatients visits and 10% and 15% of hospital admissions stem from malaria. Rwanda spent one fifth of its health budget on malaria in 1989 (51). Individuals must also spend significant amounts out of pocket. Farmers in Nigeria and Kenya spend 13% and 5%, respectively, of total household income on malaria treatment (National Intelligence Council 2000, 47). Clearly this one illness serves as a huge drag on the economies of the countries so afflicted.

Efforts to control malaria have long been hindered by the fact that, as with tuberculosis, most of those afflicted reside in poor countries. Efforts to eradicate malaria globally sputtered and failed in the 1950s and 1960s (Garrett 1994, 47), yielding to decades-long strategies of containment and case treatment in areas such as sub-Saharan Africa, where eradication proved impossible. Research efforts similarly flagged until 1997, when UNDP, WHO, and the World Bank launched the Multilateral Initiative on Malaria, providing roughly $3 million per year for research into drugs, health policies, and the pathogenesis/epidemiology of the disease (WHO 1999, 59). Similarly, the WHO, UNICEF, the World Bank, and UNDP—along with 90 other partners—launched the Roll Back Malaria Partnership campaign in 1998, with the goal of halving the burden of malaria by 2010.[10] The Global Fund also provides funds for research and control of malaria. Although these efforts hold promise for the future, they have thus far failed to halt the disease, which remains a primary killer decades after the discovery of effective drugs to treat it.

Endnotes

1. Information from the United Nations High Commissioner for Refuges web site at www.unhcr.ch.
2. Information from Michael A. Grodin, MD, from a lecture during the Intensive Course in Health and Human Rights at the Harvard School of Public Health, June 2002, Boston.
3. Information from the University of California Berkeley Museum of Paleontology web site at www.ucmp.berkeley.edu/history/malthus.html.
4. Personal observation during a visit with a delegation from Massachusetts General Hospital, December 1998.
5. Information from the Population Crisis Committee, "Human Suffering Index" (1120 19th Street, N.W. Suite 550, Washington, DC 20036).
6. Information from the Population Reference Bureau's, "Fact Sheet: Making Pregnancy and Childbirth Safer," available on the Population Reference Bureau's web site at www.prb.org.
7. I had the opportunity to visit this tribe during my time as a Kellogg National Leadership Fellow from 1994–1997.
8. Dr Edward O'Neil, Dr Peter Allen (Southern Regional Manager for Belize), personal communication, 2000.
9. Dr Edward O'Neil, Rhena Schweitzer, personal communication, May 14, 2002.
10. Information from the Roll Back Malaria web site at www.rbm.who.int.

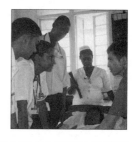

Chapter 9

Lessons from a Plague:
The History, Scope,
and Politics of HIV/AIDS

*History will judge us on how we deal with this
crisis. God will judge us even harder. We really must
make this a priority.... Charity alone will not
work. We need a new partnership based on justice
and equality.*

—Bono, lead singer of U2

*Whenever I look into the eyes of someone dying
of AIDS, I have an eerie awareness that Jesus is
staring back at me.*

—Mother Teresa

*When the University of California at Los Angeles' (UCLA's) Dr Michael
Gottlieb and the Centers for Disease Control and Prevention (CDC) first
brought to the world's attention a clustering of unusual infections in five gay
men in Los Angeles in 1981, no one could then imagine how massive and
devastating the strange new epidemic would become (CDC 1981, 250). Since
then, HIV has become history's most lethal epidemic, taking millions of lives,
destroying economies, and reversing decades of developmental progress.
If current projections hold, 250 million people will be infected by 2025.*

*To better understand the workings of HIV, we will look first at the virus
itself, from its unique biology to the distinct epidemics it has spawned, and
then quantify the wreckage in the wake of the virus in terms of lives lost,*

economies ruined, and orphans produced. The responses to AIDS have included fear, discrimination, even execution of those afflicted. We will examine the politics of fear and blame in both the United States and the world that have greatly facilitated the spread of the virus. AIDS has exacerbated pre-existing disparities between those in rich and poor countries, dramatizing the life and death differentials afforded by wealth. We will examine the reasons why. We will trace the events that led up to the US pledge for $15 billion for AIDS relief and why the response likely will prove to be inadequate.

Ultimately the best chance for salvation from AIDS will come by viewing HIV/AIDS as a human rights issue. We will track the few pioneers who coaxed world leaders to this view, strengthening the connections between health and human rights and forging a new paradigm for all who venture into health work in the new millennium.

HIV Origins and Early History

HIV is a retrovirus, a member of the lentivirus family that reproduces itself either by making exact copies in its host (the animal or human it attacks) or by combining with other retroviruses of similar genealogy to create variant strains, a process best understood as *viral sex* (Goudsmit 1997). This latter feature has allowed the virus to adapt and change, jump species, and become more widespread and lethal with time. It is one of the keys to the success of HIV and the reason that vaccines against it have proven so elusive thus far. It is also the key to understanding one of the main pathological features of HIV: it is not just one virus. Rather, the HIV family consists of at least three groups of viruses, each with many subtypes spawned by viral sexual reproduction. Each subtype in turn holds subtle differences in structure that make it more adept at exploiting certain aspects of human behavior.

Although its origins remain controversial ("How AIDS Began" 1998), considerable evidence indicates that HIV derives from a simian immunodeficiency virus (SIV) that lived harmlessly in monkeys for thousands of years in the rain forests of Central Africa. Sometime in the early 1900s, it then jumped species to humans. Earlier suspicions that HIV stemmed from a polio vaccination campaign gone terribly wrong have been thoroughly discredited ("AIDS Wars" 2000). The virus probably made the leap when a chimpanzee bit or cut a human hunter. Forest peoples have long hunted various primates for food, a practice that continues in the present day. With European invasions and conquests, people pushed farther into the monkeys' habitat, increasing the number of exposures. The reproductive nature of the virus enabled differing strains to successfully establish themselves in humans at different times. Each viral type then spawned new subtypes, a process that continues unabated.

As of this writing, HIV is composed of a family of viruses of three known types: HIV-1, HIV-2, and HIV-0 (Goudsmit 1997). These three viruses lack a common human-based ancestor; they represent three separate emerging epidemics that evolved from simian hosts in different regions of Africa. As a result, they produce varying degrees of disease severity and contagion. For the most part, HIV-0 and HIV-2 have remained smaller players on the world stage, largely confined to West Africa and a few other regions. HIV-1 is chiefly responsible for the worldwide AIDS epidemic.

The earliest cases of *suspected* HIV occurred in Europe in the 1930s and, as with a number of other modern problems, its origins can be traced to colonialism and war. Colonialism caused the mixing of diverse peoples in Africa amidst the large-scale migrations precipitated by natives' attempting to escape the violence of the invaders. European overlords kept African mistresses and commonly had sexual relations with their African subjects, which over time brought them directly into contact with the occasional HIV-infected person. The subsequent deaths of either would not have stood out amidst the enormous mortality rates from infectious disease in whites and blacks in Africa. It is likely that one or more German colonists living in pre-World War II Cameroon then acquired HIV as it began to spread through the population. In September 1939, roughly 300 of these colonialists were recalled home at the outset of World War II. Many repatriated and settled in the then-German city of Danzig, which Poland reclaimed after the war and renamed Gdansk. According to author Jaap Goudsmit, this became the probable time and place of HIV's arrival in Europe, judging by the infection clusters that soon ensued.

The clusters are not hard to spot. Because HIV attacks and depletes an important piece of the immune system, the T cells, common infections that healthy immune systems easily fight off become lethal. These infections include *Pneumocystis carinii* pneumonia (PCP), caused by a protozoan that normally lives in all of us quite uneventfully. As such, PCP infections often serve as a marker of HIV infection. Cytomegalovirus (CMV) similarly wreaks destruction when immune defenses fail, as does Candida (thrush) and other common bacteria, viruses, fungi, and protozoa.

When large groups of patients suddenly show clusters of infections like these (called opportunistic), there is a high likelihood that HIV is responsible. Such was the case in a number of European cities following the probable epidemic in Gdansk in 1939. Similar, small infection clusters soon appeared in Switzerland (1941), Austria (1942), Italy (1946), and then in Finland, Denmark, and Sweden by the late 1940s. Similar outbreaks occurred throughout the 1950s and 1960s throughout Europe. It appears that HIV did not trigger a massive epidemic at that time, probably because it lacked the aggressive traits that mark its modern descendents and it never found the right opportunity to spread widely through a society. That would come later. By the end of the 1960s, however, the European epidemic was temporarily over.

The first *proven* case of HIV infection occurred around 1966, when a well-traveled (including Africa) sailor from Norway developed a generalized swelling of the lymph nodes. He died a decade later from opportunistic infections, as did his wife and infant son. When testing for HIV became available in the1980s, frozen sera from these three cases all tested positive.

An earlier case of *suspected* HIV occurred in a sailor from Manchester, England, who died of PCP and CMV in 1959. By 1962, 33 cases of PCP had been reported in the medical literature, primarily in European men and in most instances associated with other opportunistic infections. HIV likely existed long before this, occasionally claiming lives deep in the rain forests of German East Africa at least since 1900, though mostly hidden from the outside world (Goudsmit 1997, 74). In time, a number of factors caused the virus to evolve and spread, none of which were more important than humanity's willingness to become a far more accommodating host.

The Epidemic in the Americas

It was around the late 1970s when the virus likely mutated to more virulent forms. When these combined with sexual liberation movements worldwide, large epidemics quickly followed. In North America, the gay sexual revolution served as a key cofactor in the spread of the virus. Through a "tragic accident," according to Goudsmit, HIV-1b arrived in North America just as the gay sexual revolution was under way (1997, 12). Sexual liberation in the heterosexual community, along with an increasing number of injection drug users in poor and minority populations, also contributed to the spread of HIV-1b, the subtype primarily responsible for the European and American epidemics. Because the gay sexual revolution formed a core piece of the spread of HIV-1b in North America and Europe, it warrants a brief review.

Gay men and women unleashed decades of pent-up fury on the nights of June 27 and 28, 1969, following the funeral of a beloved icon in the gay community, singer Judy Garland. For years, police had raided and occasionally beaten the various drag queens, gay professionals, and others who frequented a seedy bar called the Stonewall Inn in the Greenwich Village section of New York City. However, following a day of mourning, the gays fought back when the police from the "public morals" division raided the Village at 1:20 AM on the 28th. Hundreds rioted in the streets and the Village was soon "bleeding and burning" in a shot heard around the gay universe. One police officer summed up the day's events: "Things were completely changed. . . . Suddenly they were not submissive anymore" (Cloud 1969). The rioting continued that night.

In the midst of the chaos of the Stonewall riots, the gay liberation movement was born, radically changing the social and political landscape for gays in the United States and elsewhere. Just one year later, a commemorative parade in New York City drew 20,000 people; and just eight years later a parade in San Francisco drew 375,000 (Shilts 1987, 16). June 27 has since been remembered as Gay Freedom Day/Gay Pride Day in annual celebrations around the world.

After Stonewall, previously closeted gay men from small towns all across the United States streamed into major cities, particularly New York and San Francisco. Gay communities evolved, and from their ranks political leaders emerged to bring the power of the gay voting block to mainstream politics for the first time. In San Francisco, Harvey Milk, Cleve Jones, and Bill Kraus became dominant figures in a gay political movement that became increasingly vocal in its demands for gay rights (Shilts 1987). Simultaneously, a gay sexual revolution exploded virtually overnight. Decades of sexual repression came cascading down, and anonymous sexual encounters in bathrooms, bathhouses, and parties became commonplace for a sizable subset of gay men, some of whom counted their sexual liaisons in the thousands.

In the midst of the chaos of the Stonewall riots, the gay liberation movement was born.

Author Randy Shilts noted that "promiscuity was central to the raucous gay movement of the 1970s," and the centers of the action were the bathhouses and sex clubs that quickly became a $100 million industry (1987, 19). It was common for men to have sexual encounters with several different men during an evening in the bathhouses, where common pre-sexual formalities such as the exchanging of names were dispensed with altogether. As Shilts wrote, "It was if these people, who had been made so separate from society by virtue of their sexuality, were now making their sexuality utterly separate from themselves" (24).

Although such expressions of sexual freedom had occurred before in history, the sheer scale of "multiple-partnering" in both gay and straight worlds in the 1970s and 1980s was unprecedented (Goudsmit 1997, 12; Garrett 1994, 263). The arrival of "the pill" in the 1960s, coupled with the inception of the disco in the 1970s, propelled the heterosexual revolution forward alongside the revolution in the gay world. In developing countries, the new sexual climate coalesced with urbanization, where men commuted to cities during the week, frolicked with urban women on weeknights, and returned to their village wives on the weekends. Factoring in the rapid advancements and falling prices in air travel, the stage was set for a sexually transmitted microbe to exploit the opportunity that mankind had presented.

The party raged on with few noticing the quiet escalation of a number of sexually transmitted diseases in the health clinics throughout the United States, Europe, and Africa (Garrett 1994, 260). Gonorrhea, chlamydia, syphilis, hepatitis B and C, herpes, chancroid, warts—virtually every conceivable sexually transmitted pathogen rose rapidly through the 1970s; precursors to the coming plague. Gay men would not heed warnings to slow down, having suffered discrimination at the hands of government officials and even carrying a label of "mentally ill" until 1973.

Dr Selma Dritz, of the San Francisco Department of Public Health, noted with alarm the rapid escalation of increasingly serious infections racing through the homosexual community in the late 1970s. "Too much is being transmitted," she said in 1980. "We've got all these diseases going unchecked. There are so many opportunities for transmission that if something new gets loose here, we're going to have hell to pay" (Shilts 1987, 40).

When HIV arrived, it came with a relentless fury. Overnight, men in cities all over North America turned up with mysterious ailments such as Kaposi's sarcoma, a previously rare tumor found in elderly Greek men, as well as PCP and other infections associated with severe immune deficiency. Within a few short years, the number of known cases reached into the thousands as HIV rioted through the gay community. What remained unknown then, however, was that the asymptomatic stage lasted for years. With no blood test available until 1985, few realized the true breadth of the looming crisis.

With no blood test available until 1985, few realized the true breadth of the looming crisis.

Later studies revealed that more than 20% of San Francisco's gay men were already infected as early as the end of 1982, a year in which more than 900 identified cases of HIV already had been identified in the United States alone. The epidemic soon spread through the injection drug-using community and the blood supply. Though widely missed at the epidemic's outset, HIV quickly infected women everywhere, often taking advantage of entrenched inequalities in wealth and power (Farmer et al 1996, 3). In the United States, however, the gay community bore the brunt of the epidemic.

There is little question that the rapid spread of HIV through the gay community was aided by the multiple partnering, often anonymous, that characterized the gay sexual revolution. Some in the gay community were vocal in their opposition to the anonymous and depersonalized sexuality that defined the era. Playwright Larry Kramer, for one, in his play *Faggots* depicted a fast-paced, hypersexual culture losing its soul (Shilts 1987, 24). Some, like Kramer, understood the implications of the disease clusters early on. But few heeded the warnings and resented anyone who infringed on their sexual freedoms, which were considered at the core of the gay liberation movement. As Shilts wrote, "Self-criticism was not the strong point of a community that was only beginning to define itself affirmatively after centuries of repression" (20).

Early in the epidemic, rumors of a "gay plague" brought mostly shrugs from men hurrying off to the next dalliance on Fire Island. Others greeted early warnings with open hostility. The ennui and anger, however, quickly subsided as men began dying by the hundreds, and then by the thousands.

As the epidemic mushroomed, the shock of the rising caseloads of sick and dying men galvanized the gay community. Denial and apathy gave way to community outreach and political activism. The AIDS Coalition to Unleash Power (ACT UP) emerged in 1987 in response to widespread feelings that New York City's political leadership had been slow to respond. This group staged numerous gatherings and protests, along with radical acts that set the pharmaceutical industries and government research agencies on edge.[1] In one ACT UP tactic called the "political funeral," members held public funerals out in the open for members lost to AIDS. ACT UP members staged the funeral of one prominent activist in an open coffin in Lafayette Park, directly across the street from the White House. Other political bodies lobbied Congress and forced the reluctant hand of the Reagan and Bush administrations to channel more funding to HIV/AIDS research.

Yet HIV was hardly confined to the United States, rapidly spreading to Canada, Latin America, and the Caribbean. One of the most heavily infected Caribbean countries, also its poorest, is no stranger to blame and marginalization—Haiti. Just as in most countries of the world, it is unclear how HIV first arrived on Haitian shores. Probably, HIV arrived in Haiti from the United States, either from returning Haitian nationals or US tourists—both gay and straight—taking advantage of Haiti's entrenched poverty to indulge their sexual fantasies. Gay travel guides such as *Spartacus International* enthusiastically recommended Haiti to their readers in 1983 because of the "nominal" fees that attractive young Haitian men charged to entertain them; an advertisement in the gay magazine the *Advocate* proclaimed that, in Haiti, "all your fantasies come true" (Farmer 1994b, 122).[2] Because of the country's severe poverty, Haitian men were willing to sell sex to gay tourists for less than $5 (Garrett 1994, 308). HIV spread rapidly through Port-au-Prince and then into the countryside, flowing down economic gradients from salaried soldiers and truckers to poor and dependent women. Some inaccurately cited Haiti as the origin of the epidemic—continuing a long tradition of erroneously blaming the poor. Haiti's experience, however, reflected that of other Caribbean countries—those with the closest ties to the United States had the highest number of AIDS cases (Farmer 1994b, 125).

Within just a few years HIV had spread throughout the Western Hemisphere. Sexual tourism helped to foster the spread of HIV in many more countries in addition to Haiti. The virus was introduced to Thailand's thriving sex industry, and prostitution throughout Africa, Asia, and Eastern Europe has amplified the epidemic. HIV remains primarily a sexually transmitted disease and, no matter how uncomfortable people may be in discussing it, human sexuality—in all of its forms—will long remain the prime vehicle for the spread of the virus. Rather than castigate any specific group for fueling the spread of the

HIV remains primarily a sexually transmitted disease.

epidemic, however, it is better to try to understand the epidemic from the viewpoint of viral opportunity. To that end, humans everywhere could hardly have been more accommodating hosts.

The Epidemics in Africa (and Beyond)

In Africa a considerably larger epidemic emerged, caused mostly by HIV-1, subtypes HIV-1a and HIV-1c. The ancestral precursor to HIV-1 had remained in Cameroon in a semidormant state for decades. It then emerged in Tanzania, Uganda, Zaire (now the Democratic Republic of the Congo [DRC]), and Rwanda in the 1970s as a wasting, diarrhea-producing illness widely termed "slim disease," which is different from the clinical form in the West caused by subtype HIV-1b. These African subtypes emerged at that time, at least in part, because of the political instability of the region (Goudsmit 1997, 64).

Uganda was then in the midst of Idi Amin's long reign of terror, which claimed 300,000 lives between 1971 and 1979 (Lamb 1987, 77). Repeated clashes between Tanzanian and Ugandan soldiers continued long after the overthrow of Amin, providing an ideal opportunity for HIV transmission. Soldiers are major purveyors of sexually transmitted pathogens because they are young, sexually active, and powerful—rape and brutality often follow in their wake. Large-scale refugee movements produce starving and, hence, immune-deficient masses as health infrastructures collapse and many women are forced into prostitution as economies fail (Garrett 1994, 367). All of these factors favored the spread of the virus.

Similar dysfunction characterized Zaire, then under the rule of Mobuto Sese Seko, one of history's most corrupt rulers (Lamb 1987, 43). Tanzania stagnated under President Julius Nyere's failed socialism, and Rwanda's own dysfunction exploded two decades later. In short, HIV subtypes A and C thrived in the midst of the political and economic anarchy that characterized the region around Lake Victoria, widely considered to be the epicenter of the AIDS epidemic.

Once it was established around Lake Victoria in western Tanzania, HIV rapidly spread north and south through subtype HIV-1C and east and west through subtype HIV-1A (Goudsmit 1997, 74). Both subtypes spread largely through the backbone of Africa's commerce— the truckers. Because poverty is extreme in much of sub-Saharan Africa, many women are forced into prostitution or are in no position to refuse the advances of salaried men such as truck drivers. The main truck routes through Africa have been dubbed "AIDS highways." Along these routes, those who live closest to the highways have the highest rates of HIV infection. The same phenomena characterize AIDS in India, where the incidence of HIV mirrors proximity to truck routes ("AIDS in India" 2004).

The women have silently borne the brunt of AIDS in Africa.

Because most African women are landless, powerless, and voiceless, they can not refuse their husband's or any powerful man's sexual advances or request that they use condoms, even when the man is known to be HIV-positive. The women have silently borne the brunt of AIDS in Africa. They continue to plow the fields and rear the children until their AIDS-ravaged bodies simply give out.

Gender inequality is just one of many factors fueling the spread of HIV through sub-Saharan Africa. The civil unrest that has characterized many countries in that region after decolonization has created mass migrations of refugees and deepening levels of poverty, both of which foster the spread of HIV. Poverty's stepchild is illiteracy, and large numbers of Africans still have a poor understanding of how HIV is spread or subscribe to various myths about how to protect themselves.

AIDS in Africa comprises an epidemic that has wreaked havoc on several fronts: humane, economic, political, and strategic. The first—humane—is the most striking and potentially the most transformative for anyone who experiences it. Many prominent people, including former President Jimmy Carter, former Secretary of State Colin Powell, UN Secretary-General Kofi Annan, U2 singer Bono, Senate Majority Leader William Frist, former House Majority Leader Richard Gephardt, and Global Fund architect Jeffrey Sachs have commented on their horror at seeing firsthand the devastation caused by AIDS in Africa (Behrman 2004, 265; Eaton and Etue 2002; Stolberg 2002). The magnitude of the death toll in sub-Saharan Africa today is staggering; it is history's greatest collective dying from a single cause. Currently, infants born in seven African countries have a life expectancy of less than 40 years (Dugger 2004). By 2010, life expectancy could decrease to less than 30 years (National Intelligence Council 2000, 50).

In 1998, Catholic theologian and former Zimbabwean freedom fighter Michael Auret described the AIDS epidemic there in the starkest of terms: "Seven out of ten high school seniors in Harare are infected. We are in the midst of an ecological crisis as a result of the deforestation due to coffin construction. If there's not a major mobilization, Africa will be reduced to beach-front property for Europeans" (Behrman 2004, 87). Botswana President Festus Mogae said simply, "We are threatened with extinction" (xi).

The AIDS epidemic has also exacted a huge economic toll from sub-Saharan Africa. One World Bank official believes that HIV/AIDS represents the single greatest threat to economic growth in Africa (National Intelligence Council 2000, 46). In heavily infected countries, the economic growth likely slows by 1% per year. In the worst-hit countries, with HIV prevalence at 20% of the population, annual economic growth (gross domestic products [GDP]) has slowed by 2.6 points, a drag that even rich industrialized countries could not long tolerate ("The Cost of AIDS" 2004). When combined with malaria, several studies suggest that economic growth in sub-Saharan Africa will decrease 20% by 2010 (National Intelligence Council 2000, 46).

AIDS claims those who are in the prime of their working lives, costing the affected countries hundreds of billions of dollars each year, which represents a large percentage of their national incomes (Commission on Macroeconomics and Health 2001, 30). Families often deplete their scarce resources on the sick and end up trapped in poverty after selling off their livestock or land. Also, as workers become ill or die from any illness, tax revenues shrink, further depleting the government coiffeurs. Some South African multinational firms routinely hire three employees for every skilled position, "to ensure that replacements are on hand when trained workers die" (Sachs 2001b).

A number of workers—often female—leave their jobs for long periods to care for an ill spouse or child. Many workplaces similarly have found their staff depleted by the sheer number of funerals that take workers away from their jobs. Other skilled workers, including health workers, emigrate, leaving their communities without the talent required to reverse the illness-generated setbacks. In one stunning estimate, the net loss of productivity from AIDS alone came out to more than one third of GDP in sub-Saharan Africa (Commission on Macroeconomics and Health 2001, 31).

From political and strategic standpoints, the AIDS epidemic threatens what meager gains to overall stability Africa has made in recent decades. Even before AIDS, the continent was home to an inordinate number of wars and internal conflicts. In recent years, conflicts still raged in Algeria, Burundi, the Democratic Republic of the Congo, Liberia, Niger, Nigeria, Sudan, and Uganda, with the real possibility that new conflicts will flare in still more unstable states.[3] When a fragile base is combined with history's most destructive epidemic, the net result could be widespread political collapse, throwing many more countries into war or perpetual anarchy, as in Somalia.

AIDS has further destabilized governments through declining tax and business revenues, weakened militaries, and the loss of critical expertise in young people. The net result could produce widespread state failure, a process that has repeatedly ensnared the US military in wars and internal state conflicts. (Sachs 2001a, 187).

In 2002, a Central Intelligence Agency (CIA) advisory group called the National Intelligence Council (NIC) issued a warning that the rates of HIV infection in five populous countries—China, Ethiopia, India, Nigeria, and Russia—were rising so quickly that the epidemic posed a clear security threat to the respective nations as well as the United States (Altman 2002). An earlier NIC report in January 2000 warned that the AIDS epidemic would lead to political instability and reverse democratic gains throughout sub-Saharan Africa, parts of Asia, and the former Soviet Union (National Intelligence Council 2000, 52). It further warned that high infection rates in a number of countries would weaken national militaries and deplete peacekeeping forces given the high numbers of infected soldiers. Where the epidemic will lead Africa is anyone's guess. What is clear is that HIV/AIDS presents the most credible threat to long-term viability on the continent. Ultimately, the instability that AIDS spawns in Africa could ensnare the rest of the world.

The Scale and Impact of the Global Epidemic

During the mid to late 1980s, HIV/AIDS dominated the headlines of US and Western newspapers as the epidemic tore through homosexual, injection drug-using, and blood product–dependent communities. Over time, however, a public that was not overly interested in the problems of "fringe" groups receded. With the seemingly miraculous advent of highly active anti-retroviral (HAART) medications in 1996, death rates in the rich world plummeted and the headlines all but disappeared. Nevertheless, the epidemic rages on.

The scope of this epidemic is staggering. Estimates vary widely, and many countries are unable to treat their people, much less track the number dying from AIDS. Nevertheless, as of December 2004, the most recent year for which there are now complete data, nearly 40 million people were living with HIV/AIDS (UNAIDS 2004); 5 million people became newly infected with HIV; and 3.1 million died in 2004, the single highest yearly death total yet. Of the 3.1 million deaths, half a million occurred in children under age 15. The epidemic had claimed 28 million lives by the end of 2004, and by the end of the decade could infect 100 million people and create 25 million AIDS orphans (Behrman 2004).[4]

The region of the world hit hardest is sub-Saharan Africa. In 2004 this region had 25 million people infected with HIV/AIDS, 3.1 million new infections, and 2.3 million total AIDS deaths. The prevalence of HIV/AIDS in this region is the world's highest, estimated at 7.5% to 8.5%. Entire villages have lost their young workers and parents, and many of Africa's intelligentsia have fallen victim to the raging plague (Garrett 1994, 478). In addition, prevalence rates as high as 40% have been recorded in Botswana and Swaziland (UNAIDS 2004, 7).

Asia, where HIV has exploded in recent years, is now home to the second largest HIV/AIDS population. By the end of 2004, the region recorded 8.2 million cases and more than a half a million people had died of AIDS during the year (UNAIDS 2004, 5). And India could soon face African-sized numbers of dead and dying ("AIDS in India" 2004) unless aggressive national policies can halt the spread of HIV in that country. Other regions have similarly overwhelming HIV/AIDS statistics. In 2004, Latin America and the Caribbean accounted for more than 2 million cases and 130,000 deaths and emerging epidemics in Eastern Europe and Central Asia accounted for another 1.4 million people living with HIV/AIDS and 60,000 deaths in 2004.

After the Berlin Wall fell in 1989, Eastern European women flooded across the borders to earn comparatively high amounts of money turning tricks in Western Europe, which prompted near strikes in Western capital cities (Garrett 1994, 500). In North American countries the AIDS epidemic has slowed in recent years, and the world's largest number of HIV/AIDS patients receiving life-saving anti-retrovirals (ARVs) is in North America. By the end of 2004, 1 million people were living with HIV/AIDS and 15,000 had died.

The Faces of AIDS

What may be lost in the statistical and economic descriptions of this epidemic are its individual human tragedies, such as the one that opened this book. Since starting medical school in 1983, I have observed this epidemic while caring for distinct groups of patients on three separate fronts: homosexuals in Washington DC; predominantly black and Latino injection drug users and their sexual contacts in inner-city Boston; and the poor in developing countries in Africa, the Caribbean, and South America. On all fronts—at least until HAART dramatically changed the scene in 1996—the epidemic has been similarly depressing and frustrating.

One patient from my first encounters with HIV sticks in my mind. His name was Gary, and I assumed his care in 1986 while I was a fourth-year medical student at George Washington University Hospital in Washington, DC. Years before I had come to know him, Gary's parents had severed all contact with him because of his homosexuality. Then in his early 30s, Gary was spending the last weeks of his life in a hospital bed. In 1986 we had little to offer AIDS patients against the virus itself, and I watched Gary slowly wither away following wave after wave of infection, each more devastating than its predecessor. As HIV attacked his central nervous system, Gary slowly lost strength and his power of speech. In the end, several members from the gay community came to be with him, offering comfort and friendship to a young man—painfully alone—dying a slow and difficult death. A look of innocence mixed with incredulity and horror characterized his face when he died, an image still fixed in my mind.

Like most AIDS patients, Gary had been young and healthy when he contracted HIV. The cruelest characteristic of AIDS is that most of its victims are in the prime of their lives, physically, mentally, and physiologically. They are simply not ready to die, so they endure one horrible infection after another until the sheer volume of infectious complications overwhelms them. When CMV attacks the eyes, causing blindness, or *pneumocystis* attacks the lungs, causing the inability to breathe, or *cryptosporidium* attacks the gastrointestinal tract, causing endless diarrhea, their young bodies fight on. There is no failing heart, no renal (kidney) shutdown to bring a merciful end to the suffering as it occurs naturally in older, more infirm victims of disease. Although the victims in developing countries tend to die sooner because of their relative malnutrition, most die neither quickly nor peacefully.

By 1987 I was a resident at Boston Medical Center (BMC), where the epidemic surged through our base population of injection drug users and their sexual partners, most of whom were black or Latino. In 1988, I talked with an injection drug-using patient on the wards the morning after an HIV-positive roommate had died during the night following a particularly gruesome exsanguination from a lung infection. My patient was also HIV-positive and still shaking from the scene while an orderly mopped up pools of congealing blood from the floor. During the night she had seen frightening images of what might be in store for her. This prompted a memorable conversation in which she graphically described how difficult it was for her to overcome her addiction. She said, "Doc, you gotta understand how strong this thing [heroin] is. If I needed a fix and saw a needle in the gutter, even if someone told me that needle was covered with AIDS, hepatitis, and anything else, I'd still pick it up and stick it in my arm. I just can't shake it."

She overcame her infections and we discharged her from the hospital. I never saw her again. Like many others in the injection drug-using community, she did not return for follow-up appointments, possibly because of the other problems that preoccupied her.

While working in BMC's HIV Clinic, I cared for a long-term heroin addict who had fought off wave after wave of infections for more than two years. During a conversation in which a colleague and I were trying to get him to be more faithful in keeping his appointments, he said, "Hey, Doc, I gotta be in court tomorrow morning by 10; I got no money and they're going to kick me out of my apartment, so I don't know where I'll be living next week. AIDS is the *least* of my problems." And so it went for so many like him.

I couldn't help but feel that I had betrayed them, because AZT had been available for seven years.

While I was in Africa in 1994, we had little to offer our AIDS patients like the young girl whose story opened this book. HIV testing was available, though we usually did not inform patients of the diagnosis. Many people were shocked to hear this upon my return home. Yet, the prevailing wisdom at the time was that people would lose all hope, and possibly commit suicide, if they were to know the truth. In fact, many had done just that (Garrett 1994, 339). It was a dictum that I followed, though with considerable discomfort. However, in my experience, most people we tested already knew the diagnosis. They knew why they had been losing weight, having recurring fever, and incurring uncontrollable diarrhea. I frequently struggled not to divulge the diagnosis—one I had rendered many times in the United States. I still vividly remember the look in many patients' eyes when I told them that they should go home and take vitamins, that there was nothing more we could offer them. Most replied, quietly and simply, "Thank you, Doctor." I couldn't help but feel that I had betrayed them, because AZT had been available for seven years.

A decade later, on the wards of Guyana's Georgetown Hospital, I met AIDS patients who had been abandoned by family members, evicted, and left to die on the streets. Reminiscent of the intense stigma that characterized AIDS patients in the United States and Europe in the 1980s, the stigma remains in many locales. In India in 2004, people were stoned to death when their diagnosis was revealed. In-laws evicted women who had been infected by their husbands, and employees lost their jobs once their disease was made known ("AIDS in India" 2004). AIDS has become a modern, more lethal version of leprosy, carrying with it not just the venom of the infection itself but a host of social consequences.

AIDS: Politics, Discrimination, and Human Rights

During the early days of the HIV/AIDS epidemics in the United States, Europe, and Africa, the response consisted of avoidance, blame, and apathy. As author Garrett wrote, "*Homo sapiens* greeted the emergence of the new disease first with utter nonchalance, then with disdain for those infected by the virus, followed by an almost pathologic sense of mass denial." (1994, 10). The leaders in the 1980s bore a striking resemblance to members of the London aristocracy centuries earlier who fled a city caught in the throes of bubonic plague, leaving the poor to suffer their fate alone. None of the ranking officials in the key centers of power during the early 1980s, or many of their constituency, were homosexuals, injection drug users, Haitians, hemophiliacs, or African nationals, so they had little incentive to act. This inaction directly contributed to tens or even hundreds of thousands of lives lost.

The Politics of AIDS in the United States

The earliest phases of the AIDS epidemic in the United States came at a time when political conservatism was on the rise. There was little tolerance for flamboyant homosexuals and their openly promiscuous sexuality during the 12 years of the Reagan and Bush administrations. The Reverend Billy Graham called AIDS "a judgment of God," and the Moral Majority's Jerry Falwell cited AIDS as God's punishment for the "perverted lifestyles" of homosexuals (Shilts 1987, 347; Garrett 1994, 330). Falwell urged President Reagan to put the full might of his administration toward combating the "gay plague" so it would not break out among the "innocent American public"—an innocence apparently defined by not being included in any of the afflicted groups.

Jonathan Mann, the first director of the UN's Global Program on AIDS and the epidemic's first widely known spokesperson, wrote, "In each society, those people who before HIV/AIDS arrived were marginalized, stigmatized, and discriminated against became over time those at highest risk of HIV infection" (Mann et al 1999, 221).

Some have written that the HIV/AIDS epidemic in the United States could have proceeded quite differently had key political leaders responded sooner. Author Randy Shilts covered the epidemic for the *San Francisco Chronicle* from the beginning and meticulously documented the first five years of the American epidemic in his best seller, *And the Band Played On,* widely considered to be the best early history of the HIV/AIDS epidemic in the United States. According to Shilts, government indifference/obstructionism, delayed and paltry funding, media disinterest, and failed leadership at every level facilitated the spread of the virus during the early years of the epidemic, costing tens of thousands of lives (1987). It was, in Shilts's words, "a drama of national failure, played out against a backdrop of needless death" (xxii).

The Reagan Revolution championed less government, and the budget axes of the largest tax cut in US history fell on the National Institutes of Health (NIH), the CDC, and the other public health agencies that could have slowed the American plague. As case rates soared and deaths mounted, the federal government remained unmoved. In 1981, the total budget for research on the new disease at the CDC and the NIH amounted to less than $200,000 and Surgeon General C. Everett Koop was not allowed to make any public pronouncements about the disease for five years (Garrett 1994, 297). Koop later said, "The Reagan revolution brought into positions of power and influence Americans whose political and personal beliefs predisposed them to antipathy toward the homosexual community" (302).

Congressman Henry Waxman added,

> There is no doubt in my mind that if the same disease had appeared among Americans of Norwegian descent, or among tennis players, rather than gay men, the responses of both the government and medical community would have been different . . . . What society judged was not the severity of the disease but the social acceptability of the individuals afflicted with it. (Shilts 1987, 138, 143)

AIDS researcher Andrew Moss added, "It is inconceivable to me that we would be facing such a prospect [of scant funding] and frankly, as a society, not be alarmed about it if it were not an epidemic of a stigmatized group of people" (Garrett 1994, 332).

Government spending on HIV/AIDS research efforts reflected the disinterest shown by the administration. The federal government had spent $9 million on a Legionnaires' Disease outbreak that had claimed 29 lives in 1976; yet it spent less than $1 million studying AIDS over a similar time period, despite hundreds of deaths early on and projections of thousands more. When funding levels increased to a paltry $2.6 million in 1982, the impetus came from Congress, over the objections of the Reagan administration (Shilts 1987, 214). This was the pattern for most AIDS funding during the Reagan years. CDC researcher Joe McCormick later recalled, "By steadfastly refusing to acknowledge the true dimensions of the AIDS crisis, the Reagan administration made itself an ally of the virus" (Behrman 2004, 13).

Tylenol and AIDS

The discovery of Tylenol capsules laced with cyanide in October 1982 caused a national scare that opened a window into the curious interplay of media and power (Shilts 1987, 191). After the first few people in the Chicago area died from the tainted Tylenol, the national media responded by covering every detail of the story, often on the front page of newspapers or as the lead story on the evening news. The government reacted by sending hundreds of employees to Chicago, testing 1.5 million Tylenol capsules and developing entirely new regulations for tamper-resistant packaging, all in the span of a few weeks. Tylenol's parent company, Johnson & Johnson, spent more than $100 million during the scare. Seven people died during the episode—likely the work of a lone miscreant. By the time the Tylenol scare erupted, 634 Americans had been stricken with AIDS, of which 260 had already died (191). The *New York Times* had written only three stories on HIV/AIDS in 1981 and another three in 1982, despite the growing numbers of dead and dying homosexual men and projections from government doctors that the epidemic would claim tens of thousands of lives. By contrast, the *Times* had written a story on the Tylenol scare every day of the month of October 1982, including 4 on the front page and 23 more during the following two months. The national media reflected the *Times'* coverage. While homosexual men sickened and died by the hundreds and then thousands, the nation's watchdogs exuded a collective yawn. Scores of deaths among gay men and the occasional "junkie" did not seem to interest readers—or the media's sponsors—while few in the media were comfortable discussing matters of gay sexuality or addiction.

Awakening the Media

The Wall Street Journal did not publish its first story on the epidemic until February 25, 1982, when the first cases of heterosexually transmitted AIDS appeared. By that time, 251 Americans had become infected and 99 had died (Shilts 1987, 126). Once large numbers of heterosexuals became infected, the national media finally took an interest, prompting Dan Rather to comment that AIDS was the epidemic that "you rarely hear a thing about. . . ."

As author Shilts wrote, "Three years later, television commentators would still be talking about AIDS as that disease you rarely heard anything about, as if they were helpless bystanders and not the very people who themselves had decreed the silence in the public media" (1987, 172). By December 1982, the national media had descended on the blood transfusion-related aspect of AIDS and began to cover the epidemic broadly, albeit superficially. The number of AIDS stories in the nation's newspapers quadrupled between the last quarter of 1982 and the first quarter of 1983. Reporters descended on Castro Street in San Francisco and studied gay men like a newly discovered tribe of exotic "cave dwellers" (268). Nevertheless, the expanding coverage goaded the federal government to increase its level of research funding for AIDS.

On April 11, 1983, the National Cancer Institute (NCI) held its first meeting of the Joint Task Force on AIDS, rededicating itself to uncovering the cause. The day was later seen as a turning point in the epidemic, the day the federal government got serious about AIDS. Nearly two years after the first published reports on AIDS, 1295 Americans had contracted HIV/AIDS and 492 had died. Not until July 25, 1985, did a slumbering American public finally awaken. That was the day the world learned that Rock Hudson had AIDS. Soon AIDS was on the front page of every newspaper in the nation.

The Rock Hudson announcement was the single most important media event in the early history of the US AIDS epidemic.

To the physicians and researchers on the frontlines, the Rock Hudson announcement was the single most important media event in the early history of the US AIDS epidemic (Shilts 1987, 578). Something about the actor's revelation deeply moved the American public. Though many in Hollywood had known of Hudson's homosexuality for decades, none had disclosed it. In the end, Hudson was a reluctant pioneer, agreeing to disclose his diagnosis only after he had collapsed in the lobby of a Paris hotel. Yet his disclosure held sufficient potency to displace all events before it. From that point on, the response from the lay public, media, and government would never again return to the complacency and ignorance that had preceded it. Funding levels increased immediately, and the nation for the first time became united in the fight against HIV/AIDS. By the time Hudson's diagnosis was revealed, 12,067 Americans had been diagnosed with AIDS and 6,079 had died.

Like many of the activists and leaders in the gay community during the early years of the epidemic, Randy Shilts died of AIDS, at age 42. In perfect predatory fashion, the virus consumed those who were most active in the fight against it. Yet, in a fitting summary of the early years of an epidemic that both divided a nation and united a community, Shilts wrote, "The United States, the one nation with the knowledge, the resources, and the institutions to respond to the epidemic, had failed. And it had failed because of ignorance and fear, prejudice and rejection. The story of the AIDS epidemic was that simple" (1987, 601).

Yet the epidemic in the United States comprises just a small piece of the whole. While researchers found treatments able to hold the virus at bay for a select few, the virus surged through the world, ravaging one country after another. It is that story that will leave its mark on history and perhaps become an emblem of shame for a generation.

AIDS in the World: Inertia, Blame, and Failed Politics

AIDS is the greatest adversary humanity has ever faced. History shudders in its wake. While the world's wars have claimed 149 million lives since the first century, projections are that 250 million people will be infected by HIV by the year 2025, with the real possibility that AIDS will claim more lives than all of the wars throughout history combined. The *Washington Post* has called this "the most underestimated enemy of all time" (Behrman 2004, xiv). HIV's predatory masterstrokes were to select the most marginalized populations in the world, impose a long, silent incubation period, and primarily transmit sexually, encouraging those in power to ignore it.

Despite the lethality and magnitude of the HIV/AIDS epidemic, world response has been surprisingly weak for a number of reasons, most significant of which has been the failed leadership of the world superpower, the United States. Other factors include infighting within multilateral agencies, particularly the UN, and early silence on the part of AIDS activists, black leaders, and heads of state in the countries that were the most affected. A final reason—perhaps the most difficult to perceive and understand but equally pernicious—is a racist view of Africa as being beyond hope, blinding people to the harsh realities facing its people. We'll start by looking more closely at Africa.

Passive Racism and the Relevance of Africa

If AIDS has a face, its features are distinctly African. Nearly two thirds of the world's HIV-infected people live in sub-Saharan Africa, which should come as no surprise. No other continent registers as many countries at the bottom of the UN's human development index. Rife with poverty and disease, entrenched inequality, and abysmal governance, Africa in the age of HIV is slowly receding backward in time. Its economies are contracting, and its more precarious states face collapse if current trends continue. By 2010, it will be home to 20 million of the world's 25 million AIDS orphans who, reared in poverty and lacking parental guidance, constitute "an army in search of a leader" (Behrman 2004, xii).

It would be wrong to say that the world has little noticed Africa's plight. The world has always noticed Africa's plight, though in a way that hurried office workers notice a rumpled homeless man sleeping on a grate in winter. Rather than prompt moral outrage or goad us into action, the presence of Africa reminds us that, by comparison, our lives aren't that bad. That Africa turns to the United States for help is a given, a certainty of life as much as rain or next Thursday. But images of AIDS-afflicted Africans resurrect long-held Western stereotypes of suffering and starving Africans. These images feed deeper, darker beliefs in the rich world that Africa is simply hopeless and beyond help. We may give a little, but we have never gotten the response right. According to author and aid worker Michael Maren,

> The starving African exists as a point in space from which we measure our own wealth, success, and prosperity, a darkness against which we can view our own cultural triumphs. And he serves as a handy object of our own charity. He is evidence that we have been blessed, and we have an obligation to spread that blessing. The belief that we can help is an affirmation of our own worth in the grand scheme of things. (1997, 2)

How much we help is another matter. Because we have long viewed the agony of Africa through the lens of charity, not justice, any amount of aid we render is sufficient. Charity requires neither commitment nor understanding, so we can give what we please. As such, the global response to AIDS in Africa is the same as the response to every prior African problem: very little. From the days of European colonization to more recent infusions of foreign aid used as weapons in the Cold War, Africa has long served the interests of the powerful; its issues have been put off until later or ignored entirely. The US response to Africa for most of the epidemic has languished in a toxic brew of receding geopolitical relevance, overriding fatigue with AIDS and foreign aid in general, and subconscious racism.

During the height of the Cold War, the two world superpowers flooded African capitals with aid and arms, competing for influence amidst the perceived strategic relevance of the continent. When the Soviet Union dissolved, Africa lost its appeal to the United States, which quickly began to disengage from the continent. During the 1990s, the US government pulled back diplomatic missions, cut personnel, and reduced foreign aid precipitously. A *New York Times* columnist called Africa "the neglected stepchild of American diplomacy" (Behrman 2004, 72). The late 1990s were a time of fierce Republican-generated attacks against foreign aid, citing a long history of abuse and futility. As mentioned previously, African leaders had committed some of the worst abuses, and aid projects on the continent set the bar for efficacy quite low. For many powerful leaders in governments in the United States and abroad, it was simply the wrong era to initiate massive aid projects in Africa—no matter what the reason.

Yet the most dominant feature of the global response to AIDS in Africa remains the most difficult to see. Although overt racism is rare at the policy level at the highest levels of the US government or other world bodies, a more passive form of racism is undeniable. Activist Jamie Love proffered "a thirty million white person test," in which he said, "we'd move kind of like it was an emergency" (Behrman 2004, 67). Reflecting a thought pattern held in far more circles than many would admit, a senior military official at the National Intelligence Council commented that the AIDS epidemic actually would be good for Africa because "Africa is overpopulated anyway" (Gellman 2000). The World Bank later concluded that the HIV-mediated slowing of the population growth rate would increase per-capita income, as had occurred when the bubonic plague devastated 14th-century Europe. It is hard to imagine a similar analysis extended to, say, Wisconsin, without generating considerable outrage.

In reviewing the history of the US response to the HIV/AIDS epidemic for his outstanding book, *The Invisible People*, author Greg Behrman interviewed more than 200 people. Two of these interviewees had telling remarks concerning racism and the nonresponse to Africa. "It's not that US policy makers, the media, or the public at large wished death upon black Africans," argued Mark Schneider, a former Peace Corps director and US Agency for International Development (USAID) deputy, "it was that it simply 'made it easier to look away'" (Behrman 2004, 68). A former US AIDS czar, Patsy Fleming, recalled feeling the initial stirrings of hope when the epidemic appeared in Eastern Europe because "I thought, well, maybe now they'll pay attention to it; these are white people" (68).

The Failure of the UN

If ever an emerging epidemic could benefit from the leadership, funding, and global reach of the UN, it was AIDS. During the early years of the epidemic, however, the UN's response consisted mostly of confusion and lethargy. Then, in January 1986, Jonathan Mann, one of the world's foremost authorities on HIV/AIDS, assumed control of a fledgling operation at the World Health Organization (WHO) called the Global Program on AIDS (GPA), and everything changed. Between 1983 and 1985, Mann had headed Project SIDA in Zaire, where his team gathered useful early data on the heterosexual spread of HIV. He arrived in Geneva, Switzerland, with a missionary's zeal, and an intellect and charisma to match.

Over the next few years, Mann and his GPA staff vaulted global AIDS onto the international radar screen, raising funds, increasing awareness, and instituting national programs in countries throughout the world.

In Mann, global AIDS victims had found their most eloquent and impassioned advocate. He soon descended on Washington and other world capitols to sound an alarm while gaining praise and wide recognition for his efforts. His face regularly graced newspapers and magazines worldwide. The AIDS epidemic, he would say, will eclipse all other issues confronting humanity. Only through leadership, action, and advocacy would humanity stand a chance. Speaking in London at the historic World Summit of Ministers of Health on Programmes for AIDS Prevention in 1988, Mann said,

> Our opportunity—brought so clearly into focus by this Summit—is truly historic. We live in a world threatened by unlimited destructive force, yet we share a vision of creative potential—personal, national, and international. The dream is not new—but the circumstances and the opportunity are of our time alone. The global AIDS problem speaks eloquently of the need for communication, for sharing of information and experience, and for mutual support; AIDS shows us once again that silence, exclusion, and isolation—of individuals, groups, or nations—create a danger for us all (Garrett 1994, 461).

From a meager budget of $5 million and a personal salary borrowed from the CDC in 1986, Mann and the GPA staff quickly raised awareness of the growing epidemic. Mann increased the agency's funding dramatically and gained the ear of WHO Director-General, Halfdan Mahler, whose own speeches soon regularly included dire warnings about the rise of HIV/AIDS. In May 1987, Mann and his staff prompted the World Health Assembly, the legislative body of the WHO, to adopt the GPA's Global Strategy for the Prevention and Control of AIDS. Just five months later, Mann became the first WHO functionary ever to address the General Assembly of the United Nations. The UN then passed—for the first time in its history—a resolution against a specific disease. By 1989, the GPA was working with more than 80% of the world's countries, and Mann's budget had increased to $92 million, a rise considered "meteoric" by WHO bureaucratic standards (Garrett 1994, 462).

Unfortunately, the string of successes for the GPA simultaneously sowed the seeds of its demise. Mann's success spawned jealousy among those in other programs at WHO, and when Mahler retired in 1988, his replacement wasted little time reining in the GPA. Japan had met US demands to pay a higher share of UN dues but had demanded something in return—the replacement of Mahler with a long-time WHO bureaucrat named Hiroshi Nakajima.

When asked early in his tenure about AIDS, Nakajima replied, "Ah, don't talk to me about AIDS; I have malaria, which is a much bigger killer of people, on my hands" (Gellman 2000). Nakajima felt uncomfortable addressing sex or AIDS in general. He shared with others at WHO a general resentment for Jonathan Mann's celebrity status, unorthodox style, and privileged position. Above all, Nakajima was interested in consolidating his own power—a position threatened by no one more than Jonathan Mann. Nakajima cut back the GPA budget and limited Mann's influence. On March 23, 1990, the French newspaper *Le Monde* published Mann's resignation letter, in which he blistered Nakajima and the senior leadership at WHO, accusing them of "paralyzing our efforts completely" (Gellman 2000). In the end, the best and brightest hope to stem the inexorable tide of HIV/AIDS in the world succumbed to envy and petty politics.

Without the brilliant leadership of Jonathan Mann, the WHO effort sputtered. The GPA lasted just six more years, giving way to the United Nations Programme on HIV/AIDS (UNAIDS) on January 1, 1996. Mann's replacement, Michael Merson, had WHO credentials and offered no challenge to Nakajima's hold on power. Under Merson's leadership the GPA slowly sank into obscurity and irrelevance and he turned his attention to crafting the GPA's successor. Once established, UNAIDS would require two full years to ramp up to full speed. Because of Nakajima's failed leadership, substantial donors such as the United States and the United Kingdom wanted the new entity separate from the WHO. Subsequently, UNAIDS became a stand-alone secretariat, sponsored by various UN agencies. As a result of the political infighting, the UN and WHO lost eight years, between 1990 and 1998, during which time the world was left with no leadership against its most important infectious epidemic. During that time, HIV infected nearly 33 million people and claimed 10 million more lives.

Failed Leadership of Activists, African, and African-American Leaders

Among US activists, African leaders, and African-American leaders in the United States, a coordinated and effective response, or even an audible advocacy campaign, was slow in coming. Although activist groups such as the New York-based ACT UP and others deserve credit for goading the US government into increasing its funding levels for domestic-centered HIV research and care, they and other groups failed to grasp the significance of the global epidemic early on. Not until December 1, 1990, did ACT UP stage the first US-based protest against the WHO, the UN, and the US government to demand global access to drugs and treatment.

In general, the domestic activists targeted domestic concerns. Then, at the Eleventh International AIDS Conference in Vancouver in 1996—ironically called "One World, One Hope"—the world learned about the miraculous new drug "cocktail" called HAART (highly active antiretroviral therapy), which caused emaciated, dying AIDS patients to recover fully. *Newsweek* trumpeted the end of AIDS that year, while the US public, already weary of the epidemic, turned its attention elsewhere. For many activists, however, the Vancouver conference was a watershed event, clearly delineating to them, for the first time, those who could benefit from the new treatment and those who could not. As scholar and internationalist Nils Daulair recalled, "It really pointed out the growth in inequity more than before, and it served as a mobilizing factor for activism around HIV internationally"(Behrman, 2004, 134).

By 1999, activists had joined the fight for global access to treatment, and they began to target the large pharmaceutical companies in earnest. Eventually they formed a key entity responsible for the decrease in prices for antiretroviral medication in the new millennium.

Meanwhile, many African leaders were so mired in problems of their impoverished states that AIDS remained a distant concern. During the 1990s, as millions of Africans became HIV-positive, African leaders spent much more on arms than on preventing HIV/AIDS. Zambian President Frederick Chiluba cited AIDS as God's punishment for "irresponsible behavior," while Zimbabwe spent 70 times more on a war with the DRC than it did on HIV prevention among its citizens, 20% of whom were then infected (Behrman 2004, 196).

Each African country held its specific rationale for not addressing the epidemic—corruption in Mugabe's Zimbabwe; corruption and deference to the will of the Church in Moi's Kenya; a pathological and somewhat bizarre leadership in Mbeki's South Africa. Still, the denial and aversion to AIDS served political purposes both in the African countries and in the capital cities of rich countries that were willing to look the other way. Neither had to spend money on the AIDS crisis. African American leaders similarly said little about the epidemic, and the Congressional Black Caucus did not take on the issue seriously until 1999 (Behrman 2004, 89).

The Failure of US Leaders

Rocked by its own AIDS epidemic and vaulted into a position of concentrated global power by the collapse of the Soviet Union, the United States found itself in an ideal position to lead the response to AIDS. Those in power certainly knew the extent of the epidemic. In 1991, the CIA's Katherine Hall and Walter Barrows issued an intelligence briefing titled "The Global AIDS Disaster," which predicted 45 million HIV infections by 2000, with the likelihood of claiming more lives than the combatants killed in World Wars I and II, Korea, and Vietnam combined (Gellman 2000). The report claimed that the response of most African and foreign governments had represented a "modest level of effort," which would have "only a marginal effect."

Although its authors expected that findings such as these would generate a considerable response, the reaction from the White House and Cabinet agencies was indifference. According to *Washington Post* reporter Barton Gellman, the political response in Washington and other centers of power is a story of "willful ignorance and paralysis in the face of growing proof" (Gellman 2000).

When the US Congress finally did respond to increased media coverage and an energized activist community, it, too, directed its efforts internally. NCI researchers including Robert Gallo turned billions of federal research dollars into uncovering—along with the French—the viral cause of AIDS. Other research efforts led to the antiretrovirals that halted the epidemic for those who could afford it; these antiretrovirals only now are reaching more people in poor countries. There is no question that the epidemic could have proceeded differently had US funding sponsored more prevention success stories like those in Uganda and Thailand. In the year after release of the CIA report, the United States spent only $124 million on AIDS control overseas. From the time of the report until spending levels finally increased in 1999, nearly 18 million people became infected.

> *Research efforts led to the antiretrovirals that halted the epidemic for those who could afford it; these antiretrovirals only now are reaching more people in poor countries.*

The hardest-hit countries lacked the will or the means to respond, even as their citizens became infected and died by the millions. In 1997, sub-Saharan African governments spent only $145 million—mostly from foreign aid—for its millions of new infections, while the United States spent $8.5 billion for its 44,000 new infections (Behrman 2004, 196).From the earliest days of the epidemic, US leaders responded with indifference and discomfort in addressing the myriad of issues the AIDS epidemic had raised. Neither Reagan nor Bush had shown much interested in the global epidemic. The religious conservatives who formed a core constituency for both men had remained uncomfortable addressing issues involving condoms and sexually transmitted disease.

Although US funding levels for global HIV did rise during the Bush I administration, from $2 million in 1986 to $120 million by 1993, these increases are attributed largely to Congressional leaders such as Washington state's Jim McDermott (Behrman 2004, 31). When McDermott and other legislators including Senator Patrick Leahy, Congresswoman Nancy Pelosi, Congressman David Obey, and others tried to rally support, they found no interest at the White House and little support from their Senate and Congressional colleagues. As McDermott painfully recalled, the issue of global AIDS did not affect his colleague's districts, so they had little incentive to act. One UN official put it more bluntly: "The bottom line is, the people who are dying from AIDS don't matter in this world" (Gellman 2000).

In his first inaugural address in January 1993, Bill Clinton mentioned global AIDS, offering real hope to the global AIDS community. However, from the beginning, Clinton focused on domestic issues, notably the economy. Foreign policy, which had been the main interest of George H.W. Bush, failed to pique Clinton's interest. Worse, Clinton's first foray into foreign matters proved to be a debacle when a Somali mob dragged a mutilated corpse of a US Ranger through the streets of Mogadishu in full view of an enraged American public. The events forced the United States out of Somalia and inflicted the new administration with a colossal black eye. Under the leadership of its new president, the United States had become a meek giant and would refrain from intervention in Africa thereafter—even the genocide that engulfed Rwanda just over a year later.

Domestic events imposed even more reluctance onto Clinton officials, who already were hesitant to engage in the global fight against AIDS. Early efforts to enforce equality for gays in the military and a politically naive attempt to reform the US health care system backfired,[5] forcing the administration into a defensive mode that continued for the remainder of Clinton's presidency. When Newt Gingrich assumed control of the House of Representatives in 1994, following stunning mid-term defeats for the Democrats, AIDS activists braced for the worst. Gingrich's ally in the Senate, Jesse Helms, set his sights on foreign aid, and US funding levels subsequently plummeted to an all-time low by 1997. USAID Director Brian Atwood remained preoccupied with fighting a desperate battle to stave off elimination of the agency by Jesse Helms. What little funding USAID had was, by necessity, to be corralled. There would be little left over to fund Jonathan Mann's GPA or bilateral efforts to slow the epidemic in Africa. Coupled with the president's stated objective to reduce the deficit, global AIDS levels remained static during both Clinton terms.

For the global AIDS community, things began to change at the Geneva Conference on AIDS in June 1998.

For the global AIDS community, things began to change at the Geneva Conference on AIDS in June 1998. UNAIDS finally emerged as the new global leader in the epidemic and presented to the delegates, for the first time, comprehensive and accurate data on the true scope of the global epidemic. The data were clear and shocking—8 million AIDS orphans already, with 16,000 new infections every day. This information galvanized the world community and US leadership. Before the Geneva Conference, US diplomat Sally Grooms Cowal recalled, "Everybody was looking at one piece of the elephant and deciding that was the elephant" (Behrman 2004, 175).

Over the next two years, major news sources devoted increasing coverage to the epidemic. As the scope came more clearly into view for the public at large and government officials in the United States and abroad, people were aghast. Activists peppered presidential candidate Al Gore's various campaign stops, further raising the issue in local and national newsrooms. Gradually the public began to awaken and politicians started to hear much more about the issue from their constituents. The initials stirrings of a real US response had been set in motion.

President Clinton and officials in his administration also responded with alarm to the 1998 UNAIDS numbers and recognized the security threats the epidemic posed. With a popular president, the country riding an historic wave of prosperity, and attention increasingly turning to the epidemic—particularly in Africa—1998 was the year in which Clinton could recalibrate the US response to global AIDS and become the global leader on AIDS that the world so desperately needed (Behrman 2004, 224). Clinton did move on the issue: Spending on global AIDS increased from $120 million in 1999 to $450 million by 2001, and under Clinton's direction the United States dropped its opposition to the South Africa Medicines Act, which precipitated the falling prices of AIDS medications. Unfortunately, the Monica Lewinsky scandal consumed the president after it broke in January 1998; political issues—including global AIDS—became secondary to his political survival.

The pandemic demanded a response in billions, not millions, of dollars, and Clinton failed to meet the challenge, partly because of failed policy decisions early in his presidency, partly because of the Lewinsky scandal, and partly because of the intransigence of Jesse Helms and his allies in the House and Senate. Surprisingly, Clinton would do far more to combat global AIDS after he was out of office than during his presidency. When he left the White House, he relinquished power to a man widely viewed as the AIDS activists' worst nightmare. Activists began to regret their decision to constantly picket and harass Gore during his presidential run. The future for a US-led response to global AIDS looked grim.

Finally, a Glimmer of Hope

At first blush, George W. Bush seemed the least likely candidate to alter the course of the global AIDS epidemic. Embraced by the Christian Right and a stated devotee of Ronald Reagan, Bush's razor-thin election victory evoked dread from the global AIDS community. Memories of 12 years of Reagan and Bush I policies served to deflate all hope of an effective response from the US government. An unusual set of events and personalities, however, combined to alter the terrain and finally pull the United States back into a position of leadership on global AIDS, albeit ineffectively.

A beginning of sorts came in 1999 when economist Jeffrey Sachs accepted the offer by the WHO to chair the UN's Commission on Macroeconomics and Health—a group that would examine the nexus of health and poverty and make policy recommendations to the UN. Already a widely respected internationalist, Sachs had shown proficiency and growing concern for global poverty and the toll exacted by poor health. When the commission finished its work two years later, it recommended that the world donor community should increase its official development assistance (ODA), or foreign aid, for health by $22 billion annually by 2007, of which $8 billion would be earmarked for a new Global Fund to fight AIDS, malaria, and tuberculosis (Sachs 2001b, 13). With such an investment, Sachs argued, the global community could save 8 million lives per year by 2007. The world should act now, he argued, because the resources were there and the rich countries had a moral imperative to do so. The Global Fund became enshrined in the millennium development goals (MDGs), and UN Secretary-General Kofi Annan began to push the Global Fund at every opportunity, as did Sachs.

When Sachs joined the UN, it was a huge boon to the global poor, most of whom reside in the path of the AIDS cyclone. Sachs is widely viewed as one of the world's most respected and influential economists. His op-ed articles are printed in *The Economist*, the *New York Times*, and other influential media throughout the world. Allied with Kofi Annan, Sachs began to change the terms of the debate on global AIDS. No longer asking the world community for incremental increases in funding, Sachs was out front, demanding billions. During a conference at the American Academy of Arts and Sciences on May 2, 2002, he said, "We have faked it for a generation. Rich people do everything to say, 'It's not about money.' But the whole international debate is about money. It's *all* about money" (United Nations, 2002c). An unlikely ensemble of supporters soon joined Sachs to push the president and other prominent Republicans to action.

Tennessee Republican Senator Bill Frist had moved from his Harvard-based practice as a cardiothoracic surgeon to politics, becoming the first physician to be elected to the US Senate since 1932. As a surgeon, Frist had volunteered in Africa and was well acquainted with AIDS and its potential impact there. Following impassioned pleas from Frist, Annan, Colin Powell, and Condoleezza Rice, President Bush announced in May 2001 that the United States would be the first to contribute to the Global Fund, pledging $200 million. Microsoft magnate Bill Gates soon followed, with a pledge of $100 million. The Global Fund had begun, but at funding levels far short of what Sachs and others deemed necessary to affect change.

After terrorists hijacked four planes on September 11, 2001, the response to the global AIDS crisis seemed to have lost any real possibility of receiving attention. Mired in a recession, burdened by a huge tax cut, and facing an unheralded threat from global terrorism, the United States seemed to be the most unlikely country to lead the fight against HIV/AIDS. Yet, the attacks on September 11, 2001, turned everything around. Bush was transformed and sported a more confident look to match the spike in his approval ratings. The neoconservatives around him caught his ear, and plans to invade Iraq hatched even as US forces invaded Afghanistan. While most of those around him supported the era of unilateral, US hegemony, one strong personality bucked the trend. Colin Powell had been described as the administration's "odd man out," yet he continued to hold influence over the president on one issue in particular—AIDS. Powell had been to Africa and, like many before him, had been transformed by the experience, vowing that he would not forget what he had seen. Just one week after September 11, Powell had pushed his ambassador on global AIDS to continue to develop the Global

Fund, saying, "Regardless of what happened last week, you guys have to drive ahead and create this Global Fund" (Behrman 2004, 268).

Turning the Tide

It is still hard to imagine such opposites as conservative Senator Jesse Helms and rock star Bono sitting down together to discuss policy. During a luncheon at the Capitol building for Bono hosted by Helms, Bono quipped that the appearance wasn't good for either of their images. The results of their coming together, however, held extraordinary significance for the future of AIDS. No one had obstructed US efforts to engage internationally more than Jesse Helms. Yet a combination of advancing age, illness, and effective persuasion by the Christian group Samaritan's Purse, their leader Franklin Graham, and U2 singer Bono, had opened Helm's eyes to the problems of the world. His conversion came through faith—but only after he made the connection between AIDS and the teachings of Christ. Bono recalls meeting with Helms,

> He's a religious man, so I told him that 2300 verses of scripture pertain to the poor and Jesus speaks of judgment only once—and it's not about being gay or sexual morality, but about morality. I quoted that verse of Matthew chapter 25: "I was naked and you clothed me." He was really moved. He was in tears. Later he told me he was ashamed of what he used to think about AIDS" (Jubilee 2002).

Helm's conversion was both shocking and of profound importance, moving the religious conservatives toward poverty eradication, and toward the prevention and treatment of AIDS. Watching Helms cry and embrace Bono, a rock star, Republican Congressman John Kasich said, "I thought somebody had spiked my coffee" (Traub 2005). In an extraordinary speech in February 2002, Helms told those at a Samaritan's Purse conference that he was "ashamed" that he had not done more concerning the world's AIDS pandemic. He later wrote, "In the end, our conscience is answerable to God. Perhaps, in my eighty-first year, I am too mindful of soon meeting Him, but I know that, like the Samaritan traveling from Jerusalem to Jericho, we cannot turn away when we see our fellow man in need" (Eaton and Etue 2002, 60).

From the beginning, Bono has played a major role in both debt relief and AIDS relief. Other music stars, such as George Harrison, Elton John, Bob Geldof and Willie Nelson, had raised money and awareness for favored causes before him, but no one has approached the dedication, skill, and effectiveness of U2's Bono. Writing in the *New York Times Magazine*, author James Traub called him, "the most politically effective figure in the recent history of popular culture" (Traub, 2005). One of rock's most successful and popular singers transferred the idealism in the music to real-world political activism. Bono first signed onto the Jubilee 2000 Debt Relief campaign, sponsored by Jubilee 2000 and Fifty Years is Enough. (See Chapter 5.) He then dove into the issues, taking World Bank policy papers to bed with him and learning the nuances of third world debt and development (Jubilee 2002). He recruited Jeffrey Sachs as his teacher, and the two became fast friends, crafting political strategy and lobbying influential politicians. Sachs then pushed Bono to take on the AIDS crisis. Following a meeting with the Pope, the two raced off in a van while fans swarmed them "like in a Beatles movie." Sachs leaned over to Bono and said, "Look, they always do that with macroeconomists" (Barrett 2002).

Bono successfully lobbied Jesse Helms, and then President Bush, to increase levels of foreign aid and debt relief for third world countries (Council on Foreign Relations 2004). In a March 14, 2002, speech at the Inter-American Bank in Washington, DC, with Bono seated on the stage behind him, the president announced America's largest increase in foreign aid since the Kennedy era. Just one week later, Bush repeated the pledge at a meeting of world leaders to discuss global poverty in Monterrey, Mexico. But Bono wanted more and recruited US Treasury Secretary Paul O'Neill to tour Africa with him in a highly publicized tour in May and June of 2002. O'Neill later described the tour as "the most intense" 12 days of his life (Donnelly 2002b). Like so many before him, the experience transformed him, and he agreed to push for even further aid than what Bush had pledged in Mexico. As a *New York Times* reporter termed it, Bono was able "to package such aid . . . as a moral undertaking that should be a natural goal of religious conservatives" (Stevenson 2002).

During the "Odd Couple" tour, as the Bono and O'Neill trip was billed, the two visited Sowetto, South Africa, and some of its 4.7 million HIV-positive citizens. Bono's voice cracked as he decried the lack of treatment for HIV-positive women, saying, "I'm dumbfounded by the stupidity of a world that says this is OK," while O'Neill said simply, "For God's sake, what are we doing?" (Singer 2002).

The goals include preventing 7 million new infections while caring for 10 million people in the selected countries.

Many echoed O'Neill's frustrations with the rich world response to AIDS. But few anticipated that President George W. Bush would be the one to change the landscape. Widely ridiculed by the political left, taken to task for a unilateralist approach to an unpopular war, and criticized for tax policies that heavily favored the wealthiest Americans (Andrews 2004), Bush was the last man from whom anyone could have anticipated such far-reaching changes to both foreign aid and AIDS policy. Yet it was Bush who pledged the first major grant to the Global Fund, gradually increased funding levels for global AIDS, and increased US foreign aid by 50% through the Millennium Challenge Account. Then, in his 2003 State of the Union address, Bush shocked the world by announcing PEPFAR, his five-year, $15 billion commitment to combat AIDS in Africa and the Caribbean. The goals include preventing 7 million new infections while caring for 10 million people in the selected countries. He said, "As our nation moves troops and builds alliances to make our world safer, we must also remember our calling as a blessed country is to make this world better" (Behrman 2004, 306). His announcement was greeted by a standing ovation from both houses of Congress.

Because this pledge was delivered just months before the invasion of Iraq, some viewed Bush's commitment to AIDS prevention in Africa with cynicism, a humanitarian gesture offered to the world to take some of the sting out of a unilateral and widely unpopular war that was coming in Iraq. Still, a long series of events, of which Iraq was just one, had led to the policy shift. Bush might not have come to embrace AIDS were it not for the tireless lobbying of an unusual group of people, including Bono, Sachs, Powell, Rice, Helms, and Frist. The timing was also right. The price of AIDS drugs had plummeted, making large-scale treatment possible, and the scope of the epidemic had continued to grow unabated, creating more vocal demands for action. Countries including Uganda and Thailand had shown that AIDS could be corralled, and leaders such as Paul Farmer and Jim Yong Kim had proven that AIDS patients could in fact be treated in "resource-poor" settings.

The media had caught onto the story, increasing their coverage in the late 1990s and placing the issue onto the radar screens of national politicians, albeit as a low-priority item. The growing pandemic had begun to touch nerves in the national security nexus, with the expanding threat to Africa and, even more alarmingly, to the "next-wave" countries such as Nigeria, Ethiopia, China, Russia, and India—home to 40% of the world's population (Altman 2002). In the end, Bush's prime rationale may have come from his regular readings of the Bible. Seen as a moral mission, Bush decided to act on AIDS, and many other factors simply fell into place at the right time.

Although $15 billion represents a landmark policy shift for which the administration deserves credit, it is not the solution the world needs, for a number of reasons. First, only $1 billion of the total is dedicated for the Global Fund, widely viewed as the most effective vehicle to deliver AIDS funds. Mirroring Bush's unilateral approach to the Iraq War, an open disdain for the United Nations could prove to be the Achilles' heel of PEPFAR. Bilateral efforts have long surrendered efficacy to political will, and PEPFAR is in no way protected from political subversion, some of it from the same far right political lobbies that have long derailed efforts to target population growth and sexually transmitted diseases.

The plan also will require a wasteful duplication of bureaucracy, as poor countries run parallel programs from the Global Fund and PEPFAR. The plan also targets $9 billion against AIDS in 15 countries in Africa and the Caribbean while spreading $5 billion to 100 other countries, including the burgeoning epidemics in the "next wave" countries that comprise major humanitarian and security threats for the decades to come (US Department of State 2004). Thus, it is not a strategic solution to the problem.

PEPFAR also requires that one-third of prevention funds go toward programs (many run by faith-based groups) that stress abstinence until marriage and sexual fidelity; but many of these groups avoid discussions of condom use. While abstinence until marriage holds merit as a public policy in HIV endemic regions, marriage offers no guarantee of protection from HIV, either from a partner previously infected, or infected during the marriage through infidelity. Further, unlike the successful HIV-prevention strategies used in Uganda, PEPFAR does not promote condom use in young people, which many view as having been critically important in slowing the epidemic's spread there.[6] Ultimately, PEPFAR's reduced emphasis on condom use could cost tens of thousands of lives.

Finally, there is no guarantee that the funds will be released. Given the record budget deficits induced by tax cuts, recession, and the Iraq War, many in Congress may view $15 billion as excessive and reduce funding levels, as occurred in 2004 (McLure 2004). The estimated $200 billion price tag for cleanup of the Gulf after Hurricane Katrina will no doubt cut PEPFAR funding further.

The failings of four separate US administrations to effectively meet the challenge may well comprise the legacy of this generation.

In the final analysis, despite some well-intended but shortsighted efforts thus far, the response from the US government to the epidemic remains wholly inadequate. As it continues its riotous spread, threatening to infect 100 million people by the end of the decade, toppling nations, and greatly increasing global instability in the process, the US government has failed to devise a sound strategy or to work with those who already have, such as the architects of the Global Fund. The failings of four separate US administrations to effectively meet the challenge may well comprise the legacy of this generation. The political and moral failings of the government reflect wider failings inherent in human nature that have characterized the AIDS epidemic from the beginning.

Ultimately the story of AIDS reflects wider patters in human history, and the lessons it teaches us have broad repercussions. The virus has tracked along steep gradients of power in which those at the bottom are targeted en mass and eliminated. The response has reflected all prior efforts to deal with crises in poor countries—apathy, indifference, political infighting, and an inability to focus on what is important in a broader scheme. When the response finally came, it was largely as a result of faith-based convictions that coerced the hand of those in power. Yet, the final response to date has been largely shackled by overriding political concerns that threaten to allow the epidemic to spread to even greater proportions. The story of AIDS holds all the ingredients of human frailty that have served so long to keep us from attaining the promised land that our forefathers dreamed of. We still lack the maturity, political fortitude, and moral will to combat the epidemic effectively. Perhaps we are still missing the key baseline premise from which we should proceed.

Jonathan Mann, the man widely agreed to have had the most success in mobilizing against the epidemic thus far, realized early on that the platform from which the attack against AIDS was launched was of the utmost importance. For Mann, as for a small band of dreamers meeting in the aftermath of history's worst war, that platform was based on humanity's most basic and important aspirations, aspirations that became enshrined in national and then international law. Those aspirations were codified in a fundamental document on basic human rights called the Universal Declaration of Human Rights.

AIDS and Human Rights

Author Laurie Garrett wrote that as the HIV/AIDS epidemic spread throughout the world in the early 1980s, it became clear that a predictable pattern of societal responses followed the arrival of HIV in a new country, reminiscent of the responses to the plague in the 14th century (1994, 457). As Garrett describes it, there were "three different social epidemics within the larger biological epidemic" (472). The initial reaction, and first social epidemic, was *denial*; people simply ignored the threat or took false assurance that only certain groups would be afflicted. Even gay men living in the epicenters of the epidemic at its peak ignored the risks, demonstrating the power of this most primitive of human defenses. Pat Robertson stated that scientists were "frankly lying" when they said HIV could be transmitted heterosexually (469). Similar patterns of denial played out in Africa, Asia, and Eastern Europe as HIV spread relentlessly. During a London summit in 1988, the Chinese delegate denied the existence of homosexuals, injection drug users, and prostitutes in the People's Republic, and the Soviet Minister of Health proclaimed that the genetic superiority of Slavic peoples rendered them immune to HIV (476).

The second social epidemic was *fear*, often triggered by a public display of the disease. In the United States, the death of Rock Hudson in 1985 was one such trigger, as was the announcement by Magic Johnson of his HIV-positive status in 1991. Predictably, people responded as they often do when confronted by the unknown—they lashed out. AIDS patients in the United States were summarily fired from their jobs and were denied bank loans and health insurance; students were attacked in schools; and homes were burned. People who were already marginalized sank even lower in the societal ranking, acquiring pariah status. Some attacks were vicious, with the same rationale that had characterized prior attacks through history. The 14th-century equivalent of homosexuals, injection drug users, and Haitians were Jews, whose burnings became a regular feature of plague-torn medieval Europe (Cantor 2002, 147). In Strasbourg around 1349, residents burned more than 900 Jews, allegedly for "poisoning the wells"—the prevailing belief of the plague's cause. Rationality never caught up with the hysteria and remains a distant dream to AIDS sufferers in many of the world's hardest-hit countries.

The third social epidemic was by far the most deadly—*repression*, typically consisting of government policies based more on irrational fears than hard science. The responses were directed more at the individuals with the disease than the virus itself. As Jonathan Mann told attendees at the Third International Conference on AIDS in June 1987:

> AIDS is a touchstone of politics, of racism, of bigotry. We see a rising wave of stigmatism around the world. . . . People are promoting sex cards, tattoos, quarantines, police lists, deportations, home burnings, incarcerations of select population groups. How our societies treat HIV-positive individuals will test our collective moral strength (Garrett 1994, 471).

In the late 1980s, country after country passed laws restricting the rights of the afflicted or the social groups to which they belonged. In 1987, the US Senate voted 96–0 to mandate HIV tests for all applications for immigration, and Cuba quarantined all HIV-positive patients for life. A German judge sent tremors throughout the world when he suggested that Germany tattoo and quarantine all HIV-positive patients—practices not seen on German soil since the Holocaust. Officials from the repressive Burmese junta injected 25 Burmese HIV-positive prostitutes with cyanide and then set their bodies floating down a border stream as a warning to Thailand that it would keep AIDS out of Burma.

In most countries, the typical AIDS sufferer is a person divorced from the traditional culture and the least likely to pay attention to government pronouncements or warnings; most people with AIDS were alienated even before their illness. According to the WHO's Manuel Carballo, if the society at large reviled a particular group, that marginalization would comprise a significant risk factor, as great as any other (Garrett 1994, 475).

Jonathan Mann watched the rise of the policies that further stigmatized and isolated high-risk groups and felt a sense of impending doom. "Discrimination," he said, "simply drives AIDS underground. The epidemic doesn't go away; it simply becomes harder to see. If you drive it underground, you guarantee its spread" (Garrett 1994, 464). As an illness associated with homosexuality, promiscuity, and drug addiction, HIV pitted public health against organized religion and the "moral pillars of society" (464). The task of combating HIV/AIDS had rapidly overcome the collective powers of even the sharpest minds of the global public health community. The epidemic raged on, with projections that sobered all who ventured to discern them. Together with his expanding staff at the GPA, Mann began to study international human rights law as a nontraditional way to combat the spread of HIV.

For the previously staid WHO, the human rights agenda represented a new direction. As one WHO insider said, "We really didn't get moving on human rights until it was thrust upon us. . . . What thrust human rights up to WHO's front burner was AIDS" (Garrett 1994, 477). Jonathan Mann soon focused his considerable energies on the link between human rights and HIV. Increasingly he issued pronouncements from Geneva following precepts culled from the large body of international law. Many of the more repressive laws that governments passed against HIV-positive individuals had been in violation of charters to which they previously had been signatories. In pursuing this line of thought, Mann had a vehicle through which his staff at the GPA could finally target the real drivers of the epidemic. He wrote of an "inextricable link" between health and human rights: The former simply could not exist without the latter.

Whether those who are inflicted with HIV/AIDS are homosexuals or injection drug users in the West or poor women with no title to land or legal recourse in the developing world, what most AIDS victims share is a lack of individual human rights. Prior to the AIDS epidemic, the two fields had remained mostly separate, despite considerable efforts by groups such as Amnesty International, Médecins Sans Frontières, and the Red Cross. Jonathan Mann and his GPA staff, however, thrust human rights into the mainstream. After leaving WHO in 1990, Mann joined the Harvard School of Public Health and later became the dean of Harvard's François Xavier Bagnoud Center for Health and Human Rights. Mann dedicated the remaining years of his life to promoting human rights—more specifically to "his vision of a world where HIV/AIDS would be recognized and responded to through a combined, largely expanded health, social, and economic development strategy firmly grounded in human rights" (Mann et al 1999). Though he suffered an untimely death at age 51 aboard the Swissair Flight 111 that crashed on September 2, 1998, Mann's legacy endures.

Since Mann's tenure, each graduating student from Harvard's School of Public Health receives two documents—a diploma and a copy of the Universal Declaration of Human Rights. This document and the values it enshrines represent for each of us a moral beacon on which we can set our collective sights for the future. It may hold the key for the global response to AIDS.

Endnotes

1. For more information, see the ACT UP web site at www.actupny.org.
2. Farmer is careful to point out that such connections do not prove causality. However, Garrett (1994, 308), offers evidence to support the case that HIV did come to Haiti primarily through gay sexual tourism.

3. For more information see the Peace Pledge Union's web site at
   www.ppu.org.uk/war/countries/africa/africa_index.html.
4. Behrman noted 25 million deaths by March 2004, while UNAIDS calculated 3.1 million
   deaths during 2004, making a rough total of 28 million by March 2005.
5. For a compelling summary of the political downside of 1994's health care reform
   attempt, see *Boomerang, Clinton's Health Security Effort and the Turn against
   Government in U.S. Politics* by Theda Skocpol (W.W. Norton & Company, 1996).
6. Information from "The ABC of HIV Prevention," from the Avert.Org web site at
   www.avert.org/abc-hiv.htm.

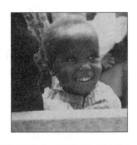

Chapter 10

Ethics, Human Rights, and Religion

A human being is a part of the whole that we call the universe, a part limited in time and space. He experiences himself, his thoughts and feelings, as something separated from the rest—a kind of optical illusion of his consciousness. This illusion is a prison for us, restricting us to our personal desires and to affection for only the few people nearest us. Our task must be to free ourselves from this prison by widening our circle of compassion to embrace all living beings and all of nature.

—Albert Einstein

If I am hungry it is a material problem.
If someone else is hungry, it is a spiritual problem.

—Gustavo Gutierrez

Get up, stand up: stand up for your rights
Get up, stand up: don't give up the fight
                    (Life is your right)

—Bob Marley

Sounds of laughter shades of earth are ringing
Through my open views inviting and inciting me
Limitless undying love which shines around me like a
Million suns, it calls me on and on Across the universe

—John Lennon and Paul McCartney

World War II and its aftermath comprised a pivotal period in human history, forever changing the underlying economic and political orders that spawned it. Well before the death of President Franklin Roosevelt in April 1945, planners began to articulate a dream founded on FDR's Four Freedoms. Under Eleanor Roosevelt's leadership, a United Nations (UN) committee formed in 1946 drafted the Universal Declaration of Human Rights (UDHR), forming a basis for international law and initiating current movement toward international human rights for all people. States, civil society, and nongovernmental groups have all embraced the UDHR. Through this document and the conventions it spawned, the world took a tentative step closer to realizing an ideal that had been dreamed of since antiquity. It was at that time that the earliest religious leaders first expressed concern for the poor and articulated the dream of a just world order.

In Judaism, Catholicism, and Islam, as well as many other religions, such a vision is attributed directly to God. In one branch of Catholicism, called liberation theology, adherents read scripture from the standpoint of the poor, deconstruct the forces that propagate poverty, and challenge all of us to act directly to create a just world order. Through these various congruent perspectives, we can revisit the story of the 10-year-old girl at the beginning of this book. All of the prior analysis bears directly on her fate, even as deeper moral and religious undercurrents challenge—in fact, demand—that we pay far greater heed to those like her.

The Birth of Modern Human Rights

Human rights have long been but a dream to the vast majority of the world's people. Throughout recorded history, most people have endured repression of some type, whether political, economic, or religious, to name a few. Yet through time and across all cultural divides, people have expressed universal desires—for freedom and security, the ability to choose one's governance, the freedom to choose one's form of worship, freedom from hunger and want, and the right to work.

Societies have attempted to legislate these desires in the Magna Carta, the US Declaration of Independence, and the French Declaration of the Rights of Man, among others. Yet it took history's worst calamity, World War II, to prompt world leaders to compile these collective yearnings into one document, which served as a basis for legislation that followed decades later. Ratified by the UN General Assembly on December 10, 1948, the Universal Declaration of Human Rights is one of the world's most impressive achievements, comprising the best collective efforts at defining the universal aspirations of humanity.

World War II and Its Aftermath

To grasp the potency of the document, we first must recall the desperate times that spawned it. World War II claimed 50 million lives, the highest toll in history. Within that number were 14 million Allied combatants, who gave their

lives to offer a better life for a people trapped by tyranny ("The Human Toll" 1995). Sixty years later, the world still traps far too many people in tyranny, poverty, and early death–the soldiers' noble cause remains partly unfulfilled.

Recent years have seen a newfound interest and much deserved respect for World War II veterans including those who stormed the Normandy beaches on D-Day, June 6, 1944. Popular movies and books about the "greatest generation" instilled more than a little awe at what those who fought in World War II accomplished. People who have seen the movie *Saving Private Ryan* (1998) cannot forget the opening scenes that depict the first few hours of the attack on D-Day, which claimed more than 2,000 US servicemen in a matter of hours. These men died while storming heavily fortified beaches, as machine guns and mortar rained down upon them. One soldier summed up the days events, "Amidst the twisted wreckage and the many bodies, we all had the feeling that democracy itself hung in the balance" (Sublett 1994). The principles upon which the current world order stands were threatened during that war and did, in fact, hang in the balance on that day.

What the men did on that day typified what men did throughout World War II. Private Felix Branham stormed Omaha Beach with the 116th Regiment, which took the highest casualties of any Allied regiment on D-Day. He later recalled, "I have gone through lots of tragedies since D-Day. But to me, D-Day will live with me till the day I die, and I'll take it to heaven with me. It was the longest, most miserable, horrible day that I or anyone else ever went through" (Ambrose 1994, 582). Author Stephen Ambrose wrote about the magnificent performance of the Allied soldiers during the war. "None of them wanted to be part of another war," he wrote. "But when the test came, when freedom had to be fought for or abandoned, they fought" ("Charlemagne" 2004).

> *Many historians believe that D-Day was the most important day of the 20th century; World War II could have turned out differently had the Allied landings at Normandy failed.*

Many historians believe that D-Day was the most important day of the 20th century; World War II could have turned out differently had the Allied landings at Normandy failed (Patsilelis 1995). Hitler had bet that the disciplined Wehrmacht troops would destroy the "comfortable and lazy" citizen soldiers of the American democracy and its allies.

Eisenhower, with FDR behind him, bet otherwise. Despite considerable advantages in firepower and troop strength, the Allies still had to storm a heavily fortified beach with German reinforcements, including armor, within a short distance. Ultimately, it was the grit, heroism, and sacrifice of ordinary "citizen soldiers" that effectively changed history.

On June 7, 1944, the *New York Times* opined, "We go forth to meet the supreme test of our arms and of our souls, the test of the maturity of our faith in ourselves and in mankind . . . . The cause prays for itself, for it is the cause of God who created man free and equal" (Ambrose 1994, 494). Following the successful landings at Normandy, the Allied forces launched massive troop movements through France, which eventually turned the direction of the war in their favor. But the Normandy victories came at an enormous cost. Although no one knows the actual number of Allied casualties on D-Day, estimates hover around 10,000, which include those killed, missing in action, or wounded.[1] Of these, the United States lost 6,600—nearly a third at the horrific Omaha Beach landings. The British lost 2,700, mostly on Gold and Sword Beaches, and the Canadians lost 946, mostly at Juno. German casualties are estimated at 4,000 to 9,000.

The aggressive Allied campaign through Europe that began on D-Day led directly to Germany's surrender on May 8, 1945, less than one year later, helped considerably by the Russians along the Eastern Front (Endy 2004). The United States suffered more than 1 million casualties, including 407,316 killed, 671,846 wounded in action, and 78,751 missing in action, at a cost of $4.53 trillion, in 1997 dollars (Center for Defense Information 2002, 47).

In many ways, the World War II period was a "watershed" for mankind (UNDP 1994, 5). This war changed history as profoundly as any event that preceded it, leaving countries in Europe, the Pacific, and North Africa in ruins. Tensions between the former allies—the United States and the USSR—escalated, reaching a peak with Stalin's blockade of Berlin in 1948. The Berlin Airlift presaged the Marshall Plan, and Cold War tensions forced countries to align themselves with either the Americans or the Soviets.

Between 1945 and 1950, enormous changes occurred throughout the world. In Asia and the Pacific, World War II had effectively ended with the detonation of nuclear weapons in Hiroshima and Nagasaki on August 6 and 9, 1945, ushering in the nuclear age. Courts in Tokyo tried those guilty of Japanese war crimes, from the 300,000 civilians killed during the "Rape of Nanking" to the tens of thousands of prisoners of war killed in Bataan (the Philippines) and elsewhere. In China, tensions between Mao Tse Tung's communists and the US-backed forces of Chiang Kai-shek erupted into a full-scale civil war, which by 1947 swung in favor of the communists, altering history for the world's most populous country (Glendon 2001, 102). Korea split along the 38th parallel, igniting a war in 1950 that claimed the lives of 36,570 US servicemen and 500,000 North Koreans and Chinese (Center for Defense Information 2002, 47).

A "Glimmering Thread" of Hope: A Prelude to the Declaration

Franklin Delano Roosevelt had guided his nation through the war and led the efforts to establish a post-war peace. As much as anyone, FDR believed in the promise of a United Nations and pushed hard for its creation. He hoped to resurrect the earlier optimism of Woodrow Wilson's League of Nations, which sank after the US Senate failed to ratify it in 1920. Seeking to avoid Wilson's mistake, he actively courted Republicans for prominent positions in creating the UN. FDR had long championed the cause of the downtrodden, both at home and abroad. During a 1943 radio address to the US public about the fledgling UN, he said, "The doctrine that the strong shall dominate the weak is the doctrine of our enemies—and we reject it" (Glendon 2001, 4).

Although the year 1945 brought good news from the European and Pacific war fronts, it brought with it images of an increasingly frail president. When the Big Three leaders met at Yalta in February 1945, Roosevelt looked tired and sick. Just two months later he died in Warm Springs, Georgia.

With Roosevelt's passing, the UN lost its most powerful supporter.

With Roosevelt's passing, the UN lost its most powerful supporter. Stalin had no intention of sharing power with smaller nations, and Churchill, presiding over a tenuous but expansive empire, had no intention of losing the crown's colonies. Still, the impetus to form the UN gained momentum. The international financial institutions and the UN's security council had concentrated power in Allied hands, while the ideals of human rights, long championed by Roosevelt, had been shuttled to the rear. In truth, these ideals had never factored heavily in the formation of the UN, because national sovereignty had long trumped any ideas regarding individual human rights. Such rights existed or did not exist not solely at the discretion of a nation's governing body. All other considerations were secondary.

Then the Allies knocked open the gates of Dachau, Sobibor, and Auschwitz, and the world saw for the first time the true extent of the Nazi reign of terror.

The Nuremburg Trials

The Allies placed the Nazis responsible for "crimes against humanity" on trial in the German city of Nuremburg between 1945 and 1947, with judges from the United States, United Kingdom, USSR, and France presiding (Mann et al 1999, 281). During these infamous proceedings the world learned about gas chambers, appalling human experiments, mass killings, and the utter disregard for human life shown by the Nazis. This also was the time when the victorious powers decided to put the first chink in the armor of sovereignty. The trials established the Nuremberg Principles, which defined for posterity war crimes and crimes against humanity. From that point on, individuals would be held individually responsible for their actions during war, just as their leaders would be. Peacetime atrocities, however, were left uncovered. The Nuremberg trials set the precedent for the International Criminal Court, established more than 50 years later in 1998; a separate tribunal tried the Nazi doctors and established the principle of *informed consent* (UNDP 2000, 3).[2]

Euphoria over the Allied victory on V-E (Victory in Europe) Day, May 8, 1945, combined with the shock of seeing the first photos from the concentration camps provided impetus to ratify the UN Charter. Human rights language found its way into the all-important preamble to the charter, signed in San Francisco on June 26, 1945, by the 50 original member states. At its outset, the charter stated two core goals of the new organization:

> to save succeeding generations from the scourge of war . . . and to reaffirm our faith in fundamental human rights, in the dignity and worth of the human person, in the equal rights of men and women and of nations large and small. . . .[3]

The Four Freedoms

Amidst the deliberations at the UN in its earliest days, a movement born of Allied war rhetoric began to gain momentum. Throughout the poor countries of the world, Allied talk of freedom and liberty for all caused long suppressed dreams to emerge and challenge the colonial world order. At the time, 250 million people still lived under colonial rule, and many more, such as blacks in the United States, lived under oppressive conditions. People everywhere believed the Allied leaders when they said they fought the war for freedom and democracy.

As FDR had inspired a nation through soaring rhetoric, he had also inspired the world. During a State of the Union address to Congress on January 6, 1941, he proposed that the new world order should be based on "four freedoms"—freedom of speech and expression, freedom to worship God in one's own way, freedom from want, and freedom from fear. "That is no vision of a distant millennium," he said. "It is a definite basis for a kind of world attainable in our own time and generation."[4]

Though FDR targeted his remarks at a nation gearing up for war, his words reverberated throughout the developing world. In 1942 the Allies issued a joint declaration to elucidate the reasons for the war—among them, "to defend life, liberty, independence, and religious freedom and to preserve human rights and justice in their own lands as well as in other lands" (Glendon 2001, 11). Three years later the UN delegate from the Philippines, General Carlos Romulo, summarized the hopes of the developing world in an address before the first delegates gathered in San Francisco:

> Mr. Chairman, the peoples of the world are on the move. They have been given a new courage by the hope of freedom for which we fought in this war. Those of us who have come from the murk and mire of the battlefields know that we fought for freedom, not for one country, but for all peoples and for all the world (12).

Harry Truman gave his first address as president after the signing of the United Nations Charter. "Experience has shown how deeply the seeds of war are planted by economic rivalry and by social injustice," he said. The UN would offer the world a new opportunity and he looked forward to an "International Bill of Rights" that could address these problems.

Author Mary Ann Glendon writes that the incorporation of human rights into the UN Charter and initial agenda was but "a glimmering thread in a web of power and interest" (Glendon 2001, 19). The dominant countries had

maintained their hold on power through the political and economic structures of the Security Council and the Bretton Woods Institutions. There was no guarantee that human rights would receive more than its inclusion in the UN Charter's preamble and first article. But an eclectic group of world leaders, intellectuals, and diplomats soon gathered to place human rights high on the UN's agenda, with repercussions that even the most idealistic could not then have imagined.

The UN Committee on Human Rights

From the beginning, Eleanor Roosevelt had garnered praise for her unconventional stands on human rights issues, from race to suffrage to the problems of the poor. FDR had long relied on her firsthand reports from the domestic and international front to inform his decisions, and the two developed a productive working relationship despite a marriage strained by FDR's infidelity. When the UN formed their Committee on Human Rights, Eleanor was elected chair. The illustrious committee included members from 18 countries, including Lebanon's Charles Malik, China's Peng-chun Chang, Canada's John Humphrey, the Philippines' Colonel Carlos Romulo, and France's René Cassin. The diversity of people and experiences represented within the committee ensured that broad representation of human values would be voiced.

Without Eleanor Roosevelt's leadership and critical input from Malik, Chang, Humphrey, and Cassin, the committee might not have completed its work. Strong personalities clashed early and often, but each member sensed the importance of their task. The committee decided that their first and most important objective would be to draft an international bill of rights, starting with a nonbinding, universal declaration of human rights. In *Foreign Affairs,* Eleanor Roosevelt wrote, "Many of us thought that lack of standards for human rights the world over was one of the greatest causes of friction among the nations, and that recognition of human rights might become one of the cornerstones on which peace could eventually be based" (Glendon 2001, 31).

As the committee members deliberated, however, tensions between the United States and the USSR continued to escalate. In February 1946, Stalin proclaimed that it would be impossible for capitalist and communist societies to peacefully coexist; Churchill responded with his famous "Iron Curtain" speech just weeks later. The committee thus had a narrow window to complete its work—from the end of the war in 1945 to the start of the Cold War in 1948.

Canadian lawyer John Humphrey and a large staff researched and complied an extensive list of "every conceivable right" into a first declaration draft that the UN subsequently proclaimed was "the most exhaustive documentation on the subject of human rights ever assembled" (Glendon 2001, 57).

He and his staff had researched all existing constitutions and instruments for human rights and consulted world experts from many cultures and societies through history. When a committee from the United Nations Educational, Scientific and Cultural Organization sought to include important human rights ideas from philosophical and religious perspectives, it found that it could add nothing to Humphrey's draft. René Cassin then applied the touch of an experienced legislative draftsman by improving the flow and internal cohesion of the document while maintaining Humphrey's content. Once Cassin's revisions were in place, the full committee met to debate the preamble and each article in turn, a process that took two full years.

The Universal Declaration of Human Rights

The best way to appreciate what the commission accomplished in 1947–1948 is to simply read the UDHR; it is reprinted in full in Appendix A of this text. Within just two pages of its preamble and 30 articles, the declaration concisely expressed centuries of human aspirations. In its opening strains, the declaration states:

> Recognition of the inherent dignity and of the equal and inalienable rights of all members of the human family is the foundation of freedom, justice and peace in the world. . . . All human beings are born free and equal in dignity and rights.

These rights are a birthright "without restriction of any kind," whether attributable to race, color, religion, gender, politics, social status, or country of birth. In subsequent articles, the Universal Declaration establishes the rights of all individuals to be recognized before the law, to be free from arbitrary arrest, and to have a right to a fair trial. It prohibits slavery and torture while ensuring equal access to work, education, and the right to participate in the cultural life of a community. It demands equality for women and protection for children, while stating that all individuals have a right to "freedom of thought, conscience, and religion." Of particular importance to health providers is Article 25, which reads:

> Everyone has the right to a standard of living adequate for the health and well-being of himself and of his family, including food, clothing, housing, and medical care and necessary social services, and the right to security in the event of unemployment, sickness, disability, widowhood, old age, or other lack of livelihood in circumstances beyond his control.

The Universal Declaration of Human Rights remains a beacon for oppressed peoples everywhere. Following its adoption by the UN General Assembly on December 10, 1948, it influenced the new constitutions of Germany, Italy, and Japan. It became a "polestar" for thousands of human rights activists and articulated the fundamental principles through which

Jonathan Mann and his staff at the UN's Global Program on AIDS launched their campaign. Movements inspired by the Declaration ended European colonialism in Africa and Asia, brought down repressive regimes in Eastern Europe, and ended apartheid in South Africa. The declaration remains the primary source and guiding document for most of the world's human rights instruments and has served through the years to "amplify the voices of the weak in the corridors of power" (Glendon 2001, xvi). Conceived at the apex of human folly, it represents a monumental change in moral and political thought, where the ancient paradigms of power and strength begrudgingly cede turf to conscience and morality.

Even though the Declaration holds great promise for the world's down-trodden, it has its limitations. On the Declaration's 50th anniversary in 1998, Amnesty International called the UDHR "little more than a paper promise" for most of the world's people (Annas 1998, 1778). And in truth, its demands simply exceed the capacity of many governments in poor countries. They can't afford the health care, education, and basic services demanded by the covenants to which they are signatories. Many countries signed, ratified, and then ignored the treaties that the UDHR spawned, despite an ever-growing core of UN monitoring bodies and nongovernmental organizations (NGOs) that make it increasingly difficult to do so. Still, the UDHR spawned several core legal instruments that hold the promise of a better life, and recent developments such as the UN millennium development goals (MDGs), the Global Fund, the President's Emergency Plan for AIDS Relief (PEPFAR), and the Millennium Challenge Account signal a growing effort by the major world powers to help poorer countries comply. In other areas that have less to do with finances than political repression, such as torture, imprisonment, and armed insurrections, NGOs including Amnesty International, Physicians for Human Rights, Médecins Sans Frontières, among others, have led an exponential growth in the "human rights" NGOs, as reviewed in Chapter 3.

Not even the most optimistic framers in 1948 could have then imagined the importance the UN Declaration would come to assume in broadening human rights for billions of people. Yet the Declaration itself contained no binding legislation; it could do little more in practice than inspire. By definition, a declaration is nonbinding and contains no legal force on its own, though, as with the US Declaration of Independence, it can take on a life of its own as an inspirational document. Rather it is the covenants, conventions, and treaties (terms used interchangeably) through which nations undertake legally binding obligations. Following completion of the declaration in 1948, it would take nearly 20 years before the first covenants were drafted, and each would become legally binding only after a host country had signed and then ratified it. After that, nations, UN monitoring bodies, and NGOs could monitor compliance with the new and ambitious agenda.

Expanding Civil and Political Rights

The first two covenants enacted reflected the ideological divisions of the Cold War. Adopted by the General Assembly in 1966, the International Covenant on Civil and Political Rights (ICCPR) championed a wide range of civil and political rights for all people, expanding the principles from the UDHR and making them law. Core components of the ICCPR are equality; freedom of religion, movement, and association; equality of the sexes; and freedom from torture or slavery. These positions reflected core US concerns, and the United States was 1 of 144 countries to ratify this document by 2000 (UNDP 2000, 45).

From the other side of the Cold War divide came the International Covenant on Economic, Social, and Political Rights (ICESCR), also adopted in 1966 and ratified by 142 nations by 2000—the United States not among them. As suggested by its title, the ICESCR advocates goals more in line with socialist or communist societies, goals that are somewhat at odds with the stated goals of capitalist systems such as the United States. The ICESCR advocates work and wages for all, health care, education, a right to be free from hunger, and "the right of everyone to the enjoyment of the highest attainable standard of physical and mental health" (Annas 1998, 1778).

As a group, the UDHR and these first two covenants comprise the International Bill of Rights. Most of the UDHR's core rights find expression in these first two covenants, and most of the world's countries already have signed one or both. Yet there are many more conventions that have amplified pressing concerns, with four in particular that have emerged since the UDHR was adopted.

In 1965, the UN adopted the International Convention on the Elimination of All Forms of Racial Discrimination (ICERD), which outlaws discrimination whether based on race, color, descent, or national or ethnic origin (UNDP 2000, 44). By 2000, 155 countries had ratified the ICERD. Following the rise of women's movements in the 1970s, the Convention on the Elimination of All Forms of Discrimination Against Women (CEDAW) became an international bill of rights for women when it was adopted in 1979, and 177 countries had ratified it by March 2004.[5] The General Assembly adopted a Convention Against Torture (CAT) in 1984 and a Convention on the Rights of the Child (CRC) in 1989. The latter convention, which seeks to protect and promote the rights of children, has become the most ratified of all the conventions—192 countries by 2004. As the United Nations Children's Fund (UNICEF) director Carol Bellamy said, "A century that began with children having virtually no rights is ending with children having the most powerful legal instrument that not only recognizes but protects their human rights."[6] Only the United States and Somalia have signed but not yet ratified this convention.[7]

However, laws mean nothing without enforcement. For each of the six major conventions, a corresponding committee is charged with monitoring signatory nations for compliance, with periodic reports made widely accessible. Following 50 years of efforts, the International Criminal Court (IIC) became a reality in July 1998.[8] The court holds jurisdiction over "crimes against humanity," including genocide, war crimes, and aggression, and greatly expanded its reach by including criminal acts that occur during peacetime (UNDP 2000, 124). The United States, however, has refused to endorse the court or become a "party to the treaty."[9]

The Status of Human Rights Today

In addition to the UN system, there are regional organizations, national governments, and NGOs that enforce human rights. The Council of Europe, Organization of American States, and Organization of African Unity all have their own human rights documents that focus on the culture and law of the regions (Mann et al 1999, 22). Many countries have adopted human rights language into their constitutions and laws. NGOs such as Amnesty International, Human Rights Watch, the International Federation of the Red Cross, and Physicians for Human Rights monitor human rights abuses, raise awareness, and challenge responsible governments.

Although the ideal of human rights has value in of itself, the rights are most useful in the world when they are put into direct action. Increasingly, UN bodies, governments, and NGOs are framing their missions and operations in the context of human rights. Perhaps the most obvious example is the MDGs. Each goal can be linked directly with economic, social, and cultural rights elucidated in the UDHR (UNDP 2003, 28). Developing specific targets has long been a successful strategy, as has occurred with smallpox, polio, malnutrition, child mortality, and life expectancy (31). Human rights-based goals overlap considerably with development goals, with one reinforcing the other. The CRC has had such an impact, with 22 countries incorporating children's rights into their constitutions (UNDP 2000, 116).

As discussed in Chapter 3, NGOs have been successful in targeting their efforts directly at human rights violations. Global Witness, a human rights-oriented NGO, exposed the complicity of conglomerate De Beers in purchasing diamonds from Angolan rebels. This led De Beers to terminate its relationship with the rebels (UNDP 2000, 126). Physicians for Human Rights has trained the international media spotlight on abuses in Argentina, Guatemala, the former Yugoslavia, Kurdistan, Haiti, and Iraq (Geiger and Cook-Deegan 1993, 616). NGOs focusing on human rights were partly responsible for ending apartheid in South Africa. An NGO called the Movement for Survival of Ogoni People launched a campaign of shame against Shell Oil's operating practices in Nigeria, prompting it to adopt a human rights code (UNDP 2000, 58).

For the global poor, human rights hold great promise for a better life, and the UDHR remains a blueprint for human aspiration. Nevertheless, the declaration was not created out of whole cloth; many of its core principles came from prior national constitutions that had borrowed heavily from principles articulated first in organized religion.

The Religious Origins of Human Rights and a Just World Order

The earliest foundations of human rights lie in organized religion. Although the subject of religion may seem, at least to some, a digression far from the realm of international health service or an understanding of global poverty, religion provides a clear moral direction for many of the world's people. As such, it provides the backbone of human rights. Ultimately, the ills of the world stem less from preconceived orders of nature than the willful intentions of man. Thus, it is incumbent upon us to understand the moral and religious underpinnings that form the core tenets of human rights. Only through morality, often rooted in religion, can we hope to change many of the themes spelled out in earlier chapters.

More than 3,000 years ago, the authors of the Jewish Torah and Hindu Vedas first recorded the themes of equality, dignity, and a collective moral responsibility to help others (UNDP 2000, 27). Around 2,500 B.C.E., Buddha and Confucius set forth their considerable insights. Then, 500 years later came Jesus and the prophets of the New Testament, followed by the Prophet Muhammad roughly 600 years afterward. Another 1,300 years went by before the UDHR offered the first chance to codify their moral views in a prelude to more far-reaching international law.

Even though the various faiths diverge on a range of subjects, they share common foundations in humanity, ethics, and concern for the poor. Religious scholar and former nun Karen Armstrong said, "Compassion . . . goes right across the board in all the world religions. Compassion is the key in Islam and Buddhism, and Judaism and Christianity. They are profoundly similar" (Solomon 2004, 17). To this, former President Jimmy Carter added, "There are many faiths in this world with which we're familiar, but I think there is one common commitment, whether you are Hindu, or Buddhist, or Christian—Protestant or Catholic—and that is we pledge ourselves to have mercy and compassion and to alleviate the suffering of the poor" (Eaton and Etue 2002, 48).

Organized religion claims more than 4 billion adherents, including at least 2 billion Christians, 1.2 billion Muslims, 815 million Hindus, 355 million Buddhists, and 14.5 million Jews (Johnson 2003). This number comprises the overwhelming majority of the world's people. That the beliefs articulated by these faiths share moral terrain with human rights is obvious. Yet we must conclude that there exists in our world a status quo that is far removed from the teachings of our most important world religions. If people

truly believe in the teaching of these varied faiths, it remains difficult to understand why we have not arrived closer to the utopian ideal that most of these faiths prescribe. Still, the ethical roots of human rights lie here, and their shared features offer further proof of a collective ideal.

Judaism

Sometime around 1800–1600 B.C.E. ("before common era," a modern and more egalitarian equivalent to "B.C.") the Jewish patriarchs Abraham, Isaac, and Jacob lived, followed around 1250 B.C.E. by Moses (Gafni 2003, 8, 58). Their stories comprise much of the early chapters of the Hebrew Bible, also known as the Torah, the Five Books of Moses, and the Pentateuch. The second book, Exodus, tells the story of how God chose the Israelites as his own people. God could have chosen a ruling, powerful elite, but instead chose a community bound as slaves to the Egyptians for 350 years. He orchestrated their release and deemed that they construct a just society built on the laws he gave them. Many of these laws surface in Genesis, Exodus, Leviticus, and Numbers, but most reside in Deuteronomy, the fifth and final book of the Pentateuch. Like Islam that followed it centuries later, the Jewish faith is grounded in law called the Torah..

When asked by a convert for a "crash course in Judaism," the sage Hillel replied, "What is hateful to you, do not do to your fellow man" (Gafni 2003, 1). Many Jews would say that their religion is a way of life, proscribing a manner of conduct for all daily activities. The Ten Commandments, which God revealed to Moses at Mount Sinai (Exod. 20:2–27; Deut. 5:6–21) form core principles of the Jewish faith. The first four address humans' relationship with God, ordering people to worship no other gods, make no craven images before God, take not God's name in vain, and honor the Sabbath. The last six commandments address people's relationship with others, commanding them to honor their parents and to avoid murder, adultery, theft, lying, or coveting their neighbor's things. These may seem obvious to us now, but, given the barbarity of the times, were most likely revolutionary when first revealed. The commandments represent early efforts, divinely ordained, to raise the standards of human behavior.

In reading the Old Testament today, many of the laws described seem antiquated, relating to rituals or modes of behavior long out of practice, such as how to conduct sacrifices, cleanse lepers, govern slaves, or punish unacceptable behaviors such as "lying with animals." Some of the writing reflects political and economic concerns of the day, particularly those of the four authors believed to have composed it (Friedman 1997). Much of the Old Testament, however, speaks to early attempts to structure a society around a higher, moral standard, believed to be delivered by God. People were told to tithe, setting aside produce from their harvest every three years and share it with "the stranger, and the fatherless and the widow who are within your gates" (Deut. 14:29). People were further instructed to cancel debts every seven years, and to care for the poor. Deuteronomy 15:7 reads, "If there is among you a poor man of your brethren, within any of the gates in your land which the Lord your God is giving you, you shall not harden your heart nor shut your hand from your poor brother, but you shall open your hand wide to him and willingly lend him sufficient for his need, whatever he needs."

Every 50th year was to be a Jubilee year in which slaves would be freed and debts forgiven (Lev. 25:8). From Leviticus 19:18 came a core teaching that Jews as well as Christians embraced: "You shall love your neighbor as yourself." In short, Judaism represents one of the earliest and most successful attempts to prescribe a law-based society through which individuals would worship God and care for each other. It continues today as one of the world's oldest and most important faiths. But Judaism was just one of the major faiths to emerge from Eurasia.

Hinduism

Around the same time as the Jewish prophets were revealing their instructions from Yahweh, Hindus (people from the Indus Valley, or Aryans) were constructing a set of principles that would govern life for people in the Asian peninsula that comprises modern India (Muesse 2003). The oldest and most sacred of Hindu texts, the Veda, which literally means "wisdom," contains a polytheistic view of life that is quite different from that of Judaism, Christianity, and Islam. In classic Hinduism, karma is a fundamental principle of justice in which one's actions in life have direct consequences on one's station in future lives. Karma can be either good or evil and is believed to attach itself directly to one's soul. Only through good karma can one improve one's station in the next life.

The unfortunate consequence of this system is the belief that all people are not created equal—people are born into their social position, or caste, as a direct result of their actions in previous lives. Those who suffer most in this system do not warrant inclusion in even the lowest order of the caste system. They are outcastes or "untouchables" and suffer the consequences of their social ordering as retribution for the sins of past lives. They call themselves *dalits,* or "oppressed ones" (Muesse 2003, 18). Although the caste system is in direct opposition to the human rights-based notion of egalitarian birthright, it does provide a moral framework through which people are instructed to conduct themselves in a manner consistent with overriding principles of justice.

Buddhism

Buddhism teaches its adherents to achieve *nirvana,* and thereby abort the painful cycle of rebirth and suffering, by following three pathways—moral conduct, mental concentration, and wisdom. Buddhism teaches the means to live a "contemplative and serene life" (Eckel 2003, 24). It instructs its adherents to refrain from killing, stealing, lying, abusing sex, or drinking intoxicants. Although not a fundamental moral precept, generosity is considered a "fundamental virtue," which explains in part why Buddhist monks throughout Asia are typically well cared for. A Bodhisattva ideal for Buddhists holds that one helps others along the path to nirvana, chiefly through attaining wisdom and by showing compassion. An oft-quoted Buddhist text summarizes the ideal as follows: "For as long as space endures/ And for as long as living beings remain/ Until then may I too abide/ To dispel the misery of the world."[10]

Islam

The world's 1.2 billion Muslims find clear moral direction from their faith (Esposito 2003; Armstrong 1993, 132). From its origins in the birth of the Prophet Muhammad in 570, Islam has become the world's second largest and the fastest growing religion. Like Christianity and Judaism, Islam is a monotheistic faith that compels its adherents to care for their brethren. In its idealized form, Muslims are called to serve God's (Allah's) will on earth. The term *islam* literally means "submission" or "surrender." The God of Islam is the same God as that of Abraham, Moses, and Jesus, and people of all three faiths trace their ancestry to Abraham and his two sons, Ishmael, the father of all Muslims, and Isaac, the father of Jews and Christians. Islam preaches religious tolerance, recognizing the prophets in both the Torah and New Testament. Yet, in Muhammad, Muslims see a prophet that they believe heard the word of God directly and then spread this word through a series of recitations over 23 years, later recorded as the Koran (Quran).

Muslims accept and follow the Five Pillars of Islam, which include: (1) declaring one's faith in Allah by accepting Mohammad as God's messenger and the Koran as the true Word of God, (2) praying five times daily; (3) following *zakat*, or a tithe, to support the poor; (4) fasting from dawn to dusk during the holy month of Ramadan annually; and (5) making a pilgrimage or *hajj* to the Mecca in Saudi Arabia at least once during one's life if one's health allows (Esposito 2003, 7). The third pillar requires all Muslims to contribute 2.5% of their total wealth, not just income, to support the less fortunate. It is not considered charity; rather it is seen as an obligation—a core tenet of the faith.

Islam arose at a time when Muhammad's home of Mecca was emerging as a major center of commerce and political power. The infusion of wealth dramatically altered life for the previously nomadic tribes and fueled a growing disparity between rich and poor. In the midst of such change, Muhammad, a deeply reflective man, first heard the voice of an angel of God named Gabriel around 610 C.E., commanding him to "recite" the first of many revelations from Allah. The recitations denounced the order of the day, calling for social justice for the poor and most vulnerable—women, children, and orphans. It also called for greater equality between the sexes. Like Christ before him, Muhammad attracted underprivileged and marginalized groups, as well as those who had grown disillusioned with the capitalistic ethos of Mecca (Armstrong 1993, 146). His ideas were radical for that time and place and posed an immediate challenge to the leaders of business, politics, and religion.

In essence, Muhammad's message was that people had to submit to the will of God, which meant creating a moral society grounded in social justice. In short, "the purpose of all actions is the fulfillment of God's will to create a socially just society, not following the desires of tribes, nations, or the self" (Esposito 2003, 16).

Although the Western view of Islam has been colored by proclamations of terrorists such as Osama bin Laden and radical Iraqi clerics, the overwhelming majority of Muslims are neither extremists nor terrorists. A particularly apt analogy holds that Islamic terrorists are to Islam as members of the KKK are to Christianity. Similarly, it is a mistake to judge Islam by the failing societies that live under it. The separation of church and state has freed the West in ways that much of the Middle East has not yet grasped. Most Muslims strive to live God's will on earth and practice complete submission to his will, as evidenced by their prostration in prayer before him five times daily, their annual Ramadan fast, *hajj*, and concern for the poor.

In her brilliant book *A History of God,* author Karen Armstrong summarizes Islam in this way:

> In practical terms, *islam* meant that Muslims had a duty to create a just, equitable society where the poor and vulnerable are treated decently. The early moral message of the Koran is simple: It is wrong to stockpile wealth and to build a private fortune, and good to share the wealth of society fairly by giving a regular proportion of one's wealth to the poor. . . . As in Judaism, God was experienced as a moral imperative (1993, 142).

Muhammad's life and moral precepts continue to fuel Islam's spread through the world. His advocacy for the marginalized and the ideal of a new world order based on social justice is reminiscent of Jesus, who preceded him by 600 years.

Christianity

Jesus Christ gathered the disenfranchised around him while preaching a message of love and compassion. His bent toward social justice threatened the political and religious order of the day and ultimately cost him his life. The faith he spawned, Christianity, currently has more adherents than any other faith, though it has splintered into many denominations. The three primary denominations—Catholicism, Orthodox, and Protestantism—reflect schisms that date back to the 11th century (Orthodox) and 16th century

(Protestant Reformation). Within the broad tent of Christianity are found Lutherans, Anglicans, Baptists, Methodists, Episcopalians, and many others.

One of the most recent and relevant groups for our purposes is *liberation theology*, which we will discuss shortly. What unites all Christians, however, is the belief that Jesus, the Christ, or Messiah, brought about deliverance to the world through his suffering and death, as prophesized in the Old Testament.

It must seem odd to non-Christians that a young carpenter, whose ministry lasted just one to three years, and then was put to death as a common criminal, could have had such a profound impact on the moral terrain of the world. Yet the historical Jesus and his main teachings are worth reviewing—for believers and nonbelievers alike—to better understand the core moral tenets of the wider Christian faith he spawned.

Jesus was born in Nazareth and probably spent much of his life working as a carpenter. At the time, carpenters and other artisans occupied a low status—just below the peasant class and just above the "expendable class" —on the economic ladder (Crossan 1989, 23). Little is known about most of Christ's early and adult life. Following his baptism by John the Baptist, Christ ventured out to become a rabbi, basing his teachings on the Jewish Torah and preaching a faith based on love. His methods and means were radical for the time. He shared meals with lepers, prostitutes, and tax collectors; healed the sick; and traveled continuously throughout the Middle East, preaching a then radical vision of social justice. His talk of a coming "Kingdom of God" posed an immediate threat to the Roman authorities, who were constantly crushing revolts throughout Judea at the time.

In addition to the fishermen who became his disciples, Jesus's adherents included the downtrodden of the ancient Middle East. His was truly a revolutionary perspective for the times—and remains so today. From my perspective as a Catholic, the core of his teaching reduces to a simple phrase: "Love one another as I have loved you." That he willingly gave his life for his core beliefs has inspired Christians for centuries and simultaneously elevates the power of his words.

A core tenet of Christian belief comes from Christ's Sermon on the Mount (Matthew 5:1, and Luke 6:20), in which he told his followers that those who were truly "blessed" were the poor, the hungry, the mourners, the meek, the persecuted, and those who "thirst for righteousness," among others. Essentially, he preaches a "subversive" message in which the rich and the traditional winners are left out and the marginalized are elevated (Wright 1997, 50). Author John Crossan states that by blessing this group, Christ argued against the very structures of a society that excluded so many. About Christ's famous saying in Luke 6:20, "Blesses are you who are poor, for yours is the kingdom of God," Crossan writes:

> If we think not just of personal or individual evil but of social, structural, or systemic injustice—that is, of precisely the imperial situation in which Jesus and his

fellow peasants found themselves—then the saying becomes literally, terribly, and permanently true. In any situation of oppression, especially in those oblique, indirect, and systemic ones where injustice wears a mask of normalcy or even of necessity, the only ones who are innocent or blessed are those squeezed out deliberately as human junk from the system's own evil operations. A contemporary equivalent: only the homeless are innocent. That is a terrible aphorism against society because . . . it focuses not just on personal or individual abuse of power but on such abuse in its systemic or structural possibilities—and there, in contrast to the former level, none of our hands are innocent or our consciences particularly clear (Crossan 1989, 62).

In another message that is no doubt unsettling to many Christian readers in the lucrative medical profession, Christ is particularly clear about people's relationship to wealth. In Matthew 6:24, he says, "No one can serve two masters; for either he will hate the one and love the other, or else he will be loyal to the one and despise the other. You cannot serve God and mammon." In Mark 10:24, he adds, "Children, how hard it is for those who trust in riches to enter the kingdom of God! It is easier for a camel to go through the eye of a needle than for a rich man to enter the kingdom of God."

In the manner in which he led his ministerial life, the manner in which he died, and the moral teachings he left behind, Christ's message is also one of service. In Mark 10:43, he says, "but whoever desires to become great among you shall be your servant. And whoever of you desires to be first shall be slave of all. For even the Son of Man did not come to be served, but to serve, and to give His life a ransom for many."

Christ's most telling parable regarding our relationship with the poor, marginalized, or disenfranchised comes from Matthew 25:31. "Assuredly, I say to you, inasmuch as you have done it unto one of the least of these my brethren, you have done it unto me." Christ tells his followers that when he was hungry, they fed him, when he was thirsty they gave him water. When he was a stranger, they took him in. When he was naked they gave him clothes, and when sick or in prison they visited him. For such actions, they gain access to the kingdom of Heaven. He then tells them that those who failed to do so face "everlasting fire . . . and everlasting punishment."

For some Western Christians, religion has evolved into an entity of convenience, heeded when it suits their political and personal choices; ignored or discarded when it imposes uncomfortable doctrine or intrudes on comfortable lives. Many have cherry-picked selected passages in the Bible that support a political viewpoint. Examples include Leviticus 18:22, in which God calls men lying with men an "abomination," which is an oft-quoted line used politically against homosexuals. Those seeking to justify the acquisition of wealth commonly cite the parable of the talents in Matthew 25. There, Jesus tells of a master who gives money to three servants, two of whom invest it, thereby increasing its value, while the third buries it in the sand. The master scolds the third, leaving a message, according to some, that one should make money. Yet the very next passage is the above-cited Matthew 25, commanding us to care for the poor.

The tendencies to cherry-pick certain passages causes one to miss the larger picture. Commentary on poverty and social justice consistently runs throughout the Bible. The Bible contains more than 2300 scriptural verses about poverty (Eaton and Etue 2002, 81). This is not an aberrant theme in the Bible. It is a core message, one that, depending on one's views, is a clear message from God. It reverberates throughout the Jewish and Christian faiths and it occupies a central place in the Koran.

Christ's message is clear: Care for the downtrodden of the world as you would care for him; failing to do so brings eternal damnation. Judging by Christ's comments and parables, one can assume that if he were alive today, he would conduct his ministry with the marginalized peoples of today's world, including those with AIDS, the poor, and the oppressed. Christ's teachings reflect a core morality as radical then as it is now.

Although many things have changed since Christ's death almost two millennia ago, the core strengths and failings in the human character remain constant. There is every bit as much greed now as there was in Herod's time. The poor remain with us, and in ever-increasing numbers in some world regions. Yet while many branches of Christianity advocate charity for the poor and right living with God, one branch in particular takes Christ's lived experience and teachings a level higher. Born of the barrios and slums of Latin America, liberation theologians, starting in the 1960s, applied Christ's essential message of social justice to the oppressive structures around them. Theirs is a quest that has fueled revolution and impels those of many faiths to listen to the factual and theological arguments they raise.

Liberation Theology

On March 24, 1980, an assassin shot and killed San Salvador's Archbishop Oscar Romero as he said mass. Many of those fleeing the church in the ensuing confusion met similar fates, gunned down by paramilitary death squads that claimed more than 70,000 lives during El Salvador's civil war; a war fueled by American aid. The United States gave $6 billion in military aid to El Salvador during its civil war, making it second only to Israel in military aid received from the United States during the 1980s ("Enemies of War" 2001).

Romero's death triggered worldwide condemnation and caused many to ask just what Christian message could be so threatening to government officials that it would warrant assassination—particularly during mass? The reason was that Archbishop Romero had forcefully challenged the order of the day in El Salvador and had publicly asked the US government to stop sending military aid. That posed a sufficient threat to those in power. Yet Romero's larger views were based on a revolutionary interpretation of the Bible called liberation theology. In fact, he had been one of its main architects at a regional bishops meeting in Puebla, Mexico, just six months earlier.

Liberation theology grew out of the stark inequalities of Latin America, both historic and modern. Gustavo Gutierrez, a Catholic priest who lives among the poor in the Rimac Slum of Lima, Peru, has been called the "father of liberation theology" because of the leading role he has played in pushing the movement forward. In 1971, Father Gutierrez published his classic text, *A Theology of Liberation*, in which he argued that the Church in Latin America had coddled the rich and ignored the poor since its arrival in the New World (Gutierrez 1995). Statements such as, "Blessed are the poor" (Luke 6:20), and "You have the poor with you always" (Matthew 26:11) lent those in power overt support from the all-powerful Church. As long as the poor could look forward to an eternal reward in heaven for their suffering on earth, they would offer no resistance to their entrenched poverty.

This support from the Church allowed governments throughout Latin America to exploit the poor while those in and close to power shored up considerable personal wealth, widening the gap between rich and poor. The Church proved "useful" to the powerful and became fully aligned with the wealthy. Author Robert McAffee Brown wrote, "For centuries, the church taught such acquiescence, passivity, and resignation in the face of poverty and injustice—a political message that the rulers and rich found ideally suited for keeping the masses docile" (Brown 1990, 5). Gutierrez argues that this has been the case for centuries. The conquistadors tortured and killed the native Amerindians on the grounds that they were "heathens" and, thus, deserving of their fate. But brave men such as Bartolome de Las Casas, discussed in Chapter 7, stepped forward to stand with the victims. Las Casas risked his life, becoming a "traitor to his class" to speak out against the European atrocities. While contemporaries saw the Amerindians as "infidels," Las Casas saw them simply as "the poor." He saw the barbaric actions of the Spanish as invalidating their claims to the legacy of Christ and claimed that the Spaniards, not the Amerindians, were risking their salvation.

Gutierrez resurrected Las Casas's writings, seeing in them clear parallels between the Amerindians of the 16th century and the Latin American poor of the 20th century. Both groups, Gutierrez argued, had suffered at the hand of a powerful elite that used religious doctrine to support its tactics. A closer reading of the Bible, however, forced different conclusions, which increasingly found voice in large gatherings of the Catholic Church's hierarchy. At regional Latin American bishops' meetings held in Medellin, Columbia, in 1968, and Puebla, Mexico, in 1979, key themes of liberation theology emerged, first generating strong opposition, but then gaining wide acceptance. At Medellín, the Church was finally "listening to the cry of the poor and becoming the interpreter of their anguish" (Boff and Boff 1998, 76). McAfee Brown writes,

Medellín has become known as the conference in which the church chose to stand with the oppressed, attacked the political and economic structures of Latin America as purveyors of injustice, pointed out the unjust dependency of Latin America on outside powers, and called for radical changes across the continent. Medellin saw clearly that the present order guarantees that the rich will grow richer at the expense of the poor, with the inevitable result that the poor will grow poorer in relation to the rich. And the bishops refused any longer to bless such an order (Brown 1990, 13).

At Puebla, the bishops rededicated themselves to offering a "preferential option for the poor"—a clear indication that they no longer saw the current order in Latin America as tolerable for the multitudes living in back-breaking poverty. The bishops offered support to the poor, who had begun to "reclaim their rights," and challenged the Church to "understand and denounce the mechanisms that generate this poverty" (Brown 1990, 19).

As expected, those in power did not take well to priests challenging the long-held power dynamics that maintained entrenched inequalities. As Paul Farmer said,

> What happens when the destitute in Guatemala, El Salvador, Haiti, wherever, are moved by a rereading of the Gospels to stand up for what is theirs, to reclaim what was theirs and was taken away, to ask only that they enjoy decent poverty rather than the misery we see here every day in Haiti? We know the answer to that question, because we are digging up their bodies in Guatemala (Kidder 2003, 195).

When poor people organize, demand essential human rights, and agitate for change, they pose a threat to foreign business interests and local, powerful elites often in their debt. Many Latin American states responded to the threats of liberation theology by escalating levels of violence against the poor.

Less than six months after the bishops left Puebla, the Sandinista forces overthrew the US-backed Somoza family that had ruled Nicaragua for 43 years. The Church played a key role in fueling the revolution, and three priests assumed prominent roles in the new Sandinista government (Brown 1990, 19). Under the Sandinista regime (1979–1990), public health dramatically improved while infant mortality plummeted. Even the World Bank called the Sandinista social programs "extraordinarily successful . . . in some sectors, better than anywhere else in the world" (Werner and Sanders 1997, 153). Despite this, the Reagan administration helped to bring it down, imposing a crushing trade embargo and funding counterrevolutionary forces (the Contras) by illegally diverting arms sales from Iran. Elsewhere in Latin America, similar themes played out.

The Teachings of Liberation Theology

For Gustavo Gutierrez as for other adherents, the "first act" of liberation theology is to embrace the poor by living among them. More specifically, the first act is not a "head trip" into academic or theological studies on poverty but, rather a "foot trip" to "engagement and identification with the poor, the victims, the marginated" (Brown 1990, 51). Only through such a perspective, Gutierrez argues, can we fully understand the poor and the various structures that so constrain their lives. By undertaking such a venture, many of the false understandings of poverty fall away. Poverty becomes anything but the "virtuous" state depicted in certain biblical passages. Instead, it is revealed as a "subhuman condition" in which its inhabitants are widely viewed as "non-entities." Those who want to make a "virtue" out of poverty invariably want to make it a virtue for someone else (56).

Gutierrez argues that by living among the poor, he has learned many lessons—first among them that material poverty is "a scandalous condition inimical to human dignity and therefore to the will of God" (Brown 1990, 56). Anyone who so ventures, Gutierrez argues, is forced to conclude that, quite simply, "the world should not be the way it is" (51). For liberation theologists, the next logical step is to analyze the factors that foster such an unjust world order. We already have undertaken such a journey, having viewed the components of structural violence, the failings of development, and the forces of disparity that continue to enslave the poor.

The observation of poverty and the understanding that the poor are largely not to blame for their condition forces one of the main tenets of liberation theology—direct action. In Gutierrez's words, "True reflection leads to action." Following a deeper understanding of the forces at work in the world, we are forced to conclude that the world order is horribly broken. Only through the direct action of service or participation in the political process can we hope to effect change. Gutierrez terms this work "praxis for the poor." *Praxis* is a term borrowed from Paulo Freire meaning an ongoing interplay between theory and practice—one informs the other. Gutierrez writes, "It is not enough to know that praxis must precede reflection; we must also realize that *the historical subject of that praxis is the poor*—the people who have been excluded from the pages of history. Without the poor as subject, theology degenerates into academic exercise" (Brown 1990, 67).

The "second act" of liberation theology is to review this praxis "in light of the word of God." This comprises a secondary reflection informed by Biblical teachings. There, Gutierrez and other liberation theologians see a God committed to relieving the suffering of the poor (Brown 1990, 56). The story of Job is particularly instructive. In the Bible, Job is a prosperous man from whom God removes wealth, house, family, and all Job holds dear, ultimately leaving Job destitute and forced to beg for food. While Job's friends judge Job harshly and believe that he must have committed some sin to incur God's wrath, Job sees—for the first time—the innocence of the poor, whose ranks he has now joined. Job turns aside the ancient doctrine of retribution, recognizing that many of the poor around him arrived in their deplorable state through no fault of their own. In its stead he embraces an ethic of compassion for the poor and suffering. In so doing Job adopts God's love for the poor, not because they are good but because they are poor and most often victims of forces beyond their control.

Liberation theology focuses on the non-persons, the poor, and the marginalized. It stands solidly with them and directs attention to the forces that constrain them. It forces a rereading of the Bible from the perspective of the poor, with an emphasis on social justice and the stated priorities of God through history. Finally, it forces its adherents *to act*. It is not enough to merely interpret, study, or conclude. One must act and do so *with* the poor, not *to* or *for* them. Ultimately, one must use the experiences gleaned to inform theory and practice in an ongoing, interactive fashion, always informed by the word of God.

For health providers, liberation theology offers important lessons. First, as this text has attempted to show thus far, we must understand the forces that constrain the poor. Only through this understanding can we get beyond the simple and erroneous explanations that too often pass as rationalizations for poverty. Through these understandings our responses to such large-scale inhumanity should evolve beyond the charitable act of sending our surplus and used items. We should be willing to go ourselves, and to provide the same high-quality care we provide in the United States and other rich countries.

Second, liberation theology advocates solidarity with the poor. According to Virchow, health providers are the "natural attorneys of the poor," so we should find ourselves siding with the poor and against those seeking to exploit them (Kidder 2003, 61). This may entail badgering our congressional representatives about aid programs or working within a civil society organization.

Third, as we have seen throughout this text, health is directly related to human rights, and liberation theology challenges the current world order that elevates some at the expense of the many. It clearly reinforces the belief that health is a "right" and not a privilege. Ours remains a profession that should safeguard that right to the last.

A Return to the Beginning

Before we turn to the individuals who have dedicated their lives to work in international health service, we should briefly take stock of where we are now. Through a modern paradigm of human rights and the ethical traditions of many world religions, we have compelling reasons to act in our world, bringing our considerable gifts as health providers. When we return to the story of the 10-year-old Kenyan girl at the beginning of this book, we should be able to better understand the varied, complex and hidden forces that conspired to rob her of her hopes, dreams, and ultimately, her life.

From all of the forces outlined in this section, it should be clear that this 10-year-old girl would have no options other than to turn to prostitution for survival. And how imminently predictable it was that AIDS and an early death would follow. As a female AIDS orphan in one of Nairobi's harsh slums, she had precious little hope. Larger forces, mostly invisible to her and many of those in the developed world, conspired to rob her of any chance to have a decent life. How do we justify it or even begin to blame her for her poverty? From the perspective of human rights or any of the world's major religions, it is clear how wrong her life was, just as it is for so many millions like her. We live in a world abounding in the wealth, knowledge, and ability to change the lives of people like her the world over. The fact that we consistently fail to do so speaks volumes about our spiritual shortcomings, to the distance between human rights on paper and their existence in our world.

But we can effect change. By insisting that all people attain the fundamental human rights that are both their birthright and a demand of virtually all of the major world religions, we can improve health for the world's people. By taking action ourselves, we can directly affect change. We can take the critical first steps required to engage the problem, to find a reason to care. By not engaging, we run the risk of keeping things as they are for yet another generation. Part 2 of this book provides the inspirational models. The companion text to this one, *A Practical Guide to Global Health Service* (American Medical Association 2006), provides the specific means to get started.

Charles Dickens once wrote of a miserly old man in 19th-century England, oblivious to the poverty and suffering around him. When the Ghost of Christmas Present opened his robes, two small, pathetic urchins named Ignorance and Want stared back at Ebenezer Scrooge. Appalled by their appearance, Scrooge asked, "Spirit, are they yours?" "They are Man's," the Spirit replied. "And they cling to me, appealing from their fathers. This boy is Ignorance. This girl is Want. Beware them both, and all of their degree, but most of all beware this boy, for on his brow I see that written which is Doom, unless the writing be erased" (Dickens 1893).

Well over a century after Dickens wrote these words, we find ourselves in a world still characterized by Want, along with enormous disparities in health and health care. Yet, as Dickens's Spirit stated, it is Ignorance that should most concern us. Ultimately it is our ignorance of what comprises life for most of the world's people and our aversion to directly tackle its root cause that most threatens humanity. We are a strange people, abounding in the wealth and technologies and skills to solve all of these problems, yet we engage them with only a fraction of our potential. Ultimately, we reap what we sow, and if current dichotomies of wealth and health continue, ours will indeed be a bitter harvest. We are all connected far more than we are inclined to think. No amount of prayer, no matter how thoughtful in its intent, will save us from ourselves.

Endnotes

1. For more information see the D-Day Museum web site at www.ddaymuseum.co.uk.
2. During a different phase of the Nuremberg trials, 15 of 23 German physicians were tried and convicted of war crimes; 7 were hung. From the "Doctors' Trial" at Nuremberg, grew the now established principle of informed consent, designated by the tribunal in a "Nuremberg Code" which defines 10 essential points for the moral and legal use of humans in experimentation (Mann et al 1999, 281).
3. For more information see the United Nations web site at www.un.org/aboutun/charter.
4. Information from the "Four Freedoms Speech" delivered by Franklin Delano Roosevelt, available online at www.libertynet.org/~edcivic/fdr.html.
5. For more information see the United Nations Division for the Advancement of Women web site at www.un.org/womenwatch/daw/cedaw.
6. For more information see the UNICEF web site at www.unicef.org/crc/crc.htm.
7. US opposition was based on several reasons: The CRC forbids military recruits younger than age 18, but the United States signs up recruits at age 17 and takes ROTC members as early as age 8; the CRC forbids juvenile executions, which until March 2005 were legal in the United States; many in the United States see the CRC as an instrument that would require the United States to cede sovereignty and may erode parental authority; and finally, some countries that use child labor are US economic partners, which might be problematic if the United States were to ratify the CRC. The United States does have some of the world's most progressive child protection laws and has become an early signatory in subsequent child protection treaties (Mettimano 2002).
8. For more information see the United Nations International Criminal Court web site at www.un.org/law/icc/general/overview.htm.
9. The United States has refused to become a "party to the treaty" creating the ICC, insisting that US soldiers be exonerated from crimes committed while abroad, a position the ICC has naturally refused to accept. The court has ongoing tribunals for war crimes from Rwanda and the former Yugoslavia. (For more information see the ICC link at http://untreaty.un.org/ENGLISH/bible/englishinternetbible/partI/chapterXVIII/treaty10.asp#N6.)
10. Excerpt from the *Bodhisattvacharyavatara* by Santideva, written in the 8th century. For more information see the Essortment web site at http://kyky.essortment.com/whatisbodhisat_rfld.htm.

Part 2

Icons and Inspirations

Of all the will toward the ideal in mankind only a small part can manifest itself in public action. All the rest of this force must be content with small and obscure deeds. The sum of these, however, is a thousand times stronger than the acts of those who receive wide public recognition. The latter, compared to the former, are like the foam on the waves of a deep ocean.

—Albert Schweitzer

Having just reviewed the forces that propagate poverty and ill health for so many, we now turn to some health providers who have chosen to respond. Of the thousands of health providers who have undertaken this work, I selected a handful of those whose stories may be particularly instructive to highlight in this part. I tried to incorporate their own voices whenever possible and refrain from inserting my own interpretations for their actions.

I arrived at the following group mainly because I knew many of them, or could find a lot written about them. Tom Dooley comes mainly through his own beautifully written books and several other books written about him. I lived with Father Bill Fryda in Kenya, and talk with him regularly.

Jim Yong Kim and I were Kellogg Fellows together, and through Jim I got to know his colleague and friend, Paul Farmer. I know Peter Allen from regular visits to Belize, while Tom Durant was a friend and mentor. Although Albert Schweitzer died when I was just five years old, I have read much by and about him, and have come to know his daughter, Rhena, well. During many phone conversations and a few meetings, she has helped me to better understand who he was and why he made such extraordinary choices.

In viewing the individuals as a group, I am struck by how themes of justice and ethics run through each of their life stories. While some like Schweitzer, Fryda, and Dooley have followed their chosen paths out of clear religious convictions, others like Farmer, Kim, Durant, and Allen talk of an ethic that resonates with faith-based teachings, lending credence to Schweitzer's talk of an "ethical imperative" to serve. All speak of larger social justice concerns and have endured some hardships in following their passions. I chose Schweitzer's concept of "Reverence for Life" as a fitting conclusion to this section, as well as a means of tying some seemingly unrelated concepts throughout Part 1 together. While Reverence for Life is secular in of itself, it derives from a number of philosophical and religious traditions, particularly Christianity. Schweitzer's life and worldview force us to contemplate what we covered in Part 1 and apply it—directly—to the world. Reverence for Life does not allow you to sit back and let others do the work for you; it forces you to take action.

Taken together, the examples of each of these men offer compelling testimony to the power of direct action. Their stories of transformation, and the incredible legacies they have left or are still crafting, offer us a precious commodity in choosing our own courses—inspiration. The word itself comes from the Latin, *inspirare* meaning "in" and "to breathe." The *spirare* comes also from the Latin *spiritus* for spirit, and the modern English hints at but does not convey the full derivation of the term, which would say more accurately, "to take in to the spirit, to draw breath into the soul as from a deity." Such figures as these provide us with a moral road map toward a better world. There is a tendency to view the lives of men like these as extraordinary and to rationalize away their accomplishments by viewing them as being simply beyond the reach of the average person. Further, many people read about Paul Farmer, Bill Fryda, or Albert Schweitzer and conclude simply that they are/were "obsessed," or so far outside society's norms that they should be disregarded completely. Yet such views directly contradict all that we have just covered in Part 1. In a world in which 27,000 children die every day of treatable illness, and 2 billion people live on less than $2 per day, isn't it more bizarre that people spend millions of dollars on yachts and luxury second homes? Isn't it more likely that we got the "norms" of society backwards? After reading the following, ask yourself whether each of the life stories that follow resonate more with the teachings of Christ than any of our most fêted celebrities.

Some who read the following will rightly ask why certain people are not included. Larimer and Gwen Mellon spent most of their lives in Haiti and built one of the developing world's best hospitals, L'Hôpital Albert Schweitzer (HAS), in Deschapelles, Haiti. I left them out mainly because I never met either one and had insufficient material to work from, though I recognize that the Mellons' story is an inspirational one, and a tremendous source of pride to all those who serve at HAS. Similarly, Dr Margaret Hamlin founded a "fistula hospital" in Addis Ababa, Ethiopia to care for and surgically repair the fistulas that develop as complications of pregnancy and lead to a constant leaking of urine—and outcast status for the women so afflicted. Although Dr Hamlin's also provides a truly inspirational story, there is little I could find about her, through no fault of her own (Kristoff 2003). Perhaps these and other inspirational figures I will no doubt meet over the coming years will make subsequent editions of this book.

I realize that I have included seven males, all but one of whom are white. I did not leave out women or people of color deliberately. Rather, I selected out those whose stories I knew best, and offered the most poignant lessons to our purposes here. Similarly, I also selected out those who came from the United States and the United Kingdom only. I did not deliberately slight the multitude of talented health providers I have come to know in Belize, Kenya, Tanzania, and Guyana. Rather, this book is about getting health providers from rich countries to travel to the developing world. As such, the stories of those already there, though similarly inspirational and impressive, simply lack relevance to our purposes here.

Some may criticize inclusion of one or more of the following, or certain aspects therein. For example, Tom Dooley's alleged role as a "pawn" for the Central Intelligence Agency. Yet, we must recognize that we live in a society of talkers, those who stand on the sidelines and criticize, never considering for a moment just how difficult life may be for those who are the target of their accusations. While criticism is welcomed, even important here, we should stay focused on the fact that our central task here is to leave the sidelines, to join in the fray and possibly transform our world in the process. Far too many people feel they have done enough by simply raising their voices in protest. Paul Farmer once commented that some people "feel that all the world's problems can be fixed without any cost to themselves. We don't believe that. There's a lot to be said for sacrifice, remorse, even pity. It's what separates us from roaches" (Kidder 2000). Much more is required of us—politically, economically, and directly through service—if we are to truly change things; but we can't affect change without action, often at a price. While few of us can hope to attain even a fraction of what these figures have done, as I have repeatedly alluded to throughout this text, we can all do our share.

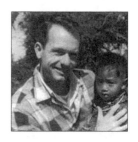

Chapter 11

Thomas Anthony Dooley, MD

I was able to see the filth and wretchedness and stink and misery of these people and was able to learn their fineness, their magnificence, and their valiant, valiant faith.

—Dr Tom Dooley,
> on Vietnamese refugees during Operation Passage to Freedom, 1954

Thomas Anthony Dooley was born in 1927 in St Louis, Misssouri, to wealthy Irish-Catholic parents. In his brief life he caught the world's attention and, for however briefly, redirected that attention to the plight of the poor of Southeast Asia. For many, he was the US physician who most closely approached Albert Schweitzer. Following US Navy work with refugees in Vietnam, Dooley built a small medical clinic in northern Laos, ministered to the poor of the surrounding community, and went on to inspire a generation of people to service through his example. By the time of his death, he had started rural clinics all over the developing world, primarily in Southeast Asia under the umbrella of his nonprofit organization Medico. Dooley had a gift for story telling, all the charm of his Irish ancestry, and the drive of a man transformed by his life's experiences. He used this combination to sear an imprint on a nation's conscience that it could—and must—address the unnecessary suffering of so many, half a world away. Dooley brought the daily lives of remote villagers into American living rooms and water cooler conversations. He and his small band of US Navy corpsmen became healers for and members of these small, rural villages in Laos, Burma, and Vietnam. For the first time, these places and the people in them mattered to ordinary Americans.

Tom Dooley remains relevant to anyone considering service in international health today. Through the methods he used, the stunning personal transformation he underwent, and the international attention he garnered, Dooley warrants a second look by the medical profession. He selflessly dedicated his life to those who had transformed it and reflected the international attention he attracted on those who, years later, still suffer in obscurity, out of the glare of the klieg lights. Though largely unknown to most under the age of 50, Tom Dooley was one of the most sought after speakers and most admired men of his generation. In a life spanning only 34 years, he became an American icon and the most visible American-born proponent of international health service. Dr Schweitzer wrote to Agnes Dooley upon her son's death, "Madame, your son was one of the great personalities that have appeared in the world" (Fisher 1997, 152).

Early Years

Tom Dooley's early life showed few signs of the promise that lay ahead of him. He aspired to maintain the opulence he had known all his life, displaying a brash arrogance and aloofness that earned him both envy and disdain from his schoolmates. Some who knew him in his early years rather unflatteringly recalled him as egotistical, arrogant, and tending to be somewhat of a loner. He used his abundant charm to cozy up to wealthy socialites, perfecting his ability to "travel in first-class splendor on virtually no money" (Fisher 1997, 29). In striking contrast to his later years, he once upgraded a return ticket home on an ocean liner departing Europe, "to avoid the 'many DPs' [displaced persons] fleeing those parts of Europe not on the itinerary of indomitable young Americans" (30). Still, there were glimpses into a more compassionate and serious side. He spent a considerable amount of time with a young girl suffering from a progressive form of rheumatoid arthritis and evolved a deep faith, once describing Notre Dame's famous grotto as "the rock to which my life is anchored" (28).

Dooley enrolled at the University of Notre Dame in the winter of 1944. After only two semesters there, he enlisted in the US Navy as a corpsman, served two uneventful years mostly in the Philippines, and returned to Notre Dame (Fisher 1997, 25). He left Notre Dame in 1948 prior to receiving a degree and enrolled at St Louis University Medical School. This was not an uncommon practice at the time, particularly when the applicant had the social connections that Dooley did. He failed to distinguish himself as a medical student, having to repeat his senior year. He was said to have "spent more time lining up wealthy female St Louisans as future patients as a 'society obstetrician' than in fulfilling his clinical duties" (30).

He was a charming nonconformist, routinely ignoring rules that had, in his mind, been developed for others. He once brought his new horse into the hospital to show patients (Mahon 1998, 18). His flamboyant personality and abundant humor earned him friends whom he curiously kept at arms length, rarely allowing anyone to know him well. Some of these personality quirks may have been due to awkward attempts to hide his homosexuality, which in the 1950s was not afforded even the begrudging tolerance it receives in the United States today. Dooley died long before the dawn of the US gay liberation movement that began with the riots at New York's Stonewall Inn in June of 1969 (Cloud 1969). At Catholic Notre Dame and in the US Navy, it is unlikely that Dooley shared his "secret" with many.

At St Louis University Medical School, Dooley was anything but a disciplined student. He spent more of his abundant energies pursuing elite social gatherings with wealthy friends than on his medical studies. According to biographer James T. Fischer, Dooley once phoned a professor asking to be excused from a final examination the next day. "Once he had talked his way out of taking the test, Dooley reportedly exulted, 'It's a good thing, since I'm calling from Paris'" (Fisher 1997, 30).

Vietnam

Dooley's medical school performance did not impress the St Louis University faculty. Deemed "too immature to begin a residency," he was ordered to extend an internship from the customary 1 year to 18 months (Fisher 1997, 35). Dooley declined the faculty's offer and rejoined the Navy instead. Assigned to the USS *Montague* in July 1954, Lieutenant Dooley became part of the US government's Operation Passage to Freedom, during which the US Navy transported more than 600,000 heavily persecuted Catholic Vietnamese from Communist North Vietnam across the demarcation line into the south. Dooley's role was to oversee the camps that housed most of these Vietnamese refugees. In the process, he began to see them in a new light. "I was able to see the filth and wretchedness and stink and misery of these people and was able to learn their fineness, their magnificence, and their valiant, valiant faith," he later recalled (Mahon 1998, 19).

He received the Legion of Merit—the Navy's highest award—for his efforts. Later he oversaw Catholic Vietnamese refugees at Haiphong, a US Navy evacuation point in North Vietnam near the Chinese border. These experiences became the subject of his first book, a national best seller titled *Deliver Us from Evil*:

> I could tell that the newcomers would be like all the rest—filthy, starving, diseased, and maimed in God knows what manner. Groping for a flashlight and pushing my swollen feet into a pair of muddy boondockers, I instinctively began murmuring the Our Father, as I had every day since childhood: "And deliver us from evil." I had to pause in the darkness. Yes, O God, that is the people's

prayer—to be delivered from evil. At that moment I think I sensed, however dimly, the purpose behind my being in Indo-China" (Dooley 1956, 25).

Dooley's book was published by *Reader's Digest* and introduced a genera-tion of Americans to Vietnam. The "evil" Dooley referred to in the book's title was the "godless communists," the great fear of Americans in the era of Sputnik—at the height of the Cold War. Two themes, which became Dooley trademarks, ran through *Deliver Us from Evil* and his two books that followed: his strong Catholic faith and fervent anticommunism. He wrote of commu-nists torturing Catholic priests, maiming teachers, and jabbing sharp wooden chopsticks into the ears of young children who had made the mistake of listening to Catholic doctrine (Dooley 1956, 98). In so doing, Dooley helped set the stage for initial US interests in Vietnam and contributed to the strong anticommunist sentiment that dominated the Eisenhower era. Dooley became a spokesman against communism and received considerable help from the Central Intelligence Agency (CIA) in publicizing his beliefs and activities. Edward Lansdale, a CIA operative, frequently pulled the right strings for Dooley's continual ascension to star status in the American media galaxy (Fisher 1997). Dooley also befriended and aided the rise of a fellow Catholic and up-and-coming US Senator John F. Kennedy (264, 209). Dooley was an enormously popular Catholic at a time before the country had elected its first Catholic president, JFK, in 1960.

Dooley enjoyed phenomenal success with *Deliver Us from Evil*. He toured the country telling stories from Operation Safe Passage and dramati-cally recounted the atrocities and religious persecution of the Vietnamese by the communists. Many claimed that Dooley greatly exaggerated both his own role in the relief operation and the true amount of atrocities the com-munists had committed. However, the criticism did not deter him, for he had the raw material, passion, and charisma to become a national sensation. His stories of Laotian people mauled by bears captured a sympathetic public's attention. When he described the same innocent people being tor-tured and murdered by the communists, always peppered with patriotic and anticommunist rhetoric, he captured their hearts and minds. Tom Dooley was made to order for a Cold War–era US public that was already fearful of foreign threats. The final *Reader's Digest* condensed version of *Deliver Us from Evil* was "a virtual gift from heaven," as Heidenry [of the *Reader's Digest*] called it—an "idealistic, devoutly religious American . . . who was single-handedly holding back the Red Sea in Southeast Asia with his thumb" (Fisher 1997, 78).

Although the US government supported his widely read works, Dooley ultimately became too large an icon for those in power to control. His brash attitude and antagonism toward all forms of authority became too much for the more rigid elements within the military. In the end, the Navy looked less than favorably on his homosexuality and gave him a General Discharge Under Less Than Honorable Circumstances in 1956 (Mahon 1998, 23).

Undeterred, Dooley put the proceeds from his book into the founding of Operation Laos, starting a small clinic in Vieng Vang.

Transformation

Dr Dooley evolved from an aspiring society obstetrician to a self-described "jungle doctor." It was an evolution that many Americans felt a part of through Dooley's books and his many radio and TV appearances. He came to admire Albert Schweitzer, modeling himself after him. Dooley's writings reveal a man transformed by his experiences, no longer interested in status or the acquisition of wealth. He was moved by what he saw and, in time, came to see the struggle of the Vietnamese refugees as his own. He saw for himself what Dr Schweitzer had termed "the brotherhood of those who bear the mark of pain." Dooley closed *Deliver Us from Evil* with the following:

> This was the last day of the last loading. Some 3,600 refugees would take the trip, first to the bay and then on to Saigon, huddled together with their cloth bags, their balance poles with household possessions at each end, their babies on mothers' hips. They were as desolate a slice of the human race as any that had preceded them. They walked slowly in line to be dusted with DDT, to accept a loaf of bread, or perhaps a few diapers and small bags of clothing. But to me they were not a mere mass of wretchedness. I had come to know their valiant hearts and stout spirit. Somehow, over the bitter months, without knowing how it happened, I had identified myself with their dream of life in freedom and their tragic destiny. They had become my suffering brothers.

> I had been taught to believe in and do believe in God's love, His goodness, His mercy. And I knew that in some small degree at least these qualities can be shared by man. But I had seen very little of them in the last year.

> 'I must remember the things I have seen,' I said to myself. 'I must keep them fresh in memory, see them again in my mind's eye, live through them again and again in my thoughts. And most of all I must make good use of them in tomorrow's life' (Dooley 1956, 117).

Dr Dooley had truly evolved and realized that he had to follow this new path. He left the Navy and set out on his own, starting a small hospital in Muong Sing, Laos. "I'm putting up $39,000 to go back [to Southeast Asia]," he said. "My own money. It all came from my book, *Deliver Us from Evil.* I got it from the Indochinese. I'll take it back to them" (Mahon 1998, 19). As had happened to Schweitzer before him, Dooley's family and friends questioned his motives. They reminded him of the importance of "all the things I [he] had always wanted, and now might have. A home, a wife, kids, a nice medical practice, maybe a few fine hunting horses" (Dooley 1958, 134). Yet Dooley had irrevocably changed. He wrote, "How could I make them see that things would never be the same?" (134).

Dooley, the wealthy socialite who barely passed his medical exams, had been touched by the needs of those he served in the refugee camps in

Vietnam. That experience had forever changed his life. He discussed his transformation in the beginning of his second book, *The Edge of Tomorrow*,

> Yes, cocky young Dooley, whom the profs at medical school had ticketed as a future "society doctor," was learning things the hard way, but he was learning at last. At Notre Dame they had tried hard to teach me philosophy. Now out here in this hell-hole I had learned many profound and practical facts about the true nature of man. I understood the inherent quality that enables tough, loud-mouthed sailors to become tender nurses for sick babies and dying old men. I had seen inhuman torture and suffering elevate weak men to great heights of spiritual nobility. I know now why organized godlessness never can kill the divine spark which burns within even the humblest human (Dooley 1958, 24).

Dooley had witnessed the human misery of war and obscene poverty. He saw the world through the lens of his religion and was able to connect his deeply held spiritual beliefs to his immediate life's work. In the process, he evolved to a higher place. He stated his reasons simply, "Since I had served in Southeast Asia and had seen the need, the duty for me as an individual was inescapable" (Dooley 1958, 135). Dooley had found his life's purpose,

> We had seen simple, tender, loving care—the crudest kind of medicine inexpertly practiced by mere boys—change a people's fear and hatred into friendship and understanding. We had witnessed the power of medical aid to reach the hearts and souls of a nation. We had seen it transform the brotherhood of man from an ideal into a reality that plain people could understand. To me that experience was like the white light of revelation. It made me proud to be a doctor. Proud to be an American doctor who had been privileged to witness the enormous possibilities of *medical aid* in all its Christ-like power and simplicity (Dooley 1958, 133).

The transformation was not lost on Dooley's friends and colleagues. Several commented on how he had become a changed man. Dr Melvin Casberg, dean of the Christian Medical College in Ludhiana, a city north of the Punjab part of India, wrote:

> Letters [from Dr. Dooley] began to arrive from across the Pacific. As the correspon-dence focused on his activities in North Vietnam, it was evident that Tom had been shaken to the very depths of his being. There came an awakening to the desperate needs of people in that part of the world. I knew that Tom would never be the same carefree young man again. The story of his transformation was vividly told in his book, *Deliver Us from Evil.* . . . The big question in Tom's mind was, "How can I do the most with my life for those in Southeast Asia who have so little?" Deluged with advice, his mind was in a state of confusion. It was evident that his heart would never be satisfied without an opportunity to serve his newly found friends in Southeast Asia. I urged him to follow his heart (Monahan 1961, 173).

Medico

Dooley brought a few Navy corpsmen with him and started a small clinic in Vang Vieng, Laos. Contrary to popular expectations, he did not make "a white man's hospital with a few Asian assistants, but rather an Asian hospital with three Americans working in it" (Dooley 1960, 357). He understood the importance of building from the ground up and of working with local people, not lording over them. Still, he and his corpsmen were often criticized for the level of services they provided. "They accuse me of practicing nineteenth century medicine," he would say. "They are absolutely correct. I do practice nineteenth century medicine, perhaps seventeenth century medicine, and it doesn't trouble me. And when I turn over a station to Laotian personnel I am sure it will be eighteenth century medicine. This offers at least a little service to people who are living in the fifteenth century" (Monahan 1961, 274). He later expanded to other sites closer to the Chinese border—and closer to the considerable dangers posed by Communist China. When asked why they were going to Laos in the first place, Navy corpsman Norm Baker replied, "Aw hell, sir, we just want to do what we can for people who ain't got it so good" (Dooley 1958, 135).

Dooley's teams became an integral part of the communities they served, living among the local villagers and engaging their traditional care providers; " . . . each team is an intimate part of the village life; each team doctor goes to the weddings and to the funerals. Each team doctor is a part of that community life. We don't come in, spend a few weeks and then pull out—we are a part of the community" (Monahan 1961, 119). He emphasized, "We belonged" (Fisher 1997, 145). He insisted that all patients pay a fee, often only a coconut or an egg. He did this to raise needed food for his hospital and to preserve the dignity of the local villagers. Dooley's men respected local customs and actively engaged the local witch doctors, splitting the two-coconut fee with them for various procedures. The local witch doctors had been there before Dooley and his corpsmen and would remain long after they left. People turned to them because they had been the only source of care available.

> *Dooley rejected the concrete building the villagers had offered, because this would set them apart from the villagers they had come to serve.*

Dooley made sure that his team's accommodations were no different than those of the people they served. His team lived in a three-room hut, made of bamboo. Dooley rejected the concrete building the villagers had offered, because this would set them apart from the villagers they had come to serve. He turned the concrete structure into a hospital (Monahan 1961, 137). Despite prior service in the refugee camps of North Vietnam, Dooley and his men had to adjust to rural Laos. "Never in the thousands of hours that I had devoted to thinking about and planning for this mission in Laos did I anticipate the depths of misery in which we would have to work and eat and sleep and live. . . . I was completely stunned by the conditions that existed in the village of Vang Vieng" (Dooley 1958, 154).

Ever clear on the purpose of his mission, Dooley shared his thoughts with an adoring public through a weekly radio show. Dooley made tape recordings at his clinic in Vang Vieng, then shipped them to a radio station in St Louis, which then broadcast the recordings to homes across the United States (Fisher 1997, 128). "In place of specific discussions of fleeting political issues in Laos, Dooley provided his listeners with a feel for commonalties they shared with these heretofore unknown peoples" (129). Through the radio broadcasts, millions of Americans came to know and admire Tom Dooley. People sent money, conducted "dollars for Dooley" campaigns, and began to elevate him to icon status. "He was an enormously gifted communicator who reached into the hearts of his audience with a rare power" (129). Dooley's star was rising fast.

Tom Dooley captured the people's imaginations through the stories of local village life and the horrendous conditions of poverty that ruled their lives. In one of the many stories he recorded from his clinics in Laos, Dooley described a young Lao hideously burned when his clothes caught fire while he was sleeping too close to the fire on a cold night. His condition worsened after the local witch doctor covered the wounds with "pig grease, betel-nut juice, and cow dung" (Dooley 1958, 175). After a treacherous trip through the jungle to get the child to their new clinic in Nam Tha, Dooley and his corpsmen spent the night debriding necrotic tissue, administering penicillin, and injecting subcutaneous fluids into what remained of the young boy's flesh. Dooley later reflected on the night,

> After the operation I walked slowly back to our hut. My boys all voted to sit up the rest of the night with [the young patient] Ion. Seeing these young men devoting their most tired hours to that child seared something into me. It is the simple clear-cut realization that the brotherhood of man does exist, as surely as does the Fatherhood of God. Indeed we are our brothers' keepers (Dooley 1958, 176).

Dooley spent one year in Nam Tha and later established clinics in Muong Sing and other locales in Laos. In late 1958, he founded Medico, Medical International Cooperation. He partnered with George Washington University physician Peter Commanduras and established Medico as a division of the International Rescue Committee. Dooley explained the structure of the fledgling organization in a press release in 1958. "Teams of doctors and medically trained assistants will be sent into underdeveloped areas of the world where they will build, equip, and staff medical clinics and small hospitals . . . and after 18 months to two years, withdraw, leaving behind all their equipment and self-sufficient local staffs" (Mahon 1998, 19).

Dooley became synonymous with Medico, which grew rapidly in the late 1950s. He was its principal fund-raiser and official spokesman. Dooley earned large amounts of money from public speaking tours and book royalties; he turned all of his earnings over to developing Medico. According to Notre Dame alumnus Frank Mahon, "Every nickel he earned, including over a million dollars in book royalties, went into his medical programs. He saw every speech, every book signing, every camera focused on him as an opportunity to promote Medico: and people all over the world responded" (Mahon 1998, 20). He also repeatedly turned down offers of federal funding for Medico, including one directly from President Eisenhower (20). He felt strongly that aid should remain on a person-to-person basis and resisted any governmental or religious affiliations.

The Ugly American

In 1958, Dooley's form of international "aid" received a boost from two friends who wrote the best-selling book, *The Ugly American*. In it, William Lederer and Eugene Burdick painstakingly exposed US Foreign Service ineptitude in the fictitious country of Sarkhan. The authors based the novel on factual experiences but created fictitious characters to boost readership and general appeal. The book became an enormous success, selling more than 4 million copies and spending 78 weeks on the *New York Times* best-seller list (Fisher 1997, 175). According to author Robert Kohls, "The novel . . . struck the Americans of the late 1950s like a thunderbolt. . . . [It] held a mirror up before us and it was with a distinct shock that we recognized the reflection we saw. We were embarrassed by the behaviors and attitudes Americans displayed as guests in other countries" (Kohls 2001, 13). James Fisher adds, "*The Ugly American* accused the diplomatic establishment not of communism but arrogance, sloth, wastefulness, and a moral softness that threatened to deliver Southeast Asia to the Reds with nary a shot being fired" (Fisher 1997, 209). In effect, Fisher continues, "*The Ugly American* recast the debate over American foreign policy so dramatically that it could very nearly be described as the Uncle Tom's Cabin of the cold war" (175).

The term ugly American *remains and now conjures up images of the typically "loud, insensitive, exploitative brand of overseas American" (Kohls 2001, 13).*

The physically ugly American of the book was actually the book's hero, Homer Atkins, an engineer who related well to the local Sarkhanians. He respected their culture, learned their language, sought out their ideas, and worked on projects that *they* valued. His actions sharply contrasted with the state department representatives who locked themselves in luxurious gated compounds, failed to understand host culture, and generated hatred for the United States through their callous treatment of locals (Lederer and Burdick 1999, 174). The book served notice to an unsuspecting American public that their foreign service personnel were defeating the national ideal of a *pax americana*. Even worse, this occurred at a time when the Soviet propaganda machine was in full swing throughout Southeast Asia. The term *ugly American* remains and now conjures up images of the typically "loud, insensitive, exploitative brand of overseas American" (Kohls 2001, 13). This was not the image people in the 1950s associated with Tom Dooley.

Dooley was the inspiration for a central character in *The Ugly American*. Father John X. Finian was a tough and thoughtful man who ventured deep into the jungles of Sarkhan to work with the local villagers, learn their ways, and develop deep trusting relationships through shared adversity (Lederer and Burdick 1999). Lederer and Burdick admired Dooley's work in Laos and used this central character to promote Dooley's model "as the prototype for the next generation of American foreign aid providers" (Fisher 1997, 175). Through the book's wide success and the firestorm it generated, Dooley emerged even larger than he had been before. He became increasingly popular on the lecture circuit, sold millions of books, and emerged as a cultural icon for the late 1950s. In December 1959, Dooley was selected for "the Gallup Pole's annual Christmastime ranking of the 'most admired' men in the world. . . . Dooley's name occupied seventh place, just below such towering figures as Winston Churchill, Pope John XXIII, and Dooley's official idol and fellow "jungle doctor," Albert Schweitzer" (4).

The Night They Burned the Mountain

In the summer of 1959, Dooley was in the process of opening yet another clinic in Laos, this time in Muong Sing, a small village close to the triangle where Laos, Burma, and China all meet. Medico was expanding, Dooley had a strong core of personnel, and the clinic was developing well. The future looked bright for Tom Dooley. Then on August 15, he received a message that would change his life. Dr Peter Commanduras ordered him back to the United States "immediately." His local staff, the embassy personnel, and countless others in Medico offices in the United States knew why Dooley was summoned home, but he did not. During a stop in Bangkok en route home, Dooley's close friend Hank Miller told him. Several weeks previously, a visiting surgeon, Dr Bill Van Valin, had removed a suspicious lump from Dooley's chest (Dooley 1960, 346). He had sent it to a pathologist in Bangkok and the results were in. Young Tom Dooley, only 32 years old, had malignant melanoma, a particularly aggressive form of skin cancer with an abysmal prognosis. "I had no reaction," he said. "The words entered my head like a fist jammed into a pillow. I felt nothing" (261).

Dooley returned to New York's Memorial Hospital to undergo extensive resection of the tumor. He agreed to have the operation filmed for a *CBS Reports* documentary called, "Biography of a Cancer" (Fisher 1997, 204). Dooley saw the experience as both an opportunity to help others better understand cancer and an opportunity to promote Medico to an audience of millions. The program was a success, winning a prestigious journalism award in the process. After a quick recovery period, Dooley spent the next seven weeks touring the country. He gave 49 speeches in 37 cities and appeared on some of the most popular television shows of the day, including *This Is Your Life* and Jack Paar's *Tonight Show*. The tour raised more than

$1 million, including a check for $500 from then vice president Richard Nixon (219).

Dooley maintained a frenetic pace throughout his tour. Then, in November 1960, despite the increasing danger posed by Communist Chinese forces, he returned to his beloved Muong Sing, the place he had come to call home. He began to feel increasing amounts of pain from the cancer, which had widely metastasized before resection. He lost weight and constantly worried whether he would live to see the future of his clinic in Muong Sing and other Medico clinics around the world. The Pathet Lao communist forces operating within Laos were conducting more frequent raids on the villages in the north of Laos near the Dooley clinic. Villagers were killed and atrocities became a regular occurrence. One visiting pilot approached a landing strip only to find that ". . . many people had been beheaded. Their heads were stuck up on posts along the side of the strip. As the plane came to land, the pilot spotted this atrocity, pulled back on the stick and flew away. The Communists fired on his plane with small weapons" (Dooley 1960, 365). The US Embassy urged Dooley and his men to evacuate their clinic, which was in a region where the communists had been active. After much deliberation, Dooley and his corpsmen decided to remain in Muong Sing, despite the considerable risk. "I knew my refusal not to evacuate was right. . . . We would not abandon these people; we would stay here as long as we were needed" (365).

One night, Dooley walked out into the dark to see people with lanterns setting fire to the mountains around Muong Sing. He was soon reassured that it was not an attack by the communist forces. Rather it was an ancient Lao ritual they called "the night they burn the mountain" (Dooley 1960, 340). This was the one night of the year—before the rains came—when the local villagers burned trees and vegetation in the surrounding mountains to provide fertilizer for the rice crops. While watching the fires burn, Dooley reflected on his life, his battle with cancer, and the fate of the people he had come to see as his family.

> Earl, Dwight and I watched the mountain burn for many hours. The strange, vague foreboding feeling that I had had in the house seemed all the stronger now. What would become of these mountains and these tribes? What would happen to their Kingdom of Laos? Would the flames of Communism conquer it? Would the flames of disease destroy the people? Would there ever be another free May when the people would burn their mountains and plant their rice in this blackened earth? (Dooley 1960, 341).

As in Vietnam before, Dooley had become far wiser through his experiences in Laos. His approaching death had forced him to become more reflective, to look deeper into his soul for answers to the increasingly difficult questions his ever-searching mind posed. The constant pain in his arm and chest reminded him that his time was short and he had much to accomplish before he would be unable to continue.

Dooley had undergone an extraordinary transformation in a short period of time, no doubt fueled by the difficulties of his experiences. His three books traced this remarkable personal growth. In *Deliver Us from Evil*, he merely chronicled his work, sometimes with humor, often with compassion. In his final book, *The Night They Burned the Mountain*, Dooley described– in a clear and compelling voice–his spiritual and personal evolution. He wrote about his transformation in language that was attainable to all. He was a doctor serving in a poor community and one who had both a healthy respect and a deep concern for the villagers he had come to adopt as his own family.

> The people of our valley were completely the victims of external circumstance. They could not control the rain coming, nor the bacteria that flooded their lives, they did not know how to improve their plows, they lacked so much. Those of us in the world who have these things must not ignore the essential needs of human nature the world over. I used to think: These people will die of misery. I have learned something, an unpalatable truth: No one ever dies solely of misery. I wondered how these people would live on. . . . (Dooley 1960, 343).

After being diagnosed with malignant melanoma, Dooley wrestled with a natural fear of dying and the frustration of not being able to see his life's work through. He wondered whether he should continue, whether he would be able to continue. Weeks after first learning of his illness, he dreamed of the burning mountain. For young Dr Dooley, it was a dark night of the soul in which he found the answers to his most difficult questions.

> One night I dreamed I was walking up a steep trail, leading across my valley floor and weaving its way through the high rain-forest onto the mountaintop just east of us. My boys were with me, and some of my Lao students. And in the vivid flash of the moment, in my dream, I saw a century-old pagoda that nestles on this mountain slope. The pagoda is made of mud stones and is crowned by a high spire. Hanging from the spire are long white banners, the streamers of Buddhist prayers. There are miniature bells that tinkled in the wind. . . . As I looked around through the eyes of my dream I saw many areas of land around this moun- tain slope, where the jungle had been burned and the mountain's naked ground was dull black. I also saw tiny insignificant little figures of men on these patches of brown earth. The month of my dream must have been May, the time of lilacs at my beloved Notre Dame. But in Laos, May is a time when the season is driest. These are the nights that they burn the mountain.
>
> The mountain in my dream was burned, and now they were planting the new life into the near dead soil. I dreamed this clearly and when the blue turquoise of morning came, though perhaps neither ear could hear nor tongue could tell, I knew the meaning of my dream. . . .
>
> From my hospital bed in New York, with the same white light of revelation I had known once several years before, I saw what I must do. After Communion that morning, Tuesday, the first of September, my God and my dream com- manded me. I must, into the burned soil of my personal mountain of sadness,

plant the new seedlings of my life—I must continue to live. I must cultivate my fields of food, to feed those who cannot feed themselves.

The concept came to me as strongly and as powerfully as if a peal of bronze bells proclaimed it. There was no more self-sadness, no darkness deep inside: no gritty annoyance at anyone or anything. No anger at God for my cancer, no hostility to anyone. I was out of the fog of confusion—standing under the clear light of duty.

The jagged, ugly cancer scar went no deeper than my flesh. There was no cancer in my spirit. The Lord saw to that. I would keep my appetite for fruitful activity and for a high quality of life. Whatever time was left, whether it was a year or a decade, would be more than just a duration. I would continue to help the clots and clusters of withered and wretched in Asia to the utmost of my ability. The words of Camus rang through, "In the midst of winter I suddenly found that there was in me an invincible summer."

Maybe I could now be tender in a better way. I was a member of the fellowship of those who know the mark of pain. The philosophical concept of Dr. Schweitzer that he used to talk to me about years ago was now a more vivid thing—I bore that mark (Dooley 1960, 376).

Before I Sleep

Dooley spent the rest of his life advancing Medico, fund-raising, and working briefly in Muong Sing. Even when not there, his thoughts often returned to the "high valley." He wrote in his last book, "I could close my eyes and conjure up the village placidly floating before me like a Chinese landscape wrapped in a fine blue mist. . . . I could see once again the mountains of my beloved northern Laos, its gulfs and gorges, the hosts of billowing clouds that roll off the slopes of the high rain forest. I could see the green lush valleys, and see huddled in their thatched huts, the sick of Laos" (Dooley 1960, 378). His final days were characterized by a restless energy born of the passion of his personal mission and the certainty of his impending death. Dooley's energy and level of activity surprised even those who knew him well. A senior editor from the *Reader's Digest* wrote,

> What impressed me most, and particularly during the last fifteen months of his life, was the relentless drive and the sense of urgency that characterized his activities. . . . It seemed that he must have been aware that his days were few, and that he was determined to complete his work or, at least, to put Medico's house in order before his time ran out (Monahan 1961, ix).

Dr Estelle Hughes, a Howard Medical School graduate, had first heard about Medico through a talk Dr Peter Commanduras had given at Howard. She joined Medico and served in Ban Souei Sai in Laos. In the summer of 1960, she met Tom Dooley in California:

> He seemed so vigorous and active, and he had the kind of infectious enthusiasm that made everyone associated with him want to work as hard and devotedly as he did. Of course, I didn't know him well at that time. Later, I began to see that

he was putting up a brave front and concealing his true condition. He was driving himself relentlessly, and inspiring rather than depressing his co-workers was part of his job. But then the days came when he could no longer feign good health, and when those remarkable stores of energy were exhausted. Those are the days which I never shall forget (Monahan 1961, 135).

When he returned to Muong Sing in November 1960, he was able to stay only a few short months. The pain from the cancer had become unbearable and he decided to return home to New York. En route to the United States, he attempted to visit one of his favorite places, the An-Lac Orphanage in Saigon. Too ill to make it to the orphanage, he instead met one of his few close friends, the orphanage curator, Madame Ngai in his hotel room. She recalled their last visit together:

> He was in very low spirits. I had never seen Tom Dooley really depressed before. . . . He admitted to me, for the first time, that his hours were numbered. He kept saying, "But somehow I must go on. I simply must. I must go up to Quang Ngai tomorrow. Then I must fly up to Muong Sing and Ban Houei Sai and get things settled there. The hardest part of it is going to be to conceal the condition I am in." There were real tears streaming down his face. He said: "The others must never see me like this. It would destroy everything" (Monahan 1961, 219).

Dooley continued to push himself to the end, convinced that he should devote all of his remaining strength to the unfinished business of his work in Laos. His cancer had metastasized to his spine and virtually every organ system. Wracked with constant pain, he received the last rites in the Erawan Hotel in Bangkok before embarking on an agonizing trip back to New York. He arrived there on December 27 and returned to Memorial Hospital. There he spent his 34th birthday, on January 17, slowly succumbing to the inevitable. Cardinal Spellman visited him there and "tried to assure him that in his 34 years he had done what very few had done in the allotted scriptural lifetime" (Mahon 1998, 21). The next day, his conditioned deteriorated sharply. By that night, Father FX Finegan was summoned to again administer the last rites, after which he bent down and whispered into Dooley's ear, "Son, go now and meet thy God" (Fisher 1997, 261). Following Father Finegan's words, a peaceful countenance overtook Dooley. He died soon after, at 9:40 PM on Wednesday, January 18, 1961, with his secretary and devoted friend Theresa Gallagher at his side. Two days later the *New York Times* editorialized, "He couldn't be patient or diplomatic with sorrow or death. He couldn't be patient with the disease that finally came over his own strong frame; he fought it and went on doing his work, and his spirit was like a flame in the dark jungle" (Mahon 1998, 18).

His body lay in state in St Louis Cathedral where thousands paid their respects. Dooley's friend Bob Copenhaver recalled the outpouring at the funeral:

> I accompanied the body to the Cathedral, and watched the thousands and thousands file by the bier. Many times that evening I thought, Tom, this is the best performance you've ever given. I watched the faces of the thousands who passed by, and I saw almost every emotion in the human heart—anger that he should die, pity, sorrow, tears, and the puzzled expressions of little children. I wasn't the only one who watched the spectacle and was deeply moved. One prominent newscaster fought back the tears and then just gave up and cried until his TV makeup washed away (Monahan 1961, 263).

In his short life, Dooley accomplished what few had before him. President Kennedy, inaugurated just three days after Dooley's death, cited "the selfless example of Dr. Tom Dooley in Laos" as the inspiration for the US Peace Corps (Fisher 1997, 267) and posthumously awarded him a Congressional Medal (Mahon 1998, 18). Although Medico lasted only two more years before becoming part of CARE, Dooley had established a form of secular, nongovernmental, person-to-person aid that remains an ideal model for rendering health care internationally. He influenced the lives of thousands through the direct patient care and health education his clinics provided. The care came not through high-tech US-style hospitals but through local clinics that incorporated host personnel and trained them to eventually take over the entire operation. The fact that many later failed says more about the void Dooley left after his untimely death than any real flaws in the approach. More important, he left a legacy of service for the health profession, establishing himself as a role model we can turn to all these years later. Dooley saw the medical profession as a unique instrument for spreading goodwill and felt that all physicians had an obligation to care for those who "ain't got it so good" throughout the world.

Still, he had his faults. Many thought that he exaggerated his feats. He had a particularly abrasive temperament, expected perfection from those around him, and relentlessly drove others as he did himself. Many disliked his allegedly huge ego. He spent much of his life as a loner and never seemed to be able to develop many close friendships. In the end, however, his insight and deep spiritual devotion led him to a life that helped many.

Dooley was a wealthy individual who experienced first-hand the poverty and misery that defines existence for much of the human population. That experience was enough to redirect his life course from society physician to advocate and healer of the poor. His personal transformation has relevance for all of us. Equally relevant is the fact that he was an ordinary man—flawed, conflicted, and inspired. For this reason, his personal odyssey is that much more extraordinary. The experience of working with the poor holds sufficient power to change the lives of those who are open enough to allow the transformation to happen. And this holds true for each of us. Dooley's legacy speaks to us through the years and challenges us still. If one can be open to the transformation that comes through working in the depths of human misery and hardship, one can make a real difference in the world.

Perhaps Dooley's greatest legacy is the passion he brought to his quest and how that, in turn, inspired people. He popularized the idea of bringing health care to the world's poor and elevated it to a status it has not seen since. Average Americans began talking about poor people half a world away. "I had never thought of all those suffering people until I read your books," wrote one 14-year-old girl (Fisher 1997, 223). Dooley painted beautiful, compassionate pictures of people otherwise unseen by the American public. The Laotian poor became closer and more real. Dooley showed how similar these people were to Americans, rekindling earlier notions of what Lincoln once called the "family of man." In this way, Dooley helped to redirect a nation's energy, for however brief a time, to that which it should always prioritize. It is unfortunate that Dooley, who was such an inspirational figure for his generation, has largely been forgotten. He warrants a reexamination, particularly by those of us who share his vocation. His words remain compelling and his long-silent voice speaks clearly to us today. If only we can still find within us a reason to listen.

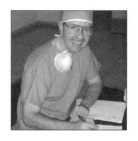

Chapter 12

Father Bill Fryda, MD

God speaks to us through the patterns of our lives.
—Father Fryda

Father Bill Fryda is a Catholic priest and Mayo Clinic–trained oncologist who has spent the past 25 years working in East Africa. Over the past seven years, he built St Mary's Hospital in Nairobi, Kenya, into one of the premiere hospitals in East Africa. St Mary's primarily serves the poor of greater Nairobi and does so in a medical ministry setting that preserves patients' dignity while providing competent, affordable care. I had the good fortune to live with Father Fryda for three months in the winter of 1994, while he was running Nazareth Hospital in Nairobi. During that time, I got to know him quite well. Our dinner conversations ranged from politics to religion to corruption to disease. He was never one to hold back his strong opinions or to tow anyone else's line. Father Fryda has followed a faith-based drive to provide care for the poor of Kenya, following in the example of Christ. His views on poverty, international donor organizations, and his own reasons for service provide an interesting and inspirational story.

"Being a Hospital:" St Mary's

Perhaps the best way to understand Father Fryda is to understand St Mary's, the hospital that he helped create, the one that will one day become his legacy. After working for 18 years in various hospitals in Tanzania and Kenya, Father Fryda decided that his efforts would best be channeled into designing, building, and running a hospital that would serve the poor of greater Nairobi. He joined the Maryknoll Fathers with the Assumption Sisters of Nairobi to see it through. As he said, "During my time here in East Africa, it became apparent to me that there was a crying need for lower-income people to have access to good, affordable health care within a Christian environment." Starting in 1998, the founders raised $3.2 million (and counting) and purchased 10 acres of Karen Blix's (*Out of Africa* fame) old coffee plantation, abutting the Ngong Forrest and across the street from the enormous Kibera slum. Every large organization Father Fryda approached rebuffed him, saying it would be impossible to develop a self-maintaining hospital in such a location. They were wrong. St Mary's was designed to be self-sufficient once bed occupancy reached 70%; it has run at above 100% occupancy (320 beds as of 9/05) since shortly after it opened. Its success has spawned plans for similar hospitals at two additional sites, which could ultimately bring 40% to 50% of Kenya's population under St Mary's expert care, truly a revolutionary model for health care in Africa.

From the vantage point of the catwalk around St Mary's water tower, one can peer across the road to a sea of tin-roofed, closely huddled shacks that comprise Kibera, one of the world's largest slums. This sea of poverty stretches for miles, overflowing with violence, illness, and despair at levels incomprehensible to most Westerners. Four million people call greater Nairobi home; nearly half live in its ample slums. Kibera is the largest, where 800,000 people live with no electricity, running water, or basic sanitation. Because it is far too dangerous to leave one's shack at night, people often defecate in plastic bags and fling them outside, contributing to the overall stench of the place. One BBC reporter wrote of Kibera, "This place is like an island—it's not really part of Kenya at all. The state does nothing here. It provides no water, no schools, no sanitation, no roads, no hospitals" (Harding 2002). AIDS, tuberculosis, malaria, violence, and malnutrition run rampant; concocting a potent stew that cuts short many young lives. Kenya's average life expectancy of 45 years is probably longer than most of those trapped in Kibera could hope for. Little health care is available and few can afford the scant, though decent, care available in the private sector. As such, people rely on the depleted services from the cash-starved government hospitals, where pharmacies are bare and health care staff demoralized by corruption and inefficiency. Most people have no other option than to simply bear their fate. That they do so with such grace reflects their strong spirits.

Father Fryda has long maintained that caring for the people of East Africa in and of itself offers the most bounteous of rewards.

Father Fryda has long maintained that caring for the people of East Africa in and of itself offers the most bounteous of rewards. Although the people of Kibera are materially poor, they are rich in other ways. During one of our conversations, Father Fryda commented that people in East Africa are much better at living than those of us are who live in the West, where we become caught up in wealth and the pursuit of ever more "stuff," much of which we don't need. "In Africa," he says, "people are far better at living in the moment and are far better at living right in the conditions in which they find themselves. Those who are not resource rich are better at living life." In my experience, people there are respectful without being subservient and they exude a natural warmth and beauty. Most seem to conform to a custom of civility—they are not rude. They do not push doctors to see them quickly and they accept clinical decisions with stoicism and gratitude. The word that these people most often bring to mind is grace. It defines them. If God has overlooked their need, he has not overlooked their character.

When asked why he chose to build a hospital at the edge of a dangerous Nairobi slum, Father Fryda replied simply that here is where the greatest need lies. He had worked in a number of rural hospitals in Tanzania and Kenya and observed that, due to urbanization of Africa, the old, rural model of providing care in the bush was dying. "Here [in East Africa]," he says, "people come to where the working relatives live who can afford to pay hospital bills. People go to the cities where there is better transportation, good facilities, and the best doctors." Also, most of the doctors gravitate to the cities, making the worker supply more readily available. "Most doctors don't want to raise their kids in the bush, they want to live in Nairobi," he says, making it far easier to recruit St Mary's high-caliber staff. Father Fryda has observed that many rural hospitals don't survive the death of their founders and benefactors. St Mary's won't face that dilemma, being largely Kenyan-run and staffed.

Father Fryda incorporated the better design elements of other East African hospitals into St Mary's. Noting the flawed leadership that doomed other hospitals to stagnation and internal ruin, he purposely created a board that included hospital employees. The board is comprised of five Assumption Sisters and four hospital employees who are elected by their peers. Father Fryda insisted on an inclusive model in which all invest personally and have a say in how things are run. He intentionally avoided the "boss man" mentality that has ruined other mission hospitals. As such, the employees really "are" St Mary's. At St Mary's, he says, "Young Kenyans come up with their own ideas, shaping the hospital." Deflecting suggestions that his own design is responsible for their early success, he says, "St Mary's is not about any one individual; it is about a like-minded group of people, working together on common problems. The people here *are* St Mary's." Although many outsiders have assisted St Mary's, Father Fryda insists, "Outside help should never supplant what Kenyan staff are doing." St Mary's does not get involved with anything that is not "primarily rooted" in their staff. Though still a young 54, Father Fryda plans to step aside as director in 2006, turning over control to a board-appointed successor. "Nothing could make me feel happier," he says, "than to see the place continue to evolve without me."

The staff at St Mary's represents the best and brightest from Kenya's ravaged medical system. A recent government initiative markedly increased the class size of Nairobi Medical School, increasing government coffers, though making effective learning difficult. While those at government hospitals languish in poorly equipped, low-morale centers of mediocrity, the staff at St Mary's sees itself as part of a vibrant, highly competent health center. It is common for some of the best and brightest in Kenya to escape the system and emigrate to the West, called "brain drain," and it leaves many who do not escape trapped in a dysfunctional system. A common expression at St Mary's is, "The worst tragedy is not the brain drain; but the brains that are left in the drain." To be left to fend for oneself in a government hospital or clinic strikes many as a dead-end job, with little hope for self-improvement or professional advancement. Some very bright and promising careers fall into cycles of substandard practice, occasionally involving bribes for care. St Mary's presents a viable alternative to such waste.

While treating some of the world's poorest people, St Mary's has turned a profit every year since it opened in 2000.

During a visit to St Mary's in 2001, Dr Ed Wyman, a friend and Massachusetts General orthopedic surgeon who has worked in developing countries for many years, found St Mary's to be "the best-designed and best-run hospital" he had ever seen in the developing world. He is, no doubt, right; Father Fryda and colleagues overlooked nothing. The hospital drilled its own wells, freeing it from the frequent disruptions in the public drinking water supply. The sewage lines have frequent and large traps for easy retrieval of the things people inevitably throw away. All the switches are hidden, to prevent those unfamiliar with technology from playing with the buttons and causing, for example, a water heater to remain on continuously. The cost of care at St Mary's is just 10% over cost, resulting in an affordable hospital that can continue indefinitely. Given the employee ownership, the staff is motivated to see that the hospital runs efficiently. The pay-as-you-go system ensures payment receipts, and the affordable, high-quality care ensures an ever-increasing volume. While treating some of the world's poorest people, St Mary's has turned a profit every year since it opened in 2000, and in a short time, it has become the preeminent hospital in East Africa. Its outpatient departments increased their volume by 150% and 186% in the past two years to 1000–1200 patients per day in late 2005 while the number of HIV-positive patients receiving antiretroviral drugs by this time has increased to 2000.[1] Every conceivable volume chart shows dramatic growth.

The hospital's location allows many of Nairobi's slum dwellers to easily reach the hospital through the extensive *matatu* system, the local transport system of fast-moving vans tightly packed with people. And the low cost of the pay-as-you-go system, including doctor visits, diagnostic tests, and drugs, make the hospital affordable to most of the local poor. It costs just $1 to see a doctor at St Mary's. There is a fund to help cover the costs of the truly needy, so no one is turned away. The beautiful, open design affords the poor an opportunity to enjoy grass and beauty instead of the fetid surroundings of the slums that are home for most. A hospital chaplain or a *mzee,* an elderly man, greets each visitor to the hospital, recognizing the inherent dignity of each person. Father Fryda states, "At St Mary's, we want to do ordinary things extraordinarily well." Patients won't receive hemodialysis or coronary bypass surgery here but they will receive competent, compassionate, affordable medical care in the context of a Christian hospital.

During one morning staff meeting I attended in April 2001, Father Fryda set the tone for the day by asking everyone to pray with him. "Please Lord," he said, "help us see every person who comes here today as an individual, and let us see your face in each one of them. Let us show them a little of our love as you have shown us yours." An awning above a central walkway bears a crucifix and the statement, "I have loved you with an everlasting love." While the staff at St Mary's excels at putting their Christian faith into action, they do not exclude anyone based on faith. Mormons, Jews, Protestants, Hindus, Muslims, and others comprise the larger St Mary's family.

St Mary's is more of a pastoral medical community than a traditional hospital. It is this concept of living one's faith through clinical service that defines St Mary's. Father Fryda has termed this "being a hospital." He explains that the vision included bringing "doctors, nurses, priests, brothers, sisters—bringing all these people of different talents together in a place where we would live together, work together, the children would grow up together, where we could create a faith-based community together, sharing and living the concept of medical ministry." In short, he adds, "St Mary's is a tangible experience of the combined power of love. . . .We're trying to, as ordinary people, be the channel of the dream of love that God has put into each of us." That channeling translates into "a very demanding type of love" for all involved.

These Christian sentiments are widely shared by the staff. Sister Monica, one of the founding Assumption Sisters, says, "We follow the example of Jesus Christ, who was meek, poor, and humble. This helps us to give good service." A favorite saying among staff comes from Ephesians 5:2, "And walk in love, as Christ has also loved us and given Himself for us. . . ." Those who initially recoil at the thought of being steamrolled by excessive proselytizing should take comfort that such is not the case at St Mary's. These are people of faith who are accustomed to getting dirt under their fingernails. They live and work at the place where faith collides with the harsh realities of poverty. Such places do not suffer fools gladly nor long sustain those of little substance.

In 2002, Father Fryda purchased an adjacent 10-acre plot of land, making St Mary's a 20-acre campus with more than 40 buildings and room to grow. Recent additions include a three-story medical education complex that will soon house East Africa's first family practice residency, a nurse anesthetist program, and a program through which clinical officers can become medical students. A dental clinic was started in 2002, and plans are underway for transitional internships. Another program started in 2005 allows hospital employees to attain their high school equivalency degrees, affording them greater opportunities for work. Father Fryda says, "So many of the hospital's janitors, ward attendants, etc, never had a chance to finish high school, as they came from poor backgrounds and they had to drop out of school." Most are "quite bright and motivated" and now have the chance to earn high school degrees and apply for other degree programs in lab, pharmacy, X-ray that will soon start. They get a second chance at a "decent life career," and, Father Fryda adds, "they deserve it." St Mary's will also offer pastoral education on site. Other buildings house a large and expanding AIDS treatment program, additional accommodations for hospital staff, and additional obstetric wards. As of late 2005, the hospital staff was on a daily basis, delivering 27 babies, and performing 25 major and 25 minor surgeries in one of East Africa's busiest operating rooms. Employees work hard but are paid higher salaries compared to those at other comparable hospitals—they have no incentive to leave. In 2005, St Mary's purchased 72 acres near Lake Elementita, in Western Kenya; construction of a 350 bed "St Mary's West" has already begun.

Staff surgeons at St Mary's perform between 6 and 15 Cesarean sections per day in what has become the largest obstetrics practice in Kenya. The C-section rate is high because women from all over Nairobi come to St Mary's for planned C-sections or show up from other hospitals—often at the last minute—to avoid paying the much higher fees elsewhere. Pregnant HIV-positive patients receive nevirapine to reduce likelihood of maternal-fetal transmission, at a cost of 40 cents per tablet. The hospital also subsidizes antiretroviral treatment for HIV-positive parents, preventing children from becoming AIDS orphans. Father Fryda has developed some protocols for cervical cancer, lymphoma, and several other solid tumors. One fortunate patient received a stem cell transplant for a myelodysplasia, something not commonly seen in these parts. The "ordinary" frequently exceeds locally defined norms.

A Collar and a Stethoscope

Bill Fryda is not your average man and far from your average priest. Brilliant, pious but irreverent, funny, organized, visionary, driven, and confident are among a few adjectives that come to mind when describing him. He radiates a faith-based inner peace, which he shares both clinically and pastorally. He seems perfectly at peace where he is, and he seems to really love his life and his work. He quite comfortably says that he has "never gotten up for a day of work" as long as he's been in East Africa. He handles an enormous work burden in what seems like effortless ease. I have never heard him complain of either his workload or the shortcomings of any of his staff. He is selfless without being deferential.

When a generous Kenyan donor offered a house on a 4-acre plot in the country north of Nairobi for Bill's personal use, he accepted it on the condition that the donor change the title for the land from "Father Bill Fryda" to "St Mary's Hospital," which he did. Father Fryda and his staff are now together designing a St Mary's retreat center, where "doctors, nurses, and janitors can all sit together and talk about our future." The compound will have several cottages where people can escape the bustle of Nairobi; spend time in the scenic, beautiful countryside; and meet in a communal house, designed with plenty of open space to foster discussions while sitting around a central fireplace. The staff also has plans to build a riding stable. "Imagine," Father Fryda says excitedly, "how some of our employees will feel to be able to take their kids up country to ride on a horse, just like the English gentry used to do. What kind of a psychological lift will that give them? Many of these people had previously been scrounging in fetid slums for their very existence. Now they can really feel part of something special." Father Fryda is always quick to point out how so many people previously "written off" in the slums blossom when given the opportunity. "They have their dignity back," he says.

Despite such accolades, I would be remiss not to mention that Father Fryda has his faults. Due to his own quick thinking, he sometimes chafes at the slower pace of others. He can be impetuous and brusque during a full day of clinical work. In a culture that demands that the personal relationship trumps all, his headstrong ways remind locals that he is American by birth. His overall temperament conjures up written depictions of Schweitzer, a deeply religious man who was as hard on his staff as he was on himself. It is not the prototypical image of the kindly minister that either Fryda or Schweitzer summons. To get results in Africa, or within any culture accustomed to failings on every front, one has to maintain a certain toughness. It was only through the enormous demands that both of these visionaries made on themselves and their staffs that ultimately brought the true dream of Christ to fruition in some of the harshest environs anywhere.

Yet Father Fryda's path did not lead directly to Kibera or to East Africa. Born the son of a "dirt farmer" in rural Armour, South Dakota, he grew up a world away from the congestion and squalor of Nairobi's slums. He recalled seeing a newsreel about Albert Schweitzer as a boy. "A seed was planted," he says. He saw something he knew in Schweitzer and "from the earliest days I knew that this was what I wanted to be."

His roots and intellect prepared him for the challenges that lay ahead. Father Fryda worked on the farm with his father, learning how to "fix things with chewing gum and bailing wire." He recalls, "Growing up on a farm was an important influence. I never felt a need for money—it never had a big appeal." He has noticed that many missionaries grow up in rural, impoverished areas, something that ideally suits them for life in Africa. Growing up in impoverished settings, "frees the mind up to think outside the box," he says. Father Fryda's rural upbringing gave him both the real-life experiences and the outlook that helped him years later to found and run a mission hospital. St Mary's and other such hospitals have little funding, requiring their founders to develop ready-made solutions to problems. There is rarely someone who will come in and fix problems for you. Father Fryda later excelled in school, graduating with honors from Baylor Medical School in Houston, Texas. He then went on to the Mayo Clinic in Rochester, Minnesota, for a residency in internal medicine and a fellowship in hematology-oncology.

During medical school and the beginning of his residency, he noted that "something was missing" from his life. He was a self-described "born again pagan" for a long time prior to his awakening while at Mayo. During his residency and fellowship, he did short-term medical work in Haiti, Guatemala, and Nigeria with Southern Baptist, Catholic, and Anglican missionaries. At the end of his training in 1980, he joined Maryknoll as a lay missioner and spent the next three years in Tanzania, just south of Kenya in East Africa. There he worked as a physician, upgrading medical education, setting up a medical supply system, serving as famine relief director, and directing clinics throughout the Diocese of Shinyanga.

In 1984, he undertook seminary training at Maryknoll, New York, working clinically in both Sing Sing and Walpole prisons. He still exchanges letters with one of Sing Sing's more troubled prisoners, who was released in 2002. Although Father Fryda has maintained relations, he has politely declined a visit. Following his ordination in 1988, Father Fryda returned to Tanzania, this time as medical director of Sengerema Hospital, a 250-bed mission hospital in Geita. While there, he developed a shallow well project using locally available materials and technology that gave the community and hospital access to clean water. He also developed clinical protocols for Burkitt's lymphoma, sickle cell disease, and tropical splenomegaly. This was also the time he began hosting visiting health personnel from the United States. During his off time, he served as chaplain to hospital workers and religious staff.

In 1991, Maryknoll transferred him to Kenya, where he served as chief medical officer in charge of Nazareth Hospital, a 220-bed mission hospital outside Nairobi. I worked with him there in the winter of 1994. While at Nazareth, Father Fryda ran the gamut of activities, though he rarely showed signs of stress. Following our nightly dinners, he would write a host of letters to supporters, then retire to bed with a full cup of black coffee. In addition to saying daily mass at 6 PM for staff, he somehow managed to juggle full-time clinical and administrative roles. He oversaw one or two of the inpatient wards, kept a full stable of outpatients, and spent a considerable amount of time refining his surgical technique. A volunteer Dutch surgeon taught him how to do C-sections and he later developed his own approach to performing prostate surgeries. ("It's the same incision," he says.) Elderly men still travel great distances to see the "Prostate Padre." On many evenings at Nazareth, he would call me over to his special section of the male ward to show me the red rubber tubes flushing boiled water and salt through the bladders of the quite relieved elderly men whose prostates he had just resected; he developed quite a following. To urinate well is one of life's essential functions.

He also hosted medical volunteers from the United States and Europe, primarily those interested in his form of Christian medical ministry. There were six volunteers while I was there, all sharing a small house with Father Fryda. We took turns cooking, though Father Bill did all of the shopping and general upkeep. Doctors do not make the easiest of guests, but Father Fryda kept things running smoothly, helping each of us with our various adjustment issues. Our nightly dinner conversations were memorable, providing each of us a glimpse into a world many would consider utterly surreal, so far removed from life in the industrialized West. Years in East Africa had taught Bill some hard lessons about the essential workings of larger political structures, governments, and world bodies. He had grown to distrust most large governmental and multilateral entities working in East Africa, having seen their failings at one time or another. Time and again he had seen corrupt government officials exploit the poor in lieu of helping them. He had similarly witnessed abuse at the hands of United Nations (UN) agencies and some nongovernmental organizations (NGOs). He resolved to pave his own way free of a dependence on any of them.

Father Fryda stayed at Nazareth until 1997 and worked in a rural hospital in Kenya's famed Rift Valley in 1997 before undertaking construction of St Mary's in 1998. His career has not been without its share of honors. He was a commencement speaker at the Mayo Clinic in 2000 along with Elizabeth Dole. In October 2003, the Mayo Clinic brought him back to Rochester for a three-day ceremony in which they bestowed upon him the honor of Mayo Clinic's Most Distinguished Alumnus. Upon first learning of the award, Father Fryda cracked that he would be immediately recognizable in the sea of tuxedos as the one wearing brown sneakers. (October is the short rainy season around Nairobi.) Vice President Dick Cheney, noticeably not wearing brown sneakers, was among the dignitaries present.

Personal Motivations and Ideas

During his residency, Father Fryda began to go overseas. Initially, he went for the adventure and then found that he loved Africa—the people, the wildlife, the mystique. It was the beginning of a life in East Africa, a life that began with the seed planted by Albert Schweitzer. Father Fryda now recalls, "That seed was always there, though I ran from it for a while." He was offered a position at Mayo Clinic and was poised to become a monoclonal gammopathy (IgM) expert with laboratory space and considerable opportunity for career advancement. Instead, he followed his passion.

Looking back, Father Fryda now recognizes a Divine hand in his decisions. "God speaks to us through the patterns of our lives," he often says. By this he explains, "We need to pay attention to what motivates us, to what fires us up. That's not just coincidence; that's God speaking to us. God calls each of us by name." He stresses that he has to actively listen and keep himself open to hear the voice of God. His personal evolution involved a number of "tough years" that included constant soul-searching amidst a number of challenges. Yet he persisted in the belief that he was right about his direction and motivation. In the end, it led him to help create St Mary's.

Ultimately, he says, it was the influence of Jesus that put him on his current path. "On a good day," he says, "that is the core." Not the historical Jesus but, as Bill says, "the dream" that Jesus so well articulated. The Catholic faith for Bill offers great theology, though suffers in its practice.

> For Father Fryda, faith is personal, and the poverty of East Africa has presented him with ample opportunity to live out his creed, seeing God in the faces of the poor.

Unlike its Mormon counterpart, there is not sufficient emphasis, he says, on reaching out into the world and sharing the love bequeathed by Jesus. In Father Fryda's eyes, St Mary's is the very manifestation of that love. "The dream" that Christ spoke of is, for Father Fryda, at the core of his Christian faith. It drives and sustains him. This dream is not an abstract concept but rather a "lived experience." For Father Fryda, faith is personal, and the poverty of East Africa has presented him with ample opportunity to live out his creed, seeing God in the faces of the poor. "At the end of all this, the face we see should be a familiar one," he says.

He is dismayed at the insular qualities he sees in some people of faith. He doesn't see much value in forming clusters or sequestrating oneself from the world. "You have to live in it," he says. It is through the direct, personal interactions that we can grow a relationship with God. "It is when you work in the trenches that the hierarchical stuff falls away." Again, he says, "God speaks to us through the patterns and fabric of our lives. It is necessary not just to listen to and hear God but to experience God." Working in the clinics and wards of St Mary's Hospital, just across the street from one of the world's largest collections of entrenched poor, he says, "God is here."

It is Father Fryda's challenge, as he says, "to live in right relationship with Yahweh." Jesus was never hung up on heaven and hell, he says. Rather, he spent his ministry encountering God in the living. Talking about two young AIDS orphans that St Mary's took in, Father Fryda says, "The smile on the four- and six-year-olds with no parents . . . these kids—that's where your faith is lived, through direct action." He has trouble relating to the larger systems and more abstract theoretical connections. "How do you love a system or a concept?," he asks. He doesn't put much into "isms" or "collective anythings," particularly the concept of a collective church. "Godness is in each of us," he says. It is through the individual encounter that he feels the most excitement and the closest encounter with God. "You gotta keep it personal," he says. Making the link between his ministry and medical practice, he adds, "It is in the touching, the being with that you encounter the ministry of healing. Over 20% of the Gospels were about Jesus touching and healing people."

I once heard him say, "Happiness is living in the right place and knowing it." After living with him for a while and talking with him regularly for several years since, I can say that for Father Fryda, this is certainly true. Bill Fryda is exactly where he should be and, likely, where he is most needed.

Aid and the Personal Approach

Bill Fryda has spent a lifetime working among dire conditions in Tanzania and Kenya, two countries that are no stranger to foreign aid and the larger multilateral organizations that have tried to "help" the poor of the continent. Like many others who have worked in East Africa, Father Fryda has little use for the large organizational approach. (See Chapters 5 and 6 on foreign aid.) In his opinion, these larger, organizational responses have claimed far too many African lives. For example, he cites the anemic international response to AIDS in Africa. "Twenty years later and nothing has happened. All the money is spent on baseball hats and conferences." He cited a November 2003 AIDS conference held in Nairobi and noted the "palpable anger" among local people, fully aware of the cost of the flights, hotel rooms, meals, and shopping for 7,000 delegates and of how many lives those funds could have saved if only more wisely spent. He expected little from the AIDS conferences in Barcelona and elsewhere because "high-paid consultants will squander it all before any of it ever reaches the poor." He adds, "Such conferences have nothing to do with the world I live in." Admittedly cynical when it comes to AIDS, Father Fryda has as much disdain for the "AIDS parasite" and for those who make their livings off of AIDS, as the AIDS virus. I once e-mailed him after attending a local conference on the Global Fund in 2002. In it, I saw an opportunity for St Mary's to seek support for its huge AIDS population. His reply reflected his years in East Africa, living quite apart from those in the wealthy countries:

> Thanks for the news about the large funds going out. It seems the larger the organization and budget (UN or USAID), the less that actually gets done. I'm sure these funds will feed many salaries, meetings in resort hotels, provide vehicles, T-shirts, and baseball caps, etc. It's "the business of Aid." Sorry to sound so cynical about it, but I honestly doubt that a single person with HIV will ever receive any direct help from any of this money. AIDS is a big business and honeypot for lots of bureaucracies and the people who staff these organizations. Sorry, but we're not in that world. Asking for practical help from such organizations is useless. We've reached the point here at St Mary's of being very tough with these endless

"AIDS parasites," organizations demanding we fill out their forms, give them time-consuming hospital tours to their useless personnel who arrive in fancy vans from luxury hotels, etc. We ask these organizations to make a $250 dollar donation to the hospital's care of AIDS patients, before we fill out their forms or provide tours, etc. None have ever responded, preferring to keep their funds for cocktail hours after their conferences, etc. Sorry, Ed, but the reality is that such organizations and their big budgets are useless in making any inroads in the battle against HIV. A lot of people live off AIDS, in a different world from those who die of AIDS or the medical personnel on the ground.[2]

Further, he says, there are specific reasons for such aid programs. "Aid money," he says, "is specifically designed to court relationships between the ruling people of the United States and the ruling people of Kenya, under the theoretical auspices of HIV. The money goes straight into the pockets of the ruling elite here. And it is a success; it accomplishes just what it seeks." I mentioned during one conversation that St Mary's would be the perfect model for President Bush's 2003 State of the Union $15 billion pledge of funding (PEPFAR) for HIV/AIDS, given its huge AIDS population. In fact, Senator Bill Frist had actually visited St Mary's while in East Africa in 2002. Confirming Father Fryda's dire predictions, none of this money had gone out a year later (McLure 2004). As of July 2005, the sites designated to receive some of these funds, St Mary's included, had received relatively small amounts, given the numbers presented to the American public. The funds had also come with the stipulation that the recipients purchase more expensive US-made drugs and use US-manufactured machines to run the CD4 counts (the diagnostic tests essential to managing HIV). The imported US drugs will ultimately cripple the local industry, driving up the price of the antiretrovirals. It remains unclear at this time how much of the funds will actually make it to the patients or their caregivers. Like many other large programs, the Bush money is well intended but may well be doomed by the political, institutional, design, and economic factors that undermine its ultimate impact. Having been involved with PEPFAR since its African beginnings, Father Fryda wrote the following about it, "The amounts of funding that actually goes into treatment is small, compared to the amount of money spent on top-heavy administrative bureaucracy structures. PEPFAR is a very good case study of how **NOT** [emphasis in original] to conduct an efficacious, affordable, locally-appropriate assistance program."[3]

Father Fryda's harsh assessment of the larger world bodies that respond to HIV/AIDS and other health issues is not unique. Many others with long-term experience in East Africa hold similar views, as do those in Guyana, Belize, and other places I have worked. It is important to keep in mind that the World Health Organization (WHO), other UN agencies, and large NGOs often work closely with host governments to distribute funding and create policy change. For years under Former President Daniel arap Moi's rule, funds came in and simply disappeared. No matter how well intended the donations were, little of the money ever made it to the poor. The NGO Transparency International rates Kenya the world's sixth most corrupt country, a factor of enormous importance to anyone who tries to help Kenya's poor.

Corruption in Kenya is more than a problem reserved for the higher levels of government. It is, in fact, rampant through all levels of government and has been in place so long that is has become a way of life. The police are notorious for extracting bribes from anyone they can. At the higher levels, it is far more dangerous. Father Fryda has developed relationships with those in government who can keep less scrupulous officials from harassing him and his staff. One particularly outspoken priest was found in his car with a shotgun wound to the head. When the US Federal Bureau of Investigation later ruled it a "suicide," it found an incredulous audience in Kenya. Corruption factored in heavily to the country's downward spiral, which has been going on since the late 1970s. It was not until the International Monetary Fund (IMF) withheld significant loan money in 1997 and again in 2001 that anyone from the donor community seemed to care.[4]

Given the climate in the Kenyan government and the larger aid agencies, it is no wonder that Father Fryda evolved a personal, direct, patient-focused approach. Almost all of the funds that built St Mary's and its expansion came from private funds. "Mostly from people sitting at their kitchen tables, writing checks for $25," he says. By staying private and separated from the government, St Mary's now has the freedom to expand its scope, free from the corruption of government and the political exigencies of the bilateral and multilateral donors. He has little tolerance for those who profess to help the poor, yet do little more than make bold pronouncements. "Many in those organizations," he says, "look for a means to justify their own existence. Their funds are not meant for what we're doing at St Mary's. They spend their time looking for an overarching solution, which so often is a cop out for dealing with the difficulty of the reality of what's directly in front of you." It is far more comfortable to work in well-compensated positions in New York City or Geneva, Switzerland, than to routinely confront the stink, misery, and filth that define the poverty of Kibera.

That poverty can be particularly difficult to confront on a daily basis. "So many people who come here and see this poverty," he says, "are disgusted by it and want to immediately get away from it. Peace and justice become excuses for not getting your hands dirty." Father Fryda has long advocated changing the glossy brochures of the large UN agencies and NGOs to include a "scratch and sniff" section. "Because poverty stinks," he says. It is offensive and people immediately put up defensive shields when confronted by it. A scratch and sniff section would remind people more forcefully what the work really entails.

I once asked Bill about the inherent frustrations he encounters in treating poor people trapped in impossible circumstance, something I got just a small taste of while working with him at Nazareth Hospital more than a decade ago. There, we saw many patients who suffered from societal and economic calamities that manifested clinically. Horrible road traffic accidents would send critically injured people our way. After weeks of hard work, we would discharge the survivors back onto those same deadly roads. Starving children would return to the very environment that caused their hunger and generated their illness. Malaria, tuberculosis, AIDS, diarrhea, and respiratory illness—indeed all infectious pathogens—thrive in the squalor, congestion, and malnutrition so abundant around greater Nairobi. Didn't Father Fryda ever tire of putting Band-Aids on a seemingly interminable tide of suffering, borne of larger forces well beyond his control?

No, he replied, because he has seen the value of the care rendered. He also has repeatedly seen people blossom when given an opportunity to better themselves. St Mary's may be one of the more ambitious plans for health care in Africa. Instead of relying on decrepit government hospitals, people now have a place where they can receive affordable, competent health care. If plans for expansion to two other sites come to fruition, St Mary's could become the main source of health care for half of Kenya's population. That would represent incredible progress for Kenya's poor. Also, things are getting better on a macro level. As Bill terms it, "I think there has been a gradual evolution with our relationship with God." Barbaric practices considered the norm during medieval times are now rare. Although genocide is still tolerated, at least the world condemns it and prosecutes its chief progenitors. No, Father Fryda says, there is progress in the world.

The Future

Despite frustrations at what he sees as repeated failings for the poor of East Africa, Father Fryda long ago decided that he could best use his talents to minister and heal the poor. He has no grandiose visions of healing the world; he sees the limits imposed by the larger global structures for what they are. Yet, through the model he and his Kenyan colleagues have developed at St Mary's, he may leave a sustainable model of medical ministry, affording competent medical care to the poor in a setting that preserves their dignity while addressing their spiritual needs.

Despite lavish praise heaped upon him, Father Fryda refuses to see anything he has done as extraordinary. He likely prefers having teeth pulled to talking about himself. He does not write books and has not, at least until recently, delivered many lectures. Yet his story warrants telling.

Father Fryda's is a story of sheer perseverance motivated by a living faith. He admits that he would not have been ready to build St Mary's until recently, and he freely weaves the various strands of his life's contacts into the functional tapestry that serves as the ideal model for health care for the poor of Africa. For hundreds of people, God has helped direct their actions to what is now a living entity at the edge of Kibera. Given its sustainable design, both financially and operationally, St Mary's should be around long after current staff members have passed on. Perhaps there could be no better legacy for Father Fryda than that.

Endnotes

1. Personal communication from Father Bill Fryda, September, 2005.
2. Personal communication from Father Bill Fryda, November 2002.
3. Personal communication from Father Bill Fryda, September, 2005.
4. Data from the Central Intelligence Agency *World Fact Book*, available online at www.cia.gov.

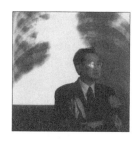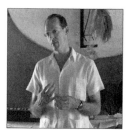

Chapter 13

Paul Farmer, MD, PhD, and Jim Yong Kim, MD, PhD

Never underestimate the ability of a small group of committed individuals to change the world. Indeed, they are the only ones who ever have.

—Margaret Mead

Paul Farmer and Jim Yong Kim are the twin engines behind a revolutionary Boston-based nongovernmental organization (NGO) called Partners In Health. Together with philanthropist Tom White and director Ophelia Dahl, these two enterprising physicians were able to bring high-quality health care to one of the most impoverished areas in Haiti. From there, they expanded their work to Peru, Guatemala, Russia, Mexico, Rwanda, and inner-city Boston. From their liberation-theology–inspired practice, they revolutionized the approach the world takes to treating poor people with tuberculosis and are evolving similar methods for treating AIDS. Both Farmer and Kim have received the coveted MacArthur "genius" award and achieved even wider fame after Pulitzer prize–winning author Tracy Kidder wrote a 2004 bestselling book about their work and lives, Mountains Beyond Mountains: The Quest of Dr. Paul Farmer, a Man Who Would Cure the World *(Random House, 2003). By forcing those of us in the comfortable "developed" countries to confront underlying issues of poverty and illness causality, they and their academic peers have forcibly pushed the medical profession—at least those who are listening—to reconsider why the world is as it is. By accepting all challenges and refusing to accept second-class status for their poor patients, they have raised the bar in delivering a "preferential option" for the health care of the global poor.*

In the Beginning

Paul Farmer strode into the Au Bon Pain restaurant just off the lobby of the Brigham and Women's Hospital, where he was spending the month as an attending with the Infectious Disease Service. "Step into my office," he said, extending his right arm in a broad sweep, rather theatrically, toward the assorted baguettes within. "Coffee?" he asked. "No, tea." He paid, insisting on doing so. From the worn look on his thin face and the rumpled black suit, I suspected that coffee sustained him. He looked like he hadn't slept in days, though as we sat down, I felt the immediate warmth and full attentiveness that made me feel that, at that moment, I was the only thing in the world that mattered to Paul Farmer.

I had heard about Paul through a mutual friend, Jim Kim. Paul and Jim, along with Tom White and Ophelia Dahl, had built Partners In Health, the Harvard-based NGO that had achieved astronomical success in just 12 years. In the fall of 1999, they had projects serving the poor in Haiti, Peru, Mexico, and just down the street in Roxbury, close to where Paul and I sat. Paul had referred Jamie McCabe to me, the first student I had ever hired for my NGO Omni Med, so we had some history. But this was the first time I had ever sat down with him. I felt strangely nervous, sitting face to face with someone who had been such an important influence on me through the written word. I had read several of his books, *The Uses of Haiti* (Common Courage Press, 1994), *Women, Poverty and AIDS* (Common Courage Press, 1993) and *Infections and Inequalities: The Modern Plagues* (University of California Press, 1994), as well as several of his articles in medical and anthropology journals.

I started, "First off, I want to thank you for all that you have written and done. You've been a great inspiration to me and, I think, have best articulated the things that so many people need to hear." I could see by his expression that he was moved. His eyes momentarily revealed an almost innocent vulnerability, as if he really wasn't sure that he had been doing quite enough or that it was unusual for him to hear such things. "Did my mother tell you to say that?" he asked. His comment disarmed me, and he quickly turned the conversation to lighter things, away from him and his accomplishments. We talked for a while about different aspects of international health work and made tentative plans for me to visit him in Haiti, though I never did. I have talked with Paul a few times since, recognizing each time that this was someone special, someone who had fused passionate service work for the global poor with an academic approach to understanding causality.

Some have compared Paul with Albert Schweitzer, but such a comparison is inexact, because Paul has forcefully pushed the envelope in a different direction. While Schweitzer personified the "moral imperative" that is a necessary motivation for many to undertake such work, Paul combined the moral with the analytical, using his anthropology training to unearth root causes of poverty and disease. His is a worldview that is profoundly disturbing—it forces us to reexamine that which we have always assumed to be true. Are we, in fact, not complicit in a global order that renders unimaginable riches to some and unbearable poverty and illness to many? His story, like that of the others depicted in this book, demands that we ask ourselves such difficult questions. Most of what follows comes from the available print literature about him, his own extensive writings, and the insights I have gleaned about both Paul and Jim through my friendship with Jim. On a personal level, I am deeply indebted to Paul and, even more so, to Jim for changing the way I see the world. My hope is that by understanding their story and their motivations, others will begin to ask the difficult questions that lead to deeper levels of understanding.

Paul Farmer's accomplishments are many and his life story unique. He received a full scholarship to Duke University where he graduated summa cum laude. After a year learning about poverty and inequality in Haiti, Paul started class at Harvard Medical School, from which he graduated near the top of his class. He earned a PhD in anthropology along the way and then split a residency in internal medicine with Jim Kim, before completing a fellowship in infectious disease. Among his many honors are a MacArthur "genius" award for $240,000, which he donated to Partners In Health, and a $250,000 Heinz Humanitarian Award, with which he did the same. He received both the American Medial Association's Nathan Davis Award for international work and the Margaret Mead Award from the American Anthropological Association. According to the Partners In Health web site, he has published more than 100 "scholarly publications," including four books, and also served as editor on two others. His curriculum vitae is longer than 20 pages and included almost every conceivable humanitarian, public health, and medical award.

In September 2003, Pulitzer prize–winning author Tracy Kidder profiled Paul and, to a lesser extent, Jim Kim in the book *Mountains Beyond Mountains: The Quest of Dr. Paul Farmer, a Man Who Would Cure the World*, deriving the title from the Haitian expression that says, beyond the immediate problems in front of you, there are others, and one simply has to go and solve each one in turn. The title quite aptly describes Paul's life and much of what follows here comes from Kidder's beautifully written text. My conversations with Paul have been occasional and brief; however, Kidder spent a considerable amount of time with him over a few years. His insights proved invaluable. Like several others depicted elsewhere in this section, both Farmer and Kim are still very much alive and very active—their story is just beginning to be told. I suspect Paul dislikes the idea that someone would be putting into print the very motivations that drive him. He would rather talk about the poor and the unequal global structures that propagate their world. Yet when Kidder pressed to learn why Paul chose to eschew the comforts that so many of his professional colleagues see as a right of passage, Paul's response was clear and direct, "I feel ambivalent about selling my services in a world where some can't buy them" (Kidder 2003, 24). In fact, he lives most of the year in Cange, Haiti, in a small house with cold water and few conveniences. He turns over all of his earnings to poor patients through Partners In Health; he once signed over a Brigham paycheck to an AIDS patient who was about to be evicted. Yes, Paul is a physician with radically different perspectives and lives life in such a way as to fully back them up.

Paul's incredible life story occasionally eclipses the considerable academic work that would make any other Harvard professor proud.

Paul's incredible life story occasionally eclipses the considerable academic work that would make any other Harvard professor proud. Paul's family of eight lived first in North Adams, Massachusetts, then in a bus in a south Florida campground/trailer park, and subsequently on a houseboat in a bayou along Florida's Gulf Coast. Farmer never wanted for anything when he was young, feeling fully secure with his somewhat eccentric father at the helm. Reflecting on his early years, living with a family of eight on a bus and a houseboat, he concedes, "It *was* pretty strange" (Kidder 2003, 52). While picking citrus alongside Haitian workers and sleeping in a mooring under the stars in the bayou, Farmer's early years instilled within him a distinct lack of respect for conventional boundaries. Anything was possible, and the young, gifted boy from the large family in the boat soon graduated valedictorian of his high school class. From his father he gained, among other things, a distaste for those who put on airs and a sympathy for the truly poor, to whom his father regularly gave away some of the family's scarce money.

In 1983, Farmer was just out of college and arrived in Port-au-Prince to spend one year learning about Haiti. He latched on to a charity called Eye Care Haiti, based in the town of Mirebalais in Haiti's Central Plateau. From there, he made trips throughout the country, soaking up the culture and history and gaining insight into the underlying structures, hidden from most, that propagate the unforgiving poverty that has always been the central feature for Haitians. For Farmer, it was a year of revelation that foreshadowed his life's work. Didn't it mean something that most voodoo ceremonies, which he had found rather long and boring, were held to ward off illness? It was the experience of Haiti that propelled him forward to his present life, not the large number of scholarly texts that he poured through. In fact, as he learned more about Haiti and the global structures that created so much of its misery, he realized that much of what was written about Haiti was inaccurate. "I would read stuff from scholarly texts and know they were wrong," he said. "Living in Haiti, I realized that a minor error in one setting of power and privilege could have an enormous impact on the poor in another. For me it was a process, not an event. A slow awakening, not an epiphany" (Kidder 2000).

If there was an epiphany, it occurred when Paul talked to a conscientious American physician who was leaving Haiti after serving there for a year. Would it be hard to leave, Paul asked? "No," the physician replied. "I'm an American, and I'm going home." Paul wrestled with this response for the next few days. What did that mean, to be an American? And how does one see all this and then just forget it? He did not challenge this physician's response, finding him a compassionate and sensible individual. Yet he had no answer of his own. How do people classify themselves? Later that same night, a young mother of five came into the clinic with the unfortunate combination of pregnancy and bad malaria. Lacking a blood transfusion to save her from overwhelming infection and red blood cell destruction, the woman soon became comatose and agonal. Her sister was crying, "This is terrible. You can't even get a blood transfusion if you're poor." Then, over and over she repeated, "*Tout moun se moun.* . . . We're all human beings. . . . We're all human beings" (Kidder 2000). Paul had his answer.

"My big struggle" he says, "is how people can not care, erase, not remember. I'm not a dour person. But I have a terrible message" (Kidder 2000). That message is that much of history has been "erased" to serve the interests of the powerful. We must consider the version of history that is told by the poor, challenge the global structures that propagate their poverty, and use our considerable knowledge and resources to bring about justice in a working partnership with the poor. Farmer's message is "terrible," chiefly because it demands that we follow up such valid concern not with talk but with decisive action. Ultimately, that requires a certain sacrifice from each of us.

As author Tracy Kidder so well described, Paul learned the lessons of Haiti very well. In his early descriptions of Haiti to companion Ophelia Dahl, who has remained with Paul since the inception of Partners In Health, "Paul laid out a comprehensive theory of poverty, of a world designed by the elites of all nations to serve their own ends, the pieces of the design enshrined in ideologies, which erased the histories of how things came to be as they were" (Kidder 2003, 73). The Haitians were fully aware of the process, reflected by a common saying, "God gives but doesn't share." In other words, God does supply all that each of us needs to thrive, but humans are responsible to see that it is shared equitably. That's where the problems come in, and this vastly unequal global order comprises the realm within which Farmer makes his most passionate arguments.

During his early explorations of Haiti, Paul discovered a branch of Catholicism called liberation theology, which brought core Christian principles to bear on the lives of the poor. Liberation theology preaches that it is all of humanity's duty to bring a "preferential option for the poor," a view that Farmer embraced. (See the section on liberation theology in Chapter 10.)

He called it "a powerful rebuke to the hiding away of poverty" (Kidder 2003, 78). Perhaps the most crystallizing summary of liberation theology comes from Gustavo Gutierrez, widely recognized as its father. At a 1995 Harvard conference by Partners In Health, Gutierrez said, "If I am hungry, it is a material problem; if someone else is hungry, it is a spiritual problem." In short, we need to care for each other. Not just the Americans, not just the wealthy. Everyone.

In May 1983, Paul met an Anglican priest named Fritz (Père) Lafontant who, along with his wife Yolande, ran a small clinic and built and administered local schools in Haiti's Central Plateau. Paul started by surveying the births, deaths, and causes of morbidity and mortality for the area, quickly concluding that the health of the surrounding environs was atrocious. Yet for the local residents, it was not hard to discern the origins of their ill health. In 1956, the US Export-Import Bank sponsored a large development project that included damming the Artibonite River (Farmer 1994a, 321). When the engineers completed construction of the Peligre Dam, the waters flooded previously productive farmland and forced the residents onto the surrounding desolate terrain. Old-timers lamented about the idyllic life in the days before the dam. Although the residents were promised electricity and water, neither came. What came in their place was backbreaking poverty— their livelihoods and prospects for a better life submerged beneath the flooding waters and never returned. Farmer called them the "water refugees," and they all knew who benefited from the dam—the agribusinesses downstream and the wealthy elites who controlled these businesses along with their American backers. Such a contrast became the emblematic case study for Farmer, who saw in the dam the perfect symbol of power politics that benefited the rich and, once again, screwed the poor (Kidder 2003, 37).

Before he began his medical studies, Farmer had gained considerable experience from Haiti and had already identified prominent 19th century physician Rudolph Virchow as his role model. "The physicians are the natural attorneys of the poor,"

Health care for the poor struck me, early on, as the noblest goal a physician could have.

Virchow had famously said, "and the social problems should largely be solved by them" (Kidder 2003, 61). Farmer followed Virchow's path to study social medicine, anthropology, and the larger political forces that constrain the agency of the poor. Farmer later wrote in *Infections and Inequalities,* "Health care for the poor struck me, early on, as the noblest goal a physician could have" (Farmer 1994b, 24). As such, he ordered every fiber in his being around understanding the causes of poverty and figuring out how he could best position himself to help the poor. In his idealized vision, Paul would become their doctor.

He began Harvard Medical School in the fall of 1984, where he soon became known as Paul Foreigner, for his tendency to pick up his books and catch the next flight back to Haiti, returning just in time to take exams or lab practicals. He spent most of his first two years of medical school in Haiti, supplementing his book knowledge with a vigorous practice as a rural physician-in-training. After Lafontant built the medical clinic, Paul provided its first microscope, freshly stolen from Harvard Medical School. "Redistributive justice," he had termed it. "We were just helping them not go to hell" (Kidder 2003, 90).

In 1984, Paul wrote an essay that caught the eye of Boston construction magnate and philanthropist Tom White, who had graduated from Harvard and built his father's construction business into the largest in Boston. White had parachuted into Normandy the night before D-Day and later served as an aide to General Maxwell Taylor. Now in his sixties, he was looking for the right cause to latch onto. When he tried to reach Farmer, he received this reply, "If he wants to meet me, tell him to come to Haiti." White did, dressed in his plaid golf pants and handing out cash to the beggars around the airport. The two connected during the visit, and White decided that Paul would be the means through which he would dispense with his considerable wealth. White had this to say of first meeting Paul Farmer, "He appealed to me immediately. So intelligent, so dedicated to his work. . . . I really can't explain it. I probably was also looking for somebody to hang my hat with" (Kidder 2003, 94). White immediately began to funnel funds toward Cange, and the clinic slowly evolved into a center of health for the entire area. In 1987, Tom White had an attorney draw up the papers for the founding of Partners In Health, the Boston sister affiliate of Zanmi Lasante (Creole for Partners In Health) in Cange. White donated $1 million, which he quite understatedly called "seed money," just to get things started. Most of the building blocks for the organization were already in place, consisting of Tom, Paul, Ophelia, and a growing core in Haiti. But there was one more key player yet to call Partners In Health his home.

The Other Half: A Perfect Match

In the combined anthropology–medical program at Harvard, Paul met an intense and brilliant Korean-American named Jim Yong Kim. Jim shared Paul's passion for social justice and, following lengthy conversations with Paul, Ophelia, and Tom, grew interested in the project in Haiti. A few months after Partners In Health began, Jim joined in earnest, becoming the other half of a unique physician pairing. Together, the two show a rare combination of intelligence, dedication, and passion to make a difference. Together, they represent a new paradigm for doctors. Instead of focusing the energies of the best and brightest on the molecular basis of disease or on developing new treatment modalities, these two turned their considerable talents to developing ways to bring health care to the poor. Certainly research is important, but the profession desperately needs more like Farmer and Kim. From the very beginning, this was a winning combination. While Paul became the spokesman and the articulate and prolific writer, Jim focused on building Partners In Health in Boston, helping to write grants, hire staff, solicit donations, run the organization, and eventually pursue new clinical projects.

I had the good fortune to share a fellowship with Jim starting in the summer of 1994. Jim and I had both been selected as Kellogg National Leadership Fellows in Group XIV, along with 43 others from a wide variety of professions. Over the next three years, I got to know Jim well and feel fortunate to have been in a position to watch the meteoric rise of Partners In Health from a close vantage point.

After just a few conversations with Jim Kim, I concluded that he was, in fact, the smartest human being I had ever met. The son of a periodontist and Confucian scholar, Jim's energy seemed limitless and his mind fully engaged. In those days, Jim was a piston, pushing ever forward, relentless, driven, and fueled by a passion that seeped through his entire being. Jim was far removed from the cold, godless pragmatism of certain intellectuals. Emanating from him was a very clear "moral clarity" that suffused all he said and did. I learned a lot from Jim, only a handful of others have imparted more wisdom to me. It is Jim who led me to liberation theology and Gustavo Gutierrez, challenged me to think more deeply about underlying causality, and painted a vision of moral clarity. This book strongly reflects a worldview that Jim and Paul fashioned together; I feel fortunate to have been the beneficiary of that collective wisdom.

During one memorable Kellogg seminar, Jim spoke to an audience on diversity and the "identity politics" he despised. Growing up Korean-American in lily-white Iowa, Jim had received more than his share of racial insults. But he rejected the idea that all members of a certain racial class suffered equally. Class-based inequalities dominated his worldview, no doubt based on experiences in Haiti. "Is it worse," he asked, "to be starving and white in Appalachia or for Professor Cornel West (who is black) to have a hard time flagging a cab in New York City?" In other words, racism is bad, but all suffering is not equal. Those from a certain racial group who suffer the inequalities of global poverty pay a far steeper price than many who suffer the indignities of racism in the developed world, particularly those in upper classes. Paul Farmer once taught a course at Harvard called Varieties of Human Suffering. The staff at Partners In Health had grown to recognize the hypocrisy in some of the race debates, in which politically correct speech allowed certain people to erroneously feel they had adequately addressed far deeper and more complex issues of race and class. For Farmer and Kim there was "just the one thing," meaning to remain fully engaged in the real problems of suffering in the world.

Jim speaks often of "first principles," by which he means the moral basis for our actions. Like Paul, he ascribes to liberation theology and refers often to the "moral clarity" that it demands. In describing his worldview to a group at one seminar, he said, "There are two types of simplicity, the one on this side of complexity and the one on that side of complexity." In other words, there is a lot of work that one has to do to really understand matters that quite often appear differently. For example, Haiti is frequently misrepresented by the press. The people are characterized as ignorant voodoo-practicing peasants who have somehow earned their fate. The reality, however, is far different and infinitely more complex, having far more to do with global power structures, history, racism, trade, and political elitism. To reach the simplicity on "that" side of complexity, we have to invest our time and energies to decipher complex realities. The "simplicity on that side of complexity" requires an often arduous journey, but only through such expeditions do we find ourselves closer to the truth.

Growing Partners In Health

During the early years in Haiti, Paul witnessed a country in turmoil and he befriended the one person capable of bringing deliverance to the Haitian poor. That person was a young priest named Jean-Bertrand Aristide who had spoken at the pulpit about liberation theology. During the late 1980s, Haiti was primarily under the rule of the Haitian army. Following democratic elections in 1990, Aristide became president, capturing two thirds of the vote. It was a brief period of hope for Haiti's poor, and Cange found significantly more cooperation from the Ministry of Health. Unfortunately, it didn't last. On September 29, 1991, the army overthrew Aristide in a violent coup. Thousands were killed and Farmer lost several close friends in the escalating violence that gripped the country. While Paul was back at Harvard, the new junta blacklisted him. Then, in 1992, Père Lafontant paid a Haitian army colonel "an insultingly small bribe" that allowed Paul back into the country.

During the early 1990s, Paul's visits to Haiti were dangerous. He smuggled $10,000 from Tom White into the country and gave it to the underground and he had many run-ins with soldiers. Once, when Farmer told a soldier he could not bring a gun into the Zanmi Lasante courtyard, the soldier replied, "Who the fuck are you to tell me what I can do?" A crowd gathered, raising the stakes for both. Farmer's quick reply, "I'm the person who's going to take care of you when you get sick" (Kidder 2003, 116). The crowd anticipated the worst, but the soldier left, recognizing the truth in the statement. Farmer lowered his profile afterward. During the time of the military junta, which lasted until 1994, the United Nations (UN) estimated that more than 8,000 people were killed, in addition to the hundreds, perhaps thousands, of "boat people" who drowned trying to escape. The number who died from the military repression and devastation to the public health system was, in all likelihood, considerably higher; it usually is (Farmer et al 2003, 420).

Despite the dangerous times in Haiti, Partners In Health began to expand its roles, clinically and academically. They broadened the reach of their programs in Haiti, physically expanding the Clinique Bon Saveur in Cange and increasing its services. In 1994, they began a program in Peru based on the Cange model. Other programs in the United States, Mexico, and Guatemala followed. In 1993, Paul published his award-winning book *The Uses of Haiti*, written in 10 days in a Quebec City hotel room. Using $240,000 prize money from his MacArthur Award, Paul started the Institute for Health and Social Justice at Harvard, designed to serve as the academic arm of Partners In Health. In 1996, the fledgling institute published its first book, *Women, Poverty and AIDS*, which won the Eileen Basker prize from the American Anthropological Association. It then took on the global economic order in 2000 with the book *Dying for Growth*, edited by Jim Kim, which is widely cited throughout this text.

Partners In Health then expanded to a staff of volunteers and nominally paid employees, working from a deep blue painted house on River Street in Cambridge. The group shared a clear purpose, a "pragmatic solidarity," as they termed it, with those who struggled alongside the poor. Farmer published *Infections and Inequalities* in 1999, followed by *Pathologies of Power* in 2003. Interspersed in between the many books were scores of articles in journals of anthropology, religion, public health, and clinical medicine. The group also coordinated large conferences at Harvard that opened up topics from their books for general discussion. Past speakers include Jean Bertrand Aristide, Jeffrey Sachs, Eric Sawyer (cofounder of the global activist group, AIDS Coalition to Unleash Power [ACTUP]), as well as Farmer and Kim.

Partners In Health held a particularly memorable conference in 1995. The featured speakers were Gustavo Gutierrez, a priest known as the father of liberation theology, and Noam Chomsky, an intellectual best known for taking controversial though well-documented positions on US foreign policy. Prior to the conference, Jim Kim told me that the Partners In Health's philosophy was perhaps best represented by wedding these two great thinkers together. From Gutierrez, they took the foundation of liberation theology and its preferential option for the poor, or "O for the P" as they called it. During the conference, Gutierrez said, "We need to enter the world of the poor to help . . . we must know them intimately. If we don't really *know* them, we are not really committed. We must try to enter the world of the poor and remain there." He had done just that for years, living as a priest in a poor barrio in Lima, often carting home large bags filled with books from his many lectures abroad. He emphasized the moral obligation that we all have to understand the larger, structural reasons for poverty and to struggle alongside the poor. "We must respect the dignity of every person," he said. "The love of God is universal—no one is outside of this love. Poor persons are first in the eyes of God according to the Bible. Don't be committed to the poor because they are good. They are not all good. Be committed because God is good. We are compelled to act by what our faith says. We must act against poverty and the *causes* of poverty. If we aren't against this, we aren't truly committed to the poor." Recognizing the tendency of many academics to read broadly but then fail to act, he added, somewhat tersely, "Forget the head trip and take a foot trip."

Noam Chomsky represented the other half of the Partners' philosophy. He is one of the most widely quoted individuals ever, and a hero to the left. Chomsky's many books extensively cite US government sources to make the case that the United States plays a far different role in the world than most of its citizens believe. Chomsky reeled off fact after fact about US intervention in Latin America, Southeast Asia, and elsewhere. His essential message was that much of US policy, representing the interests of entrenched elites, had directly supported the structures that propagate global poverty, reinforcing a world order against which Gustavo and others rail. From Chomsky, Partners derived a rigorous and reproducible academic approach to deciphering the underlying reasons for common problems. As in Chomsky's writings, all of Farmer's and Partners In Health's writings are heavily referenced, assuring that arguments that seem at first implausible become difficult to disprove. Just as many of the US government's more damaging global policies have escaped most US citizens' notice or been portrayed and perceived differently than they are, many factors in global health are not as they appear and our collective role far from helpful. Partners In Health set out to study such questions and document, as best it could, that which its various scholars, activists, and clinicians could collectively agree was the truth. That truth reads like a disturbing, even incredulous, narrative of our times. It is impossible to view our world without considerable unease after wading through Partners' various texts.

Tuberculosis and Socios en Salud

In 1994, Jim Kim planned to create a version of Zanmi Lasante in the Carabayllo slum of the Peruvian city of Lima. A close friend of Paul's, Father Jack Roussin, had moved there from Roxbury, where the two had formerly shared living space in a rectory. Father Roussin had repeatedly asked Partners In Health to start a clinic in Carabayllo, citing the overwhelming need. Enticed, Jim had planned to recreate the Haitian model, complete with young community health workers and a clinic. Tom White backed it with $30,000 and Jim drew some additional funds from the Kellogg Fellowship. The program became known as Socios en Salud, Spanish for Partners In Health. Paul came out to help Jim conduct a survey similar to the one he had first done in Cange 11 years earlier. Things progressed well, despite a bombing that destroyed the pharmacy Partners In Health had built there. In Peru at the time, warring factions between the government and the guerrillas, known as the Shining Path, fought for the hearts and minds of the citizenry. The Partners In Health staff simply rebuilt the pharmacy elsewhere and continued their work.

Kim was pleased with the progress they had seen in Carabayllo and envisioned a model that others could replicate in poor communities around the world. Then, Father Roussin got sick. He had been working in these same slums when he developed a hacking cough with weight loss and fevers. He returned home to Boston on the eve of Mother's Day in 1995. Jim picked him up from the airport and brought him straight to the Brigham and Women's Hospital, where both he and Paul were on staff at the time. Despite aggressive therapy with four different drugs, Father Jack died from tuberculosis one month later, in one of the world's best hospitals. Tuberculosis, an ancient scourge, was clearly the pathogen responsible, but something unusual had killed Father Jack.

As many health providers know, tuberculosis is caused by the bacterium *Mycobacterium tuberculosis*, transmitted from one person to the next through "droplet nuclei," essentially airborne packets of infective bacteria that remain suspended in the air for days. Inhalation of a single droplet is sufficient to cause disease, earning tuberculosis the moniker "Ebola with wings." Most people infected by tuberculosis don't realize it, just as I didn't when I became infected while on the wards of Boston City Hospital in 1989. An extensive literature demonstrates *M. tuberculosis'* highly infectious nature. For example, during a flight from Honolulu to Chicago, one passenger infected between 6 and 15 people with a multidrug-resistant form of tuberculosis (Kenyon et al 1996, 933). In most healthy people, the lungs wall off the bacillus and keep it locked there permanently in 90% to 95% of cases (Strickland 2000, 491). In a less fortunate 5% to 10%, age, disease, or starvation cause the walls to break down, allowing the organism to spread through the lungs, bones, and solid organs, reaping destruction and eventual death.

From our clinic in central Haiti, it is impossible not to regard the notion of 'tuberculosis resurgence' as something of a cruel joke—or yet another reminder of the invisibility of the poor.

Given the importance of host immune competence, it is readily understandable why tuberculosis is not as much of a problem for those in industrialized countries who are healthy. Like HIV, it prefers those immunologically suppressed by poverty, hence its predilection for developing countries and the poor within the industrialized ones. In fact, despite occasional outbreaks in inner city shelters and immigrant communities, most in the industrialized world don't hear very much about tuberculosis, thinking of it as an old scourge. Many journals and press reports have mistakenly described "resurgent TB" as the cause of a rise in case numbers in developed countries following the spread of AIDS. The only real resurgence has been in the realm of the privileged; the poor have never seen it recede. As Paul once wrote, "From our clinic in central Haiti, it is impossible not to regard the notion of 'tuberculosis resurgence' as something of a cruel joke—or yet another reminder of the invisibility of the poor" (Farmer 1994b, 47).

To the *M. tuberculosis* bacillus, the poor have been anything but invisible. The hospitals where I have worked in Tanzania and Kenya have all had isolation wards filled with tuberculosis patients and many more treated as outpatients. A full one third of the world's population is likely infected with tuberculosis and 10% of them will die from it (Strickland 2000, 491). It still kills 2 million people per year, more than any other pathogen until HIV overtook it in 2001. As a disease entity, tuberculosis accounts for a full one quarter of the developing world's preventable deaths; during the 1990s, it claimed 30 million lives. As far back as 1993, the World Health Organization (WHO) declared tuberculosis a "global health emergency," though the world has mustered little additional funding against it (491). The Global Fund targets HIV, tuberculosis, and malaria, but, as of this writing, remains hopelessly under funded.

Treating tuberculosis in poor countries is fraught with problems. Because *M. tuberculosis* is a very slow-growing bacterium, cultures that reveal drug susceptibilities may not return until it is too late to help the afflicted. Many poor locales lack the laboratory structure to perform such cultures, making appropriate treatment difficult. It is also highly prone to develop resistance to the various drugs used against it, even under ideal circumstances. Drug-resistant strains rapidly proliferate in poor countries, where many simply cannot afford all medicines, health systems cannot support tuberculosis programs, or people simply fail to take the full, long course of therapy. To combat such problems, many countries have standard programs for treating tuberculosis patients, often at costs substantially reduced by the state. Further, health providers have evolved a method that ensures patient compliance, called "directly observed therapy," or DOTS, with the "S" for "short course." This means that a health worker directly observes patients taking every single dose of medication for the entire treatment period, often for one year.

Until recently, most tuberculosis has been treated with standard mixtures of first- and second-line drugs. Father Jack's case was no exception. He received four first-line drugs as standard treatment. It was not until the slow-growing *Mycobacterium* cultures returned following his death that Farmer and Kim realized that a multidrug-resistant form of tuberculosis had taken Father Jack's life. By convention, any *M. tuberculosis* that proves resistant to isoniazid and rifampin, the two most important first-line drugs, warrants the description "multiple drug resistant," or MDR-TB (Partners In Health 2002, 3). Father Jack's tuberculosis had proven resistant to all four drugs he had taken. Following the considerable shock and grief that followed their close friend's death, Farmer and Kim realized that they faced quite a dilemma. If Father Jack had contracted a multiple-resistant strain of tuberculosis in the densely packed slum on the outskirts of Lima, how many others in that city of 8 million carried such a lethal bug?

Father Jack's case raised alarm, particularly in light of the moral compulsion of "O for the P," which demanded that these patients get treatment. However, given the intense poverty of the region, how could the Partners In Health team possibly afford to treat their clinic patients adequately to eradicate this MDR-TB? The first-line antibiotics were affordable, but the second-line agents were extremely expensive. These agents offered the only hope of a cure for thousands of patients in Lima and many times more patients in other countries. When a previous MDR-TB epidemic struck New York City from 1989 to 1994, it cost more than $1 billion to rein it in (Garrett 1994, 523). In another case cluster, reported by the Centers for Disease Control and Prevention (CDC) in 1990, it cost $1 million to treat just 10 patients in Texas, California, and Pennsylvania (Farmer 1994b, 243). Partners In Health had pledged itself to the poor, no matter the obstacles, but how could its founders actually take this on and prevail?

Both Jim and Paul worried about taking on MDR-TB, particularly because the WHO at the time recommended against treating the resistant strains given the cost of the drugs required. According to its official policy, "MDR-TB is too expensive to treat in poor countries; it detracts attention and resources from treating drug-susceptible disease" (Kidder 2003, 146). The health providers in Peru at the time followed WHO convention by adding one drug to the standard two-drug regimen when treatments failed, virtually guaranteeing that resistance would spread, a process Farmer called "amplification." Jim had recruited a bright, energetic Peruvian health worker named Jaime Bayona to direct Socios en Salud. Jaime set out to track MDR-TB cases around Carabayllo and found many.

The group decided to treat a small number of patients with MDR-TB. Initially, Jim and Paul loaded their briefcases with drugs, courtesy of the Brigham and Women's pharmacy, and brought them to Peru. Tom White later wrote a $92,000 check to cover the cost of the "borrowed" drugs. In fact, according to the *Boston Globe,* most of the cost for treatment came directly from Tom White, "He gave about $12,000 per patient per year, an almost unheard of sum for treatment of the poor in the developing world" (Donnelly 2000). The group then assembled a team of health workers who could "directly observe" their patients taking every dose. Paul had already treated tuberculosis patients for years in Haiti, including some MDR-TB cases, so he designed regimens for each patient. To the surprise of many in the global tuberculosis community, they achieved a cure rate of 85% (Farmer and Kim 1998, 671).

Spurred on by such heartening results, Howard Hiatt, the former dean of the Harvard School of Public Health and a long-term advisor to Partners In Health, convened a meeting of 50 global leaders on tuberculosis, including representatives from the WHO, the American Academy of Arts and Sciences, and Partners In Health. Arata Kochi, who was among them, at the time served as the head of WHO's tuberculosis program. WHO had long opposed treating MDR-TB, citing the lack of "cost-effectiveness" in resource-poor settings, a euphemism for poverty. The underlying tensions at the meeting stemmed chiefly from opposing philosophies. The WHO, recognizing the realities of global health scarcities, had staked out a reasonable position. Simply stated, poor countries could not spend scarce resources on the expensive medications required to treat MDR-TB, which still constituted just a small percent of the global tuberculosis case burden. Jim and Paul, however, argued the opposite. Jim pointed out the striking surge in global wealth that characterizes our current era, "We are talking about wealth that we've never seen before. And the only time that I hear talk of shrinking resources among people like us, among academics, is when we talk about things that have to do with poor people" (Kidder 2003, 164).

Jim further responded to earlier charges that Partners In Health—a small organization with limited resources—had been somewhat reckless in taking on such a monumental task in Peru. "We took on this project," he said, "because we thought that by proving that one could do community-based treatment of multidrug-resistant TB, that we might have the opportunity to work with a roomful of people like you. To actually *expand* resources to a problem that afflicts the populations we serve" (Kidder 2003, 163). The participants discussed the various "hot zones" of MDR-TB and debated potential responses. Arata Kochi introduced the term *DOTS-Plus*, a term that encompassed the standard approach of directly observing the therapy but including the necessary additional drugs to cover the MDR-TB strains. It seemed a winner, though the debate was far from over. Partners In Health had demonstrated to the world that, even in a "resource-poor" community, cure rates of 85% were achievable, and the WHO had at least accepted the possibility that MDR-TB should be taken on. Yet, cost remained the key barrier. The world could not responsibly reproduce what Tom White had financed in Peru under the current restrictions. He had already spent $3 million on less than 200 drug-resistant tuberculosis patients (Donnelly 2000). Something had to give.

Jim Kim set out to find the breaking points with "an assault on several fronts." He convened a meeting of pharmaceutical representatives to try to undermine the considerable "price gouging" that caused the second-line agents to cost so much. Jim had done his doctoral thesis on pharmaceuticals in Korea and was well prepared for the challenge. During the meeting, Guido Bakker, a young man who worked for the NGO International Dispensary Association (IDA), informed the gathering that IDA was pursuing the small, independent drug manufacturers that specialized in making generic copies of off-patent drugs for which the larger pharmaceuticals charged much higher prices. IDA and Doctors Without Borders had combined forces to buy shipments of drugs for their programs in a number of countries.

Jim then lobbied the WHO to include second-line tuberculosis drugs on their "essential drugs" list. By such inclusion, the WHO would essentially tell generic manufacturers that it would be worth their while to manufacture these drugs because many health NGOs and country health ministers would start purchasing them. Jim had long been aware of patients with strains of tuberculosis resistant to all known tuberculosis drugs. It would not suffice to simply make more tuberculosis drugs available; the WHO had to simultaneously come up with a means through which the drugs would be used effectively, so as not to spur further resistance. A Partners In Health employee sent to work for WHO in Geneva, Switzerland, found the precedent, the "Green Light Committee" to distribute meningococcal vaccine. Under such an initiative, only programs that could prove that they could reliably supervise treatment would be allowed to purchase drugs at the reduced rates. Soon, Jim became the "founding chairperson" for the WHO's Green Light Committee for the procurement and control of MDR-TB medications, in addition to chairing the WHO's Working Group on DOTS-Plus for MDR-TB.[1]

Soon, the cost for tuberculosis drugs, many of which had been off patent for decades, plummeted. By July 2000, the cost had fallen by more than 90% in just one year (Donnelly 2000). The combination of Tom White's generosity, Paul Farmer's tuberculosis knowledge, and Jim Kim's dogged persistence had helped change the manner in which the world's leading infectious disease body treated tuberculosis. Although Howard Hiatt, Doctors Without Borders, the International Dispensary Association, and a host of others played important roles, one person closely involved ascribed the bulk of the credit to one person. "I really see Jim as the one who did this. He just pushed and pushed and pushed. Eighty-five percent of it was Jim" (Kidder 2003, 173).

MDR-TB remains an ongoing and critical problem for a number of countries. A global survey published in the *New England Journal of Medicine* in 2001 found MDR-TB prevalence rates among those previously treated (for at least one month) of 36.9% in Estonia, 28% in Guinea, 34% in one province in China, and 48% in Iran (Espinal et al 2001 1294). For new cases of tuberculosis, ie, those who had not previously been treated with any drugs, the MDR prevalence averaged just 1%, though some spots were high, eg, 14% in Estonia, 9% in Latvia, 8% in Israel, and 6.5% to 9% in the Tomsk and Ivanovo oblasts (administrative provinces) of Russia. Five countries in Asia account for 75% of the world's tuberculosis cases, and it is in this region that the MDR-TB epidemic remains at its worst. Most countries showed trends of slowly increasing resistance. In many areas in Africa, rates of resistance have remained low, chiefly because so few patients receive any treatment at all. Considering the fact that significant percentages of tuberculosis strains in some "hot spots" are MDR, the ramifications of the changes introduced by Kim and Partners In Health cannot be understated (Farmer and Kim 1998, 671). The entire diaspora of the poor may ultimately benefit. As Howard

Hiatt summarized, "Paul and Jim mobilized the world to accept drug-resistant TB as a soluble problem" (Kidder 2003, 181). When the WHO adopted the prescriptions derived by Partners In Health for treating MDR-TB in June 2002, Jim Kim e-mailed Partners In Health from Geneva, "The world changed yesterday."

Growing Pains

By 2003, the staff of Partners In Health was able to report in the *New England Journal of Medicine* that 83% of their 75 patients in Peru had been cured of MDR-TB, though it had cost the group an average of $15,681 per patient (Mitnick et al 2003, 119). They had demonstrated that properly structured health programs could effectively treat MDR-TB, even in the poorest settings. However, the needed finances had stretched Partners to the breaking point. Jim and Paul devised a plan to keep their various operations afloat, to avoid lapsing into a downsized version of Partners In Health or, as Jim termed it, "screaming into the wilderness" (Kidder 2003, 176). They would do so by expanding their tuberculosis model, starting with Peru. Although they would be redirecting their focus to a specific infectious disease entity, they would be taking on an illness that attacked primarily the poor. They applied to all the major foundations for funding. Following Howard Hiatt's introduction to Bill Foege, who would later move to head up the global health efforts at the Gates Foundation, Jim put a grant proposal together. On July 28, 2000, the *Boston Globe* announced that a group of "Harvard doctors" had received a $44.7 million Gates grant for a tuberculosis program in Peru (Donnelly 2000). Partners In Health had just reached a new level.

I had lunch with Jim Kim just after Partners received the Gates grant. Jim looked haggard as always and seemed more tense than usual. I congratulated him and asked how it felt to receive a multimillion-dollar grant, one of the most elusive prizes available to those doing NGO work. "Like a kick in the gut," he replied. I was surprised by the response, but Jim explained, "Sure, it's nice to have the money, but with it comes incredible responsibility. We now have to replicate our model for an entire country." True enough, Partners In Health, along with colleagues at Harvard Medical School and WHO, had accepted the responsibility of implementing the Partners plan for the entire country of Peru, a five-year project that began in 2000. To Tracy Kidder, Jim later described the ongoing workload, "At times I feel like my head's going to explode," though he assured Kidder that he felt certain they would succeed (Kidder 2003, 241). Peru, however, was not the only pressing tuberculosis project they faced.

During meetings in Boston in April 2000, a Russian named Alexander Goldfarb challenged the group with descriptions of the MDR-TB outbreak in a prison in Tomsk, Russia, which he was charged with managing with some help from the Soros Foundation. Goldfarb pointed out that he had a limited budget of $6 million to treat 5,000 inmates. He simply did not have the resources that Partners had in Carabayllo. When Paul Farmer learned that Goldfarb had been treating these patients following standard WHO recommendations, he quickly realized that a disaster loomed. Economic downturns had, as they always do, swollen Russia's prison population, and "amplification" by current tuberculosis regimens would only cause the percentage of resistant tuberculosis in the overall pool to grow exponentially. MDR-TB in Russian prisons was well characterized as "an epidemiological pump," because the infection spread rapidly through vulnerable prisoners who cycled back out into society to infect others. Still worse, Goldfarb said, "The pump is replaced every three years," as new prisoners rotate through the system (Kidder 2003, 232). The implications were obvious.

Farmer quickly wrote George Soros to tell him why the current treatment design in Tomsk would fail. Soros summoned Farmer and Goldfarb to his office in New York; soon after, Partners In Health had a new project, the MDR-TB outbreak in Russia. Soros arranged a meeting at the White House with Hillary Rodham Clinton. Instead of getting the foundation support they had requested, Clinton pressed the World Bank to give Russia a loan worth $150 million to fight the epidemic. Farmer and the Partners In Health staff spent months developing a useful guide called *A DOTS-Plus Handbook, Guide to the Community-Based Treatment of MDR-TB*. Money from the Gates Foundation allowed them to offer it free from their web site.[2] Farmer convinced the World Bank and other competing groups within the Russian government to keep half of the grant money within the prison system, where the epidemic raged.

Along with the projects in Peru, Haiti, and now Russia, several other important projects continued to percolate along at Partners In Health. One in Boston trained health workers to apply DOTS with antiretroviral medications to local AIDS patients. The Institute of Medicine had previously shown that poor, uninsured HIV patients were 85% more likely to die prematurely of their disease. Once again, the Partners now-familiar model of employing trained community health workers served a community well, this time in Boston. In the border province of Huehuetenango, Guatemala, Partners In Health financed a project for local community health workers to help the local Mayan Indians. They provided legal, mental health, and logistical assistance for the Mayans to dig up the bodies of their relatives who had been slaughtered by the Guatemalan army and buried in mass graves during the 1980s. Partners In Health later funded a film about the exhumations, called *Voices from the Earth: The Dirty War in Guatemala*, which screened to an audience of more than 650 in Boston in 2002. In the poor state of Chiapas, Mexico, Partners In Health has been involved for years in community health training and has written more than 20 different manuals on health-related subjects. In 2005, the group partnered with the Clinton Foundation to open a new site in Rwanda.

As their work expanded to several other countries, Paul never let his focus drift from Haiti, which he continues to call home. At Zanmi Lasante, he developed protocols for treating AIDS patients in the poor Central Plateau region with another version of DOTS, this one for antiretrovirals. In May 2003, the *Lancet* published preliminary findings from this effort (Nierengarten 2003, 266). The issue reported that the Zanmi Lasante group had treated 100 HIV patients with a directly observable, highly active anti-retroviral therapy (HAART), which they called DOT-HAART. As in other Partners In Health models, community health workers delivered most of the therapy. Early results showed 0% mortality and a significantly reduced number of opportunistic infections in these patients. Haiti, which received $66 million from the Global Fund over five years, will put "a significant portion of it" toward HAART. The article concluded, "With the good results from the DOT-HAART programme, Farmer and his colleagues are showing that bringing antiretrovirals to the poorest people in the poorest areas of the world is feasible" (266).

Advocacy

Jim Kim often said the world's response to AIDS and tuberculosis would define the moral standing of his generation (Kidder 2003, 299). In his eyes it was everyone's responsibility to forcefully advocate on behalf of those long silenced by their poverty. He had once told me he thought the world needed an "AIDS Marshall Plan." Although still reluctant to declare an even modest victory over the ennui that has historically enveloped such ideas, Jim cited reason for optimism. He feels that he has witnessed a significant change in thinking in recent years. More medical students are now interested in international health work (a full 30% of Harvard Medical School's entering classes wanted to work with Partners In Health as of 2004, according to Jim) and more people than ever before seem committed to taking on AIDS. Even Jesse Helms has come around. Both Jim and Paul have taken on both challenges and developed models that offer hope to those in even the poorest places.

Partners In Health's work has had repercussions well beyond their ever-expanding programming parameters. Jeffrey Sachs has testified with Jim Kim in front of Congress on a number of occasions. In response to a question about Paul's work in Haiti, he said, "Paul's work (and his concept of high-quality medical care for the poor) has had a *huge* effect. I was able to use the example of his work in many key forums around the world in the past few years, with the US Congress, the WHO Commission on Macroeconomics and Health, the White House, the US Treasury, United Nations Secretary-General Kofi Annan, etc. When I worked with the secretary-general to help launch the Global Fund to Fight AIDS, Tuberculosis and Malaria, Paul's work was a key example" (Kidder 2003, 257).

As part of their own personal evolution, both Jim and Paul have taken on more and various political powers in their work. Haiti has offered the best instruction on the importance of global political decisions and the direct impact they have on the poor. Paul chronicled this sad story well in his book, *The Uses of Haiti*.[3] Paul in particular has written more editorials in both mainstream newspapers and medical journals in recent years, including several on the impact of the long US embargo on the Haitian poor. History teaches that embargoes always hurt the poor while having little effect on their leaders. Iraq, Cuba, the former Yugoslavia, Nicaragua, and Haiti all bear this out. In editorials published in both the *Boston Globe* in 2002 and the *Lancet* in 2003, Farmer and others pointed out how much poor Haitians suffered during the military coup and subsequent embargo: infant mortality doubled between 1991 and 1992, in part due to a measles outbreak fueled by markedly decreased availability of vaccines and food; life expectancy dropped to 49.6 years, the lowest in the hemisphere; poliomyelitis, long thought eradicated from the Western hemisphere, has resurfaced; maternal mortality increased to 450 deaths per 100,000 births in 1994, nearly 29% higher than in 1989 (Farmer et al 2003, 420; Farmer et al 2002, A15). Not all of these health measures can be traced directly back to the embargo, but it logically follows that $500 million in well-targeted aid toward health, water, and education could make a substantial difference for a country as small as Haiti. This belief was presented by Farmer and Mary Smith Fawzi in the *Boston Globe* editorial, prior to President Aristide's forced removal from power in 2004.

The public holds physicians in great esteem. When physicians like Paul Farmer make strong pronouncements on public policy, people listen. History is replete with examples of the poor suffering at the hands of the empowered elite. It is up to those of us who serve as the advocates of the poor to rise to their defense.

Divergence and Motivations

As Partners In Health grew and developed, the two engines most responsible for driving it diverged. Jim Kim found his work with the WHO exhilarating and rightly felt that he could exert a far greater impact on the poor by influencing larger health policy, as happened with MDR-TB. Jim campaigned heavily for Dr Lee Jong-Wook to take over the WHO as its next director-general for a five-year term starting in July 2003. Jong-Wook and legendary AIDS guru Peter Piot were deadlocked for two rounds of voting until one country changed its vote to Jong-Wook (Vogel 2003, 809). Once elected, Lee tapped Jim Kim as an adviser in his inner circle. Accepting the position required Jim and his family to move to Geneva and put physical distance between Jim and Paul and the Partners staff, yet all recognized this as a great opportunity to continue the "O for the P" on a larger stage. Jim said to Paul, "Political work is interesting to me, and it has to be done. . . . But didn't we always say that people who go into policy make a preferential option for their own ideas? For their own sorry asses?" Paul replied, "Yeah, but Jim, we trust you with power. We know you won't betray the poor" (Kidder 2003, 174).

Dr Lee Jong-Wook went before the UN General Assembly in September 2003 to announce that the WHO was scaling up its AIDS operations to provide antiretrovirals to 3 million people by the end of 2005, most of whom were in sub-Saharan Africa (Altman 2003). He charged Jim Kim with overseeing the AIDS program. Quite predictably, the program immediately reflected Jim's vision and sense of urgency. Although widely respected, the WHO has long had a reputation for slow, deliberate steps that achieve results over long periods of time. Following their actions over the SARS (severe acute respiratory syndrome) epidemic and the infusion of new leadership, the organization finally, some would say, began to treat AIDS as an emergency. Jim said to the *New York Times*, "From a public health perspective, we need to treat at least three million people by 2005 to avert an enormous catastrophe. We cannot wait any longer" (Altman 2003).

Falling prices for antiretrovirals has markedly broadened their availability. Chiefly because of this, developing countries, along with foundations and multilateral donors, can now revamp their AIDS programs and actually treat patients, not just preach abstinence and condom use. As Harvard School of Public Health Dean Dr Barry Bloom said, "Addressing HIV/AIDS in resource-poor settings will be the defining issue for WHO and its new leadership." Given AIDS' dramatic rise in recent years, it is clear that we are at a critical juncture. "The next 10 years will be the most important years for public health in history," Jim told *Science* magazine. "We're going to be able to tell whether we will be able to take on HIV or not" (Vogel 2003, 809). Despite many limitations from the political, the bureaucratic, and the inevitable inertia endemic to such large organizations, Jim will have to find a way to prevail. But, he always has. To add additional luster to his already impressive rise, the MacArthur Foundation recognized Jim with a "genius" grant in October 2003 (Lee 2003).

Jim once mentioned that he ended most of his talks to medical students citing two major historical entities—the Civil Rights Movement and the Space Program. The Civil Rights Movement had galvanized a country and had created unusual alliances to work toward the higher principles of racial equity and social justice. The Space Program was important because we as a nation had accepted a challenge from President Kennedy that had been previously thought impossible—and then showed we could do it. "Whatever it takes" was the attitude that prevailed. In Jim's view, if we could combine the missionary zeal of the Civil Rights Movement with the "whatever it takes" attitude from the Space Program and apply it to global health inequalities, we would truly witness a global health revolution. These health inequalities could be solved in a generation, he says. Jim added that he thought we would know we were advancing when children started to ask their parents, "Mommy, why don't I die when I'm 40 like they do in Africa?" Jim concludes his talks to medical students along a similar line: "The task for every generation is to find out what is primitive with the current generation and fix it. For our generation the task is the lack of equity in global health care." Jim's passion, zeal, and idealism resonate most clearly with his visionary partner from Partners In Health.

More than one person has called Paul Farmer a "saint," a term seemingly well earned. A wise friend once told me that the best ways to judge someone is by where he spends his money and his time. On both counts, Paul Farmer walks the talk. He works every day, almost all day, sleeping just three to four hours per night. All of his energies go toward patients, the bulk of them poor. He has turned over all of his prize money, speaking honoraria, and book royalties to Partners In Health. He receives a salary from Harvard Medical School and the Brigham and Women's Hospital of more than $100,000 per year, but he never sees it. A bookkeeper pays his family expenses, his mother's mortgage, and then puts the rest into the Partners treasury. Once in 1999 Paul tried to use a credit card but was told he had reached the limit. The bookkeeper told him, "Honey, you are the hardest workin' broke man I know" (Kidder 2003, 23).

It is difficult to summarize just what drives Paul to maintain such incredible levels of sacrifice in his pursuit of social justice and improved health for the poor. To Tracy Kidder, Paul once said, "The problem is, if I don't work this hard, someone will die who doesn't have to. That sounds megalomaniacal. I wouldn't have said it to you before I'd taken you to Haiti and you had seen that it was manifestly true" (Kidder 2003, 191).

Kidder concluded the following about Paul Farmer, "In his mind, he was fighting all poverty all the time, an endeavor full of difficulties and inevitable failures. For him, the reward was inward clarity, and the price perpetual anger, or, at best, discomfort with the world, not always on the surface but always there. . . . Farmer wasn't put on earth to make anyone feel comfortable, except for those lucky enough to be his patients" (Kidder 2003, 210). Farmer terms it this way, "When others write about people who live on the edge, who challenge their comfortable lives—and it has happened to me—they usually do it in a way that allows a reader a way out. You could render generosity into pathology, commitment into obsession. That's all in the repertory of someone who wants to put the reader at ease rather than conveying the truth in a compelling manner. I want people to feel unhappy about Lazarus and all the others who are shafted" (207).

Giving the "shafted" people of the world an option for reasonable health care has been a driving passion for the Partners In Health staff for years. They have succeeded at bringing high-quality health care to those living in extreme poverty. In 2002, the Clinique Bon Saveur in Haiti performed the first open heart surgery with visiting doctors from Boston and North

Carolina. In an editorial published in the *New England Journal of Medicine* in 2001, Paul wrote,

> Although science has revolutionized medicine, we still need a plan for ensuring equal access to care. As study after study shows the power of effective therapies to alter the course of infectious disease, we should be increasingly reluctant to reserve these therapies for the affluent, low-incidence regions of the world where most medical resources are concentrated. Excellence without equity looms as the chief human-rights dilemma of health care in the 21st century (Farmer 2001, 208).

In his acceptance of the Heinz Award, Paul reminded us all that "as members of the world community, we must recognize that we can and should summon our collective resources to save the countless lives that were previously alleged to be beyond our help."[4] He believes we can do no less than this. But in order to proceed, we need to reexamine history and the global structures that render so much of the world vulnerable and in abject poverty. Farmer says that erasing history has always served the interests of power. It is up to us to examine our own understandings of global power structures and bring pressure to those whose decisions so greatly affect the poor.

In a number of conversations, Jim Kim has accepted that few people can hope to accomplish what he and Paul have thus far together. Few have the resources that Tom White and Harvard have made available to them and few have the intelligence and passion that have allowed them to achieve so much so quickly. Neither is ordinary, and both push themselves considerably, often at the expense of time with family. Jim once e-mailed me, "For better or worse, Paul and I are both outliers—politically, psychologically, and personally (as our respective wives would attest)." Theirs is certainly not the traditional path, nor is it for many of the people they have pulled into this with them. We should recognize that considerable credit must go to the efforts of the rest of the Partners In Health team; the scholars, students, and doctors in Boston; and the dedicated employees in Peru, Haiti, Roxbury, and in other countries. When I talk with Jim about how extraordinary their trajectory has been, he modestly replies that they have been "lucky." Yet, he also shares Paul's concern that people occasionally feel that to achieve something in international health, they must follow their path.

Jim said this to Tracy Kidder, though he could just as easily have been describing himself, "Paul is a model of what should be done. He's not a model for how it has to be done. Let's celebrate him. Let's make sure people are inspired by him. But we can't say anybody should or could be just like him. Because if poor people have to wait for a lot of people like Paul to come along before they get good health care, they are totally [screwed]" (Kidder 2003, 244). Paul echoes these sentiments, as illustrated by an e-mail from a student that upset him. The student had said that he believed in Paul's cause but couldn't do what Paul did. Paul replied aloud, with an edge,

"I didn't say you should do what I do. I just said these things *should* be done" (244). He then sent a kind response.

As both Paul and Jim have clearly shown, it will simply not suffice to wage this battle on global health inequality on one front. We must engage, as health providers, on a number of fronts simultaneously. In addition to taking on the challenges of caring for poor people in their home settings, we must take on global power structures and find the breaking points, whether they exist in the political, public health, academic, or other realms. Fully embracing the tenets of liberation theology and pushing forward in the belief that we are, in fact, "all human" leaves us with little choice other than to rededicate ourselves to this quest. In time, all kinds of barriers, previously thought unassailable, may well come tumbling down.

Endnotes

1. Taken from Jim Yong Kim's curriculum vitae, courtesy of Michele Welshhans, assistant to Jim Yong Kim at Harvard Medical School.
2. For more information, see the Partners In Health web site at www.pih.org/library/books/MDRTBguide.htm.
3. Much of the dates here come from the Haitian Embassy in Washington DC web site at www.haiti.org/keydate.htm.
4. Information from the Partners In Health web site at http://network.twii.net/publish.sps?syndicatorguid={8BA31799-FED2-4A67-BCAE-7808F2194E6C}&rmasiteinstanceguid={46B96458-4E96-4103-9CF1-785A00B582E2}&rmapageid=27&sectionID=5456.

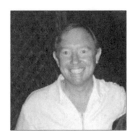

Chapter 14

Peter Allen, DMD

When living in a developing country, you get so much more out of it than what you put in.
—Dr Peter Allen

Dr Peter Allen went to Belize through a British volunteer organization nearly 20 years ago. Leaving a comfortable dental practice and life in England, he fully made the transition to Belizean. He radiates a sense of satisfaction and happiness that so many of his colleagues in the United States and United Kingdom lack. His message is simple: life in a developing country need not be thought of solely in terms of sacrifice and altruism. While working toward larger social justice concerns, it can also be fun and fulfilling. Peter Allen embodies a Caribbean persona while maintaining backbreaking work hours, all the while helping Belize build its health system. He has risen to a lead position in the Belize government through dedication and hard work. His story offers a different perspective on living and working abroad, and his insights over the years answer many questions about a different approach to life for health providers.

Peter Allen is immediately recognizable in the old hospital pickup truck that sputters along the edge of this southern town in Belize, Central America. He beams as several people along the sparsely paved streets of Dangriga call out to him, which seemingly everyone does. His fair English skin often assumes a reddish hue from the sun, faring less well in the subtropical climate here than his personal warmth and good nature. Because Dangriga is comprised predominantly of Garinagu, the descendents of Caribs and runaway African slaves, Peter's look is that much more distinctive. His smile radiates, not an uncommon finding among dentists. Peter knows most of Dangriga's 10,000 people, having lived there for 15 years and becoming, in the process, a very public and popular individual. While accompanying him around town, one is struck by how happy he seems with his work and his life. One gets the impression that Peter Allen is exactly where he ought to be.

"I feel great sympathy for many of the doctors in the States and in England," he says, "because health care seems to have moved away in many ways from being a vocational profession towards being a business." In lieu of treating caries and dental decay in his home in England, Dr Allen opted for an approach in which he could make a broader impact. He liked the clinical work enough, still does. But he had always been interested in the broader health of the public and he searched for a place where he could treat the larger issues that so commonly breed poor dental and general health. Along the shores of the Caribbean, in a laid-back community plagued by disease and unacceptable levels of poverty, he found it.

Transitions

Peter Allen came to Belize in 1987 as he terms it, "by accident." Following four years of practice in Merseyside and Liverpool, England, he responded to a call from the private Volunteer Service Organization (VSO), the United Kingdom's large, service organization that predates the US Peace Corps. He went to Belize to help establish dental public health programs in the Stann Creek and Toledo districts, the poorest in Belize. After completing his two-year term of service, he signed on as a district dental officer for the Belize Ministry of Health, finding the larger public health issues to his interest. He conducted research on Xylitol, a sugar substitute, and developed public dental health programs for southern Belize. He sought to reduce the far too frequent dental extractions—the dental equivalent of euthanasia—and sought to bring people "better options." Preventing dental disease rather than sacrificing complete sets of teeth seemed a far more effective use of his time and skills.

Life in Dangriga immersed him in the poverty and ill health that inexorably stalk the local population, pushing him far beyond the realm of dentistry. Observing that the population in his district was "terrorized" by HIV, hepatitis, sexually transmitted diseases, malaria, and tuberculosis, he began to study the broader public health of the area and to design solutions with other like-minded people. In 1996, he became the district medical officer for the Stann Creek District and later the Toledo District, a region virtually covering the lower half of the country. Three years later, following a huge investment of time and energy, he and his staff opened the Southern Regional Hospital (SRH), a modern hospital funded by a loan to the Belize government. SRH replaced the ancient structure that had housed the sickest of the poor of southern Belize since the 1940s.

I have met with Peter Allen once or twice yearly since 1997 and have come to know him reasonably well. During many of my visits, we would go to a local diner or talk in his office for a few hours. He is perhaps best described as a committed man who seamlessly mixes serious work with good fun, all the while pushing himself to do more. Accomplished though self-effacing, he has never been one to put on airs about his position or closeness to those in power. Rather, he tends to downplay what he does. Following a suspected outbreak of hemorrhagic dengue fever in Belize, he e-mailed me to say that the outbreak had them all "a bit concerned." "Somewhat odd circumstances of course," he continued, "but 'the authorities' are investigating–am never quite sure what that phrase means–I've a sneaking feeling that somehow it's supposed to involve me in some way."

One can easily understand how Peter, or anyone else for that matter, could be drawn to Belize, a country situated in Central America but with a far more Caribbean feel. Here, one is seduced by the culture, the palm trees, and the unhurried pace to life. These aspects draw thousands of tourists each year, though mostly to the offshore Cayes, separated from the mainland by a few miles and an enormous economic differential. On the Cayes, one finds all-inclusive resorts and diving tours; the impoverished residences of immigrant workers are tucked neatly out of view. On the mainland, there is incredible beauty and warm people, though far too many of them live in poverty. The bulk of the population lives amidst the factors that places Belize at the highest ranking of lower-middle income countries, as designated by the OECD (Organization for Economic Co-Operation and Development 2002, 300). It is easy for a visitor to be fooled into thinking that life here is easy–particularly if one only visits the areas that tourists typically see. For the poor of Belize, as everywhere, life is hard and often subjected to capricious visitations by debilitating illness, sometimes beyond the reach of their caretakers.

Health providers here typically work long hours. The starting salary for physicians in the public sector is $12,500 (US) per year in a country that is not inexpensive by Central American standards; that is why many also work in the private sector. For those who venture to advance public health in this country, life is difficult–particularly given the invariable paucity of funds. Such is life for Peter Allen. One evening, I came to see him shortly after the new hospital had opened in 2000. Busy developing a presentation on a new prevention of mother to child transmission of HIV program (PMTCT), he had forgotten to eat dinner. When we left his office it was close to midnight. I asked him how often he kept such hours. "Too often," he replied. "If days were only 12 hours long it would be a blessing." Most of his days, it seemed, were 14 hours–often seven days a week for long stretches.

"I feel lucky," Peter says. "I am part of a process that moves this country forward."

The enormous workload, however, never seems to bother him–he still relishes his work and life. Laughter follows him to staff meetings, dinners out, and on casual drives through town. In Dangriga Hospital and later the

SRH and Ministry of Health, he created a thriving work environment where he was very popular with his staff, finding some success in getting them to join in a vision for a healthier community. "I feel lucky," Peter says. "I am part of a process that moves this country forward." The process is slow and required considerable work on the part of Pete and many others for a number of years.

Despite his workload, however, he has seen much of the Central American region and found a favorite Caye to visit with friends. "I love it here," he says. "I live in a beautiful country—I wouldn't want to live in a place that I didn't like, no matter how much I liked the work."

On only a few occasions have I known his boundless enthusiasm to founder. The first was when a close friend of his was killed on one of Belize's still-dangerous roads. The episode shocked Peter, and his subsequent grief was understandable, particularly after losing a young friend so tragically. The second occurred in December 2000, when a local 17-year-old was stabbed in a street fight. The victim was taken to Dangriga Hospital, where the treating physician sewed over the stab wound, not recognizing the risk. The young man returned to the hospital, complaining of pain and fever and was again treated and released. On his next return, he had become quite ill. He was emergently transferred to a larger regional hospital where he underwent emergency surgery. But it was too late. He died from the septic complications of a perforated bowel.

Peter had known the family for years and now had to respond to an angry community that wanted to string up one of his staff. I saw him just a few weeks after this event. He looked tired, and talking about the episode brought tears to his eyes. It was not his fault and he could have done nothing administratively to prevent it. Yet he felt it as intensely and as personally as if he had been the treating physician. Talking with him after this event reinforced for me just how much a part of Dangriga he had become and how much Dangriga had become a part of him. He was no visitor. His work in Belize had become the dominant piece of his life. Here was a man grieving the tragic loss of a family friend and member of the community—his community. It was both humbling and instructive to see.

It is readily apparent to anyone who knows him that Peter has become Belizean; what is less readily apparent, at least to me, is why he has made the choices he has. During our many conversations, I repeatedly asked him why he lives where he lives; with no malice intended toward Dangriga, which is a decent enough place. The people and the weather are warm and there is plenty to do during time off. But Dangriga is still racked by poverty and the problems that invariably accompany it. Many of the conveniences of his birthplace in England are missing and the living standard is quite austere when compared to the United States or the United Kingdom. Peter's own modest home is one of many row houses up on stilts, packed in so tightly together that neighbors' conversations are certainly not private. Naturally, he was reluctant to answer most of my questions, preferring to talk about politics, health, or just about anything else.

However, I persisted in my questioning—interrogation is a more apt description—because Peter had made such a rare choice. He didn't have to be there and this was no brief volunteer stint. This was a life choice, one that he had followed for nearly 20 years. I guessed that every other member of his graduating class was practicing dentistry in the United Kingdom or North America, earning five times his salary. Few, if any, were driving around in old pickup trucks with temperamental clutches and loud, clanking noises that erupted at speeds over 15 mile per hour. Fresh from explorations of Schweitzer, Dooley, and others, I was ready to hear of a deep religious calling or a "reverence" for humanity that compelled him to serve.

A Natural Choice

Although Peter's motivations do echo those of Schweitzer and others, his rationale always seemed far more practical and grounded, exuding common sense. To hear Peter discuss his rationale, one would quickly agree that for him to do anything else would be just a little bit crazy. He had gone to Belize to do interesting public dental work and found that he really liked it—not just the work but the life that went along with it. In Belize, he found the opportunity to work with, in his words, "great people with shared ideals." In England, he could influence the lives of individual patients as a solo provider, certainly a meritorious pursuit. In Belize, however he could affect 10 times that number through larger public health initiatives that would have been much harder—if not impossible—to achieve at home. He once told me, "I have always felt that, here, we are making a difference. There are very few days when you can't feel good at the end of the day, and that's very valuable to me. Not that we don't have our share of frustrating days—we do. But here we get to contribute in a sustainable way for people to better look after themselves." And that matters. He has collected the data to show that some of his interventions have directly improved the public's health.

When pressed to talk about some of his deeper motivations, Peter readily says that his progression to a life in Belize came through the convergence of several factors: a strong ethical foundation laid by his parents, a larger awareness of unfairness in the world, a regular commitment to service, and a choice to follow his ideals to the Caribbean.

Pete was raised in what he describes as the "perfect family." His father was a trade unionist in the British car industry and his mother stayed home to raise the kids. His parents taught their kids strong values, gave them education, religion, and full, happy lives that included community service from a young age. This "idyllic" life continued for the Allen family until seemingly distant events came home to England. The slowing of the global economy in the 1970s caused the local auto plant to lay off workers. Charles "Chris"

Allen, Peter's dad, was among them, and a young Peter watched his idyllic family life suddenly and radically change. His mother Lucy went to work and "did an outstanding job in a non-traditional role," while his father collected benefits and all learned to get by with considerably less. As Pete recalls, "If I look at how families should prosper, this was it—accept sacrifice, spend time with kids, get kids educated, church on Sundays, Boy Scouts, sports, friends, extended family, volunteering together. And then, due to the economy, their lives got screwed up."

The episode reinforced for a young Peter Allen how unfair life could be. He wondered how others were similarly affected by distant events. "Things happen on a macro level, and people are incredibly impacted by things utterly beyond their control," he said. If distant forces could produce economic calamity in his stable family, what effect would those same forces have on those who were even more vulnerable? "If it's not fair in the UK," he reasoned, "how much more unfair is it in developing countries?"

He says he would probably have come to a developing country even if his father had not been laid off. It is hard for him to discern now whether this event triggered his decision to go abroad. But it certainly affirmed his ideas on inequality and service, in lessons learned since his youth. He had always done volunteer work in the United Kingdom, motivated by a deep awareness of general unfairness in life for so many people. He worked with mentally retarded individuals, the visually impaired, and abused kids. About his own volunteer work he adds, "the chief motivating factor was that I enjoyed doing it. People fall through the cracks," he continues. "There will always be a need for community-based organizations that try to find ways to plug those gaps. I've always felt that I had a responsibility to assist in any way that I can."

In moving from the local to the international stage, he noted, "the gaps in the developing countries are just that much larger." Moving to a country like Belize became a natural progression based on his concepts of fairness. "I am a little bit outraged," he says, "at how much rests on where people are born and the circumstances they are born into." Echoing Schweitzer, he adds, "It's not quite fair that I had the good fortune to be born into a place where I received better health care, education, and the opportunity to have a happy and successful life."

Perspectives

Reflecting back over the years, he finds that the motivations that first brought him to Belize through VSO differ from those that keep him here now. He remains committed to principles of social justice and sees no real change in the reasons for his efforts. However, as he succinctly puts it, "The list of reasons people first come down are rarely the reasons they stay or return." People evolve and change. Peter is ever aware that he lives in a place that is "incredibly beautiful, where people enjoy themselves so much." Despite his own recent "workaholic ways," he has changed. Things he used to value in England, he values considerably less now. He has become a part of a community that is important to him and has evolved his innate cultural views to those that put more emphasis on relationships between people and less on things. It is those relationships amidst the general flow of life that have kept him in Belize. Combine that with a fulfilling job that offers the opportunity to improve life for many and you have, at least for Peter Allen, a formula that makes for a happy and rich life.

Perhaps the most valuable cultural lesson he has learned along the way, he says, is "to give up the chase." Recalling his early years in dental practice in England, he says, "My perception of what was a good standard of living then is other than what it is now. As that expression goes, 'happiness isn't having what you want, it's wanting what you have.' I now live in a wonderful community of people who have allowed me to become a part of this fabulous environment where concepts of what is desirable are simpler. It doesn't have to be a new Rolls Royce—it can be a bicycle. Motivations are just different now."

Accompanying his personal evolution has been an evolution of his worldview. While still an "Anglophile," he now finds himself, for example, more cynical about the reasons donor governments do what they do, seeing many self-serving actions thinly cloaked under the veil of humanitarianism. "I'm less confident," he says, "that they do things out of humanitarian reasons or out of goodness or fairness." His experiences with "aid" in a number of forms have affirmed his suspicions. Although he finds most projects well intentioned, he is struck by how much those directly involved in their planning gain from them "on both sides of the Atlantic" and at how frequently these programs "miss their marks." Seeing the "largesse" of the wealthy world from the perspective of one living amidst the poor seems to have a way of altering one's views. Peter's views in this regard echo those of many other people with similar experiences in the developing world.

> *No matter how simple things appear from a couple of thousand miles away, here one finds that they are infinitely more complex.*

Regarding health service, Peter has seen a lot of well- and ill-intentioned people come to Belize through the years. There are, he says, a "million reasons why" people come, and he feels it is not for him or anyone else to judge. Some come to enhance their curriculum vitaes, others to work in a place with "rum and coconuts," and others to do good and effective work. His only criterion is that those who come do no harm, as some occasionally do. In his experience, many of those who come to Belize for short periods tend to require more time and resources than they are able to give in return. Exceptions include those who train local providers and those who provide a specific, needed service such as cataract resections, cleft palate repairs, etc.

For those who stay longer, he says, "Those who get the most out of it are the ones who are flexible and are able to compromise without losing sight of their targets." For those who come to "save the world by Christmas," he says, "it doesn't take long to figure out that's not going to happen. No matter how simple things appear from a couple of thousand miles away, here one finds that they are infinitely more complex."

That complexity has consumed Peter Allen for a number of years. He has learned to begrudgingly accept the things he can't change, be they for political, financial, interpersonal, or other reasons. Horizons seem longer here and change is best viewed over years. To help him better adapt to his increasing role in public health, he completed a "distance learning" masters in public health (MPH) program based at the University of South Florida. In 2002, Belizean Prime Minister Said Musa appointed him as director of the [Health] Policy Analysis and Planning Unit for Belize, essentially the position that plots the future course of health care for the country. It was a job he accepted with relish and his characteristic enthusiasm. Requiring him to leave his beloved Dangriga became the price for his ascension, but the opportunity to make a difference on a considerably larger scale was, in his mind, worth it. He now holds one of the most influential health positions in the country, with an opportunity to influence national health policy until at least 2008, when the next round of national elections occurs.

Following a particularly long meeting in March 2003, Peter Allen walked back to his car for the long ride from Belize City to Belmopan, his new home. Elections just completed, he had a new slate of issues to tackle. He was working as hard as ever, though still seeming to enjoy it. During our lunch meeting, he naturally knew several others in the dining room, glad-handing like the politicians he now works with so closely. As he walked away, my colleague Dr John O'Brien commented, "There goes one incredible guy."

Peter's life is not for everyone, and though he makes an ideal role model for anyone considering service in a developing country, the ingredients that make up the man have not been reproduced on a large-scale basis. Few are so equipped as to get past the ubiquitous obstacles that life in a poor region holds, to get to the beauty of what lies behind them. This is why people like Peter are so uncommon, though not exactly rare. His life is not unique—many have done what he is doing before and will again in the future. Yet the joy that he gives and receives through his work and his life choices remain instructive for us all. When his friends and family come to see him, he says, they look around and see the dilapidated homes, the dirt, and the bugs and wonder why he's here. But after a few days, he wryly notes, "they usually leave thinking I'm the lucky one."

In perspective, what Peter does is neither charity nor development. Nor, in his mind, is it sacrifice. Work in a developing country has its own rewards and need not be viewed solely through the lens of service. As he readily admits, his early motivations have changed. Social justice concerns remain but have become secondary to the overall satisfaction he finds living and working in Belize. Peter echoes many I have talked with through the years, "When living in a developing country," he says, "you get so much more out of it than what you put in." As he walks away laughing, perfectly content in his life and world, one gets the impression that he has found the right place and will never find a reason to leave.

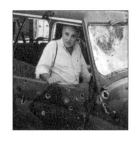

Chapter 15

Thomas S. "Doc" Durant, MD

It's the proof of Original Sin, of good vs. evil, of man's inhumanity to man. But the most striking thing is that this shows the resiliency of the human spirit. Despite all you see here, there are still people who can laugh, who can show kindness to others.

—Dr Tom Durant,
in a refugee camp in Macedonia, April 1999

For more than three decades, Dr Tom Durant worked through the worst calamities humanity has faced. Genocide, war, and natural disasters have caused millions to become dispossessed, sick, and vulnerable. To so many of these people, Tom became the reassuring voice and source of laughter amidst their sorrow. Tom's international service included the most dangerous and difficult work. He probed the nexus where bad politics collides with health. Most of his patients were refugees, and most of his study was of modern history's worst tyrants. "Doc" shed light on why we must broaden our worldviews to include the larger political realm. Genocide in Cambodia, hurricanes in the Caribbean, and massive refugee movements in the Balkans all impact the health of hundreds of thousands. Through such events, seemingly distant worlds become intimately connected to the very core of our health profession. Tom's world is shared by those from Médecins Sans Frontières (MSF), Physicians for Human Rights (PHR), Amnesty International, CARE, and countless other nongovernmental organizations (NGOs) that work in the darker corners of the world. In viewing his life's work, we gain a window into a world that most consider the realm of others. Yet it affects us all and demands that we, as health providers, see it as our own.

I first met Dr Tom "Doc" Durant on a warm night in May 1977, the day I graduated Boston Latin High School. My classmate Sean Durant, Tom's third son, held a graduation party at his family's home on Melville Avenue in Dorchester. At the time,I had no way of knowing how important that night would later become. Later in the evening, I came across three men singing rugby songs and hoisting glasses of beer, laughing and carrying on as though they had just graduated themselves—though they looked considerably older. Dr Durant was among them. I really did not know who he was, I only knew him as Sean's dad. But I knew that this was a man who fully enjoyed life, while staying tough enough to play rugby long after most had hung up their cleats.

Almost 20 years passed before I saw Dr Durant again. In the intervening years, I had gone through medical school and a residency and had twice worked as a doctor in East Africa. I had started to write this book when Joe Callahan, another friend from high school, mentioned that Sean's father had worked internationally and would be a good person to meet. I called Massachusetts General Hospital (MGH) to find him, only to learn that he was the assistant director. Maybe Had I mistaken "Doc" for someone else singing rugby songs on Melville Avenue? I introduced myself, outlined what I was doing, and asked him for advice. He said he would be happy to talk with me and invited me to meet him for lunch.

I met him in the MGH lobby and we walked outside. It was *him*. Several people stopped him along the short walk from the lobby to the corner of Cambridge Street. He greeted each one warmly, leaving them laughing following a stinging, pithy remark. We had lunch in a nearby restaurant. He ordered in Thai and, in the process, said something to the waitress that produced a stream of embarrassed giggles. I did not know Tom at all then, but could only assume that he had told the waitress, in Thai, that he loved her last movie. Soon other waitstaff, seemingly drawn to this compelling man, came to our table to hear Tom's stories of working near their homeland. The bill came and he insisted on paying—a habit I later saw him repeat many times. In the way he talked, the manner in which he carried himself, and the way he greeted people, it quickly became clear that here was a gem of a man.

Over lunch, we talked about service, the conditions of poverty, and the incredible suffering that so many of the world's people continually endure. He railed against both the political left and right, deriding the shortsightedness of some of President Clinton's foreign policy decisions and the isolationism of the Republican opposition at the time. Tom had seen thousands of people suffer and die needlessly in several wars and their aftermath. These images never left him and forever shaped his views.

During that first memorable encounter, it seemed that an immediate bond formed between us. Maybe it was because our roots were similar—we were both half-Irish and had roots in Boston's neighborhoods. Maybe it was our connection through Sean. Maybe it was the genuine passion we shared in wanting to alter the plight of the poor. Maybe it was the transformations we had undergone, mine while working in Tanzania in 1987 and Tom's under much harsher conditions in Vietnam 20 years earlier. Whatever it was, the connection seemed real enough to me and I soon began calling on Tom for advice. He readily complied, usually leaving me with a line or two that would keep me chuckling for days. About one local politician, Tom said, "Deep down, he's a very superficial guy."

Tom became a mentor for me—always available, always insightful, and always ready to comment on whatever political or societal event graced the front pages of the newspapers. He possessed a rare combination of biting wit and intellectual fire, grounded in tough experience. When I talked of Schweitzer and an ethical imperative to serve, he talked of death camps and neighbors killing neighbors in Bosnia. His worldview was tempered by harsh experiences that revealed the absolute worst in human nature. I tried to understand this man, but he remained sphinx-like about his deepest motivations. He never spelled out the reasons why he traveled to so many troubled regions of the world. He would typically shrug off my inquiries with references to others whose sacrifices were, in his mind, far greater than his own.

I later learned that my relationship with Tom was far from unique. Dr Jim O'Connell, the acclaimed founder and director of Boston's Healthcare for the Homeless, had also benefited from Tom's counsel. Jim had been my attending/preceptor during part of my first year on the medical wards of Boston City Hospital, where Tom had also trained. I was unaware that the two had known each other for years. Jim credits Tom with first sending him off to Pine Street, Boston's largest homeless shelter where it had all begun for him many years before. A host of others have similar stories.

An Extraordinary Life

Tom's life story reads like a Tom Clancy novel, though he always denied any Central Intelligence Agency ties. His international career began when he ran the civilian medical clinics in Saigon and the Mekong Delta in Vietnam for US AID from 1966 to 1968, and he survived the shelling of one of his clinics during the Tet Offensive in 1968. He set up a clinic in the Holy Rosary Church in Saigon, South Vietnam, to care for limbless children and parents who, in the words of Doc's long-time friend Mike Barnicle, "had lost half their families to war yet never knew what an aspirin was" (1995). Tom also treated Vietnamese patients in a nearby cemetery, turning a former mausoleum into a treatment room. Tom's experiences in Vietnam never left him, and he vowed to commit his life to helping those affected by war and natural disasters. When he returned home, he joined MGH as assistant director, a position he held for more than 30 years. He also joined the American Refugee Committee and over the next 35 years saw first-hand humanity's worst events.

During the height of the Khmer Rouge genocide in Cambodia, Tom spent eight months working in refugee camps along the Thai-Cambodia border; joined by his sons Sean and Joe. When Rwanda exploded in 1994, Tom worked in the refugee camps in nearby Goma where, he said, "We had 70,000 dead in two weeks from cholera. We counted 2,000 dead the first day we were there" (Barnicle 1995). He also worked in the refugee camps in Macedonia in 1999 (Cullen 1999, A13) and in the Kurdish camps on the Turkish-Iraqi border just after the Persian Gulf War (Mooney 2001). In Africa, he worked in Sudan, Ethiopia, Somalia, Mozambique, and Rwanda. In the troubled Balkans, he served in Bosnia, Macedonia, Albania, Croatia, and Kosovo. He also worked in Afghanistan, Iraq, Honduras, and virtually every other hot spot since Vietnam.

Tom became a celebrity in Boston and internationally among the roving band of humanitarian workers. He became friends with local politicians including Joseph Moakley, Ted Kennedy, and William Weld. Columnists Mike Barnicle and David Nyhan were also friends. Pulitzer Prize-winning author David Halberstam wrote of "a lifelong friendship with a man who was as close to becoming a contemporary saint as any man I've ever known" (Halberstam 2002). For his work, Tom received a bevy of awards, including the Joseph Moakley Award for Distinguished Public Service in 2001. His greatest honor came in 1995 when he received the Humanitarian Award from the United Nations, along with such celebrities as Jacques Cousteau, Ted Turner, and Trudie Styler, Sting's wife. To that Tom said, "Imagine that! Me from Codman Square with people like that" (Barnicle 1995). Such responses were typical. Tom always deflected any praise or attention toward others.

Doc was never one to boast of his credentials, including Harvard, MGH, or simply being a physician. He had worked in too many dire situations and seen too many "ordinary" people perform heroic acts that many of the more widely cited measures of success simply lost their appeal to him. In Honduras, the doctors groups had not made the biggest difference to those devastated by Hurricane Mitch; lay Rotarians had. After the 1994 Rwandan genocide, it was not the doctors, nurses, or large international relief organizations that turned the tide on cholera in those infamous death camps in Goma; it was a group of firemen. Tom told the story to columnist Mike Barnicle,

> Let me tell you who did the most good in Rwanda. Five firemen from San Francisco and San Diego. These five guys saved more lives than all the doctors combined. They were retired and they volunteered to come over with a brand new pumper. They were flown in on a C-5A. First day there, they had to push bodies away from the shore of a lake to begin pumping water. They got the water chlorinated in tank trucks and finally people had water to drink that wouldn't kill them. The point is, those five guys were just ordinary guys. Wonderful, ordinary folks who came over on their own to help out and they ended up being more valuable than doctors (1995).

No doubt Doc's lack of appreciation for his badges of social acclaim stem directly from his roots. Tom lived his entire adult life in the house in Dorchester near where he grew up. Dorchester is Boston's largest neighborhood, comprised of working class people, ethnically diverse, and with its fair share of crime, drugs, and racial tensions. His son Stephen described it as a place that "does not suffer fools, phonies, or cowards gladly." Not many physicians call Dorchester home. Most of his colleagues lived in pricey homes in Newton, Wellesley, or other wealthy suburbs. I once asked Tom about it, and he replied that he thought one of the great domestic policy mistakes in US history was FDR's decision to segregate the classes. He had recalled growing up with both rich and poor in the same neighborhood in Dorchester. Doctors lived with janitors and teachers and cops and lawyers. All their kids played together and got to know their role models well. In Tom's view, that was the way it should be, though it changed for most people in the 1930s. But Tom was not one to follow belief with inaction. He and his wife Fredericka raised their three sons in Dorchester; no gated community there.

Tom readily shared his opinions on a range of issues through the years. As we were traveling on a bus through rural Belize, I asked him why he thought so few doctors volunteered internationally. He rather dramatically outlined a man being nailed to a cross. He threw one arm back to the right, "the house." He threw the left arm back, "the schools." He then crossed his legs, "the summer home, the car, the boat. . . ." "Too many doctors," he said, "get caught up in the money, and become prisoners." He thought more doctors should be out serving, but he was not one to waste his time arguing with them. "Ninety percent of them tell me they'll go with me 'next time,'" he said. "But they never do." To him, the discussions became pointless; so he continued on his own way, as he always had.

Travels with "Doc"

In mid-1997, Tom raised my interest in international health to a more pragmatic level. He introduced me to a group of Rotarians from Hingham, Massachusetts, including Sheldon Daly, Richard Bridges, Harold Lincoln, and others who had been donating medical equipment to Belize. They invited me to join Tom and a few others on a tour of Belize to advise them on their program. That was the start of the Omni Med health education program.

In late October 1998, Hurricane Mitch devastated sections of Honduras, Nicaragua, and El Salvador. Soon after, Tom invited me to go with him with two others from MGH to Tegucigalpa, Honduras, to see how we could help the local Rotarians in their outreach efforts. Tom and I had been talking about poverty and international health, and I think he had wanted me to see another side of this work. We toured the capitol city Tegucialgalpa and the surrounding areas, seeing up close the incredible damage Mitch had inflicted on so many people. War, natural disasters, and the resultant mass movements of humanity cause tremendous upheaval, sickness, and death in the world. Tom wanted me to see this firsthand and add to my perspective on service. The lesson did not go unheeded.

During a reception in Tegucigalpa, three of us watched in amazement as Tom worked his way through a dense crowd toward the First Lady of Honduras, Mary Flores. Within five minutes of her arrival, Tom had her in the palm of his hand, charming her and entertaining her with stories about rugby and the many global adventures and misadventures of his rugby team-mates, which included his sons Joe and Steve. He later charmed two US senators and several other prominent dignitaries. I asked Tom about his ability to meet and "charm" virtually anyone. He replied, "It doesn't matter if you are the greatest guy, or have the best and most noble ideas. People put their trust in people. In the end, it's all about getting to know people." Tom's life centered on knowing and caring for people. Whether in Dorchester or Rwanda, MGH or Somalia, Tom knew people everywhere. He had seen some of the worst in man, and that left him with an unquenchable thirst to be there for those who suffered under less caring hands.

Tom was the consummate world traveler, cursing in many languages, ("it gets you instant credibility") and raising the level of basic humanity all around him through laughter and goodwill. He had a stable of lines: "Was it love at first sight or should I walk by again?" "I loved your last movie." "The water in my knee is boiling." "I'm tired of being right, I just want to be obeyed (believed)." He had a way of bringing people to life. He always brought Swiss army knives with him and dispensed them to anyone who helped along the way, usually accompanying his gesture with a smile and a laugh. He had a keen eye for detail, often noting subtleties about people that escaped others. During our 1997 Belize trip, he commented on the eye color of one of our hosts and asked if she had some Portuguese ancestry. She had. Toward the end of that trip, we met Peter Allen, a dentist who had lived and worked in Belize for years. During a conversation with Tom, he mentioned that he used to drink Scotch but had not recently done so because it was so hard to come by. During my next visit to Belize, I delivered the bottle of single malt that Tom had handed me in Boston.

I have great memories of Tom. I can picture him laughing and buying rounds for a full table of Rotarians in Tegucigalpa. He could passionately deride the ruthless dictators of the world in one minute and tell a hilarious rugby story in the next. I remember discussing Balkan politics with him in the afternoon and turning on the Red Sox-Yankees playoff game (the Sox lost) in the evening, only to see him sitting a few rows back on the third-base side. I wasn't surprised when a surgical resident at St Elizabeth's told me he had met "the most amazing guy" in a bar (Christies) in Newport, Rhode Island, the other night. Of course, it was Tom. He lived the fullest life possible. If he had he spent his time and money on the "finer things," he would have missed the richness of the tapestry of the world's people—with their unconscionable suffering, their laughter, their humanity and love, their cruelty and compassion.

Few of us have the boundless energy that Tom had. I worked a particularly grueling overnight emergency room shift before flying to Belize with him on an early morning flight in 1997. When I mentioned that to him, he told me he had just flown straight back from Bosnia and had not slept in two days. He was 68; I was 37. That was the last time I ever mentioned my work schedule to him.

To get a sense of the man, consider that he had a heart-felt compassion, an incredible intellect, a broad historical perspective—much from having lived it, the quick wit of a stand-up comedian and the fiery passion of one transformed by what he had seen. That was Tom. During a dinner with colleagues Paula Buick and Ed Wyman in Tegucigalpa, our conversation turned surprisingly heated. Tom turned his Red Sox hat backward and zeroed in on my defense of then President Clinton. As the conversation progressed, I got the impression that one of us was about to learn something. "Clinton, like Bush before him, has blood on his hands," Tom roared. Referring to US inaction in Rwanda, he said, "All those people. He let them all die, when he could have stopped all the killing by landing one C-130 [a US military transport plane] in Kigali." And then, as if again relaying an apology to the dead, he repeated softly, "Just one C-130."

On a walk through the mud-covered streets of Tegucigalpa in the aftermath of the worst hurricane in the history of Honduras, reporter and friend Amalia Barreda asked Tom what lessons Mitch had taught us. "The response to something of this magnitude is a marathon, not a sprint," Tom said. Then he added, "It also shows you the resiliency of the human spirit." Tom's own spirit remains with us, challenging us to do more than we traditionally have for the oppressed of the world.

> *To practice medicine is a wonderful gift, but Tom Durant's legacy challenges each of us to think in the broader context.*

Tom helped shape my approach to service, infusing me with impressions of war and the ultimate medical catastrophes. Tom did not make pronouncements, preferring to lead by example. Still, I can infer the following from much of what he said: We have a duty to engage those who are suffering, both politically and personally. To practice medicine is a wonderful gift, but Tom Durant's legacy challenges each of us to think in the broader context. We may nobly heal in Boston, but if our government abandons Rwanda, leaving thousands to die, have we really served mankind well? We may develop cutting-edge treatments at our finest hospitals, but if only a small percentage of the world's people benefit, can we rightly claim success? Can we rightly claim that we have fulfilled the promise of our profession?

A Most Fitting Tribute

Tom Durant died on October 30, 2001, after a long battle with prostate cancer. (In 1999, he had gone directly from a German hospital bed, where he had received experimental immunotherapy treatment, to a squalid refugee camp in the Balkans [Mooney 2001].) On November 2, 2001, in Dorchester's St Mark's Church, Tom's son Stephen delivered the most beautiful eulogy I have ever heard. After sharing a number of funny and poignant stories about his father, Steve tried to describe who "Doc" was, first by examining the name that Steve felt "fit him perfectly." "Durant," he said, "is Old French for stubborn, but I think we'll leave that alone" ("Eulogy" 2001). "Thomas," he said, "was the name of the apostle who did not believe in the resurrected Christ. He had insisted on putting his hands into Jesus' wounds before he would believe." To Stephen, Tom Durant did the same for all of us. "My father needed to put his hands in the wounds. He was at his best when the suffering was right in front of him, demanding a response. It made him feel better too about his own sufferings. He wanted to be there. He needed to be there. When he was, his faith became strengthened and crystallized into action" ("Eulogy" 2001). Stephen continued,

> Life's not about status, it's not about money, it's not about power. It's about people. It's about loving people . . . that's it. You can do that anywhere . . . Cambodia, Rwanda, Dorchester Avenue, MGH, the rugby pitch . . . anywhere. My dad did his best to be a man for others. He wasn't perfect but he totally understood that it's about people. In our faith, we are called **not** necessarily to save the world, **not** to save lives, **not** to make all things perfect . . . we are called for one job, to witness the truth. What is the truth you ask? That was Pilate's question. The truth is this. There is a God and we are wonderfully made and LOVED. Our job is to witness that love and pass it on in our own unique idiosyncratic fumbling way. God trusts us with that task and gives us the freedom to do it, however haphazard and limited we may be in our attempt. Maybe it means we hold someone's hand. Maybe we bind their wounds. Maybe we bring them water. Maybe we work with them or for them or maybe we give them work. We put our hands in the wounds. We are called to place ourselves in the path of suffering. Take the punch. But at the end of the day do it with passion and humor and grace and hope and joy. Do NOT be afraid. The good my father did was not *in* him. It was not *of* him. It came *through* him. It comes from God. . . . He passed that love onto others and brought back love and truth to us. He was our guy in those places. He carried us with him and he carried *them* back to us. . . . Everyone is connected. What you do matters. Right now, right here. In his slide presentations and just in general, my father cried more and more toward the end of his life. I think he completely grasped the truth of what I am struggling to say here.
>
> So you want to honor my father . . . to remember him. Don't be afraid to hold someone's hand. Don't be afraid to hug someone. Don't be afraid to reach out to someone in need or in pain. Take a punch . . . maybe even throw one . . . if the cause is just. Tell the poseurs and the phonies where they can go. Don't be

concerned with your own status, your own power and your own wealth. Be grateful. Dance, laugh, play, sing, but make sure you pass on your love . . . like he did ("Eulogy" 2001).

Steve's eloquence bespeaks a deep love and respect for his father, even though his work took Tom away from his family for long stretches of time. As for me, I miss my friend, my mentor, my great teacher. Tom was such a rare gem among those who do international work, where some take themselves far too seriously. The world became a colder place when he left it. As I continue my own quest, I miss the guiding voice on the other end of the line, always available, always willing to listen and advise. For many patients and colleagues in the world's poorest places at the worst times in their histories, Tom was the laughter amidst a sea of tears.

In the months following his death, I had a recurring vision of a man in a rugby shirt, singing and laughing as if tomorrow would never come. I long to pick up the phone and hear that reassuring voice, telling a story of a recent visit to Bosnia or Honduras or railing on about some stupefying pronouncement by someone in the public eye. Like so many others, I wish I could return to the house on Melville Avenue in Dorchester and hear just one more song.

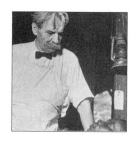

Chapter 16

The Life of Albert Schweitzer, MD

I decided I would make my life my argument.
—**Dr Albert Schweitzer**

I first met Albert Schweitzer on a crisp, fall night in Boston in 1991, some 26 years after his death. The occasion was a symposium sponsored by The Albert Schweitzer Fellowship, titled, Reverence for Life: The Importance of Albert Schweitzer's Ethic for Boston and the World Today. Through the testimony of those who knew him and the passionate oratory of those who had long followed similar ideals, a picture of the man began to emerge. Schweitzer was possessed by a divinely inspired passion to make a difference, and he followed that passion to a life of hardship in the jungles of West Africa.

Along the way, he spelled out his reasons for doing this, and the world took notice. He inspired millions and shone like a moral beacon through the decades. Lauded with honorary degrees, volumes of praise, and a Nobel Peace Prize, Schweitzer became, in President John F. Kennedy's words, "the towering moral figure of the twentieth century." He became, for me, a man to understand.

What follows is a condensed version of the life of Albert Schweitzer, one of the century's great figures. Any clinician who is thinking about working internationally to treat those who are less fortunate will benefit from knowing about Schweitzer and understanding his words. Specifically, he said that service to those in need is more than just charity; it is an ethical imperative that we all share. "My life is my argument," he explained. What exactly was his life, what argument did it make, and why should we care now, all these years later? To properly address the life and thought of Albert Schweitzer, I have separated the two. In this chapter, you will read of his extraordinary

*journey, from gifted musician, philosopher, and theologian in Europe to
minister, builder, and healer in West Africa. Of most relevance, you will learn
why he made such an extraordinary life change and what he left behind for
those interested in following—however briefly—in his footsteps. In Chapter 17
you will better understand how he developed his philosophy—"Reverence for
Life"—and how it remains relevant more than 50 years later, compelling each
of us to give part of our own lives in service to those who are less fortunate.*

Albert Schweitzer was born in 1875 in Alsace, the fertile region midway
between Germany and France. As a border territory, its population suffered
heavy casualties in a number of wars, including the Franco–Prussian War
and World Wars I and II. The region frequently changed hands between the
oft-warring colonial powers, with Alsatians' shifting political and cultural
ties between Paris and Berlin. Thus, linguistic, religious, and cultural influences from France and Germany greatly influenced the population of the
region, including young Albert. These roots later enabled the gifted young
scholar to study under the great minds in music, theology, and philosophy
in both countries.

Schweitzer spent his youth in Alsace. His family moved to Gunsbach just
a few weeks after his birth in Kayersberg. Because Germany had taken the
provinces of Alsace and Lorraine in a settlement following the Franco–Prussian
War $3\text{-}\frac{1}{2}$ years before his birth, Schweitzer was born a German citizen. This
historical occurrence would cost him dearly later in his life, as the horrors of
World Wars I and II still lay ahead. His father, Louis Schweitzer, was a strong,
articulate, and liberal Protestant minister, himself the son of a schoolmaster/
organist. Adele Schweitzer, Albert's mother, was the daughter of an organist
and organ builder, Schillinger, who also was a pastor. Intelligence and liberal
thinking characterized Albert's extended family. A much younger cousin
achieved worldwide recognition as an existential philosopher, playwright,
and novelist. His name was Jean-Paul Sartre.

Early Influences

Young Albert, along with his brother and three sisters, spent every Sunday
in church listening to his father's sermons. Albert began to study the New
Testament at age eight and soon after displayed a forceful inquisitiveness. His
mother taught him his bedtime prayers and gave her young son an appreciation for the wonder of Nature. For both mother and son, Nature offered
a soothing escape from life's troubles. She—and he in turn—developed a love
for Nature and the calm it instilled. She often took him, his brother, and two
sisters for walks in the countryside near Gunsbach. As they walked by
a much-loved lakeside, she would say, "Here I am completely at home. Here
among the rocks, among the woods. I came here as a child. Let me breathe
the fragrance of the fir trees and enjoy the quiet of this refuge from the

world. Do not speak. After I am no longer on earth, come here and think of me" (Bentley 1992, 14).Years later, after his mother's death, Schweitzer had a house built in Gunsbach and returned often to the solace and quiet of the lake to think of her.

In an early indication of his life's philosophy, Schweitzer was bothered that his prayers were always said for people only and "mostly around one's own interests" (Marshall and Poling 1971, 25). After his mother left the room, he added his own prayer: "Bless and protect all things that have breath, guard them from evil, and let them sleep in peace" (25). Photographs of Schweitzer working in Lambarene with his pet pelican, Parsifal, following behind, and photographs of him seated at his writing table with his cat, Sissy, reflect a lifelong devotion to animals. As a young child he saw two men cruelly leading an old, sickly horse through the narrow streets of Gunsbach, likely to its death at a nearby glue factory. The men pulled and beat the horse in a futile effort to urge it forward and move faster to its end.

The young Albert Schweitzer rarely revealed his brilliance or talents.

The blatant disregard the two men showed for the horse's obvious suffering made an indelible impression on the young Schweitzer. He couldn't understand how people could have such disrespect for other forms of life.

The young Albert Schweitzer rarely revealed his brilliance or talents. He did not distinguish himself academically early on—merely passing his subjects. When he recognized innate gifts in a certain area, he felt guilt, not pride, that he should be so fortunate while others were not. As a pastor's son and one of five children, Albert Schweitzer was not well off but he was better off than most. He resented any material or outward expression of affluence, even refusing to wear a new coat or hat that might set him apart from his classmates, most of whom were poor. He kept his feelings inside, a trait that continued throughout his adult life. He later commented, "I believe that no-one should force himself to show to others more of his inner life than he feels it natural to reveal" (Bentley 1992, 16). This later opened a door for those who sought to criticize him; he guarded his privacy and often did not respond even to outrageous charges.

The Musician

Music coursed through the veins of the grandson of Pastor Schillinger of Muhlbach. Albert inherited the musical passion and talent of his maternal grandfather, who was both a noted organ builder and a performer with a flair for improvisation. Early on, Albert developed a love for the organ—the instrument that was an intimate part of church services and the national instrument of Germany. By age nine, he had become proficient enough to substitute for the organist in his father's church in Gunsbach. The strong tie of the organ to religion no doubt fueled his interest. He later wrote, "The organ has in it an element of the eternal. Even in a secular room it cannot become a secular instrument" (Schweitzer 1933, 80).

He found resonance in the music of Johann Sebastian Bach, whose works, such as the "St. Matthew Passion," evoked strong religious feelings. Schweitzer later acquired a complete collection of Bach's organ works and, in the quiet of night in his study, wrote the definitive book *The Complete Organ Works of J.S. Bach.* He also wrote biographies of Bach in both French and German. Schweitzer became a Bach scholar, describing him as "a poet and painter in sound" who conveyed "the purest religious feeling" (Schweitzer 1933, 66). Schweitzer elaborates, "A soul that longs for peace out of the world's unrest and has itself already tasted peace allows others to share its experience in this music" (67). Schweitzer biographer James Bentley commented, "Lutheranism then as now was a passionately musical facet of the Christian world and Bach its demigod" (1992, 39). Because young Albert was contemplating the life of minister–philosopher, Bach's music offered the ideal complement to his coming years of rigorous study.

The Scholar

In October 1893, the 18-year-old scholar began studies at the University of Strasbourg, which then was at the height of its fame and the most liberal university in Europe. German rationalism, which later coursed through Schweitzer's writings, dominated the intellectual discourse of the faculty. German philosophers Hegel, Kant, and Schopenhauer, along with theologians Baur, Weber, Muller, and Harnack inspired and motivated faculty and students alike. Students were encouraged to pursue independent research and employ the principles of reason and inductive logic. Above all else, "the free mind was viewed as the highest achievement of intellectual authority" (Marshall and Poling 1971, 40).

Paris, Berlin, and Strasbourg served as the background for Schweitzer's philosophical study. Schweitzer thrived at the Sorbonne and the Universities of Berlin and Strasbourg. While in Paris he also devoted a considerable amount of time to the organ, studying under the renowned Widor—who recognized his pupil's great talent and taught him without charge. Schweitzer read the great philosophers, immersing himself in deep study. He later wrote, "My good health allowed me to be prodigal with nocturnal labor. It happened sometimes that I played for Widor in the morning without having been to bed at all" (1933, 19). He wrote and later published his doctoral dissertation on the religious philosophy of Immanuel Kant, the great German philosopher and theologian. From Kant, Schweitzer wrote that "the ethical is a mysterious fact within us," and that it was "ethics which frees us from the natural order of the world of the senses, and attaches us to a higher world-order" (182). In Kant Schweitzer found a thinker—much like himself—who viewed God and mankind through the lens of morality and ethics. In July 1899, Schweitzer received a PhD in Philosophy at Strasbourg.

The Theologian

Immediately afterward, Schweitzer turned his full attention to theology. Although he held a deep Christian faith, he would not let more restrictive Christian dogma obscure the clear light of reason. Unlike many of his time and most before it, he felt that a search for truth and historical accuracy in studying the life of Jesus would strengthen the Church, not weaken it. "The fundamental principles of Christianity have to be proved true by reasoning, and by no other method" (Marshall and Poling 1971, 58). He added, "Since the essential nature of the spiritual is truth, every new truth represents a gain. . . . Religion has, therefore, nothing to fear from a confrontation with historical truth" (Schweitzer 1933, 54).

As a brash young scholar, Schweitzer openly questioned the historical accuracy of some of the statements in the New Testament, leading him to his most important contribution to theology. His subsequent book, *The Quest for the Historical Jesus*, made a lasting contribution to Christian theology and became popular all over Europe. For years, this book remained an important resource for those studying the historical life of Jesus. Schweitzer's positions, however, did cause members of the Christian establishment to bristle. Many did not share his views, and he later paid dearly for challenging the Christian conservatives. He said, "I have not wished to create problems for Christianity. I have suffered deeply because some of my ideas have become problems for Christianity" (Cousins 1960, 195).

> The Quest for the Historical Jesus *made a lasting contribution to Christian theology and became popular all over Europe.*

Of all the influences on Albert Schweitzer, none was more important than Jesus, and no time more valuable than that spent studying Jesus's life. Jesus inspired Schweitzer, both through the power of his words and the example of his life. Schweitzer often referred to Jesus' saying, "Whoever would save his life shall lose it, and whoever shall lose his life for My sake and the Gospels shall save it" (Schweitzer 1933, 82). In pursuing the historical Jesus, Schweitzer followed a path of reasoned exploration. What he found was a flawed but real person. The son of the Lutheran minister challenged the established Christian theology and emerged with a far deeper conviction and faith, based on reason and the clarification of the ethical component of Jesus's life and words. "He kindles the fire of an ethical faith. The truth that the ethical is the essence of religion is firmly established on the authority of Jesus," he wrote (60).

More than Kant, Hegel, Shillinger, or any other philosopher Schweitzer had studied, Jesus offered a path to an ethical view of the world. In Jesus,

Schweitzer found a man who thought, prayed, and taught but, most important, acted on his beliefs, offering up the most precious of gifts for his most deeply held beliefs—life itself. Preaching to parishioners at St Nicholae in 1904, Schweitzer said, "Let everything else go, so long as you hold on to this one truth: Jesus is a man who demands your help in the work He Himself began" (Bentley 1992, 35). Speaking with author Norman Cousins on the significance of Jesus's teachings to his own life course, Schweitzer commented:

> New ideas in this field of thought [Christianity] are powerful things. One cannot just conceive of them as mere intellectual properties and then take leave of them. . . . This is what I mean when I say I came to Lambarene because I wanted my life to be my argument. I didn't want my ideas to become an end in themselves. The ideas took hold of me and changed my life. Resistance to those ideas would have been impossible (Cousins 1960, 195).

On July 15, 1900, Schweitzer passed the examination for the licentiate degree of theology en route to prosperous careers in philosophy, theology, and music. In September he was ordained as a curate at St Nicholae in Strasbourg, soon finding that preaching had become for him "an inner necessity." He noted, "I felt it something wonderful to be allowed to speak to my assembled fellow men and women on the deepest questions of existence" (Bentley 1992, 105). He received teaching appointments at the University of Strasbourg and the Theological College of St Thomas, where he became the latter's principal in 1903. He published books on the Last Supper, Bach, and another on Christianity—*The Mystery of the Kingdom of God*. At age 28, Schweitzer became the organist of the Paris Bach Society, and his organ recitals in the concert halls of European capitol cities secured his status as a rising star in European society. By age 30, he was widely known for his talents in theology, philosophy, and music. Successful careers in any of these three disciplines awaited him. He had only to choose.

A Restless Spirit and the Decision to Go to Africa

Despite holding two degrees and achieving near dreamlike success in three disciplines, not all was well with Albert Schweitzer. He felt restless and wondered if people really understood the meaning of his words. He worried that he understood what Jesus had said but was not fully living out his beliefs. Schweitzer's was an active faith, one that struggled with the direction of his current path: Am I supposed to devote my life to making ever fresh critical discoveries, so as to become a famous theologian, and to go on training pastors who will also sit at home? It became clear to me that this is not my life. I want to be a simple human being, to do something small in the spirit of Jesus" (Bentley 1992, 110).

On a spring day in Gunsbach, he began to think that he owed something for his good fortune and that, like Jesus, he would dedicate his life to the service of humanity. He recalled the day in his autobiography:

> It struck me as inconceivable that I should be allowed to lead such a happy life while I saw so many people around me struggling with sorrow and suffering. . . . I could not help but think continually of others who were denied that good fortune by their material circumstances or their health. One brilliant summer morning at Gunsbach, during the holidays—it was 1896—as I awoke, the thought came to me that I must not accept this good fortune as a matter of course, but must give something in return. While outside the birds sang I reflected on this thought, and before I had gotten up I came to the conclusion that until I was thirty I could consider myself justified in devoting myself to scholarship and the arts, but after that I would devote myself directly to serving humanity (Schweitzer 1933, 82).

Schweitzer had heard the call of service and decided wholeheartedly to pursue it. As he approached 30 years of age, his resolve increased. During his academic years he unsuccessfully tried volunteer work with orphans, poor families of Gunsbach, and prisoners. None had worked out well, and Schweitzer looked for an opportunity to devote himself to "an absolutely personal and independent activity," in which he could serve unrestricted by the bureaucracy of any organization (Schweitzer 1933, 85).

At age 29, he picked up a magazine that had been left on his writing table, titled, *Journal des Missions Évangélique*, published by the Paris Missionary Society, a Christian organization that had established missions throughout French Equatorial Africa. The June 1904 edition of the journal contained an article titled, "The Needs of the Congo Mission," written by then president Alfred Boegner, who (Schweitzer 1933, 85; Marshall and Poling 1971, 73) wrote that the mission did not have enough people to carry out its work in Gabon, in the Congo colony. The mission particularly needed those who could offer relief in the form of medical care. Boegner issued a desperate plea for a response from those "on whom the Master's eyes already rested" (Schweitzer 1933, 85). Schweitzer wrote, "I finished my article and quietly began my work. My search was over" (86).

Although his autobiography characterizes his momentous decision as rational and devoid of emotion, letters from Schweitzer to Hélène Bresslau at the time reveal some of the angst he clearly felt. One of the most revealing sentences comes from a letter he wrote in 1902: "There are times," the future Nobel Laureate says, "when I am afraid of my own future, it all seems so difficult."[1]

Schweitzer stressed that his decision had not come through "hearing the voice of God, or anything like that," and strongly objected to the idea that he had a "calling" to serve as a doctor in Africa (Cousins 1960, 192). To the theologians who stated they had indeed heard the voice of God, Schweitzer didn't argue the point, merely commenting that their ears were sharper than his. His decision, like everything else in his life, was a purely rational one, following the example of love shown by Jesus. Schweitzer wrote to Hélène Bresslau in September 1910, "I must carry the glow of the Christmas lights into the world . . . become simply human . . . in order to serve the one who was human and is my Lord . . ."[2] That he should find an opportunity to serve in equatorial Africa he considered his great fortune.

> In choosing Africa, Schweitzer combined his Christian ideal for an ethically motivated course of action with a deeply held sense of justice.

In choosing Africa, Schweitzer combined his Christian ideal for an ethically motivated course of action with a deeply held sense of justice. Tales of brutal oppression that seeped back to Europe from colonial Africa challenged the moral sensibilities of the young Schweitzer and many other conscientious Europeans. As a child, Schweitzer had frequently visited his grandparents' home in the Alsatian town of Colmar, birthplace of the sculptor Frederic Auguste Bartholdi, best known for creating the Statue of Liberty. In the town square there stood another Bartholdi creation, a monument to Admiral Bruat. One of the figures clustered around the admiral was that of an African slave, noble and powerful, yet wearing a facial expression that belied a deep melancholy. As a young boy, Schweitzer used to go to the square and sit, staring at the slave. He recalled, "His face, with its sad, thoughtful expression, spoke to me of the misery of the Dark Continent. If a record could be made of all that has happened between the white and the colored races, some of the pages—referring to recent as well as earlier times—would be turned over unread, because their contents would be too horrible for the reader" (Bentley 1992, 82; Schweitzer 1948a, 115). The statue was destroyed sometime during the German occupation between 1940 and 1945. Years later, the town of Colmar donated the head of the statue to Schweitzer and, according to his daughter Rhena, it still sits on his desk in Gunsbach.[3]

When Schweitzer decided upon service in the "Congo Mission," he—like the rest of the world—had only a superficial understanding of how much the Africans were suffering at the hands of their European conquerors. According to author Adam Hocksfeld, the Congo during this period was the scene of one of the century's worst cruelties. In the late 1800s, King Leopold II of Belgium transformed large tracts of land along the Congo River into enormous personal wealth, reaping profits estimated in today's terms at $1.1 billion (Hochschild 1998, 277). Under the guise of a Belgian protectorate, Leopold's soldiers slaughtered, starved, and mutilated millions of Africans while extracting first ivory, then rubber, from the area. Population surveys show that between the years 1880 and 1920, the population of the region just 100 miles south of the site of Schweitzer's future hospital in Lambarene decreased by half, or roughly 10 million people, making

King Leopold II's rule over the Congo one of the worst genocides in human history (233).

The Belgian "Protectorate" soldiers and employees of the Anglo–Belgian India Rubber Company routinely committed atrocities against their African captives in a never-ending pursuit of higher profits. Decapitations and mutilations became commonplace. Many Africans, including young children, lost hands and feet to their captors' blades. Some Belgian officers adopted the macabre habit of staking severed African heads around their living

The best and worst of man were to become neighbors near the heart of Africa.

quarters. A story printed in the *Saturday Review* of December 17, 1898, described Belgian Captain Leon Rom decorating his flower bed with the severed heads of 21 African women and children (Hochschild 1998, 145).

Into this setting sailed a young Polish merchant named Konrad Korzeniowski, later known to the world under the pen name Joseph Conrad. His descriptions of Leopold's African colony became one of the most widely read short stories of all time, "The Heart of Darkness." Captain Rom and a few other Belgian officers may have been the prototypes for Conrad's Mr Kurtz. Although Conrad's epic became "one of the most scathing indictments of imperialism in all literature," it achieved immortality through its clear description of the potential for darkness in all humans (Hochschild 1998, 146). It is hard to imagine a more stark contrast than the real-life figures who inspired Conrad's Mr Kurtz and the young German minister preparing to become a healer for the Africans. The best and worst of man were to become neighbors near the heart of Africa. European missionaries witnessed the atrocities first-hand and were familiar with the dire conditions of much of colonized Africa. Much of what they saw found its way into the daily newspapers, prompting the first international human rights campaign, led by a Belgian clerk named ED Morel. Schweitzer read the press reports that circulated widely between 1900 and 1910, which no doubt helped confirm his decision to serve where the need was greatest. He wrote, "We must make atonement for all the terrible crimes we read of in the newspapers. We must make atonement for the still worse ones, which we do not read about in the papers, crimes that are shrouded in the silence of the jungle night" (Marshall and Poling 1971, 74).

In August of 1905, Schweitzer's future wife, Hélène Bresslau, heard missionary Dr Gratton Guiness lecture about King Leopold's commercially motivated abuse of the Africans in the Belgian Congo. In summarizing parts of the lecture to Schweitzer, she wrote, ". . . It was horrifying, even if only half of the cruelties he reported are actually committed there." She then added prophetically, ". . . If the descriptions of the atrocities are based on fact, no responsible person could remain a calm observer."[4]

On the subject of race relations, the themes of atonement and justice dominate Schweitzer's writings. He was particularly troubled by the extent to which people who professed themselves Christian had brought such unrelenting misery to the Africans. He therefore viewed it not as a matter of charity that he served in Africa but, rather, as a matter of justice.

> We are not free to confer benefits on these men, or not, as we please; it is our duty. Anything we give them is not benevolence but atonement. For every one who scattered injury someone ought to go out to take help, and when we have done all that is in our power, we shall not have atoned for the thousandth part of our guilt. That is the foundation from which all deliberations about "works of mercy" out there must begin (Schweitzer 1948a, 116; Cousins 1960, 210).

In addition to his overwhelming need for justice and ethical action, Schweitzer felt increasingly distant from the religion and civilization of his birth. He believed that Christianity had become overcomplicated and had become more concerned with debating theological controversies than spreading the great and simple truths in the life and words of Jesus. He saw stagnation in the Church he so loved and he urged it forward. "Christianity must not be afraid of change," he said. "It must not be afraid to examine and reexamine and grow. Jesus symbolized change and growth" (Cousins 1960, 195). Schweitzer saw Europe in decline and civilization itself regressing. He saw a generation in decline, proud of its achievements, yet increasingly devoid of the ethical values upon which progress in any civilization rests. He could no longer remain inactive. The restless embers that simmered deep within Albert Schweitzer were about to ignite.

Chasing Hippocrates

On October 13, 1905, Schweitzer mailed letters to his parents, friends, and colleagues, informing them of his decision to become a doctor and serve in equatorial Africa. His decision to abandon a promising life and pursue uncharted territory was extraordinary. His family, friends, and the intelligentsia of his day were baffled, even upset with his decision. They found it difficult to comprehend how he could cast aside a future of remarkable promise for a task that others of less promise could easily carry out. Schweitzer wrote, "My relatives and friends reproached me for the folly of my enterprise. They said I was a man who was burying the talent entrusted to him and wanted to trade in false currency" (1933, 86). He was amazed that many who called themselves Christians could not understand that "the desire to serve the love preached by Jesus may sweep a man into a new course of life" (87). Through the many trials he endured, he learned a lesson oft revealed to those who have since followed his example: "Anyone who proposes to do good must not expect people to roll any stones out of his way, and must calmly accept his lot even if they roll a few more into it" (90).

In choosing his course, Schweitzer realized that he would have to sacrifice music, philosophy, and theology, all areas that had profound meaning and importance for him. He wrote that there were "no heroes of action, only

heroes of renunciation and suffering" (1933, 88). He soon embarked on
a path that his daughter later described as "a hard life—very much like that of
a monk."[5] After quitting his teaching positions, he found it difficult to walk past
St Nicholea's Church or the university. The thought that he might never again participate
in his beloved teaching and preaching was so painful for him that he avoided even the
sight of the places of his former activities.

> *Of all the needs of the poor peoples in equatorial Africa at that time, none was more pressing than the need for health care.*

Of particular interest to those in the health professions is the reason
Schweitzer pursued medicine. Although his commitment to service was
clear, he could have helped the world's less fortunate in many ways, including two vocations he already practiced—teacher and minister. Still, at the age
of 30, Schweitzer began studies to become a doctor. He realized that of all
the needs of the poor peoples in equatorial Africa at that time, none was
more pressing than the need for health care. Frequently, missionary writers
of the time said they regretted not being able to offer medical care to the
afflicted Africans who were in great physical pain. Schweitzer hoped one
day to become, in his words, "the doctor whom these unhappy people
needed" (1933, 92). He wanted to turn his verbal ministries into physical
and clinical ones. Thus he committed himself to an arduous course of study,
and soon found himself fighting the worst periods of fatigue of his life.
He later elaborated on his decision:

> I wanted to be a doctor so that I might be able to work without having to talk.
> For years I had been giving of myself in words, and it was with joy that I had followed the calling of teacher and preacher. But this new form of activity would
> consist not in preaching the religion of love, but in practicing it. Medical knowledge would make it possible for me to carry out my intention in the best and
> most complete way, wherever the path of service might lead me (1933, 92).

From 1905 to 1912, Schweitzer studied medicine at the University of
Strasbourg. Though he fully expected to sacrifice his music, preaching, and
writing the day he left for Africa, he continued to lecture to his theology students and preach at St Nicholae while he was in medical school. He played
the organ for the Paris Bach Society, traveling to Paris several times each
winter for performances. On the train en route back to Strasbourg, he
sketched out Sunday sermons. Because he needed income for the medical
supplies his impending African service would demand, he increased his
pace of performing concerts and recitals. Along with his music, his writing
thrived while he studied medicine. He completed the *The Quest of the
Historical Jesus* (JCB Mohr, 1906) and wrote additional books on organ
building, Bach, and Paul the Apostle. During these years the pace of life
proved difficult for the previously indefatigable Schweitzer. He recalled this
time as the "worst crisis of exhaustion that I can recall during my whole life"
(1933, 105). It is said that he regularly asked a housekeeper to leave a basin

of cold water in his room. She thought it was to wipe his brow during studies and only later realized that he plunged his feet into the basin and forcibly kept them there to keep the nocturnal fatigue from overtaking him.

In October 1910, Schweitzer took the state medical examination and qualified as a medical doctor. He subsequently completed his internship and residency, going to Paris in 1912 to specialize in tropical medicine. There he also began to acquire supplies for his pending trip to Africa. He received his MD in February 1913 at the age of 38, adding it to his PhD in philosophy and licentiate degree in theology. His excursion to Africa cost him the opportunity to earn his PhD in theology—something he had long wanted. Years later, after a host of honorary doctorate degrees, a 1947 *Life* magazine story described him as "the Greatest Man in the World." The article read as follows:

> He is Albert Schweitzer, Ph.D., Th.D., Mus.D., M.D., a 72-year-old medical missionary who lives among the wild cannibals at Lambarene, deep in the jungles of French Equatorial Africa ("The Greatest" 1947).

Schweitzer would not have described his neighbors as "wild cannibals," but his uniqueness remains. It is doubtful that the world will see a similar description applied to anyone.

A Partnership, a Wife, and the Lost Letters

While still an undergraduate student, Schweitzer met Hélène Bresslau, daughter of a distinguished professor of history at the University of Strasbourg. They met at a friend's wedding, and she had regularly attended Schweitzer's sermons. Their relationship grew as Schweitzer frequently visited Helene's father, Professor Bresslau, to discuss philosophy and religion. Young Schweitzer greatly admired Professor Bresslau, an atheist with a Jewish background. His quiet and studious daughter, however, had been baptized as a child and spent her life as a devout Christian. She had become a social worker at a time when that was a rarity for women. She came to admire and fall in love with the brilliant university student. When Schweitzer weathered the turbulence generated by his controversial theological positions and his decision to depart for Africa, Hélène stood with him. In characteristic fashion, however, Schweitzer revealed little about their relationship.

As the friendship of Albert and Hélène deepened, he came to rely on her. She became his confidante and the person who best understood his passions. They began a correspondence in 1901, which their daughter, Rhena Schweitzer Miller, discovered only recently. According to Rhena, "My father would be furious with me if he knew I had released [the letters]," since this was a side of his life that he wanted no one to see.[6] Still, in the winter of 1999, Rhena sent me copies of the English translation of more than 200 pages of his letters and approved their inclusion here.

The letters reveal a softer, less secure Albert Schweitzer and the beginnings of a loving relationship that both kept secret for as long as possible—though it is not clear why. Albert clearly loved Hélène and likely would not have become the man he was without her support and encouragement. In one of many love letters, Albert wrote:

There is now something so serene and so beautiful in you—do you know how much you give me? How easy it is to walk the good and straight path, to reach "'higher,"' if one is supported as I am through you! If you would know how freely and deeply I breathe in this air—and how grateful I am to you. You are such a wonderful woman."[7]

Despite clearly loving and needing Hélène, Albert implored her to marry someone else and have children of her own. It seems that he did not consider the possibility of having children of their own, given the path he had chosen. He acknowledged that Hélène had sacrificed "the most beautiful years" of her life waiting for him in exchange for "a life of hard work, shaken by struggles with yourself and your family, full of sadness . . . with much heavy loneliness. . . . And all that for me!"[8] In a touching letter that runs counter to the public image he portrayed, Schweitzer wrote,

> My darling, do you know how much you are giving me? Sometimes it chokes me, and I ask myself if it is right for me to accept it. What a modest and impoverished life I am offering you. . . .what a struggle for health! . . . I shudder at the thought of living on charity one day, and hardly dare to think that you will share this life. And a life in which illness and death lie in wait for us. . . .[8]

The letters written by both Albert and Hélène reveal that each realized the sacrifice at hand. But each of them did so willingly in their belief that service to Jesus took priority over all else, including their own personal happiness or material comforts. Hélène may or may not have stayed on this path had she foreseen her own future. But in 1911, she wrote to Schweitzer and admonished him for his concerns. "Don't you know that you are always, always free & would be completely free, yes, [Albert], utterly and completely free the moment you might wish for it?"[9] They married on June 18, 1912, and left for Africa less than a year later.

One Final Hurdle

A publication of the Paris Missionary Society years earlier had redirected the path of Albert Schweitzer. He had since completed his medical studies and stood ready to accept the Society's call to heal the sick in Africa. As a doctor and a minister, Schweitzer seemed the ideal candidate, one who no doubt would bring the society considerable international attention. There was just one problem: Schweitzer had articulated liberal views in his theological dissertations, and his publication, *The Quest of the Historical Jesus*, was seen as an affront to the more conservative Christians, who included members of the Paris Missionary Society. Schweitzer's application was rejected. He was not sufficiently orthodox. Then Schweitzer offered to serve as a doctor only, completely abandoning his preaching. Still the Society refused, saying that Schweitzer's radical scriptural interpretations might "confuse the natives." Schweitzer's daughter later recalled how much patience her father, an ordinarily impatient man, showed this organization.

He determined that he would strengthen his position and resubmit his application. His wife Hélène was shocked that his application was rejected but nevertheless joined him in a fund-raising campaign to build and sustain a hospital deep in the jungle of Gabon, under the aegis of the Paris Missionary Society. Schweitzer planned to reapply, after raising sufficient funds, assuring the Society that he would need no money and would remain "muet comme une carpe," or "dumb as a carp," in religious matters (Schweitzer 1933, 15). Despite some embarrassment in soliciting funds, Schweitzer found that the kindness people showed far outweighed the humiliation he had to endure during these rounds. Parishioners at St Nicholae contributed generously, as did former pupils, friends, medical school faculty, and colleagues from his other disciplines. He performed benefit concerts, collected book royalties, and soon had enough funds to run the hospital for a year.

> *He repeated his vow of silence and finally persuaded the Society to accept him.*

Then he went back to the Society and, refusing their offer to submit to theological questioning before them, met individual members one by one. With great personal charm he allayed their fears. He repeated his vow of silence and finally persuaded the Society to accept him, prompting one board member to submit his resignation. On the afternoon of Good Friday, 1913, Albert and Hélène said good-bye to their parents—it was the last time he would ever see his mother—and set off for the train station in Gunsbach. Nearly the entire town came to see them off. With tears in his eyes, Schweitzer joined his wife in the fourth-class section of the railway car, destined to write a new chapter in the text of an already extraordinary life.

Africa at Last

The Schweitzers boarded a ship at Bordeaux and sailed more than 5,000 miles south over a stormy Atlantic, hugging the western coast of Africa. After nearly three weeks, they finally arrived at Port-Gentil, a city at the mouth of the Ogowe River in Gabon, West Africa. There they boarded a steamboat to make the 130-mile trip to Lambarene. The final leg of their journey took them through miles of deep jungle, revealing to them all the beauty and splendor of their new home: "River and forest. . . ! Who can really describe the first impression they make? We seemed to be dreaming," wrote Dr Schweitzer (1948b, 15), upon seeing the Ogowe for the first time. Such was Schweitzer's introduction to the place where he would spend most of his life, beginning in the mission station in Andende, a small enclave situated along a tributary of the Ogowe River.

The Ogowe River has served as the main highway connecting African tribes throughout the region for centuries. The river is one of Africa's largest, consisting of a series of smaller tributaries that connect hundreds of square miles of dense tropical jungle. Traveling by pirogues—small, dugout canoes—the sick could reach the new European doctor. Andende itself sits a mere 40 miles from the equator and remains home to several different tribes, including some that practiced cannibalism at the time of Schweitzer's arrival. Populating the area are gorillas, leopards, elephants, and hippopotami, as well as large snakes that occasionally surprise the unsuspecting boatman.

The bungalow at Andende that became the Schweitzers' new home was just 2 miles upstream from the island of Lambarene, across from which Schweitzer would later move his famous hospital. Lambarene is a 2-mile long, oval-shaped island engulfed by the Ogowe River, which stretches for nearly a mile on either side. The area is covered by lush tropical jungle, with all the beauty and humidity that entails. As native drums spread word of the new European doctor's arrival in Andende, the Schweitzers found themselves without medical supplies, an interpreter, or a hospital. The Paris Missionary Society had kept its promise to supply living quarters but not much else. As such, Schweitzer was little prepared for the droves of patients who sought his services just after he arrived. "From the very first days, even before I had found time to unpack my drugs and instruments, I was besieged by sick people," Schweitzer wrote (1933, 136).

Initially, patients came from the two local tribes—the Galloa and Pahouin. Later they came from all over the region, some from hundreds of miles away. Schweitzer saw only the most urgent cases immediately. Then, after three weeks of preparations, he began treating all who came. Lacking a formal hospital, he saw patients on the veranda of his living quarters until the makeshift first hospital—a converted chicken coop—was ready. On August 13, 1913, he successfully conducted his first operation—repair of a strangulated inguinal hernia. Most Africans had seen the agony of those dying from the strangulated hernia and attributed these deaths to powerful spirits. The European "Oganga," or fetishman, as Schweitzer was called, could "kill" a person, cut something out of him, and then bring him back to life without the pain he had before. Such was the power of the European medicine man. None of the local talisman could match him.

Schweitzer's reputation spread, bringing in even more patients. The bulk of his clinical work consisted of cases of malaria, leprosy, sleeping sickness, dysentery, pneumonia, heart disease, elephantiasis, tumors, and hernias. Schweitzer wrote of the common cases of strangulated hernias:

> How can I describe my feelings when a poor fellow is brought to me in this condition? I am the only person within hundreds of miles who can help him. . . .

We must all die. But that I can save him from days of torture, that is what I feel as my great and ever new privilege. Pain is a more terrible lord of mankind than even death itself" (1948b, 62).

He found that he could offer a valuable service for thousands of people, even with modest equipment and medicines.

By late autumn of that first year, he had finished construction of the first real hospital in Andende, funded by his fellow missionaries. It measured 26 by 13 feet, with corrugated-iron walls, enclosed at either end by mosquito netting. It housed a small consulting room, an operating theater, and a dispensary. Schweitzer soon began work on a patient dormitory, followed by an isolation ward for infectious cases. He found that the only way to get the laborers to do the work was for him to work alongside them. Schweitzer soon spent much of his time in Lambarene remodeling and building new additions to his hospital, a pattern that persisted through most of his life there. The genius behind *The Quest of the Historical Jesus* became, by necessity, a proficient architect and builder.

[My father] had to give them a village, not a hospital.

From the first days, the villagers made themselves at home in the new hospital, and Schweitzer accommodated them. As was the tradition among the tribes, family members accompanied their sick relatives to the hospital area and stayed with them until they were well enough to leave. They cooked meals for their sick relatives, bathed them, and made the hospital grounds their home. Daughter Rhena later said, "[My father] had to give them a village, not a hospital."[5] After arriving at Adende, Schweitzer understood immediately that the traditional European model of health care would not work there.[5] The fact that families often translocated was radically different from European norms. Schweitzer was heavily criticized for creating an African village instead of the "gleaming hospital in the jungle" that some had expected. Many visitors became disillusioned upon seeing the Schweitzer hospital, a relatively unsanitary place, with no clear boundaries between hospital and village. Chickens and goats scurried about and people wandered freely in and out of the wards. Some visitors wrote scathing reports that received wide attention in the world's press. But Schweitzer's approach worked best for the Africans. He understood the culture of the local people and designed a hospital that would best address their needs.

In a surprise reprieve from their prior renunciations of Schweitzer, the local missionaries invited him to take part in preaching within a few months after his arrival. The questions of dogma that had so preoccupied the Paris Missionary Society had no place in the sermons at Lambarene. Absolved of his promise to be "muet comme une carpe," Schweitzer again found joy in the act of preaching. It added to his joy to be able to introduce the sayings of Jesus and Paul to those who had not heard them previously. In the equatorial jungle, Christianity was necessarily taught simply and as a religion based upon ethics. Issues of dogma and orthodoxy were irrelevant. In another similarity to early Christianity, Lambarene had no chapel. Like St Paul and other early Christians, Schweitzer preached outside, where all could hear. A famous picture shows Dr Schweitzer preaching to a group of patients, families, and hospital staff. In the middle of the group stand two pelicans. In Schweitzer's Africa, animals were a part of his extended ministry.

Another beloved part of Schweitzer's life accompanied him to Africa as well— his music. Upon learning of Schweitzer's planned departure, the Paris Bach Society rewarded his years of service as their organist by giving him a zinc-lined piano, fitted with organ pedal attachments. The zinc lining would protect the piano from the tropical climate and the pedal attachments would allow him to practice as if on an organ. Convinced at first that medical work in Africa meant renunciation of his life as an artist, Schweitzer gave little thought to playing this unusual piano. However, he soon found time to play in the late night hours, improving his technique and interpretation and memorizing several complete scores. When he finally returned to play in Europe, he had refined his technique and improved his interpretations of Bach, much to the delight of his many fans.

Life in the "Primeval Forest"

As a result of living in Africa for years at a time, Schweitzer came to understand the vast cultural differences between Africans and Europeans. He did not share the commonly held European belief that only Europeans had "culture," and he felt strongly that it was not his or anyone else's duty to impose this culture on the Africans. These views separated him from most of the colonial administrators, missionaries, and developers throughout Africa at the time. Through the intimacy afforded by countless clinical interactions, Schweitzer realized that Africans had evolved a strong indigenous culture, one that deserved visitors' respect. In time, Schweitzer felt closer spiritually to the local tribesmen of the Ogowe than he did to the Europeans embroiled in war. Biographers Marshall and Poling wrote:

> Schweitzer felt sadly that most Africans, including those who were pagans, were more full of love and goodwill than white Christians. They [the Africans] seemed to share a strong sense of well-wishing and concern for one another. Too often, the doctor noted, many Christian white men, including some of the missionaries and teachers, were too preoccupied with specific tasks of their professional service to take the time to express simple human interest in the African or his personal problems. (1971, 140)

In his popular book, *On the Edge of the Primeval Forest* (Macmillan, 1948), Schweitzer portrayed Africans in a way that Western audiences had not seen previously. Unlike the "savages" and "cannibals" depicted by the renowned explorer Lord Stanley, whose own writings had become international best sellers earlier, Schweitzer painted a more understanding portrait of daily life in the villages around Lambarene and his life as a doctor serving there. He chronicled how he and assorted local workers had painstakingly built a hospital in the forest and how the "magic" of Western medicine had attracted patients by the thousands. He described a simple but superstitious people with a culture radically different from that of his readers. He told of local villagers drowning their mentally ill, believing them to be possessed by evil spirits, and of local witch doctors treating illnesses with incantations or potions. He wrote: "That the diseases have some natural cause never occurs to my patients. They attribute them to evil spirits, to malicious human magic, or to "the worm," which is their imaginary embodiment of pain of every sort" (Schweitzer 1948b, 24). He described scenes of idyllic beauty and detailed the lives of a people largely filled with compassion for one another. Surprisingly, he supported the native practice of polygamy, noting that it was the bedrock of the tribal society, assuring that all women would be married and all children would have families. Schweitzer's insight and understanding of local culture and customs made the *Primeval Forest* a novelty for its time. It did not, however, ease the impact of two worlds colliding. Inevitably, the cultures of the local African tribes and that of their new resident doctor clashed. Schweitzer was an accomplished man who drove himself hard and held high expectations for everyone around him. The local tribes did not intend to suddenly change a pattern of life they had followed for centuries, no matter how much the new white doctor yelled. When they got tired, they rested. When they no longer felt like working, they went home. When they saw something they needed, they took it, as they always had shared things among extended family and the tribe.

These attitudes would not safeguard medicines or supplies or build a new, badly needed hospital. For the impatient Schweitzer, these actions led to conflict. To remain true to the ideal of Reverence for Life, Schweitzer became, out of sheer necessity, a hard-driving foreman. The ideal manifested itself in the man in a nearly unrecognizable form. The contradiction was not lost on visitors to the hospital, who expected Moses and got Patton. Rhena recalled, "He was the authoritarian and the disciplinarian. It had to be done exactly as he wanted it done. He was not a man you said 'no' to."[5] In a quote widely reported—and misconstrued—by the world press, Norman Cousins wrote, "The image of Albert Schweitzer I carried away with me was intact—fortified, if anything, by a direct view. For at Lambarene I learned that a man does not have to be an angel to be a saint" (Cousins 1960, 222).

Schweitzer became an enigma to many. To local tribesmen who had painfully learned to distrust any European, Schweitzer was a rarity, good to his word and always there to help them. To the many early 20th-century Europeans who saw the black Africans as subhuman, Schweitzer was a mystery. After all, he had abandoned prosperous careers in three disciplines to live among the "savages" in the jungle. Why would such an accomplished man take such an unprecedented step? To the modern reader, Schweitzer bears markings of the colonial era that spawned him. Some of his writings reflect a man who loved his African brethren but never fully accepted them as his equal. He repeatedly said to them, "You are my brother. But I am your elder brother."[5]

Some of his writings in *On the Edge of the Primeval Forest* sound dissonant chords to ears accustomed to our modern sanitized speech. References to Africans as "children of nature" and what were considered other derogatory comments earned Schweitzer rebukes from eminent scholars such as WEB Dubois. Dubois suggested that Schweitzer perpetuated colonialism by making life tolerable under it. Referring to the considerable crimes of the white man in Africa, he added that Schweitzer would have been better off saving the souls of white men rather than the bodies of black men. Still, DuBois recognized the enormous contribution Schweitzer made: "He saw the pain and degradation of this bit of God's earth as something he could alleviate; for many years he gave his life to it" (Marshall and Poling 1971, 289). People all over the Congo region came to rely upon Schweitzer's care and viewed him as a friend and advocate, one who would go so far as to argue on the Africans' behalf. White advocates for Africans were exceedingly rare at the time. Through his unique understanding of both European and African cultures, Schweitzer had come to a centrist position regarding African autonomy. He first expressed these views in *the Primeval Forest*, published before World War I and a full 40 years before independence movements swept across Africa. He believed that the Africans should control their own destiny, yet do so with European guidance. He disagreed with those who thought the Africans should be abandoned, and his hospital offered a clear example that this help was both welcomed and needed. Yet he railed against those he saw as hypocrites, saying: "This noble culture of ours! Speaking so piously of human dignity and human rights, it then disregards the dignity and the rights of countless millions, treading them underfoot simply because they live overseas or because their skins are of a different colour, or because they cannot help themselves" (Bentley 1992, 191).

To the local African tribes, the net impact of the European conquerors was personal, environmental, and cultural destruction.

Schweitzer had arrived in Lambarene well after the first European colonialists forever altered the culture and economy of the local tribes. Slave traders, European and African alike, repeatedly raided the villages deep in the jungle, depleting local tribes of their more robust members. European traders introduced alcohol and diseases previously unseen. One smallpox epidemic in Gabon wiped out half the people in the area around Lambarene. The lumber industry, also introduced by the Europeans, radically changed the local economy. Villagers left their lands to become salaried workers for the first time. They spent money on alcohol and European-made goods that soon became "needs" of the locals, just as they had become needs for those in the developed countries a century earlier. To the local African tribes, the net impact of the European conquerors was personal, environmental, and cultural destruction.

In the conclusion of *On the Edge of the Primeval Forest*, written in 1948, Schweitzer wrote compellingly of the need to alleviate the suffering of the Africans and attempted to erode the racial mythology that had long dominated European thinking about "Negroes," debunking views that Africans did not experience pain or sorrow in the same ways that white Europeans did:

> Physical misery is great everywhere out here. Are we justified in shutting our eyes and ignoring it because our European newspapers tell us nothing about it? We civilized people have been spoilt. If any one of us is ill the doctor comes at once. If an operation is necessary, the door of some hospital or other opens to us immediately. But let every one reflect on the meaning of the fact that out here millions and millions live without help or hope of it. Every day thousands and thousands endure the most terrible sufferings, though medical science could avert them. Every day there prevails in many and many a far-off hut a despair which we could banish. Will each of my readers think what the last ten years of his family history would have been if they had been passed without medical or surgical help of any sort? It is time we should wake from the slumber and face our responsibilities! (1948b, 115).

War and Salvation

World War I broke out in the summer of 1914. As German nationals living in French Gabon, the Schweitzers suddenly became enemy aliens and were eventually taken as prisoners of the French. Ironically, Schweitzer's family had opposed the German annexation of Alsace in 1871, though this was of little help to Albert and Hélène. French authorities initially confined Dr and Mrs Schweitzer to house arrest, forbade them to work at the hospital, and restricted them from contacting Europeans or Africans. The sick still came to the hospital in great numbers, but now armed guards informed them of the doctor's arrest and told them to leave. These guards were not popular. The doctor's confinement and the war itself made little sense to people in the local tribes. One asked, "Why, doctor, do the white men who brought us the Gospel of Love not practice it among themselves?" (Marshall and Poling 1971, 148).

Schweitzer used his "free time" to continue work on his book, *The Philosophy of Civilization* (Prometheus Books, 1949), but it didn't last long. Just three months after arresting the Schweitzers in 1917, the French government ordered all African prisoners transferred to Bordeaux. Albert and Hélène arrived there in November, and both struggled with the cold weather. Both became ill with dysentery, and Hélène again contracted tuberculosis. Already physically weakened by vertebral fractures sustained while skiing, Hélène was never again able to join fully in her husband's work at the hospital or in their collective dream in Africa.

Soon the French authorities transferred the Schweitzers to other prison camps—first to Garaison and then to St Rémy de Provence. Dr Schweitzer finally was able to resume activity as a medical doctor, caring for the many sick of the camps. He continued work on *The Philosophy of Civilization* and maintained a rigorous schedule playing Bach fugues on a table that served as an imaginary organ. While Schweitzer filled his time with his typical abundance of activities, the war dragged on, ultimately killing nearly 20 million people and destroying hope for a generation (Sivard 1996, 18). The war cost Albert and Hélène dearly. He lost his mother when cavalry horses ran over and killed her in 1916. He also lost years of productive life and faced a crippling depression in the wake of the war. Hélène never fully regained her health. The Schweitzers fought constant fatigue, illness, cold, and hunger, finally obtaining their release just before the end of the war. Their lives had been turned upside down for three long years.

Schweitzer returned home to Gunsbach to see the grave of his mother and the remnant of the man who had been his father. After his wife's senseless death, Louis Schweitzer had not even bothered to take shelter from the bombs falling all around him. He had lost his will to live, according to those who knew him best. German officers had commandeered his vicarage and reduced the venerable pastor to the role of houseboy. Gunsbach itself, situated near the border between France and Germany, was the closest unevacuated town to the trenches of the Western Front. As such, the horrors of war engulfed it. Heavy artillery rounds echoed in the surrounding hills, machine gun installations decorated the landscape, and barbed wire lined the roads.

For Albert Schweitzer, the years following the war were filled with sickness and despair. He suffered recurring attacks of fever that physically depleted him, finally ending in August 1918, when Professor Stolz of Strasbourg surgically removed a rectal abscess. Schweitzer later required additional surgeries to cure the problem. The cure for his growing depression, however, was far less attainable. The idealistic young doctor had sacrificed everything to go to Africa to treat the sick. When he returned Europe, he found all the elements of his former life in ruins. The war itself had nearly shattered his increasingly desperate hope for a civilization based on ethics. He became uncharacteristically withdrawn and depressed in response to the collection of tragic events. For nearly two years, the man who had been able to do anything was capable of doing almost nothing.

Salvation for Albert Schweitzer came in the form of a religious benefactor in war-neutral Sweden. Archbishop Nathan Söderblom invited Schweitzer to give a series of lectures, and Schweitzer gratefully accepted, visiting Sweden in the spring and summer of 1920. Schweitzer wrote that, before this invitation, he had felt "like a coin that has rolled under a piece of furniture and has been forgotten there" (1933, 185). While in Sweden, he confided to the Archbishop that he had amassed considerable debts to the Paris Missionary Society and other Parisian benefactors of the hospital.

The Archbishop arranged a series of lectures and concerts throughout Sweden for a considerable sum of money, enough to enable Schweitzer to pay off his debts and plan a return to mission work in Gabon. Speaking publicly on his philosophy, Reverence for Life, for the first time, he noted, "I was so moved that I found it difficult to speak" (186). More than his financial resurrection, Schweitzer regained his spirit and joy in his work. He later wrote, "I came to Sweden a tired, depressed, and still ailing man. . . . I recovered my health and once more found enjoyment in my work" (1933, 186; Marshall and Poling 1971, 159).

Return to Lambarene

After an additional two years of lectures and concerts to raise money for the hospital, Schweitzer planned a return to Lambarene. His books, *The Philosophy of Civilization, Volumes I & II* (Prometheus Books 1949); *Christianity and the Religions of the World* (Allan and Unwin, 1939); *Memoirs of Childhood and Youth* (Macmillan 1949); and American and European versions of *On the Edge of the Primeval Forest*, were all published prior to his return to Africa. His fame had grown considerably from his concerts and lectures, and with a proven track record in Gabon, he found it easier to solicit funds. He planned to return in early 1924. This time, however, Hélène would not go with him even though she wanted to. She had given birth to daughter Rhena on Albert's birthday, January 14, 1919, and did not think her health could withstand another rainy season in West Africa. She urged her husband to return to the work he most valued—but to make the trip without her. According to their daughter Rhena, it was "most courageous of her to let him go. She was ill with tuberculosis, had a little girl and still let her husband go away for two years—that turned into three years. Not many women would do that."[3] Schweitzer later wrote, "Unceasingly I thank her in my heart that she rose to the sacrifice of acquiescence in my return under these circumstances to Lambarene" (Marshall and Poling 1971, 163). On February 14, 1924, Schweitzer left Strasbourg for Africa.

Seven years had gone by since the Schweitzers left Gabon as prisoners of war. The years had not been kind to the hospital. All but one of the buildings had collapsed, and the path to the doctor's house was no longer visible. Schweitzer immediately began reconstructing the hospital for the patients who arrived soon after he did, dividing his time between seeing patients and repairing the various buildings on the hospital grounds. Help was sporadic and unreliable, and the basic repair work took several months. After an epidemic of dysentery swelled the patient population to more than 150, Schweitzer realized that he needed more space and a new hospital. He chose a large site named Adoninalongo (meaning "it overlooks the tribes") directly across from the island of Lambarene, just 2 miles upstream from Andende.

Over the course of the next two years, he designed and built his new hospital, with the help of many Africans and visiting Europeans. When it opened, it was a complex of more than 40 buildings, providing patient wards, staff living quarters, and dwellings for the families that would stay and care for their sick relatives. Like Andende before it, it was more of a village than a hospital. No longer dependent on the Paris Missionary Society, Schweitzer was on his own at last. After a full day transporting the patients two miles up river, Schweitzer opened the Albert Schweitzer–Breslau Hospital in January

> *No longer dependent on the Paris Missionary Society, Schweitzer was on his own at last.*

1927. Schweitzer recalled the first night there: "From every mosquito-net peered out a happy face" (Bentley 1992, 167). For the first time, he felt that his patients were housed as basic humanity demanded.

Schweitzer's fame continued to grow, and his jungle hospital attracted help in all forms. Doctors, nurses, carpenters, and tradesmen came from all over to offer their assistance. After another dysentery epidemic, construction began in yet further hospital expansion. By July 1927, the staff was sufficiently large for Schweitzer to return to his family in Europe for two years. His daughter recalled that he was so busy during these periods at home that she and her mother rarely saw him. He gave lectures and concerts, recruited people and funds for his hospital, and spent much of the rest of his time writing. Rhena later recalled, "He had to provide for mother and me and finance the hospital, so he had little time for us."[6]

In the late 1920s, publisher Felix Meiner suggested to Schweitzer that he write an autobiography. Schweitzer resisted initially, thinking that biographies were supposed to come at the end of one's life, and at age 54 his life was by no means over. Meiner warned that if Schweitzer did not write his life story, someone else would. His wife Hélène intervened and suggested that he write about the development of his thought to that point in his life. Schweitzer relented and immediately set upon a rigorous course of writing. While the hospital staff carried on the daily schedule, Schweitzer wrote all day and most of the night. He slept only two hours each day and left his study only for meals. In this fashion he finished the manuscript in less than a month. *Out of My Life and Thought* (Henry Holt & Co, 1949) became the definitive account of his life, published in England in 1932 and the United States in 1933.

Another War

The rise of the Nazis in Germany in the 1930s underscored the importance of Schweitzer's philosophy and work. A party opposed to rationalism, liberalism, and democracy, the Nazis were the antithesis of Albert Schweitzer, who became the moral authority that Europe desperately needed. Unlike most of his former colleagues, Schweitzer saw the storm clouds gathering over Germany and did not remain silent. During a centennial celebration of the death of the German philosopher Goethe on March 22, 1932, Schweitzer urged his listeners to "strive for true humanity" and to "remain men, in possession of your own souls. Do not become human beings which have offered hospitality to souls which conform to the will of the masses and beat in time with it" (Marshall and Poling 1971, 198). Referring to the bicentennial celebration of Goethe's birth two years hence, Schweitzer said, "May it be that he who gives the memorial address at that new festival be able to state that the deep darkness which surrounds this one has already begun to lighten. . . ." (199). His remarks incensed the Nazis, and several of Schweitzer's friends feared for his life.

The Nazis cast a lengthening shadow over Germany, burning the Reichstag in February 1933. One month later, Hitler became chancellor. Soon Schweitzer and his wife returned to a far more dangerous Germany. His German friends feared severe repercussions from the mere association with him. Schweitzer cancelled all of his German concerts and lecture dates, vowing not to return to Germany as long as Hitler was alive—a vow he kept.

Schweitzer spent the years of World War II in Lambarene, remaining there from March 1939 through October 1949. Hélène joined him there in 1941, making a daring trek across southern Europe after the Nazis took Paris. Before the outbreak of the war, Schweitzer had stocked up on medical supplies, but the supplies lasted only so long. A small group of Americans formed the Albert Schweitzer Fellowship in New York and provided timely relief to Lambarene when shipments from Europe stopped. As in World War I, the fighting of World War II spread to Africa and the Congo.

One morning in 1942, Schweitzer was checking his vegetables in the predawn light when he became the target of a machine-gun burst. He dove for cover as bullets sprayed around him. With each move, more shots rang out, pinning him down until it was light enough for the gunner to clearly identify him. Unhurt, Schweitzer fired off a letter to the French commander, admonishing him for his soldier's violation of the Geneva Convention provision mandating that hospitals and medical personnel be neutral: "If you shoot at me again I will prohibit your men from visiting the hospital" (Marshall and Poling 1971, 217). The commander called a cease-fire and came to the hospital to personally apologize. Ironically, later the same day he became ill and required Schweitzer's services.

The war years were difficult for Schweitzer and the hospital, forcing both to the brink. Unable to travel to Europe to gather funds, Schweitzer increasingly became unable to pay for the supplies and salaries that kept the hospital running. He turned 70 on January 14, 1945, in the midst of near-famine conditions that further strained resources. It became difficult just to feed the patients and staff. With the hospital staff depleted, Schweitzer faced the very real possibility of bankruptcy and the end of the hospital at Lambarene. He lost hope and confided to his wife and Mademoiselle

Mathilde Kottman, the sole remaining European nurse, that failure had to be faced (Marshall and Poling 1971, 219). On October 16, 1946, Schweitzer received a letter from the Banque Commerciale Africane, stating that he had overdrawn the account by $1,045. He had withdrawn the money to pay for provisions, rice, and cement for a new hospital landing, and this overdraft virtually closed the hospital.

Fate, however, had different plans for Schweitzer and his hospital. On the same day he received the letter from the bank, he received another letter informing him that the Unitarian Service Committee of the United States had deposited $4375.00 into his bank account. His wife and daughter's visits to the United States had paid off. In addition to immediate financial relief, this windfall provided a psychological boost at the most opportune time. Schweitzer immediately repaid his debts, paid the hospital salaries, and wrote a letter to Charles R. Joy of Newton, Mass. (the Unitarian minister and friend who had organized the relief effort): "I can find no words to express the extent of my gratitude. . . . You cannot know how I feel uplifted and encouraged by your kindness" (Marshall and Poling 1971, 221).

Fame, Recognition, and the Nuclear Threat

The work of the hospital went on, and Schweitzer, the celebrated septuage-narian, made his only visit to the United States in the fall of 1949. He visited Aspen, Colorado; Chicago; Boston; and New York City, meeting with his new benefactors and many fans. During portions of his visit, near mania ensued. Celebrities wanted to meet him and people everywhere wanted to shake his hand or get his autograph. He had accepted an invitation—and a considerable stipend—to speak at the Goethe Bicentennial in Aspen. His US visit was too brief to allow him to accept an invitation from his friend Albert Einstein to visit him and speak at Princeton. But he did meet Larrimer and Gwen Mellon, who later founded the Hospital Albert Schweitzer in Deschapelles, Haiti, in recognition of the principles of Reverence for Life. Schweitzer also visited the pharmaceutical company in New York City that had been so generous to him and his hospital. He met Charles R. Joy and others who built the network that formed the first Albert Schweitzer Societies in New York City and Boston. The financial base for Schweitzer's mission noticeably shifted from Europe to the United States.

In the 1950s, Schweitzer received considerable recognition for his life of sacrifice and principled action. During this decade he also secured the long-elusive financial stability that his work in Lambarene required. In September 1951, the West German Association of Book Publishers and Sellers awarded him a 10,000-mark prize for promoting world peace. In 1952, Swedish King Gustavson Adolf awarded him the Prince Charles Medal for humanitarian achievements. That same year, Schweitzer was inducted into the prestigious French Academy of Moral and Political Sciences and the American Academy of Arts and Sciences. In 1955, he received the order Pour le Merite from the West German Republic and Queen Elizabeth conferred on him the title Honorary Member of the Royal Order of Merit, joining Dwight D. Eisenhower as the only other non-Briton so honored.

The highest acclaim for Albert Schweitzer came when he received the 1952 Nobel Peace Prize. He was in Lambarene at the time, was unable to leave the hospital, and received the award *in absentia*. He later donated all of the proceeds from the prize to building the Leper Village at Lambarene. He delivered his acceptance speech in Oslo, Norway, in 1954. In a stunning departure from the political neutrality he retained most of his life, he titled his talk "The Problem of Peace in the World Today" and expressed his concern about the propagation of nuclear weapons. Norman Cousins, Pablo Casals, and Albert Einstein, among others, had persuaded Schweitzer to break his silence and speak out against nuclear weapons. His address received wide attention, and Radio Oslo broadcast three of his addresses on the subject in 1957 and 1958. In one broadcast, he commented on a near nuclear calamity precipitated by faulty radar, "Such are the heights of our civilization that a cold electronic brain rather than the moral conscience of man may decide human destiny" (Cousins 1960, 247).

The highest acclaim for Albert Schweitzer came when he received the 1952 Nobel Peace Prize.

As a doctor, Schweitzer firmly grasped the health implications of nuclear testing. "It is not for the physicist, choosing to take into account only radiation from the air, to utter the final word on the dangers of nuclear tests. That right belongs to the biologists and physicians who have studied internal as well as external radiation . . . " (Cousins 1960, 240). He continued, "Only those who have never been present at the birth of a deformed baby, never witnessed the whimpering cries of its mother, should dare to maintain that the risk of nuclear testing is small" (241).

Schweitzer became a passionate and articulate advocate for a ban on nuclear testing and proliferation. Among others, he corresponded with Prime Minister Jawaharlal Nehru of India, Soviet Premier Nikita Khrushchev, and US Presidents Dwight D. Eisenhower and John F. Kennedy.

A Long and Fruitful Life

The hospital that started in a converted chicken coop at Andende and faced bankruptcy in 1946 eventually encompassed more than 75 buildings and treated thousands of patients annually. Between 1924 and 1965—Schweitzer's tenure at the hospital—the staff admitted more than 150,000 patients and performed nearly 20,000 surgeries (Marshall and Poling 1971, 257). The Albert Schweitzer Bresslau Hospital began to attract physicians, nurses, and other volunteers from all over the world, and Schweitzer necessarily became more of an administrator than an active clinician. He learned to screen applications carefully, because so many volunteers could not tolerate the heat and general living conditions. The hospital started training Africans as nurses' assistants.

Just days before he died, Schweitzer turned over the considerable administrative responsibilities to his daughter Rhena. She did not relish her new role. "I was no administrator," she said. "I had no interest in running the hospital."[5] Although she felt in no way qualified for the job, she ran the hospital for 5 years before relinquishing control to others. She stated that she thought her father would be shocked to see the hospital still flourishing today. "Lambarene is my improvisation, and I know it will disappear one day," he had told her.[5]

Albert Schweitzer spent the last years of his life on African soil. Africa had become his home, and he would not leave those who became his extended family. His immediate family stayed with him in his final years; his wife Hélène spent the last two years of her life in Lambarene. She died shortly after returning to Switzerland in May 1957 and Albert had carried her ashes back for burial at Lambarene Hospital. Daughter Rhena also lived with him during the last five years of his life. During these years, she recalled that he continued to push himself and those around him until he no longer had sufficient energy to match his drive. He confided to Rhena of his great frustration at lacking the strength to launch one more broad appeal for nuclear disarmament. When asked if her father spent time at the end of his life reminiscing about his place in history or the considerable accomplishments of his life, Rhena replied, "No, he never spoke about it. He wanted people to know his philosophy, yes. But he spoke mostly of what he still had to do, and how frustrated he was that he no longer had the energy to do it."[5]

In late August 1965, Schweitzer asked to be driven around the hospital grounds so he could survey one last time that which he had so painstakingly created. One week later, on September 4, he died peacefully at 10:30 PM. His death triggered worldwide mourning. From presidents and kings, from the working poor, and from all those who had been moved by the man and his message, letters of sympathy poured into Gunsbach and Lambarene. The local villagers around Lambarene grieved the loss of one of their own, and festivals of mourning accompanied by singing and dancing went on for months.[3] In the end, the loss of Oganga meant as much to the Galloa and Pahouin tribesman as it did to anyone else in the world.

Epilogue

In exploring the man who was Albert Schweitzer, one finds a gifted, passionate, and venerable enigma who inspired millions through the example of his life and the power of his words. In a survey carried out in Germany in 1985—20 years after his death—Schweitzer topped the list of the 30 most admired people, both living and dead. He followed the example of Christ but devoted more time to the patients in his hospital than the needs of his family. In Lambarene, he saw the opportunity to live out a moral imperative and to breathe life into his philosophy of Reverence for Life. He often repeated, "I made my life my argument," and, as in the example of Jesus, offered his own life to service. Rhena Schweitzer Miller noted that her father found the freedom to express himself in Lambarene, unencumbered by bureaucracy or a formal organizational structure: "Lambarene gave him the opportunity to become the man he became."[5]

It is impossible to understand the man without recognizing the depth of his faith. It suffused him, inspiring much of what he wrote and thought. The letters he wrote to Hélène Bresslau between 1901 and 1910 bear testimony to the personal importance of Jesus's influence in his life. In one of the letters, he wrote of a living God within:

> When I prayed last night, the prayer of the last days to gain strength for the coming winter, I asked myself again and again: What is God? Something infinite in which we rest! But it is not a personality, it becomes a personality only in us! The spirit of the world that brings man to the consciousness of himself. Prayer: to feel the stirring of the highest being in us, to give ourselves to the divine and thus find peace.[10]

In his time, Schweitzer did find peace and created the setting through which the divine within him could emerge. Rather than teach theology and preach in his native land, he chose a more rugged path through which he could "think the thoughts I want to think" and "to live [my ideals] quietly and simply."[10] Although he wanted the hospital at Lambarene to grow and thrive, he died believing it would not. More important, he hoped his beliefs would spread and endure: "I have a certain vision of immortality, that what is immortal and immaterial in us is our thoughts. We live when our thoughts are reborn in others."[11] In a seeming epitaph to his life, he once told Norman Cousins, "No one has ever come back from the other world. I can't console you, but one thing I can tell you, as long as my ideals are alive, I will be alive" (1984, 69).

For those of us in the medical profession, Schweitzer left a clear message. Acutely aware of the suffering in the African colonies, Schweitzer probed the conscience of the European colonial powers, urging that they recognize their responsibilities and act accordingly. Schweitzer's vision extended well beyond the European nations, seeing deeper into the universal suffering of men:

> Other doctors must go out to the colonies as a humane duty mandated by the conscience of society. Whoever among us has learned through personal experience what pain and anxiety really are must help to ensure that those out there who are in physical need obtain the same help that once came to him. He no longer belongs to himself alone; he has become the brother of all who suffer. It is this "brotherhood of those who bear the mark of pain" that demands humane medical services for the colonies. Commissioned by their representatives, medical people must do for the suffering in far-off lands what cries out to be done in the name of true civilization (1933, 195).

Schweitzer became for many a symbol of hope in an imperiled world. His life spanned some of the worst acts of European colonialism, two world wars, and the dawn of the nuclear age. Yet he followed a different path and offered the philosophy of Reverence for Life as a future direction for humanity. Only through progress in ethical thinking could man move forward and create a true civilization, he said. With characteristic eloquence and fire, he added, "I want to be the pioneer of a new Renaissance. I want to throw faith in a new humanity like a burning torch into our dark times" (1933, vii).

For those of us whom Dr Schweitzer has inspired, that torch still burns. For me, he remains an important source of inspiration. In him, I see a man who risked everything for an ideal. His personal sacrifices made amends—in part—for the damages inflicted on many by an unjust world. His level of dedication to a belief is rare. In this current age of cynicism, Schweitzer and his life story are refreshing. When he talked of an "ethical imperative," he spoke to all of us in the medical profession. He forces reflection on the question of why any of us became health providers and on how much we can contribute with our extraordinary gifts as healers.

Endnotes

1. Albert Schweitzer, Hélène Bresslau, personal communication, 1902.
2. Albert Schweitzer, Hélène Bresslau, personal communication, 1910.
3. Dr Edward O'Neil, Rhena Schweitzer, personal communication, 2001.
4. Albert Schweitzer, Hélène Bresslau, personal communication, 1905.
5. Dr Edward O'Neil, Rhena Schweitzer, personal communication, 1999.
6. Dr Edward O'Neil, Rhena Schweitzer, personal communication, undated.
7. Albert Schweitzer, Hélène Bresslau, personal communication, 1903.
8. Albert Schweitzer, Hélène Bresslau, personal communication, undated.
9. Albert Schweitzer, Hélène Bresslau, personal communication, 1911.
10. Albert Schweitzer, Hélène Bresslau, personal communication, 1906.
11. Albert Schweitzer, Hélène Bresslau, personal communication, 1904.

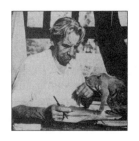

Chapter 17

Reverence for Life: The Compelling and Timeless Ideal of Albert Schweitzer, MD

Just as the wave cannot exist for itself, but is ever a part of the heaving surface of the ocean, so must I never live my life for life itself, but always in the experience which is going on around me. It is an uncomfortable doctrine which the true ethics whisper to my ear. You are happy, they say; therefore you are called upon to give much.

—Dr Albert Schweitzer

Albert Schweitzer struggled with many of the same questions posed at the beginning of this book. For him, moments of reflection came as the sun set over the Ogowe River or when the late hours afforded him time alone with the stillness of the African night. Schweitzer spent years developing a philosophy that can still help us find our own answers to these difficult questions. As a minister, philosopher, and musician, he was able to see the world through several lenses. Yet it was his vocation as a doctor in rural Africa that revealed to him the needless suffering of so many people and the need for moral clarity in our approach to the poor.

Ultimately, Schweitzer arrived at a worldview he called "Reverence for Life," in which he cited an "ethical imperative" for each of us to care for all of the life around us, including people not in our traditional realms of concern.

He explained his philosophy in the 347-page, two-volume set called The Philosophy of Civilization, *written between 1914 and 1923. In volume one, titled* The Decay and Restoration of Civilization, *he explained the decline of civilization and how removed it had become from philosophy and ethics. In volume two, titled* Civilization and Ethics, *he summarized the ethical views of the great philosophers and religious thinkers in world history. He then developed the tenets of Reverence for Life and how they could fundamentally alter the relationships among people and all of the life around them. Schweitzer compels each of us to listen not to an external summons but, rather, to an internal drive. Reverence for Life offers us profound insight into the questions that each of us must face in our lives—particularly those questions that arise while we are serving the poor.*

Wir Epigonen

In the summer of 1899, Schweitzer was talking with friends from the University of Berlin about an idea that had long disturbed him—the apparent decline of European civilization. One member of the group declared, "So we are all nothing but epigones" (Schweitzer 1933, 145)—defined as "a descendant less gifted than his ancestors, or any inferior follower or imitator."[1] Schweitzer said the comment hit him "like a bolt of lightning," substantiating views he had held in silence. He wrote in his autobiography, "My own impression was that in our intellectual and spiritual life not only had we sunk below the level of past generations, but we were in many respects merely living on their achievements, and that not a little of this heritage was beginning to melt away in our hands" (146).

Schweitzer did not share in the exuberance that many felt for the great advances in science and technology. He saw instead, well ahead of many of his time, a generation in spiritual decline. "I had grown to doubt increasingly the idea that mankind is steadily moving toward improvement. My impression was that the fire of its ideals was burning out without anyone noticing or worrying about it . . . . I noticed a number of symptoms of intellectual and spiritual fatigue in this generation that is so proud of its achievements . . . " (Schweitzer 1933, 145).

He decided to write a book—and sound a warning—about the decline of civilization. He would call it, *Wir Epigonen*, or *We Inheritors of a Past*. His study of medicine and the creation of a new hospital left him just enough time to write outlines and the beginning of the text. Then World War I intervened, ultimately claiming nearly 20 million lives. No warning of the impending collapse of civilization could save Europe from itself. His warning would come too late. By 1914, Schweitzer was a German prisoner of war under house arrest in Lambarene, with plenty of time to think about the conflict in Europe. As news of the war weighed on him heavily, he wrote, "Many a night I sat thinking and writing, overcome with emotion as I thought of those who at that very hour were lying in the trenches"

(1933, 147). He added, "I was aware of the great blessing that I could save lives while others were forced to kill, and that at the same time I could work toward the coming of the era of peace" (160). Over the next seven years he wrote and rewrote two volumes despite a number of setbacks.

The Decay of Civilization

"We are living today under the sign of the collapse of civilization" (Schweitzer 1949b, 1). So began the book, *The Decay and the Restoration of Civilization.* He was convinced that World War I did not cause this collapse, that the war was only an outward sign of it. The real collapse had occurred years earlier and was the result of far deeper failings, among them the spiritual decline of man, the decline of philosophy, the dissociation of philosophy from ethics, the rise of the unreflective natural sciences, and a host of economic and social factors produced by the Industrial Revolution. The sum of these forces, according to Schweitzer, had produced a lessened version of man capable of global war.

According to Schweitzer, the basis for civilization had always been ethical thought, whose generators and guardians were the philosophers of the ages. "Every age lives in the consciousness of what has been provided for it by the thinkers under whose influence it stands. Kant and Hegel have commanded millions who had never read a line of their writings, and who did not even know that they were obeying their orders" (1949b, 50).

The Roles of Philosophy and the Natural Sciences

Goethe, Kant, Schillinger, Plato, and many other important thinkers guided the ship of civilization for centuries. Yet, somewhere around the beginning of the 19th century, philosophy was pushed aside by the natural sciences and, in Schweitzer's words, "renounced its duty." The captain had fallen asleep at the wheel. The few philosophers who remained influential, such as Hegel, Nietzsche, and Darwin, had strayed from the ethical, transposing natural selection to humanity, in which "supermen" triumphed and the weak, naturally, suffered. All three philosophers provided compelling logic to an age in which people looked increasingly to the natural world around them for the source of their worldview. As a consequence, Schweitzer wrote, "The ethical ideas on which civilization rests have been wandering about the world, poverty-stricken and homeless" (Schweitzer 1949b, 4). Humans had lost the capacity to reflect on what true civilization was.

The Role of Science

Science, too, played a significant role in civilization's decline, according to Schweitzer. He wrote that science had regressed ethically, and, paradoxically, its great advances had "put us in a position to kill at such a distance, and to annihilate men in such masses that we sank so low as to push aside any last impulse to humanity" (1949b, 88). Schweitzer venerated earlier generations of scientists who viewed their work in a larger context. "Once every man of science was also a thinker who counted for something in the general spiritual life of his generation," Schweitzer wrote. "Our age has discovered how to divorce knowledge from thought, with the result that we have, indeed, a science which is free, but hardly any science which reflects"(44).

The Role of Urbanization

In addition to philosophy and science, many destructive forces arose when great masses of people shed their agrarian past and adopted urban, industrialized lives. In Schweitzer's view, the human spirit nearly drowned in the aftermath of the Industrial Revolution. People began to live as workers primarily and as human beings secondarily. The excessive demands of work required them to spend less time raising children, developing their spirituality, or reflecting on the deeper questions of life. The collective culture reacted to these tendencies, tending more toward the superficial and the entertaining at the expense of the serious and the fundamental. Schweitzer wrote in 1917, "The spirit produced in such a society of never-concentrated minds is rising among us as an ever growing force, and it results in a lowered conception of what man should be" (1949b, 12). Unlike the Chinese, Indian, and Jewish civilizations, which had placed the spiritual and ethical on a higher level than the material, Western civilization evolved in the opposite direction.

The increasing specialization of man, he said, caused his artistic and creative powers to atrophy. Because man was called upon to use only a fraction of his abilities to perform his job, he became stunted—myopic in his worldview and vacuous in his spirituality. The overcrowding of urban centers and the hurried pace of working life fostered a mechanical being, impersonal in his dealings with other people. That this remains an essential—though invisible—part of our Western culture becomes readily apparent to anyone who works in the developing world.

An Ethical Foundation

In realizing that he needed to do more than simply chronicle the decline of civilization, Schweitzer wrote, "At the beginning of the summer of 1915 I awoke from some kind of mental daze. Why only criticize civilization? Why limit myself to analyzing ourselves as epigones? Why not work on something constructive?"(1933, 147) He decided to research the history of ethics in civilization and offer a more solid ethical foundation for the future. Thus, he began a massive exploration of the world's great theological and philosophical thinkers. While the guns roared and the dead accumulated at Verdun, Somme, Flanders, and Marne, Schweitzer searched for the basic truths underlying man's construct of a civilization. Going beyond mere research on the political or social precipitants of war, he expanded his considerable knowledge of world philosophy and Christian theology by studying the works of great Chinese, Indian, and Hindu thinkers. Somewhere in the history of thought, he felt there must be a unifying theme to the universe.

The Restoration of Civilization

Schweitzer defined civilization as "material and spiritual progress on the part of individuals as of the mass" (1949b, 22). To him, civilization encompassed all of the advances made by mankind, as long as they fostered the spiritual perfecting of the individual and, consequently, of the society. Without the "ethical element," no lasting progress could be possible. The salvation of civilization could come only through individual pursuit of the ethical, emanating from a solid spiritual foundation. No institution would save civilization; only its individual members could. "It is the duty of individuals to rise to a higher conception of their capabilities and undertake again the function which only the individual can perform, that of producing new spiritual-ethical ideas" (45). When enough individuals collectively shared an ethical worldview, civilization would have its permanent foundation at last.

Schweitzer believed that this unifying view of the world would bind the members of civilization together. He believed that man could defy 3,000 years of history and develop a new kind of civilization, prophesized by Jesus and based on love. The key to this civilization, he said, was a unifying theory of the universe. Schweitzer pored through the philosophical writings of the world, searching for the components of that unifying theory, in what could best be termed an obsession:

> We have to stir up the men of today to elementary meditation on what man is in the world, and what he wants to make of his life. Only when they are impressed once more with the necessity of giving the meaning and value to their existence, and thus come once more to hunger and thirst for a satisfying worldview, are the preliminaries given for a spiritual condition in which we again become capable of civilization (1949b, 93).

Weltanschauung

Schweitzer defined this worldview—*weltanschauung* in German—as follows:

> It is the content of the thoughts of society and the individuals which compose it about the nature and object of the world in which they live, and the position and the destiny of mankind and the individual men within it. (1949b, 49).

Great thinkers through time had struggled with concepts of a worldview, yet Schweitzer believed that none had succeeded. Reverence for Life, which we will explore shortly, became Schweitzer's Weltanschauung, arriving serendipitously in the early stages of his voluminous study. Ironically enough, Schweitzer "discovered" his Weltanschauung not through a progression of logic but, rather, through an inspired moment of clarity, a leap in thought of the type that has visited great thinkers throughout the ages. Once he conceptualized Reverence for Life, he continued to research the history of ethics in civilization. Importing cases of books to his jungle hospital, he searched for the basis of a universal ethic, found none, and felt sure that he had broken new ground. In the end, Schweitzer was convinced that he had established a universal ethic that could guide man in his relationships with all of the life around him. Being the German rationalist that he was, he had to first build the theoretical basis for Reverence for Life.

The Theoretical Basis

In *Civilization and Ethics*, Schweitzer outlined the three conditions that would have to be part of any Weltanschauung: The theory would have to be based on thought; it would have to be optimistic and life-affirming; and it would have to be ethical.

Thought

Thought would be the first precondition—though not thought in the traditional sense. To Schweitzer, thought did not mean repeating ideas that already existed. To him, thought meant "the totality of all the functions of our spirit in their living action and interaction" (Brabazon 1975, 245). In other words, thought meant listening in on the inner workings of life. "Thinking is a harmony within us," he said (245).

In Schweitzer's view, only the reflective man could adequately address the challenges we all face. He wrote, "Nothing but what is born of thought and addresses itself to thought can be a spiritual power affecting the whole of mankind" (1949b, 53). When man based his worldview on his senses alone, he was misled. He attributed this to the characteristics of Nature, which did not model ethics or morality and showed man only a cold indifference. Life took other life out of necessity, and life was lost for no apparent reason. As a doctor practicing in Africa, Schweitzer saw this all too frequently. Despite the sense of wonder that man should rightly feel in contemplating the universe, he mused, he needed more than his senses alone. "Only where there is a constant appeal to the need of a reflective view of things are all man's spiritual capacities called into activity" (53).

Schweitzer did not encourage people to withdraw from their interactions with the natural world for the purpose of thinking. He encouraged the opposite. To him, the world was inexplicably mysterious and beyond man's understanding; yet it was still a source of profound inspiration and spiritual renewal. He wrote:

> How much would already be accomplished toward the improvement of our present circumstances if only we would all give up three minutes every evening to

gazing up into the infinite world of the starry heavens and meditating on it, or if in taking part in a funeral procession we would reflect on the enigma of life and death, instead of engaging in thoughtless conversation as we follow behind the coffin! . . . How much more is it true that the injustice and violence and untruth, which are now bringing so much disaster on the human race, would lose their power if only a single real trace of reflection about the meaning of the world and of life should appear amongst us! (1949b, 63).

The Optimistic and Life-Affirming

Schweitzer thought that man had always struggled between an optimistic and a pessimistic view of life. He defined true optimism as actively "contemplating and willing the ideal in the light of a deep and self-consistent affirmation of life and the world" (1949b, 99). His was an activist view in which man must always play a constructive role. By contrast, true pessimism meant simply letting life be. This passive view dominated early Christianity and much of world philosophy throughout the Middle Ages. It still exists in the philosophies that encourage withdrawal from the world, such as Buddhism and that of the philosopher Schopenhauer. Most important for Schweitzer was his belief that optimism and pessimism are qualities not of judgment but of will. Through optimism, people exert their will to actively shape a future of their own choosing.

Throughout his writing, Schweitzer uses the term "life affirmation" liberally. By this, he means that the individual takes a positive approach to life and believes that life is worth living and affirming. He explains, "To us Europeans and to people of European descent everywhere, the will to progress is something so natural and so much a matter of course that it never occurs to us that it is rooted in a concept of life and springs from an act of the spirit" (Schweitzer 1949b). Whether this concept is present or not depends, in Schweitzer's view, on the prevailing concept of the world. For many of the world's people through much of time, that concept has been the negation of the world and life, the idea that one should endure life to get to the beauty of the afterlife that arrives upon one's death. By contrast, Reverence for Life includes life affirmation and requires an active cultivation and nurturing of all life. It is, by its own definition, optimistic and life-affirming.

The Ethical

In *Civilization and Ethics*, Schweitzer writes, "We must pass through the whole experience of mankind in its search for the ethical" (1949b, 106). For him that meant bringing down the "artificial" wall that separated religion from philosophy. The higher people from both disciplines attempted to go in their respective searches for morality, the closer they came together. He continued, "In every religious genius there lives an ethical thinker, and every really deep philosophical moralist is in some way or other religious" (106). He read the words of the world's great thinkers, always searching for the underlying theme that would tie ethics and civilization together. "Is there a possibility of getting beyond all these contradictory convictions of the past to new beliefs which will have a stronger and more lasting influence?" he wrote (Schweitzer 1949b, 103). "Can the ethical kernel of the thoughts of all these men be collected into an idea of the ethical, which will unite all the energies to which they appeal?" (103). Schweitzer persisted in his quest, seeing the ethical as the key to man's salvation.

A Breakthrough

By the summer of 1915, Schweitzer had reached an impasse in his thinking. He could not find what he considered the essential link between ethics and life affirmation. He wrote, "I remained convinced that ethics and the affirmation of life are interdependent and the precondition for all true civilization" (1933, 153). Man had come to embrace life affirmation. In fact, Schweitzer said, because the modern view embraced life affirmation so readily, it seemed to have always been the case. In ethics, Schweitzer found the prevailing concepts "lifeless" and "so lacking in content that it was impossible to relate them to an affirmative attitude" (154). He believed that something far deeper tied ethics and life affirmation together, yet it eluded him. He wrote,

> For months on end I lived in a continual state of mental excitement. Without the least success I let my thoughts be concentrated, even through my daily work at the hospital, on the real nature of the world-and-life-affirmation and of ethics, and on the question of what they have in common. I was wandering about in a thicket in which no path was to be found. I was leaning with all my might against an iron door which would not yield (154).

Schweitzer's breakthrough came during a long trip up the Ogowe River. Called to see the ailing wife of a missionary, Schweitzer boarded a small steamer to make the 160-mile trip to N'Gomo. It was an opportunity to be alone with his thoughts, surrounded by the teeming life along the great river. He recounted the trip in his autobiography:

> Slowly we crept upstream, laboriously navigating—it was the dry season— between the sandbanks. Lost in thought I sat on the deck of a barge, struggling to find the elementary and universal concept of the ethical that I had not discovered in any philosophy. I covered sheet after sheet with disconnected sentences merely to concentrate on the problem. Two days passed. Late on the third day, at the very moment when, at sunset, we were making our way through a herd of hippopotamuses, there flashed upon my mind, unforeseen and unsought, the phrase, "reverence for life." The iron door had yielded. The path in the thicket had become visible. Now I had found my way to the principle in which affirmation of the world and ethics are joined together!

I was at the root of the problem. I knew that the ethical acceptance of the world and of life, together with the ideals of civilization contained in this concept, has its foundation in thought (1933, 155).

Schweitzer found his breakthrough and was now free to develop the support for his theory. The concept should become clear in what follows.

Reverence for Life

During his seminal trip up the Ogowe River, Schweitzer concluded his search for the elusive Weltaschuung, or worldview. Reverence for Life became that concept, grounded in thought, life-affirming, and ethical. Schweitzer said that if man wished to understand himself and his role in the world, he had to turn away from preexisting concepts. Man had to turn inward and understand the most elemental drive within his being—not the thoughts produced in the conscious state but something deeper. Schweitzer spent months looking inward, searching his own mind for the elemental, driving force in his life. During his trip up the Ogowe, the idea came to him that his driving force was his "will to live." He wrote, "Day by day, hour by hour, I live and move in it. At every moment of reflection it stands fresh before me. There bursts forth from it again and again as from roots that can never dry up, a living world- and life-view which can deal with all the facts of Being. A mysticism of ethical union with Being grows out of it" (Schweitzer 1949b, 309).

Man begins by understanding his most basic instinct—his will to live—and then recognizes that the same instinct drives all of the life around him.

For Schweitzer the "will-to-live" was the most fundamental aspect of his own nature—and that of all of the abundant life around him. Consciousness of this will to live preceded even the most basic act of thinking. He said, "I am life that wills to live in the midst of life that wills to live" (Schweitzer 1949b, 309). Such is the basis of Reverence for Life. Man begins by understanding his most basic instinct—his will to live—and then recognizes that the same instinct drives all of the life around him. Schweitzer wrote that this shared will to live should instill in us an appreciation for the mystery of life. The knowledge of his own will to live, he wrote, "forces upon me an inward relation to the world, and fills me with reverence for the mysterious will-to-live which is in all things" (309). This force, shrouded in the mystery of life, lies well beyond the understanding even of science. This fundamental shared life drive was, for Schweitzer, the bedrock of ethics. He wrote, "Ethics consist, therefore, in my experiencing the compulsion to show to all will-to-live the same reverence as I do to my own. There we have given us that basic principle of the moral which is a necessity of thought. It is good to maintain and to encourage life; it is bad to destroy or to obstruct it" (309).

In Schweitzer's view, ethics leads directly to action—action that supports and nurtures other life. His is an ideal that both logically and ethically demands action following reflection. In his autobiography, Schweitzer offers a summary of the thought progression leading from the will to live to ethical action upon the world:

> The beginning of thought, a beginning that continually repeats itself, is that man does not simply accept his existence as something given, but experiences it as something unfathomably mysterious. Affirmation of life is the spiritual act by which man ceases to live thoughtlessly and begins to devote himself to his life with reverence in order to give it true value. To affirm life is to deepen, to make more inward, and to exalt the will to live. At the same time the man who has become a thinking being feels a compulsion to give to every will to live the same reverence for life that he gives to his own. He experiences that other life in his own. He accepts as good preserving life, promoting life, developing all life that is capable of development to its highest possible value. He considers as evil destroying life, injuring life, repressing life that is capable of development. This is the absolute, fundamental principle of ethics, and it is a fundamental postulate of thought (1933, 157).

Reverence for Life demands much from man in his relationships with all living things. According to Schweitzer, "It is unceasingly compelling him to be concerned about all the life that is round about him, and to feel himself responsible for it" (1949b, 330). For virtually all of recorded history, man's behavior toward Nature is most accurately characterized as adolescent. Domination trumps harmony; exploitation trumps understanding. Most of our attitudes toward insects, plants, and animals have been shaped by consideration of our needs alone. As adolescents are prone to do, we have been painfully egocentric. We have displayed an often-fatal disregard for the intrinsic wishes of other life forms, whether those wishes are expressed or silent. In his universal ethic, Schweitzer offers insight as to what those intrinsic wishes are and challenges us to reconsider our relationships to each other and all of the life around us. Given the rapid rate with which species are being lost forever, there is no better time to reconsider our position than now.

Before moving on to the specifics required by the ethic, it is worth reviewing Schweitzer's own description of his logical progression to Reverence for Life. Biographer James Brabazon recorded a 1953 Radio Brazzaville interview in which Schweitzer clarified his theory:

> I was always, even as a boy, engrossed in the philosophical problem of the relation between emotion and reason. Certain truths originate in feeling, others in the mind. Those truths that we derive from our emotions are of a moral kind—compassion, kindness, forgiveness, love for our neighbor. Reason, on the other hand, teaches us the truths that come from reflection.
>
> But with the great spirits of our world—the Hebrew prophets, Christ, Zoroaster, the Buddha, and others—feeling is always paramount. In them emotion holds its ground against reason, and all of us have an inner assurance that the truth of

emotion that these great spiritual figures reveal to us is the most profound and the most important truth.

The problem presented itself to me in these terms: Must we really be condemned to live in this dualism of emotional and rational truths? Since my particular pre-occupation was with problems of morality, I have always been struck by finding myself forced to recognize that the morality elaborated by philosophy, both ancient and modern, has been meager indeed when compared to the morality of the great religious and ethical geniuses who have taught us that the supreme and only truth capable of satisfying man's spirit is love.

I reached a point where I asked myself this question: Does the mind, in its striving for a morality that can guide us in life, lag so far behind the morality that emotion reveals because it is not sufficiently profound to be able to conceive what the great teachers, in obedience to feeling, have made known to us?

This led me to devote myself entirely to the search for a fundamental principle of morality. Others before me have done the same. Throughout history there have been philosophers who believed intuitively that reason must eventually succeed in discovering the true and profound nature of the good. I have tried to carry their work further. In so doing, I was brought to the point where I had to consider the question of what the fundamental idea of existence is. What is the mind's point of departure when it sets itself to the task of reflecting on humanity and on the world in which we live? This point of departure, I said to myself, is not any knowledge of the world that we have acquired. We do not have—and we will never have—true knowledge of the world; such knowledge will always remain a mystery to us.

The point of departure naturally offered for meditation between ourselves and the world is the simple evidence that we are life that wishes to live and are animated by a will in the midst of other lives animated by the same will. Simply by considering the act of thinking, our consciousness tells us this. True knowledge of the world consists in our being penetrated by a sense of the mystery of existence and of life.

If we proceed on the basis of this knowledge, it is no longer isolated reason that devotes itself to thought, but our whole being, that unity of emotion and reflection that constitutes the individual (1975, 246).

Other Life

"Who among us knows what significance any other kind of life has in itself, as a part of the universe?" Schweitzer asked. Wasn't it pure hubris through which man ranked other life forms—solely on the basis of their phylogenetic closeness to man? He warned of the dangers of this view: "From this distinction comes the view that there can be life that is worthless, which can be willfully destroyed. Then in the category of worthless life we may classify various kinds of insects, or primitive peoples, according to circumstances" (Schweitzer 1933, 235).

History has proven him painfully right many times over. Schweitzer predicted that the time would come when people would be astonished at how long it took man to recognize the narrowness of his worldview. People one day will realize that thoughtless injury to any life is incompatible with ethics: He wrote:

> Until now the great weakness in all ethical systems has been that they dealt only with the relations of man to man. In reality, however, the question is, What is our attitude toward the universe and all that it supports? A man is ethical only when life as such is sacred to him—the life of plants and animals as well as that of his fellow men—and when he devotes himself to helping all life that is in need of help. . . . The ethic of the relation of man to man is nothing but a fragment of the universal ethic" (1933, 158).

The ethic of Reverence for Life naturally flows into all life, whether that life is microbial, animal, or human. Schweitzer's ethic by necessity erected a big tent, standing in sharp contrast to most of the world's religions and their emphasis on human concerns: "To the person who is truly ethical all life is sacred, including that which from the human point of view seems lower" (1933, 235). For Schweitzer, this created daily ethical dilemmas. He rejoiced over a cure for sleeping sickness, yet he wrote that "every time I put the germs that cause the disease under the microscope I cannot but reflect that I have to sacrifice this life in order to save another" (236). Schweitzer did opt to treat the humans at the expense of the microbes. As such, he practiced a ranking system for life forms. However, he made choices in the light of a deeply held reverence for all forms of life—even microbial pathogens. Therein lies the difference: Schweitzer lived and practiced ethics in all the actions of his life, establishing a model behavior for us all. Referring to the truly ethical man, he wrote,

> He tears no leaf from a tree, plucks no flower, and takes care to crush no insect. . . . If he walks on the road after a shower and sees an earthworm which has strayed on to it, he bethinks himself that it must get dried up in the sun, if it does not return soon enough to ground into which it can burrow, so he lifts it from the deadly stone surface, and puts it on the grass. If he comes across an insect which has fallen into a puddle, he stops a moment in order to hold out a leaf or stalk on which it can save itself (Schweitzer 1933, 310).

Schweitzer recognized how difficult his theory would be for most people to accept. He was mocked for his comments on insects and bacteria, yet persisted in the conviction that he was right: "It is the fate of every truth to be a subject for laughter until it is generally recognized. Once it was considered folly to assume that men of colour were really men and ought to be treated as such, but the folly has come to become accepted as truth" (Schweitzer 1949b, 310).

He shared in the laughs that his theory could invoke when pushed to the extreme. When United Nations Ambassador Adlai Stevenson swatted a mosquito on the back of Schweitzer's neck, Schweitzer told him, "That was my mosquito."

Reverence for Life's love for mosquitoes and amoebae also made Schweitzer susceptible to the charge of being overly sentimental. Yet, his actions spoke to the contrary. When hunters wounded his favorite pelican, Parsifal, Schweitzer consulted Dr Frank Catchpool, a surgeon at Lambarene. Dr Catchpool recalled, "[Dr Schweitzer] had very clearly established the priorities of medical treatment: humans first, the worst cases first, and his own pelican, which he loved very much, was not to be put ahead of even the most minor human case" (Brabazon 1975, 256). An x-ray revealed buckshot in the bird's abdomen, making multiple bowel perforations likely. Dr Catchpool offered to operate. Schweitzer refused, stating that he could not justify using the scant resources of the hospital on his pelican. Over the next five days the pelican did not eat or drink. Dr Catchpool told Schweitzer that Parsifal was dehydrating and would surely die. Schweitzer replied, "If he's not better tomorrow I'll chop his head off" (256). Dr Catchpool recalled that Schweitzer was a man who would not let sentiment overrule his reason. Reverence for Life did not preclude him from killing the pelican he loved. Instead, it compelled him to relieve its suffering, which he did.

Schweitzer held a special place for animals ever since he was a boy.

Schweitzer held a special place for animals ever since he was a boy. Animals of all kinds wandered freely about the hospital grounds in Lambarene. His pelican Parsifal followed him everywhere, and photographers filmed Schweitzer with the abundance of animal life that populated the surrounding jungle, including antelopes, wild pigs, pelicans, lizards, and monkeys. He believed that humans owed a special debt to animals, in part because of all they had endured in experiments to benefit humans. He did not take lightly man's constant cruelty to animals. He passionately decried the suffering that animals routinely endured in human hands for the most trivial of reasons. For the torture that students routinely put animals through to observe known phenomena, for brutality in the slaughterhouses, for the "intolerable" treatment from heartless men and the cruel play of children, Schweitzer said, "we all share the guilt" (Schweitzer 1949b, 319). The ethics of Reverence for Life "make us join in keeping on the look-out for opportunities of bringing some sort of help to animals, to make up for the great misery which men inflict on them . . . " (319).

Individual Responsibility: The Challenge of the Ethic

Although it may seem initially absurd that a doctor could feel pain in killing bacteria, consider just for a moment how profoundly different the world would be if each of us were to assume personal responsibility for all of the life around us. Schweitzer did not say that one couldn't kill pathogenic bacteria, dangerous animals, or someone intent on killing you. Rather, he said that we must choose. And we must weigh each of our choices carefully in light of the knowledge that all life is sacred and intimately connected through a universal will to live. How often is there another option in what we do that can save and preserve life? You may kill an animal for food, he said, but you must not hunt for pleasure or sport. A farmer may mow down a thousand flowers to feed his livestock. Yet, if on the way home he knocks the head off one more flower for pleasure only, "he thereby commits a wrong against life without being under the pressure of necessity."

> *The ethic forces individual responsibility and individual choice in the light of a deep reverence for all life.*

In Reverence for Life, Schweitzer gave us not a map but a compass. The ethic forces individual responsibility and individual choice in the light of a deep reverence for all life. Like Goethe before him, Schweitzer detested dogma in all forms and proposed no guidelines or rules for individuals to follow. That would make it easier and absolve people of the responsibility to think and act on their own: "In ethical conflicts man can arrive only at subjective decisions. No one can decide for him at what point, on each occasion, lies the extreme limit for his persistence in the preservation and furtherance of life. He alone has to judge this issue, by letting himself be guided by a feeling of the highest possible responsibility towards other life" (Schweitzer 1949b, 318).

Relationships Among People

For those interested in health service, the obligations that Reverence for Life holds for the relationships among people are by far the most relevant. Reverence for Life requires everyone to exercise personal responsibility for all of the people around them. No one is exempt, and no living person anywhere is outside our collective sphere of responsibility. Ultimately, the ethic compels all thinking people to raise their idealistic impulses to the surface and improve the lot of humanity through some form of service. The choice is not optional; it is an imperative and logical consequence of Reverence for Life. Schweitzer once told one of his grandchildren, "Find your own Lambarene." Not everyone could do what he did in Africa, but his message was clear: We all can—and should—find service in some form.

Schweitzer strongly believed in the idealism that many in our modern culture have forgotten, or have sacrificed to the gods at the altar of Wall Street. Even the word *idealism* carries a modern connotation of naiveté or conjures up images of a Pollyanna. But it didn't always. Idealism lies at the very heart of the ethic that Reverence for Life holds for people. Schweitzer dedicated his life to that idealism, and the world recognized him for it with, among many other honors, a Nobel Peace Prize. Schweitzer believed that the world was—and, I believe, it remains—full of idealistic people. He urged people to bring forth that nascent idealism and practice it—to make it part of the very fiber of their lives. In Schweitzer's view, the future of the world depends on it:

> Judging by what I have learned about men and women, I am convinced that far more idealistic aspiration exists than is ever evident. Just as the rivers we see are much less numerous than the underground streams, so the idealism that is visible is minor compared to what men and women carry in their hearts, unreleased or scarcely released. Mankind is waiting and longing for those who can accomplish the task of untying what is knotted and bringing the underground waters to the surface (1933, 91).

It is unfortunate that most of the idealistic acts performed in this world receive little recognition. I know many people who have sacrificed much to improve the lives of the less fortunate. These people have worked in obscurity, made do with less, and received only the affirmation that comes from the work itself in return for their services. Any of them would say that that is enough. Still, a culture that so profusely rewards athletes, entertainers, the wealthy, and anyone on television should pay more attention to those who work to change the world. Schweitzer recognized how unusual his own fame was, particularly given the work he chose to do. He wrote, "Of all the will toward the ideal in mankind only a small part can manifest itself in public action. All the rest of this force must be content with small and obscure deeds. The sum of these, however, is a thousand times stronger than the acts of those who receive wide public recognition. The latter, compared to the former, are like the foam on the waves of a deep ocean" (1933, 90).

The idealistic impulses for Schweitzer were synonymous with the spiritual, the windows through which one would come in intimate contact with God. Schweitzer's faith was an active one. For him, as for many others, service instilled a joy and sense of fulfillment that sustained him through the more difficult stretches of life. Schweitzer knew the hard times well, suffering through many himself during the 50 years he lived in Africa in what his daughter Rhena termed a "monk-like existence."

During a conversation with Norman Cousins at Lambarene in the 1950s, Schweitzer candidly discussed his views on God, saying, "God manifests himself through the human spirit. Insofar as the individual is able to discover and develop his spiritual awareness, he is at one with the Deity. Nothing is more wonderful or mysterious than watching the workings of the inner awareness by which man discovers his true spirituality" (Cousins 1960, 194).

Schweitzer's own awareness expanded during his medical service to the Africans at Lambarene. The work became his active spiritual manifestation and fostered a close connection with God. Maybe that can be true for us all. During a conference I attended, a friend, Mark Murphy, commented on how the service work he had been doing tied in with his own faith. "Perhaps," he said, "what we are all doing is building the Kingdom of God here on earth."[2]

To Schweitzer, spiritual evolution came not through striving for the perceived rewards promised in the afterlife of Christian belief but, rather, through actively developing the goodness that is inherently alive within us all. The individual discovers his true self when he brings his inherent goodness to life through ethical action. According to Schweitzer, God does not actively intervene on the side of the righteous, and man's role is not to sit and await Divine intervention. The horror of two world wars provided ample evidence of that. Rather, it is up to all of us to intervene on the side of the ethical, the side of God. Schweitzer wrote, "God manifests himself through the spiritual evolution of man and through the struggle of man to become aware of the spiritual nature of his being and then to nurture it and give it scope" (Cousins 1960, 192). For Schweitzer, that scope required ethically grounded action. Specifically, it meant devoting the self to others whose lives were in need. Thus, the work became the outward manifestation of the inner spiritual growth. The inner spiritual growth fueled the desire to continue the work. One infused the other. In the midst of the exchange, one could feel the presence of God. Schweitzer wrote,

> By devoting myself to that which comes within my sphere of influence and needs me, I make spiritual, inward devotion to infinite Being a reality and thereby give my own poor existence meaning and richness. The river has found its sea (1949b, 305).

Anyone undertaking the practice of Reverence for Life must first practice reverence for the self. According to Schweitzer, it is not possible to practice goodwill to others while neglecting the self or not being fully honest with oneself. He wrote, "I practice higher self-maintenance. Out of reverence for my own existence I place myself under the compulsion of veracity towards myself. . . . I fear that if I were untrue to myself, I should be wounding my will-to-live with a poisoned spear" (1949b, 314). Devotion to one's own life leads one to practice a more broad-based ethic of devotion to other life. Schweitzer said, "The ethics of sincerity toward oneself passes imperceptibly into that of devotion to others," (1933, 314). He added, "Only he who in deepened devotion to his own will-to-live experiences inward freedom from outward occurrences is capable of devoting himself in profound and steady fashion to the life of others" (1949b, 314). That devotion quite naturally includes other struggles:

> We have to carry on the struggle against the evil that is in mankind, not by judging others, but by judging ourselves. Struggle with oneself and veracity to oneself are the means by which we influence others. We quietly draw them into our efforts to attain the deep spiritual self-realization which springs from reverence for one's own life. Power makes no noise. It is there, and works. True ethics begin where the use of language ceases (Schweitzer 1949b, 315).

Although Schweitzer wrote mostly on the moral and the ethical, he also noted the unequal distribution of resources that cause so much of the world's suffering. He thus targeted those who oriented their lives around the acquisition of wealth, "They [the ethics of Reverence for Life] bid me think of others, and make me ponder whether I can allow myself the inward right to pluck all the fruit that my hand can reach" (1949b, 320). Schweitzer thought that wealth should serve the larger community, not just a few individuals within it. Everyone has a moral responsibility to contribute. Schweitzer gave most of his life's earnings, acquired through concerts, book royalties, lectures, and the Nobel Peace Prize to the hospital in Lambarene. He aimed his most jarring shots at those who still need most to hear it all these years later: those who are comfortable. Schweitzer knowingly challenged us, recognizing that we were—and are—the least likely to hear him. He said, "To the happy the voice of the true ethics is dangerous, if they venture to listen to it" (1949b, 321). He drew heavily upon the ethical teachings of Jesus in calling the comfortable forward into service. There is no clearer wake-up call to the American medical establishment of the early 21st century than this one:

> Nor will Reverence for Life grant me my happiness as my own. At the moment when I should like to enjoy myself without restraint, it wakes in me reflection about misery that I see or suspect, and it does not allow me to drive away the uneasiness I feel. Just as the wave cannot exist for itself, but is ever a part of the heaving surface of the ocean, so must I never live my life for itself, but always in the experience which is going on around me. It is an uncomfortable doctrine which the true ethics whisper into my ear. You are happy, they say; therefore you are called upon to give much. Whatever more than others you have received in health, natural gifts, working capacity, success, a beautiful childhood, harmonious family circumstances, you must not accept as a matter of course. You must pay a price for them. You must show more than average devotion of life to life (Schweitzer 1949b, 321).

For health professionals, Reverence for Life holds specific obligations. Schweitzer saw the huge disparities between the health services available in Europe and those in colonial Africa. He saw the Africans' needless suffering and dying and urged physicians to respond. Reverence for Life contained no provisions about nationalities or borders. Man was obliged to relieve suffering everywhere, even in remote corners of African jungles. As long as there was a need for their services, the ethic obliged those who had the skills to respond. "The ethics of Reverence for Life," he wrote, "demand from all that they devote a portion of their life to their fellows" (1949b, 323). As health providers, we are in a better position than most to understand Schweitzer's words. We share the same profession and understand the depth of human suffering. Most of us already carry heavy patient-care responsibilities, work long hours, and wrestle with the changing business of health care.

Still, in Schweitzer's call, we can readily identify the aspirations that guided us into the medical profession in the beginning. We got into this to care for those who need us. Reverence for Life challenges us to broaden our mandate to include those who do not pay our salaries and do not live near us. We must care for all people, whether they be victims of a tsunami in Asia or poverty in Africa. With actions more powerful than his inspirational words, Schweitzer gives us all pause for reflection. Few of us can do what he did in his life—but we all can do our part. In his autobiography, he wrote,

> It struck me as inconceivable that I should be allowed to lead such a happy life while I saw so many people around me struggling with sorrow and suffering. . . . The thought came to me that I must not accept this good fortune as a matter of course, but must give something in return. . . . I cannot help but feel the suffering all around me, not only of humanity, but of the whole of creation. . . . I have never tried to withdraw myself from this community of suffering. It seemed to me a matter of course that we should all take our share of the burden of pain that lies upon the world. . . . But however concerned I was with the suffering in the world, I never let myself become lost in brooding over it.
> I always held firmly to the thought that each one of us can do a little to bring some portion of it to an end. . . .
>
> If people can be found who revolt against the spirit of thoughtlessness and are sincere and profound enough to spread the ideals of ethical progress, we will witness the emergence of a new spiritual force strong enough to evoke a new spirit in mankind (1933, 82, 242).

Some 40 years after his death, Schweitzer continues to offer us a path to a richer, more meaningful existence. Reverence for Life holds timeless wisdom for us all, compelling us to nurture, revere, and recognize the Divine within all of the life around us. It compels us to assume responsibility for all of the people in our "sphere of influence," which includes all of humanity. The challenge for us now is to heed the call Schweitzer made to us so long ago.

Endnotes

1. *Webster's New World Dictionary, Third College Edition.* New York: Simon and Schuster; 1991.
2. The conference, Kellogg Conference on the Non-Profit Sector, was held in Washington, DC in 1998. Mark Murphy is a former Kellogg Fellow and the director of the Fund for New Jersey, a philanthropic organization.

The Universal Declaration of Human Rights

Preamble

Whereas recognition of the inherent dignity and of the equal and inalienable rights of all members of the human family is the foundation of freedom, justice and peace in the world,

Whereas disregard and contempt for human rights have resulted in barbarous acts which have outraged the conscience of mankind, and the advent of a world in which human beings shall enjoy freedom of speech and belief and freedom from fear and want has been proclaimed as the highest aspiration of the common people,

Whereas it is essential, if man is not to be compelled to have recourse, as a last resort, to rebellion against tyranny and oppression, that human rights should be protected by the rule of law,

Whereas it is essential to promote the development of friendly relations between nations,

Whereas the peoples of the United Nations have in the Charter reaffirmed their faith in fundamental human rights, in the dignity and worth of the human person and in the equal rights of men and women and have determined to promote social progress and better standards of life in larger freedom,

Whereas Member States have pledged themselves to achieve, in co-operation with the United Nations, the promotion of universal respect for and observance of human rights and fundamental freedoms,

Whereas a common understanding of these rights and freedoms is of the greatest importance for the full realization of this pledge,

Now, therefore, **THE GENERAL ASSEMBLY Proclaims this Universal Declaration of Human Rights** as a common standard of achievement for all peoples and all nations, to the end that every individual and every organ of society, keeping this Declaration constantly in mind, shall strive by teaching and education to promote respect for these rights and freedoms and by progressive measures, national and international, to secure their universal and effective recognition and observance, both among the peoples of Member States themselves and among the peoples of territories under their jurisdiction.

Article 1
All human beings are born free and equal in dignity and rights. They are endowed with reason and conscience and should act towards one another in a spirit of brotherhood.

Article 2
Everyone is entitled to all the rights and freedoms set forth in this Declaration, without distinction of any kind, such as race, colour, sex, language, religion, political or other opinion, national or social origin, property, birth or other status.

Furthermore, no distinction shall be made on the basis of the political, jurisdictional or international status of the country or territory to which a person belongs, whether it be independent, trust, non-self-governing or under any other limitation of sovereignty.

Article 3
Everyone has the right to life, liberty and the security of person.

Article 4
No one shall be held in slavery or servitude; slavery and the slave trade shall be prohibited in all their forms.

Article 5
No one shall be subjected to torture or to cruel, inhuman or degrading treatment or punishment.

Article 6
Everyone has the right to recognition everywhere as a person before the law.

Article 7
All are equal before the law and are entitled without any discrimination to equal protection against any discrimination in violation of this Declaration and against any incitement to such discrimination.

Article 8
Everyone has the right to an effective remedy by the competent national tribunals for acts violating the fundamental rights granted him by the constitution or by law.

Article 9
No one shall be subjected to arbitrary arrest, detention or exile.

Article 10
Everyone is entitled in full equality to a fair, and public hearing by an independent and impartial tribunal, in the determination of his rights and obligations and of any criminal charge against him.

Article 11
Everyone charged with a penal offence has the right to be presumed innocent until proven guilty according to law in a public trial at which he has had all the guarantees necessary for his defence.

No one shall be held guilty of any penal offence on account of any act or omission which did not constitute a penal offence, under national or international law, at the time when it was committed. Nor shall a heavier penalty be imposed than the one that was applicable at the time the penal offence was committed.

Article 12
No one shall be subjected to arbitrary interference with his privacy, family, home or correspondence, nor to attacks upon his honour and reputation. Everyone has the right to the protection of the law against such interference or attacks.

Article 13
Everyone has the right to freedom of movement and residence within the borders of each State.

Everyone has the right to leave any country, including his own, and to return to his country.

Article 14
Everyone has the right to seek and to enjoy in other countries asylum from persecution.

This right may not be invoked in the case of prosecutions genuinely arising from non-political crimes or from acts contrary to the purposes and principles of the United Nations.

Article 15
Everyone has the right to a nationality.

No one shall be arbitrarily deprived of his nationality nor denied the right to change his nationality.

Article 16
Men and women of full age, without any limitation due to race, nationality or religion, have the right to marry and to found a family. They are entitled to equal rights as to marriage, during marriage and at its dissolution.

Marriage shall be entered into only with the free and full consent of the intending spouses.

The family is the natural and fundamental group unit of society and is entitled to protection by society and the State.

Article 17
Everyone has the right to own property alone as well as in association with others.

No one shall be arbitrarily deprived of his property.

Article 18
Everyone has the right to freedom of thought, conscience and religion; this right includes freedom to change his religion or belief, and freedom, either alone or in community with others and in public or private, to manifest his religion or belief in teaching, practice, worship and observance.

Article 19
Everyone has the right to freedom of opinion and expression; this right includes freedom to hold opinions without interference and to seek, receive and impart information and ideas through any media and regardless of frontiers.

Article 20
Everyone has the right to freedom of peaceful assembly and association. No one may be compelled to belong to an association.

Article 21
Everyone has the right to take part in the government of his country, directly or through freely chosen representatives.

Everyone has the right of equal access to public service in his country.

The will of the people shall be the basis of the authority of government; this will shall be expressed in periodic and genuine elections which shall be by universal and equal suffrage and shall be held by secret vote or by equivalent free voting procedures.

Article 22
Everyone, as a member of society, has the right to social security and is entitled to realization, through national effort and international co-operation and in accordance with the organization and resources of each State, of the economic, social and cultural rights indispensable for his dignity and the free development of his personality.

Article 23
Everyone has the right to work, to free choice of employment, to just and favourable conditions of work and to protection against unemployment.

Everyone, without any discrimination, has the right to equal pay for equal work.

Everyone who works has the right to just and favourable remuneration ensuring for himself and his family an existence worthy of human dignity, and supplemented, if necessary, by other means of social protection.

Everyone has the right to form and to join trade unions for the protection of his interests.

Article 24
Everyone has the right to rest and leisure, including reasonable limitation of working hours and periodic holidays with pay.

Article 25
Everyone has the right to a standard of living adequate for the health and well-being of himself and of his family, including food, clothing, housing and medical care and necessary social services, and the right to security in the event of unemployment, sickness, disability, widowhood, old age or other lack of livelihood in circumstances beyond his control.

Motherhood and childhood are entitled to special care and assistance. All children, whether born in or out of wedlock, shall enjoy the same social protection.

Article 26
Everyone has the right to education. Education shall be free, at least in the elementary and fundamental stages. Elementary education shall be compulsory. Technical and professional education shall be made generally available and higher education shall be equally accessible to all on the basis of merit.

Education shall be directed to the full development of the human personality and to the strengthening of respect for human rights and fundamental freedoms. It shall promote understanding, tolerance and friendship among all nations, racial or religious groups, and shall further the activities of the United Nations for the maintenance of peace.

Parents have a prior right to choose the kind of education that shall be given to their children.

Article 27
Everyone has the right freely to participate in the cultural life of the community, to enjoy the arts and to share in scientific advancement and its benefits.

Everyone has the right to the protection of the moral and material interests resulting from any scientific, literary or artistic production of which he is the author.

Article 28
Everyone is entitled to a social and international order in which the rights and freedoms set forth in this Declaration can be fully realized.

Article 29

Everyone has duties to the community in which alone the free and full development of his personality is possible.

In the exercise of his rights and freedoms, everyone shall be subject only to such limitations as are determined by law solely for the purpose of securing due recognition and respect for the rights and freedoms of others and of meeting the just requirements of morality, public order and the general welfare in a democratic society.

These rights and freedoms may in no case be exercised contrary to the purposes and principles of the United Nations.

Article 30

Nothing in this Declaration may be interpreted as implying for any State, group or person any right to engage in any activity or to perform any act aimed at the destruction of any of the rights and freedoms set forth herein.

UN Millennium Development Goals

1. Eradicate Extreme Poverty and Hunger

Target 1: Halve, between 1990 and 2015, the proportion of people whose income is less than one dollar a day.
Target 2: Halve, between 1990 and 2015, the proportion of people who suffer from hunger.

2. Achieve Universal Primary Education

Target 3: Ensure that, by 2015, children everywhere, boys and girls alike, will be able to complete a full course of primary schooling.

3. Promote Gender Equality and Empower Women

Target 4: Eliminate gender disparity in primary and secondary education, preferably by 2005, and to all levels of education no later than 2015.

4. Reduce Child Mortality

Target 5: Reduce by two-thirds, between 1990 and 2015, the under-five mortality rate.

5. Improve Maternal Health

Target 6: Reduce by three-quarters, between 1990 and 2015, the maternal mortality ratio.

6. Combat HIV/AIDS, Malaria, and Other Diseases

Target 7: Have halted by 2015, and begun to reverse, the spread of HIV/AIDS.
Target 8: Have halted by 2015, and begun to reverse, the incidence of malaria and other major diseases.

7. Ensure Environmental Sustainability

Target 9: Integrate the principles of sustainable development into country policies and programmes and reverse the loss of environmental resources.
Target 10: Halve, by 2015, the proportion of people without sustainable access to safe drinking water.
Target 11: By 2020, to have achieved a significant improvement in the lives of at least 100 million slum dwellers.

8. Develop a Global Partnership for Development, With Targets for Aid, Trade, and Debt Relief

Target 12: Develop further an open, rule-based, predictable, non-discriminatory trading and financial system. Includes a commitment to good governance, development and poverty reduction—both nationally and internationally.
Target 13: Address the Special Needs of the Least Developed Countries. Includes tariff- and quota-free access for their exports; enhanced debt relief for heavily indebted poor countries; cancellation of official bilateral debt; and more generous official development assistance for countries committed to poverty reduction.
Target 14: Address the Special Needs of landlocked countries and small island developing states (through the Programme of Action for the Sustainable Development of Small Island Developing States and the outcome of the twenty-second special session of the General Assembly).
Target 15: Deal comprehensively with the debt problems of developing countries through national and international measures in order to make debt sustainable in the long term.
Target 16: In cooperation with developing countries, develop and implement strategies for decent and productive work for youth.
Target 17: In co-operation with pharmaceutical companies, provide access to affordable, essential drugs in developing countries.
Target 18: In co-operation with the private sector, make available the benefits of new technologies, especially information and communications.

Glossary

Acquired Immune Deficiency Syndrome (AIDS): A disease in which the immune system becomes severely weakened and unable to properly fight serious infections and secondary diseases. AIDS results from infection with the human immunodeficiency virus (HIV), which attacks and depletes human helper t-cells.

Acute Respiratory Distress Syndrome (ARDS): Acute respiratory distress syndrome manifests as an acute and severe injury to the lungs (often both). ARDS does not have a specific cause but is a lung dysfunction associated with a variety of diseases, such as pneumonia, sepsis, and trauma. ARDS occurs in children of all ages, reflected by the name change from "adult" to "acute" respiratory distress syndrome.

Aid to Families with Dependent Children (AFDC): Aid to Families with Dependent Children was a welfare program administered by the United States Department of Health and Human Services. It was created by the Social Security Act of 1935 as part of the New Deal under the original name of Aid to Dependent Children (ADC). In 1996, the program was revised and renamed the Temporary Assistance to Needy Families (TANF). The corresponding legislation imposes a lifetime limit of five years on the receipt of benefits.

Apparel Industry Partnership (AIP): An informal association initiated by President Clinton in 1996. The partnership is made up of representatives from consumer, human rights, and religious organizations, and footwear and apparel companies. The group is designed to develop recommendations and develop standards about working conditions in domestic and overseas apparel factories, and to provide consumers with confidence about working conditions that ultimately produces their apparel and footwear.

Asia Pacific Economic Cooperation (APEC): A membership organization made up of 21 "member economies" from the Asia-Pacific Rim. APEC is designed to promote economic growth, cooperation, and open trade and investment in the Asia-Pacific region.

Bank of Credit and Commerce International (BCCI): The Bank of Credit and Commerce International was a prominent foreign bank in Pakistan from 1972 until it collapsed in 1991. It dissolved among swirling allegations of fraud, racketeering, and laundered drug money. At the time of the shut down, BCCI reported over $20 billion in losses and was reportedly linked to the CIA and numerous alleged terrorists.

Border Industrialization Program (BIP): A program initiated by the Mexican government in 1965 with the design of stimulating the economies of the northern states on the US border. The program was intended to provide jobs for Mexican workers by allowing US companies to operate assembly factories on the Mexican side of the border. Better known as maquiladoras, the factories produce products for duty-free export and maximum profit using Mexican (and Central American) labor.

British Broadcasting Corporation (BBC): A state-owned broadcasting network in the United Kingdom that operates television and radio stations and is financed by the sale of television licenses, publishing interests, and programming. It is not allowed to carry advertisements and is controlled by a board of governors, each appointed by the government for a five-year term. A 1927 royal charter converted the BBC from a private company to a public corporation and required that news programs be politically impartial.

Centers for Disease Control (CDC): An agency of the Department of Health and Human Services that is designed to safeguard the American people's public health and safety. The CDC works towards providing credible information about current and emerging diseases in order to enhance health decisions. The CDC works with federal agencies, state health departments, and other organizations to prevent and control diseases and educate the public about infectious diseases, environmental health, and general health promotion. The CDC is headquartered in Atlanta, Georgia.

Central Intelligence Agency (CIA): An independent US executive agency formed in 1947 with the goal of conducting covert operations and gathering intelligence beneficial to the well-being of the country. The CIA reports to the president and the National Security Council and enjoys special powers uncommon to other federal agencies. The CIA may spend agency funds without accounting for them, may maintain a secret staff, and the CIA employees may be hired or fired without any adherence to civil service procedures. As a safeguard against potential abuse, the agency has no authority to conduct domestic investigations and must obtain assistance from the Federal Bureau of Investigation (FBI) in such cases.

Congressional Budget Office (CBO): A federal agency contained within the legislative branch. It is designed to provide Congress with a nonpartisan analysis of the economic impact of current and future budget decisions.

Consumer Price Index (CPI): A measure of the average change of the price paid by consumers for a representative set of goods and services (such as food, gasoline, and clothing). The CPI program generates data each month and can help identify periods of inflation or deflation. The CPI is also known as a cost-of-living index.

Convention Against Torture (CAT): A treaty that set out to establish an inspection protocol of prisons and detention centers for each country in agreement. Inspectors would monitor countries holding detainees and torture or "cruel, inhuman and degrading treatment or punishment" directed against such prisoners would be forbidden. The treaty has been criticized for lacking an enforcement mechanism, allowing even those countries in agreement to violate the basic provisions.

Convention on the Elimination of All Forms Discrimination Against Women (CEDAW): The convention constitutes an 18-member committee with the view that "discrimination against women is incompatible with human dignity and constitutes an obstacle to the full realization of the potentialities of women; therefore, the right of women to share equally in improved conditions of life must be promoted and protected." The committee is empowered to settle disputes between states regarding observance of the convention and shall also receive input from various states to aid in implementing the articles of the convention.

Convention on the Rights of the Child (CRC): A treaty that mandates that children everywhere should have basic human rights, including protection from abuse and exploitation, and have the opportunity to participate in the development of a chosen culture, familial organization, and social society. The treaty seeks to protect those rights and ensure that children worldwide receive them without discrimination.

Department of Health and Human Services (HHS): A cabinet level agency of the executive branch charged with safeguarding the health of all Americans and sponsoring health-related programs. HHS administers programs such as Social Security, Medicare, and the federal portions of Medicaid. HHS also overseas other health-related agencies such as the National Institute of Health and Centers for Disease Control.

Development Assistance Committee of the OECD (DAC): A special committee formed by the Organization for Economic Co-operation and Development. The DAC works to expand aid resources used to assist developing countries and to make sure that any such aid is used in the most effective way possible. The DAC is composed of member countries that review their own contributions to developing nations and consult with the other members on new development assistance policies. Most of the developed world, including the United States, Canada, Australia, New Zealand, the European Union countries, and more are members of the DAC.

Dichlorodiphenyl Trichloroethane (DDT): Dichlorodiphenyl trichloroethane (DDT) is an insecticide containing chlorine that had widespread use in the 1940s and 1950s until scientists became aware of its high toxicity to humans and other living organisms. DDT was sprayed to combat mosquitoes carrying malaria, although some began to show a resistance to it over time. The United States banned the use of DDT in 1972, but other countries, such as India, still depend on DDT to combat the high annual mortality resulting from malaria infections.

Disability-Adjusted Life Year (DALY): The disability-adjusted life-year (DALY) is a measure that factors in the impact of illness, disability, and mortality on overall population health. The DALY indicator considers the amount of time lived with an illness or disability and the life years lost from premature mortality. The amount of time lost due to premature mortality is calculated via reference to standard life-expectancy tables.

Drug Enforcement Administration (DEA): An agency branch of the US Justice Department with the duty to enforce federal laws and regulations that apply to controlled substances. The DEA often works together with the FBI and state law enforcement agencies. The DEA is also responsible for conducting US-related drug investigations abroad.

Environmental Protection Agency (EPA): An independent governmental agency responsible for the enforcement of environmental laws. The EPA must ensure the protection of the natural environment, including safeguarding air quality, water quality, wetlands, and monitoring hazardous wastes, and other environmental matters.

European Union (EU): A union of 25 independent states drawn from the European Community and founded to enhance political, economic, and social cooperation between members. The 1993 treaty establishing the EU expanded the political scope of foreign and security policy, and created a central European bank that adopted the euro as a common currency at the end of the 20th century.

Export Processing Zone (EPZ): Industrial parks designed by a government to encourage the development of labor-intensive exports using a large amount of imported inputs. The term "export processing" describes the labor that "processes" the imported inputs and then exports the end products. Companies working in such zones can manufacture goods with low or no taxes as an incentive.

Food and Agriculture Organization (FAO): A United Nations agency concerned with expanding a stronger world economy by promoting sustainable rural development. The FAO seeks to promote food production and self-reliance for the poorest farmers, and to raise nutrition levels worldwide The FAO works to accomplish these goals by making investigations, publishing reports, organizing conferences, and offering technical aid to improve agricultural methods and food yields.

Food and Drug Administration (FDA): A federal agency responsible for regulating the production, use and safety of food, dietary supplements, drugs, cosmetics, medical devices, and related products. The FDA is a branch agency of the Department of Health and Human Services.

Foreign Direct Investment (FDI): A cross-border investment made to establish a lasting financial stake and degree of control in an enterprise. The foreign investor usually holds an interest of at least 10% in equity capital. FDI is important for economic growth and contributes to the Gross Domestic Product (GDP) of national economies.

Free Trade Area of the Americas (FTAA): A US-led expansion of the North American Free Trade Agreement that established a trading block of the countries of North and South America, excluding Cuba. The current FTAA agreement includes 34 countries, 800 million people, and covers more than $13 trillion in annual goods and services.

Free Trade Zone (FTZ): A port or area within a country where duty-free foreign goods enter usually for purposes of additional manufacture, storage, or additional packaging. The foreign goods are subject to duty only when they leave the duty-free zone and enter other parts of the country.

Gender-related Development Index (GDI): A United Nations Development Program index based on three indicators: life expectancy measured at birth, educational attainment, and one's standard of living (real GDP per capita). For each indicator, minimum and maximum values have been established and adjusted in accordance with the disparity in expected between women and men.

Genetically Modified (GM): A technology called recombinant DNA technology that alters the genetic makeup of living organisms (animals, plants, or bacteria). The resulting organism will carry a scientifically engineered trait and will be considered "genetically modified." Current and future GM products include biological medicines and vaccines, food ingredients, and animal feeds.

General Accounting Office (GAO): An independent, non-partisan agency designed to review federal financial transactions and report directly to Congress. Upon congressional request, the GAO investigates and reports on the government's performance while using public funds.

General Agreement on Tariffs and Trade (GATT): An international agreement originally created in 1947 and amended in 1994. GATT aims to increase international trade by reducing tariffs and other trade barriers, and also sets a code of conduct for such trade. The 1994 amendment created a World Trade Organization, which oversees the implementation of the GATT and the 125 participating countries.

Global Fund to Fight AIDS, Tuberculosis, and Malaria (GFATM): An independent public-private partnership designed to attract, manage, and distribute financial resources from governments, businesses, and individuals worldwide. GFATM does not implement health-related programs but instead channels funds to organizations or local communities with experience fighting AIDS, TB, and malaria.

Global Program on Aids (GPA): A United Nations–World Health Organization program initiated in 1988 with the purpose of developing a global strategy to fight HIV/AIDS. The GPA strategy set out to prevent the transmission of HIV without the use of expensive new technologies or resources. The program had three main components: condom promotion and distribution, changes in sexual behavior, and the control of STDs that may increase the transmission of HIV.

Gross Domestic Product (GDP): The total market value of all of the goods and services produced within the national borders of a country. The GDP is the best overall measure of a country's economic output, size and annual growth.

Gross National Income (GNI): The total value of goods and services produced within a country (ie, its Gross Domestic Product), combined with income received from other countries, minus payments made to other countries. Income received or payments made are often in the form of interest and dividends.

Gross National Product (GNP): The total value goods and services produced for consumption in a society. The GNP measures economic activity based on labor and production output. GNP data figures include the manufacture of tangible goods such as cars or food, as well as allowances for depreciation and indirect business taxes.

Group of Seven (G-7)/Group of Eight (G-8): The seven largest industrialized nations that meet regularly to discuss international economic policies. The organization includes the United States, Canada, Britain, France, Italy, Germany, and Japan. When referred to as the G-8, the group also includes Russia.

Health Maintenance Organization (HMO): A health plan that provides health care services to its members for a fixed annual premium. The organization can be either for-profit or not-for-profit, and members must generally stay within a network of participating providers when seeking treatment.

Heavily Indebted Poor Country Initiative (HIPC): An international debt relief initiative for the world's poorest countries to ensure that they can fully manage their foreign debt burden. The current HIPC aims to ensure that the development of a country will not be compromised by the original debt or restructured debt burden. HIPC strategies include debt relief/cancellation and structural and social policy reform that includes protections for basic health and education. The revised 1999 HIPC allows for full debt cancellation by G7 nations for counties that face an "unsustainable debt burden, beyond available debt relief mechanisms." The HIPC remains controversial as public interest groups claim it takes too long for complete debt relief and that countries must still divert money from essential public services to comply.

Human Development Index (HDI): A United Nations Development Program (UNDP) index that measures human development according to poverty, literacy, education, life expectancy, and other factors such as GDP. HDI has become the favored standard for measuring people's well-being, especially in the case of children.

Human Immunodeficiency Virus (HIV): A retrovirus that attacks the human immune system and compromises the ability to fight off infections such as pneumonia, diarrhea, tumors, and other illnesses. HIV is the virus which eventually causes AIDS.

Human Poverty Index (HPI): A poverty index developed by the United Nations Development Program (UNDP) that does not rely on income figures. The HPI relies on human conditions associate with poverty low life expectancy, illiteracy, and lack of access to basic health services, clean drinking water, and adequate nutrition.

Import Substitution Industrialization (ISI): An economic and trade and policy advocating that developing countries substitute imported products with local alternatives. ISI often requires government subsidies and high tariff barriers to shield local industries.

Infant Mortality Rate (IMR): The number of deaths of infants under one year old per 1,000 live births in the same year.

Inter-American Development Bank (IDB): A multilateral lending agency formed in 1959 to promote economic and social development in the Americas and the Caribbean. The bank conditions many of its loans on the privatization and development of public sectors such as health care, energy, and education, but does not demand any broad-scale economic or social adjustments. The bank currently has 46 member countries.

International Bank for Reconstruction and Development (IBRD): Also known as the World Bank, the IBRD is a specialized United Nations agency dedicated to reducing international debt by providing financing, research, and guidance to developing nations to help aid their economic advancement. The IBRD also strives, through its lending practices, to encourage political actions that curb corruption and encourage democracy. The IBRD's operations are maintained by debt payments regulated by its member countries.

International Confederation of Free Trade Unions (ICFTU): An international trading body formed in 1949 to help improve the lives of the poorest workers worldwide. The ICFTU is composed in part of national organizations representing workers unions and devotes most of its work toward educational, social, and economic projects aimed to benefit those same workers.

International Convention on the Elimination of All Forms of Racial Discrimination (ICERD): A United Nations article that provides a definition of racial discrimination and seeks to end discriminatory practices worldwide, particularly in the employment and education sectors. The Convention was entered into force in 1969 has been ratified by more than three-quarters of the United Nations membership.

International Covenant on Civil and Political Rights (ICCPR): A United Nations treaty based on the Universal Declaration of Human Rights. The ICCPR is monitored by the Human Rights Committee (HRC), which meets three times annually to review and consider reports from member states detailing their compliance with the treaty. The ICCPR contains two optional protocols. The first establishes the means by which individuals from one of the 149 member states can voice complaints (communications) for review by the HRC. The second abolishes the death penalty.

International Covenant on Economic, Social, and Cultural Rights (ICESCR): A multilateral United Nations treaty committed to encouraging state parties to improve economic, social, and cultural rights for their citizens. The treaty was written in 1966 and entered into force in 1976. The ICESCR, together with the International Covenant on Civil and Political Rights and the Universal Declaration of Human Rights, comprises the International Bill of Human Rights.

International Financial Institution (IFI): A multilateral lending institution, like the World Bank or IMF, that provides resources for the development of poorer nations. Many indebted nations owe the majority to IFIs extending international credit, rather than individual governments, which complicates issues of debt forgiveness and economic moratoriums.

International Labor Organization (ILO): A United Nations agency that establishes international standards for labor rights and monitors compliance. Founded in 1919 under the treaty of Versailles and recognized as a UN agency in 1946, the ILO promotes the development of independent employers' and workers' organizations worldwide.

International Monetary Fund (IMF): A specialized agency affiliated with the United Nations responsible for stabilizing the international monetary network. The IMF provides loans to member nations (most often developing countries) when they undergo balance of payment problems. These loans often carry conditions allowing the IMF to require substantial internal economic reforms on the part of the recipients.

Joint United Nations Programme on HIV/AIDS (UNAIDS): A United Nations program designed to coordinate and manage a global response to the HIV/AIDS epidemic. UNAIDS spearheads a multinational effort focused on preventing transmission of HIV, providing care, and alleviating the worldwide impact of the disease. It was founded out of the World Health Organization's Global Program on HIV/AIDS in 1996.

Less Developed Country (LDC): A country lacking a strong industrial base that depends on other products (crops, minerals) for revenue. LDCs experience low technological development, low per capita incomes, and high population growth rates. In 1964, 77 countries were designated LDCs to pressure industrialized countries into giving greater aid.

Maternal and Child Health (MCH): A health category focusing on birth outcome and mortality data for infants and children. Measurements of maternal access to health care are included because of the high correlation between maternal care and birth outcomes.

Millennium Development Goals (MDG): A United Nations coordinated effort to define specific goals to help implement and monitor progress toward reducing poverty worldwide. The target areas include: income poverty, hunger, disease, and a lack of adequate shelter. The MDG also promotes greater gender equality, education, and environmental sustainability while reaffirming the basic human rights of health, education, shelter, and security.

Multidrug-resistant Tuberculosis (MDR-TB): A form of tuberculosis with resistance to two or more of the primary drugs used to treatment non-resistant (normal) strains of TB. Resistance can occur after the bacteria are exposed to an antibiotic and survive by developing an ability to withstand the drug (often as a result of inadequate treatment or improper use of the drugs). The MDR-TB then multiplies and passes on the resistance to their progeny.

Multilateral Agreement on Investment (MAI): A preliminary agreement that would make it illegal for signatory states to discriminate against foreign investors, specifically transnational corporations. The MAI was drafted by the 29 member countries of the Organization for Economic Co-operation and Development but was never completed or approved.

Multilateral Development Bank (MDB): An institution providing financial support and advice for economic and social development activities in developing nations. MDB usually refers to the World Bank Group and four Regional Development Banks (African Development Bank, Asian Development Bank, European Bank for Reconstruction and Development, and Inter-American Development Bank Group). The banks have members from both donor countries and borrowing developing countries. Although independent, the banks have similar mandates, many joint owners, and maintain a high level of cooperation with one another.

Multinational Corporation (MNC): *See* Transnational Corporation.

National Charities Information Bureau (NCIB): A nonprofit organization that collects data from charitable organizations and strives to improve the level of those charities' performance. The NCIB seeks to provide donors with accurate information regarding the charitable organizations it deems needy and worthy of donations.

National Institutes of Health (NIH): An independent agency of the Department of Health and Human Services with the mission to "employ science in the pursuit of knowledge to improve human health." The NIH is responsible for overseeing government-sponsored biomedical research both in its own laboratories and by non-Federal scientists funded by NIH grants. The NIH also helps in the training of research investigators and promotes the open communication of medical information.

Newly Industrialized Country (NIC): A social/economic classification status applied to several countries that are rapidly developing. Examples include Saudi Arabia, Kuwait, Taiwan, and South Korea.

Nongovernmental Organization (NGO): A civic organization maintaining its own funding and independence from any central, local, or municipal government. The term "NGO" is generally restricted to social and cultural groups with noncommercial goals.

North American Free Trade Agreement (NAFTA): An agreement between the United States, Canada, and Mexico that removed tariffs, quotas, and other trade barriers among the countries. NAFTA also included specific provisions designed to protect workers and the environment.

Occupational Safety and Health Administration (OSHA): A federal agency under the Department of Labor that drafts and enforces safety and health regulations for businesses, industries, and academic institutions. OSHA works to ensure the well-being of America's workers by monitoring and preventing work-related injuries, illnesses, and deaths.

Office of the High Commissioner for Human Rights (OHCHR): A United Nations office that works to ensure that human rights are fully respected and peacefully enjoyed. The office intervenes on behalf of victims worldwide and pressures the international community to uphold human rights standards and take steps to prevent violations. The office views the right to development as an essential human right.

Official Aid (OA): State-sponsored resources flowing to countries "in transition" (not considered developing) through grants or loans. The goals and definitions of aid are the same as those in official development assistance (ODA).

Official Development Assistance (ODA): State-sponsored aid to developing countries provided through grants or loans. The state provides the aid with the goal of promoting economic development and welfare at concessional financial terms. In addition to financial flows, technical assistance is included in the aid figures, while all assistance for military purposes are excluded.

Official Development Finance (ODF): The inflow of resources to recipient countries that includes bilateral official development assistance (ODA) and official aid (OA) and concessional and nonconcessional development lending by multilateral financial institutions (ie, World Bank and IMF), which have too low a grant element to qualify as ODA.

Oral Rehydration Solution (ORS): A solution containing salt and a form of sugar (preferably glucose) made to prevent dehydration in children suffering from diarrhea. ORS rehydrates the patient while its dissolved additives stem further fluid loss.

Organization for Economic Co-operation and Development (OECD): An international body with 29 member countries pledged to work together to promote their economies, aid underdeveloped nations, and expand world trade. The OECD's executive body is a council composed of representatives from each member country who develop policy.

Organization of African Unity (OAU): An international organization founded to promote common goals and cooperation among the independent nations of Africa. The OAU was disbanded in 2002 and replaced by the African Union.

Organization of Petroleum Exporting Countries (OPEC): An international organization made up of 11 oil-producing nations. OPEC members meet regularly to unify prices and set crude oil production quotas.

Pan American Health Organization (PAHO): The international public health agency working to improve the health and living standards of the people of the Americas. PAHO has been established for over a century and also serves as the regional office of the Americas within the World Health Organization.

Political Action Committee (PAC): A committee set up by and representing business, labor, or other special-interest groups to raise and spend campaign contributions on behalf of certain political candidates or causes. PACs permit organizations to participate in the political process at all levels of federal, state, and local government.

Poverty Reduction Strategy Paper (PSRP): Papers prepared by a country in collaboration with the World Bank and IMF. A PRSP outlines economic and social policies that a country will pursue (including further financing) to promote growth and reduce poverty. PSRPs must include host governments, members of civil societies, and affected indigenous people. PSRPs must also follow the UN's Millenium Development Goals and promote social goals such as lower infant mortality rates or better schools.

President's Emergency Plan for Aids Relief (PEPFAR): A pledge and plan by President George W. Bush to provide $15 billion over five years to fund medical aid and other efforts to combat the global HIV/AIDS pandemic. The fundamental goals of the plan are to treat those currently ill and prevent new infections. The president's plan would supply new drug therapies, and establish a more coordinated overall healthcare effort.

Primary Health Care (PHC): Defined by the WHO as the principal vehicle for the delivery of essential health care at a country's most basic health system. With an emphasis on preventing disease as well as curing it, PHC should include family planning, clean water supply, sanitation, immunization, and nutrition education. PHC should be affordable for both the people who receive it and the governments providing it.

Purchasing Power Parity (PPP): An alternative monetary exchange rate model and a way to compare the relative purchasing power of different countries' currencies. PPP uses a standard measure of currency (usually dollars), to compare the international variations in cost for the same types goods and services.

Severe Acute Respiratory Syndrome (SARS): A respiratory disease caused by a previously unknown type of coronavirus and first documented in mainland China in 2003 and characterized by fever, coughing, and difficulty breathing. SARS is transmitted by close contact with infected persons and can be life-threatening.

Severely Indebted Low-Income Country (SILICS): A region of Africa situated south of the Sahara Desert and ranging laterally from Sierra Leone to Somalia, and south to South Africa.

Structural Adjustment Program (SAP): Loans given from the International Monetary Fund (IMF) to a nation with certain conditions. The conditions often restructure the borrowing countries economies to more efficiently pay off the loans and include cutting social expenditures, devaluing currencies against the dollar, lifting import and export restrictions, and removing price controls and state subsidies

Transnational Corporation (TNC): A corporation with economic activities and operations in multiple countries. TNCs normally have a base country and affiliates overseas and are often referred to as multinational corporations (MNCs).

Tuberculosis (TB): An infectious disease caused by a bacteria (myobacterium tuberculosis) producing small round swellings (tubercles) on mucous membranes. TB can infect almost any tissue or organ but most commonly manifests in the lungs.

United Nations (UN): An international organization that includes most of the sovereign nations of the world. The UN coordinates international cooperation in promoting global peace, security, and economic development and acts through its members to respond to social, political, or humanitarian crises.

United Nations Children's Fund (*formerly United Nations International Children's Emergency Fund*) (UNICEF): A United Nations organization that provides long-term humanitarian and developmental assistance to needy children and mothers worldwide. Established in 1946, UNICEF delivers food, clothing, shelter and other assistance to wherever extreme hardships exist.

United Nations Development Program (UNDP): A UN agency that works with governments worldwide to improve areas such as health and education, and infrastructure development. It provides governments with expert advice, training, and equipment with increasing emphasis on assistance to the least developed countries. The UNDP is voluntarily funded and the world's largest multilateral technical assistance program.

United Nations Educational, Scientific and Cultural Organization (UNESCO): A specialized United Nations agency designed to enhance worldwide peace and security by promoting scientific, educational, and cultural collaboration between nations. UNESCO strives to develop universal respect for justice, rules of law, and individual human rights and fundamental freedoms.

United Nations High Commission for Refugees (UNHCR): A United Nations agency with the primary purpose of safeguarding the rights and well being of refugees at the request of a government or the UN. By its mandate, the UNHCR may lead and coordinate international action to protect refugees and resolve refugee problems worldwide.

United Nations Population Fund (UNPF): A UN fund with the goal of ensuring universal access to reproductive health care, including family planning, population, and sexual health education, to all persons regardless of race, gender, or social or religious beliefs. The UNPF began in 1969 as the United Nations Fund for Population Activities and was renamed the United Nations Population Fund in 1987.

United States Agency for International Development (USAID): The official independent federal agency responsible for supplying nonmilitary development assistance to other countries. USAID receives overall foreign policy guidance from the Secretary of State and can supply assistance either bilaterally (government to government) or through a broad range of NGOs.

Universal Declaration of Human Rights (UDHR): A 1948 United Nations declaration stating that all people had basic rights including life, liberty, equality, justice, and self-determination. The declaration was signed and ratified by most of the world's countries, although most did not rigidly follow it. The UDHR does not represent a document of international law.

Women, Infants, and Children (WIC): A program subsidizing foods intended to "supplement" participants' diets. WIC foods are rich in protein, calcium, iron, vitamin A, and vitamin C, which tend to be low in the diets of participants. WIC is run by the Food and Nutrition Service (FNS), a Federal agency of the US Department of Agriculture.

World Health Organization (WHO): An organization run by the United Nations and committed to improving worldwide public health. The WHO helps countries strengthen their health services, provides technical aid in health emergencies, promotes disease control, and helps establish food and medical safety standards. The WHO has over 190 member countries.

World Trade Organization (WTO): A global governing body for international trade that was established in 1995 as the successor to the General Agreement on Tariffs and Trade (GATT). The WTO exists to liberalize and enforce international free trade of manufactured goods, services, and intellectual property. Currently, the WTO has 148 member nations with 25 additional nations in the process of joining.

Bibliography

"A Buildup Against AIDS." 2003. *The Boston Globe*. February 3.

"A Flood of Fiascos." 1997. *The Economist*. April 17.

"A Question of Justice?" 2004. *The Economist*. March 13.

"A Regime Changes, Special Report: Paul Wolfowitz at the World Bank." 2005. *The Economist*. June 4.

"A Timely Departure." 2005. *The New York Times*. June 19.

Abelson, R. and Rosenthal, E. 1999. Charges of Shoddy Practices Taint Gifts of Plastic Surgery. *The New York Times*. November 24.

Adler, N.E. et al. 1999. Socioeconomic Status and Health: The Challenge of the Gradient. In: Mann, J.M. et al. (eds). *Health and Human Rights: A Reader*. New York, NY: Routledge.

"Africa at the Summit." 2005. *The New York Times*. July 3.

Aguayo, V.M. et al. 2003. Monitoring Compliance with the International Code of Marketing of Breastmilk Substitutes in West Africa: Multisite Cross-Sectional Survey in Togo and Burkina Faso. *British Medical Journal*. 326(7381):127.

"AIDS in Five Nations Called Security Threat." 2002. *The New York Times*. October 1.

"AIDS in India: Abating or Exploding?" 2004. *The Economist*. April 15.

"AIDS Wars." 2000. *The Economist*. September 14.

Alexander G.C. and Sehgal, A.R. 1998. Barriers to cadaveric renal transplantation among blacks, women, and the poor. *JAMA*. 280(13):1148–1152.

Altman, D. 2002. As Global Lenders Refocus, A Needy World Waits. *The New York Times*. March 17.

Altman, L.K. 2003. W.H.O., Declaring Crisis, Plans a Big Push With AIDS Drugs. *The New York Times*. September 22.

Ambrose, S.E. 1994. *D-Day June 6, 1944: The Climactic Battle of World War II*. New York, NY: Touchstone/Simon and Schuster.

Anderson, G.F. 1997. In Search of Value: An International Comparison of Cost, Access, and Outcomes. *Health Affairs*. 16(6).

Anderson, S. 1998. International Financial Flows. *Foreign Policy In Focus*. 3(41).

Anderson, S. et al. 2001. Executive Excess 2001. Institute for Policy Studies and United for a Fair Economy. Available online at http://faireconomy.org/press/2001/EE2001.pdf; downloaded 2/02.

Andrews, E.L. 2004. Report Finds Tax Cuts Heavily Favor the Wealthy. *The New York Times*. August 13.

Annas, G. 1998. Human Rights and Health—The Universal Declaration of Human Rights at 50. *New England Journal of Medicine*. 339:1778–1781.

Antonovsky, A. 1967. Social Class, Life Expectancy, and Overall Mortality. *Millbank Memorial Fund Quarterly*. 45(2):31–73.

Armstrong, K. 1993. *A History of God: he 4,000 Year Quest of Judaism, Christianity, and Islam*. New York, NY: Ballantine Books.

Baccino-Astrada, A. 1982. *Manual on the Rights and Duties of Medical Personnel in Armed Conflicts*. Geneva: International Committee of the Red Cross, League of Red Cross, and Red Crescent Societies.

Baker, T.D. et al. 1984. US Physicians in International Health: Report of a Current Survey. *JAMA*. 251(4):502–504.

Baker, T.D. and Quinley, J.C. 1987. A US International Health Service Corps: Options and Constraints. *JAMA*. 257(19):2622–2625.

Banta, D. 2002. Economic Development Key to Healthier World. *JAMA*. 287(24):3195–3197.

Barnicle, M. 1995. Humanitarian is the Real Story. *The Boston Globe*. November 5.

Barrett, A. 2002. Poor Man's Economist. *The New York Times Magazine*. December 15.

BBC News. 2001. Kenya accused over AIDs orphans. Available online at http://news.bbc.co.uk/2/hi/africa/1406628.stm.

———. 1999. World Population: Special Report. Available online at http://news.bbc.co.uk/2/hi/special_report/1999/06/99/world_population/381043.stm.

Bearak, B.F. 2002. Bangladeshis Sipping Arsenic as Plan for Safe Water Stalls. *The New York Times*. July 14.

Becker, E. 2003a. Western Farmers Fear Third-World Challenge to Subsidies. *The New York Times*. September 9.

———. 2003b. US Ready to Ease Trade Rules on Some Generic Drug Sales. *The New York Times*. August 27.

Behrman, G. 2004. *Invisible People*. New York, NY: Free Press.

Bentley, J. 1992. *Albert Schweitzer: the Enigma*. New York, NY: Harper Collins Publishers.

Bhagwati, J.N. 2002. The Poor's Best Hope. *The Economist*. June 20.

Blackhall, L.J. 1987. Must We Always Use CPR? *New England Journal of Medicine*. 317(20):1281–1285.

Bloom, B.S. et al. 1993 Revisiting US Vaccination Policies: The Case of the Hepatitis B Virus Vaccine. *Health Policy Research Quarterly*. 3(1):1–2.

Boff, L. and Boff, C. 1998. *Introducing Liberation Theology*. Maryknoll, New York, NY: Orbis Books.

Boyd, T. 2002. There's No Bridging the Hip-Hip Gap. *The Boston Globe*. October 2.

Brabazon, J. 1975. *Albert Schweitzer: A Biography*. London, England: Victor Gollancz.

Brauman, R. and Tanguy, T. 1998. The Médecins Sans Frontières Experience. Médecins Sans Frontières/Doctors Without Borders. Available online at www.doctorswithoutborders.org/publications/other/themsfexperience.shtml.

"Brazilians Find Political Cost for Help from IMF." 2002. *The New York Times*. August 11.

Brenner, M. 1996. The Man Who Knew Too Much. *Vanity Fair Magazine*. May.

Brown, R.M. 1990. *Gustavo Gutierrez: An Introduction to Liberation Theology*. Maryknoll, NY: Orbis Books.

Bruderlein, C. and Leaning, J. 1999. New Challenges for Humanitarian Protection. *British Medical Journal*. 319(7207):430–435.

Bryce, R. 2002. *Pipe Dreams: Greed, Ego, and the Death of Enron.* New York, NY: Public Affairs.

Bryden, D. 2005. Bush Overstates Africa Aid Increase. *Foreign Policy in Focus,* July 20. Available online at www.fpif.org.

Budd, W. 1931. *Typhoid Fever: Its Nature, Mode of Spreading, and Prevention,* New York, NY: Arno Press.

"Can Debt Relief Make a Difference?" 2000. *The Economist.* November 16.

Canto, J.G. et al. 2000. Payer Status and the Utilization of Hospital Resources in Acute Myocardial Infarction. *Archives of Internal Medicine.* 160(6):817–823.

Cantor, N.F. 2002. *In the Wake of the Plague.* New York, NY: Harper Collins.

Caufield, C. 1996. *Masters of Illusion: The World Bank and the Poverty of Nations.* New York, NY: Henry Holt.

Center for Arms Control and Proliferation. 2005. Highlights of House Armed Services Committee Action on the Fiscal Year 2006 Defense Authorization Bill (H.R. 1815). May 24. Available online at www.armscontrolcenter.org/archives/001658.php.

Center for Defense Information (CDI). 2002. *2002 CDI Military Almanac.* Washington, DC: Center for Defense Information.

———. 1997. *1997 CDI Military Almanac.* Washington, DC: Center for Defense Information.

Centers for Disease Control and Prevention (CDC). 2001. Influence of Homicide on Racial Disparity in Life Expectancy—United States, 1998. *Morbidity and Mortality Weekly Report.* 50(36):780–783.

———. 1999a. Achievements in Public Health, 1900–1999: Control of Infectious Diseases. *Morbidity and Mortality Weekly Report.* 48(29):621–629.

———. 1999b. Achievements in Public Health, 1900–1999: Safer and Healthier Foods. *Morbidity and Mortality Weekly Report.* 48(40):905–913.

———. 1999c. Achievements in Public Health, 1900–1999: Impact of Vaccines Universally Recommended for Children—United States, 1900–1998. *Morbidity and Mortality Weekly Report.* 48(12):243–248.

———. 1999d. Achievements in Public Health, 1900–1999: Decline in Deaths from Heart Disease and Stroke—United States, 1900–1999. *Morbidity and Mortality Weekly Report.* 48(30):649–656.

———. 1999e. Achievements in Public Health, 1900–1999: Tobacco Use—United States: 1900–1999. *Morbidity and Mortality Weekly Report.* 48(43):986–993.

———. 1999f. Achievements in Public Health, 1900–1999: Healthier Mothers and Babies. *Morbidity and Mortality Weekly Report.* 48(38): 849–858.

———. 1999g. Ten Great Public Health Achievements—United States: 1900–1999. *Morbidity and Mortality Weekly Report.* 48(12):241–243.

———. 1999h. Achievements in Public Health, 1900–1999: Improvements in Workplace Safety—United States, 1900–1999. *Morbidity and Mortality Weekly Report.* 48(22): 461–469.

———. 1999i. Achievements in Public Health, 1900–1999: Motor Vehicle Safety: A 20th Century Public Health Achievement. *Morbidity and Mortality Weekly Report.* 48(18): 369–374.

———. 1999j. Achievements in Public Health, 1900–1999: Changes in the Public Health System. *Morbidity and Mortality Weekly Report.* 48(50):1141–1147.

———. 1999k. Achievements in Public Health, 1900–1999: Family Planning. *Morbidity and Mortality Weekly Report.* 48(47):1073–1080.

————. 1988. 1988 Surgeon General Report: The Health Consequences of Smoking, Nicotine Addiction. Available online at www.cdc.gov/tobacco/sgr/ sgr_1988/1988SGR-Intro.pdf.

————. 1981. *Pneumocystis* Pneumonia—Los Angeles. *Morbidity and Mortality Weekly Report*. 30(21):250–252.

Central Intelligence Agency. 2005. *The World Fact Book*. Available online at www.cia.gov.

"Charlemagne: The Longest Day, Revisited." 2004. *The Economist*. June 5.

Chen, J. et al. 2001. Racial Differences in the Use of Cardiac Catheterization after Acute Myocardial Infarction. *New England Journal of Medicine*. 344(19):1443–1449.

Chomsky, N. 1993. *Year 501: The Conquest Continues*. Cambridge, Mass: Southend Press.

Christie, M. 1995. Wave of Suicides Sweeps a Brazilian Indian Reserve. *The Boston Globe*. December 21.

Cloud, J. 1969. Standing up for Gay Rights. *Time*. March 30.

Cloud, S. 1996. The Opportunities and Challenges of a More Diverse American Society as We Enter a New Century. Speech presented at the Lahey Clinic, North Shore: Massachusetts.

Collins, C. et al. 1999. *Shifting Fortunes: The Perils of the Growing American Wealth Gap*. Boston, Mass: United for a Fair Economy.

Colvin, G. 2001. The Great CEO Pay Heist. *Fortune Magazine*. June 25.

Commission on Macroeconomics and Health. 2001. *Macroeconomics and Health: Investing in Health for Economic Development*. Geneva, Switzerland: World Health Organization. Also available online at www.un.org/esa/coordination/ ecosoc/docs/RT.K.MacroeconomicsHealth.pdf.

"Concerns over WWII Revisited." 1995. *The Boston Globe*. August 14.

Congressional Budget Office (CBO). 1997. The Role of Foreign Aid in Development. Also available online at www.cbo.gov.

Congressional Research Service. 2004. Foreign Aid: An Introductory Overview of US Programs and Policy. April 15. Also available online at www.crs.gov.

Contee, C.E. 1987. *What Americans Think: Views on Development and US-Third World Relations*. Prepared for the Public Opinion Project cosponsored by InterAction in New York and the Overseas Development Council in Washington, DC.

Corbin, M. and Levitsky, O. 2003. Vital Statistics: The US Military. *The Defense Monitor, Center for Defense Information*. 32(5).

Corbin, M. and Pemberton, M. 2004. A Unified Security Budget for the United States. Foreign Policy in Focus and Center for Defense Information, March. Available online at www.cdi.org.

Cornelius, D. and Cover, J. 1997. *Population and Environment Dynamics*. Washington, DC: Population Reference Bureau.

"Corruption at the Heart of the United Nations." 2005. *The Economist*. August 9.

Council on Foreign Relations. 2004. Foreign Aid, Has the Debate on US Foreign Aid Shifted Since September 11? In: *Terrorism: Questions and Answers, Foreign Aid*. Available online at www.terrorismanswers.com/policy/foreignaid.html.

"Courtroom Tales of Martha's Lies . . . " 2004. *New York Times*. March 6.

Cousins, N. 1984. *The Words of Albert Schweitzer*. New York, NY: Newmarket Press.

————. 1960. *Dr Schweitzer of Lambarene*. New York, NY: Harper & Brothers, Publishers.

Crossan, J.D. 1989. *Jesus: A Revolutionary Biography*. San Francisco, Calif: Harper Collins Publishers.

Crossette, B. 1999. Rethinking Population at a Global Milestone. *The New York Times*. September 19.

Cullen, K. 1999. MGH Doctor on Night Shift in Macedonia. *The Boston Globe*. April 7.

"Damming Evidence, The Pros and Cons of Big Earthworks." 2003. *The Economist*. July 19.

Danaher, K. 1994. *50 Years is Enough: The Case Against the World Bank and the International Monetary Fund*. Boston, Mass: South End Press.

Davey, S.G. and Egger, M. 1993. Socioeconomic Differentials in Wealth and Health. *British Medical Journal*. 307(6912):1085–1086.

Deen, T. 2004. Development: Tied Aid Strangling Nations, Says UN. *Inter Press Service*. Global Policy Forum, July 6. Available online at www.globalpolicy.org.

de las Casas, B. 1965. (Orig. pub. in 1552.) *The Devastation of the Indies*. Baltimore, Md: Johns Hopkins University Press.

DeMartino, G. 1998. Foreign Direct Investment. *Foreign Policy in Focus*. 3(14).

DeParle, J. 2005. Broken Levees, Unbroken Barriers: What Happens to a Race Deferred. *The New York Times*. September 4.

Diamond, J. 1999. *Guns, Germs, and Steel*. New York, NY: W.W. Norton & Company.

Dickens, C. 1893. *A Christmas Carol*. New York, NY: Bantam Books.

Diez Roux, A.V. et al. 2001. Neighborhood of Residence and Incidence of Coronary Heart Disease. *New England Journal of Medicine*. 345(2):99–106.

"Does Population Matter?" 2002. *The Economist*. December 5.

Dolan, M. 2003. A Generation Takes a Stand. *Time*. March 30.

Donnelly, J. 2003. Study: AIDS fund in Financial Straits. *The Boston Globe*. May 7.

———. 2002a. AIDS Fund Falters as U.S. Plans Grants. *The Boston Globe*. January 31.

———. 2002b. O'Neil Sees Foreign Aid as Duty. *The Boston Globe*. June 6.

———. 2000. Gates Foundation Gives $44.7m to Fight TB. *The Boston Globe*. July 28.

Donovan, B.M. 1974. Introduction. In: *The Devastation of the Indies*. (de las Casas, B.). Baltimore: Johns Hopkins University Press.

Dooley, T. 1960. *The Night They Burned the Mountain*. New York, NY: Farrar, Straus, and Giroux.

———. 1958. *The Edge of Tomorrow*. New York, NY: Farrar, Straus, and Giroux.

———. 1956. *Deliver U.S. From Evil*. New York, NY: Farrar, Straus, and Giroux.

"Doubts Inside the Barricades." 2002. *The Economist*. September 26.

Dowell, S.F. et al. 2000. Mortality from Pneumonia in Children in the United States. *The New England Journal of Medicine*. 342(19):1399–1407.

Driscoll, D.D. 1998. What is the International Monetary Fund? Washington, DC: International Monetary Fund. Available online at www.imfsite.org/operations/driscoll998.html.

Duffield, M. 1994. Complex Emergencies and the Crisis of Developmentalism. *Institute of Development Studies Bulletin*. 25(4):37–45.

Dugger, C.W. 2004. Devastated by AIDS, Africa Sees Life Expectancy Plunge. *New York Times*. July 16.

Easterly, W. 2002. *The Elusive Quest for Growth, Economists' Adventures and Misadventures in the Tropics*. Cambridge, Mass: MIT Press.

Eaton, J. and Etue, K. 2002. *The aWAKE Project, Uniting Against the African AIDS Crisis*. Nashville, Tenn: W. Publishing Group.

Eckel, N.D. 2003. *Great World Religions: Buddhism*. Chantilly, Va: The Teaching Company.

Eckhardt, W. and Young, C. 1977. *Governments Under Fire: Civil Conflict and Imperialism*. New Haven, Conn: Human Relations Area Press Files, Yale.

Eichenwald, K. 2002. White-Collar Defense Stance: The Criminal-Less Crime. *The New York Times*. March 3.

Eisenberg, D. 2002. Dennis the Menace. *Time*. June 17.

Elliott, V.S. 2003. American MD Killed Serving Troubled Corner of the World. *American Medical News*. 46(4):1.

Endy, C. 2004. The Wrong Lessons to Learn From D-Day. History News Service. June 2. Available online at http://hnn.us/articles/5442.html.

"Enemies of War: El Salvador's Humanity and Dignity." 2001. *PBS Home Programs*. Available online at www.pbs.org/itvs/enemiesofwar/perspectivesH.html.

"Enron, and on, and on." 2001. *The Economist*. April 19.

Epstein, P.R. 1992. Commentary: Pestilence and Poverty—Historical Transitions and the Great Pandemics. *American Journal of Preventive Medicine*. 8(4):263–265.

Espinal, M.A. et al. 2001. Global Trends in Resistance to Antituberculosis Drugs. *New England Journal of Medicine*. 344(17):1294–303.

Esposito, J.L. 2003. *Great World Religions: Islam*. Chantilly, Va: The Teaching Company.

"Eulogy for Dr Tom Durant." 2001. St. Mark's Church, Dorchester, Mass. November 2.

"Executive Pay: A Special Report." 2002. *The New York Times*. April 7.

Fackler, M. 2002. Political Tensions Threaten Millions with Malnutrition in North Korea. *The Boston Globe*. November 16.

Faiola, A. 2002. Brazil's Rich Take Safety to New Heights. *The Boston Globe*. June 9.

Farmer, P.E. 2001. The Major Infectious Diseases in the World—To Treat or Not to Treat? *New England Journal of Medicine*. 345(3):208–210.

———. 1994a. *The Uses of Haiti*. Monroe, Maine: Common Courage Press.

———. 1994b. *Infections and Inequalities: The Modern Plagues*. Berkeley, Calif: University of California Press.

Farmer, P.E. et al. 2003. Unjust Embargo of Aid for Haiti. *The Lancet*. 361(9355):420–423.

Farmer, P.E. et al. 2002. Unjust Embargo Deepens Haiti's Health Crisis. *The Boston Globe*. December 30.

Farmer, P.E. et al. 1996. *Women, Poverty and AIDS*. Monroe, Maine: Common Courage Press.

Farmer, P.E. and Kim, J.Y. 1998. Community-Based Approaches to the Control of Multidrug-Resistant Tuberculosis: Introducing 'DOTS-Plus.' *British Medical Journal*. 317(7159):671–674.

Fein, O. 1995. The Influence of Social Class on Health Status: American and British Research on Health Inequalities. *Journal of General Internal Medicine*. 10(10):577–586.

Fesperman, D. 1996. In Flanders, a Deadly Crop Rises from the Soil. *The Boston Globe*. August 11.

Fidler, D.P. 2000. *International Law and Public Health: Materials on and Analysis of Global Health Jurisprudence*. Ardsley, New York, NY: Transnational Publishers, Inc.

Fisher, J.T. 1997. *Dr America: The Lives of Thomas A. Dooley, 1927–1961*. Amherst, Mass: University of Massachusetts Press.

Forero, J. 2004. In a Land Torn by Violence, Too Many Troubling Deaths. *The Boston Globe*. November 23.

Frank, J.W. and Mustard, J.F. 1994. The Determinants of Health from a Historical Perspective. *Daedalus*. Fall.

Freire, P. 1970. *Pedagogy of the Oppressed*. New York, NY: Continuum Publishing, Co.

Friedman, L.N. et al. 1996. Tuberculosis, AIDS, and Death Among Substance Abusers on Welfare in New York City. *New England Journal of Medicine*. 334(13):828–833.

Friedman, R.E. 1997. *Who Wrote the Bible?* San Francisco, Calif: Harper Collins.

Friedman, T.L. 2005. *The World is Flat: A Brief History of the Twenty-First Century*. New York, NY: Farrar, Straus, and Giroux.

Fryda, W. 2000. *St. Mary's Mission Hospital: A Catholic Center of Health Care Ministry In Service to the Poor*. Nairobi, Kenya: self-published.

Fukuyama, F. 1992. *The End of History and the Last Man*. New York, NY: Avon Books.

Gafni, I.M. 2003. *Great World Religions: Judaism*. Chantilly, Va: The Teaching Company.

Garrett, L. 1994. *The Coming Plague: Newly Emerging Diseases in a World Out of Balance*. New York, NY: Penguin Books.

Geiger, H.J. and Cook-Deegan, R.M. 1993. The Role of Physicians in Conflicts and Humanitarian Crises: Case Studies From the Field Missions of Physicians for Human Rights, 1988 to 1993. *JAMA*. 270(5):616–620.

Gellman, B. 2000. "The Belated Response to AIDS in Africa." *The Washington Post*. July 5.

"Generation Gaps: Enron in India." 2001. *The Economist*. January 11.

"Genetically Modified Food, Far Less Scary than it Used to Be." 2003. *The Economist*. July 24.

"Ghosts of Rwanda." 2004. *Frontline, PBS*. April 1. Available online at www.pbs.org/wgbh/pages/frontline/shows/ghosts/interviews/wilkens.html.

Gilligan, J. 1996. *Violence, Our Deadly Epidemic and Its Causes*. New York, NY: Grosset/Putnam Books.

Gimein, M. 2002. The Greedy Bunch, You Bought, They Sold. *Fortune*. September 2.

Glain, S.J. 2003. Land of Economic Unrest. *The Boston Globe*. August 24.

Glendon, M.A. 2001. *A World Made New: Eleanor Roosevelt and the Universal Declaration of Human Rights*. New York, NY: Random House.

Global Alliance for TB Drug Development. 2004a. A Global Threat. Available online at www.tballiance.org.

———. 2004b. No R&D in Thirty Years. Available online at www.tballiance.org/ 2_3_C_NoRandDin30Years.asp.

"Globalization and Its Critics." 2001. *The Economist*. September 27.

"Good but not Great." 2005. *The Economist*. July 8.

Goodwin, D.K. 1994. *No Ordinary Time*. New York, NY: Touchstone Books, Simon and Schuster.

Goudsmit, J. 1997. *Viral Sex: The Nature of AIDS*. New York, NY: Oxford University Press.

Grabel, I. 1998. Portfolio Investment. *Foreign Policy in Focus*. 3(13).

Griffiths, L. 2000. Hardships Plague Women Worldwide, UN Report Says. *The Boston Globe*. September 21.

Grusky, S. 2000. The Poverty Reduction Strategy Papers: An Initial NGO Assessment. *Bread for the World Institute Debt and Development DOSSIER #3.* Available online at www.jubileeplus.org/analysis/reports/bread010600.htm.

Guerrant, D.I. et al. 1999. Association of Early Childhood Diarrhea and Cryptosporidiosis with Impaired Physical Fitness and Cognitive Function Four–Seven Years Later in a Poor Urban Community in Northeast Brazil. *American Journal of Tropical Medicine and Hygiene.* 61(5):707–713.

Gunston, G. et al. 1992. Reversible Cerebral Shrinkage in Kwashiorkor: An MRI Study. *Archives of Disease in Childhood.* 67 (8):1030–1032.

Gutierrez, G. 1995. *A Theology of Liberation 15th Anniversary Edition.* Maryknoll, New York, NY: Orbis Books.

Haan, M.N. et al. 1987. Poverty and Health: Prospective Evidence from the Alameda County Study. *American Journal of Epidemiology.* 125(6):989–998.

Halberstam, D. 2002. Sports Can Distract, But They Don't Heal. *ESPN Network.* September 10. Available online at http://espn.go.com/page2/s/halberstam/020911.html.

Hancock, G. 1989. *Lords of Poverty.* New York, NY: Atlantic Monthly Press.

Harden, B. 1990. *Africa: Dispatches from a Fragile Continent.* Boston, Mass: Houghton Mifflin.

Harding, A. 2002. Nairobi Life, Kibera's Children. BBC News. October 10.

Hartmann, B. 1999. Wrong Signals on Overpopulation. *The Boston Sunday Globe.* October 10.

Health Volunteers Overseas. 2005. 2004 Annual Report. Available online at www.hvousa.org/hvoAR04.pdf.

"Helping the Poorest." 1999. *The Economist.* August 12.

Herbert, B. 2005. No Stranger to the Blues. *The New York Times.* September 8.

Hibbs, J.R. 1994. Mortality in a Cohort of Homeless Adults in Philadelphia. *New England Journal of Medicine.* 331(5):304–309.

Hitchens, C. 1997. *The Missionary Position.* New York, NY: Verso Press.

Hochschild, A. 1998. *King Leopold's Ghost: A Story of Greed, Terror, and Heroism in Colonial Africa.* New York, NY: Houghton Mifflin Company.

Hoge, W. 2005. Panel Says Annan Didn't Intervene in Iraq Contract. *The New York Times.* March 30.

"How AIDS Began." 1998. *The Economist.* February 5.

"How to Make Aid Work." 1999. *The Economist.* June 24.

Hurt, R.D. et al. 1998. Prying Open the Door to the Tobacco Industry's Secrets About Nicotine: The Minnesota Tobacco Trial. *JAMA.* 280(13):1173–1181.

Hwang, S.W. et al. 1997. Causes of Death in Homeless Adults in Boston. *Annals of Internal Medicine.* 126(8):625–628.

Institute for Health and Social Justice. 1996. The Consumption of the Poor, Tuberculosis in the Late 20th Century. September.

Institute of Medicine. 1997. *America's Vital Interest in Global Health: Protecting Our People, Enhancing Our Economy, and Advancing Our International Interests.* Washington, DC: National Academy Press.

International Bottled Water Association. 2004. Bottled Water Now Number Two Commercial Beverage in US, Says Beverage Marketing Cooperation. *International Bottled Water Association Press Release.* Available online at www.bottledwater.org/public/downloads/Bev_Marketing_2004_Release_04082004.doc.

"Investment Guide: Charity, Clarity of Vision." 2001. *Forbes*. December 10.

"Irrelevant, Illegitimate, or Indispensable?" 2003. *The Economist*. February 22.

Jackson, D. 1999. Raging Bulls on Wall Street. *The Boston Globe*. April 2.

Jacobs, C. 1996. Slavery: Worldwide Evil From India to Indiana, More People are Enslaved Today than Ever Before." Available online at www.iabolish.com/today/background/worldwide-evil.htm.

Jha, A.K. et al. 2005. Racial Trends in the Use of Major Procedures Among the Elderly. *New England Journal of Medicine*. 353:683–691.

Johnson, C.A. 2004. *The Sorrows of Empire*. New York, NY: Metropolitan Books.

Johnson, L.T. 2003. *Great World Religions: Christianity*. Chantilly, Va: The Teaching Company.

Jordan, M. 1998. Memphians Remember Martin Luther King's Final Crusade. *Memphis Flyer*. April 4.

Jubilee. 2002. The Guardian Celebrates the Bono Phenomenon. Available online at www.jubileeplus.org/analysis/articles/bono180302.htm.

————. 2000a. Background to Debt. Available online at www.jubileeplus.org/analysis/reports/beginners_guide/resisting.htm.

————. 2000b. G8 Leaders Commit a Further $1bn in Debt Relief for the HIPC Countries. Available online at www.jubileeplus.org/hipc/what_is_hipc.htm.

Kar, D. and Watkins, N. 2005. The G-8 Debt Deal: First Step on a Long Journey. Foreign Policy in Focus. Available online at www.fpif.org.

Kawachi, I. et al. 1997. Social Capital, Income Inequality, and Mortality. *American Journal of Public Health*. 87(9):1491–1498.

Kenyon, T.A. et al. 1996. Transmission of Multidrug-Resistant *Mycobacterium Tuberculosis* During a Long Airplane Flight. *New England Journal of Medicine*. 334 (15):933–938.

Kickbush, I. 2000. Influence and Opportunity: Reflections on the US Role in Global Public Health. *Health Affairs*. 21(6):131–141.

Kidder, T. 2003. *Mountains Beyond Mountains: The Quest of Dr Paul Farmer, a Man Who Would Cure the World*. New York, NY: Random House.

————. 2000. The Good Doctor. *The New Yorker*. July 10.

Kim, J.Y. et al. 2000. *Dying for Growth*. Monroe, Maine: Common Courage Press.

Kindig, D.A. et al. 1984. Share Our Doctors Abroad. *The New Physician*. September.

King, C. III and Siegel, M. 2001. The Master Settlement Agreement with the Tobacco Industry and Cigarette Advertising in Magazines. *New England Journal of Medicine*. 345(7):504–511.

Kitagawa, E.M. and Hauser, P.M. 1973. *Differential Mortality in the United States: A Study in Socioeconomic Epidemiology*. Cambridge, Mass: Harvard University Press.

Kleinman, A. et al. 1997. *Social Suffering*. Berkeley, Calif: University of California Press.

Klitgaard, R. 1990. *Tropical Gangsters: One Man's Experience with Development and Decadence in Deepest Africa*. New York, NY: Basic Books.

Kohler, G. and Alcock, N. 1976. An Empirical Table of Structural Violence. *The Journal of Peace Research* 12(4):343–356.

Kohls, L.R. 2001. *Survival Kit for Overseas Living, 4th Edition*. Yarmouth, Maine: Intercultural Press.

Koutsky, L.A. et al. 2002. A Controlled Trial of a Human Papillomavirus Type 16 Vaccine. *New England Journal of Medicine*. 347(21):1645–1651.

Krasner, J. and Lewis, D.E. 2002. Have and Have Not. *The Boston Globe*. March 17.

Krieger, N. et al. 1993. Racism, Sexism, and Social Class: Implications for Studies of Health, Disease, and Well-Being. *American Journal of Preventive Medicine.* 9(6Suppl.):92.

Kristoff, N.D. 2003. Alone and Ashamed. *The New York Times.* May 16.

Kristoff, N.D. and Wudunn, S. 1995. *China Wakes: The Struggle for the Soul of a Rising Power.* New York, NY: Vintage Books.

Kroll, L. and Goldman, L. 2005. The World's Richest People. *Forbes.* March 10.

————. 2003. Survival of the Richest. *Forbes.* March 17.

Kull, S. 2001. Vox Americani. *Foreign Policy.* Sept/Oct.

————. 1995a. Americans and Foreign Aid, A Study of American Public Attitudes. *Program on International Policy Attitudes,* University of Maryland, March 1, 1995. Available from the CISSM, School of Public Affairs at the University of Maryland.

——. 1995b. Foreign Aid Perception and Reality. *The Washington Times.* February 27.

Kuttner, R. 2001. No Escape from Money-Driven Politics. *The Boston Globe.* June 10.

Lacey, M. 2005. Beyond Bullets and Blades. *The Boston Globe.* March 20.

LaFraniere, S. 2005. Entrenched Epidemic: Wife-Beatings in Africa. *The New York Times.* August 11.

Lamb, D. 1987. *The Africans.* New York, NY: Vintage Books.

Lancaster, C. 2000. *Transforming Foreign Aid, United States Assistance in the 21st Century.* Washington, DC: Institute for International Economics.

Lawless, J. 2002. The Meal was Costlier than it First Appeared, and the Bill Topped $60,000. *The Boston Globe.* February 27.

Lederer, W.J. and Burdick, E. 1999. *The Ugly American.* New York, NY: W.W. Norton & Co.

Lee, F.R. 2003. 24 Win MacArthur 'Genius Awards' of $500,000. *The New York Times.* October 5.

Leonhardt D. 2002. Did Pay Incentives Cut Both Ways? *The New York Times.* April 7.

Lewis, B. 2002. *What Went Wrong? The Clash Between Islam and Modernity in the Middle East.* Oxford, England: Oxford University Press.

Lewis, C. 2004. *The Buying of the President 2004.* New York, NY: HarperCollins.

Leyton, E. and Locke, G. 1998. *Touched by Fire: Doctors Without Borders in a Third World Crisis.* Toronto, Canada: McClelland and Stewart Press.

Lobe, J. 2004. Foreign Aid Budget Looks Like a Retread from the Cold War. *Foreign Policy in Focus.* February 19.

Lurie, N. 2005. Health Disparities—Less Talk, More Action. *New England Journal of Medicine.* 353:727–729.

Lynch, J.W. et al. 1997. Cumulative Impact of Sustained Economic Impact on Physical, Cognitive, Psychological, and Social Functioning. *New England Journal of Medicine.* 337(26):1889–1895.

Maass, P. 1996. *Love Thy Neighbor, A Story of War.* New York, NY: Alfred A. Knopf.

MacLeod, S. 1994. The Life and Death of Kevin Carter. *Time.* September 12.

Mahon, F. 1998. The Legacy of a Legend. *Notre Dame Magazine.* 27(1).

Makua, M. 2003. Kenyans Break Free from a Corrupt Past. *The Boston Globe.* January 4.

Mander, J. and Goldsmith, E. 1996. *The Case Against the Global Economy, and for a Turn Toward the Local.* San Francisco, Calif: Sierra Club Books.

Mann, J. et al. 1999. *Health and Human Rights.* New York, NY: Routledge.

Maren, M. 1997. *The Road to Hell: The Ravaging Effects of Foreign Aid and International Charity.* New York, NY: The Free Press.

Marmot, M. 2000. Inequities in Health. *New England Journal of Medicine*. 345(2): 134–136.

———. 1993. Social Differentials in Health Within and Between Populations. *Daedalus*. Fall.

Marshall, G. and Poling, D. 1971. *Schweitzer*. New York, NY: Albert Schweitzer Fellowship.

Masland, T. 2002. We Beat and Killed People. *Newsweek*. May 13.

McCord, C. and Freeman, H. 1990. Excess Mortality in Harlem. *New England Journal of Medicine*. 322(3):173–177.

McLure, J. 2004. We're Ready. *Newsweek*. May 17.

"Measuring up for Aid." 2000. *The Economist*. January 6.

Mehta, P.S. 1994. Fury Over a River. In: *50 Years is Enough: The Case Against the World Bank and The International Monetary Fund* (Danaher, K., ed). Boston, Mass: South End Press.

Mettimano, J. 2002. Senate Ratifies Two Child Protection Treaties. *Monday Developments*. Interaction web site. Available online at www.interaction.org/library/detail.php?id=760.

"Milestones." 1994. *Time*. August 8.

"Milking Lessons, the Crisis at Parmalat." 2003. *The Economist*. December 30.

"Mired in Poverty, Kenyans Bear the Heavy Burden of Foreign Debt." 1999. *The Irish Times*. October 2.

Mitnick, C. et al. 2003. Community-Based Therapy for Multidrug-Resistant Tuberculosis in Lima, Peru. *New England Journal of Medicine*. 348(2):119–128.

Mittal, A. 2002. Giving Away the Farm: The 2002 Farm Bill. Food First, Institute for Food and Development Policy. *Backgrounder*. 8(3).

Mohl, B. 2004. It is Better to Give When Not Being Deceived. *The Boston Globe*. November 21.

"Moi, Lord of Kenya's Empty Dance: Kenya is Caught in a Vicious Circle of Corruption and Political Incompetence." 1999. *The Economist*. May 13.

Monahan, J. 1961. *Before I Sleep . . . The Last Days of Dr Tom Dooley*. New York, NY: Farrar, Straus, and Cudahy.

Moneychimp. 2004. About Moneychimp. Available online at www.moneychimp.com/about.htm.

Mooney, B.C. 2001. Dr Thomas Durant: Attendee of the Dispossessed. *The Boston Globe*. October 31.

"More Dangerous Work than Ever." 2004. *The Economist*. November 18.

Morrison, A.B. 1984. The World Health Organization and Health for All. *Health Affairs*. 4(1):102–113.

Muesse, M.W. 2003. *Great World Religions: Hinduism*. Chantilly, Va: The Teaching Company.

"Nairobbery: Lawlessness Grips the Kenyan Capital." 2000. *The Economist*. August 8.

National Intelligence Council. 2000. The Global Infectious Disease Threat and Its Implications for the United States. Available online at www.cia.gov/cia/reports/nie/report/nie99-17d.html.

National Public Radio. 2003a. *All Things Considered*. July 15.

———. 2003b. *Marketplace*. September 10.

Navarro, V. 1990. Race or Class Versus Race and Class: Mortality Differentials in the United States. *The Lancet*. 336(8725):1238–1240.

Newacheck P.W. et al 1995. Decategorizing Health Services: Interim Findings From the Robert Wood Johnson Foundation's Child Health Initiative. *Health Affairs.* 14(3):232–242.

Niehaus, M.D. et al. 2002. Early Childhood Diarrhea is Associated with Diminished Cognitive Function 4 to 7 Years Later in Children in a Northeast Brazilian Shantytown. *American Journal of Tropical Medicine and Hygiene.* 66(5):590–593.

Nierengarten, M. 2003. Haiti's HIV Equity Initiative. *Lancet.* 3(5):266.

North, F. et al. 1993. Explaining Socioeconomic Differences in Sickness Absence: the Whitehall II Study. *British Medical Journal.* 306(6874):361–366.

Noviny, N.L. 1995. *Vaclav Havel Toward a Civil Society, Selected Speeches and Writings 1990–1994.* Prague, Czech Republic: Lidove Noviny Publishing House.

"Old Battle; New Strategy." 2000. *The Economist.* January 6.

Omran, A. 1971. The Epidemiological Transition. *Millbank Memorial Fund Quarterly.* 49(4):509–538.

O'Neil, E. and Reardon, C.C. 1992. *Boston City Hospital Medical Service Chief Resident's Report: 1991–1992 Admission Diagnoses.* Self-published.

Organization for Economic Co-operation and Development (OECD). 2004. *The Development Assistance Committee Journal of Development Co-Operation 2003 Report (Vol 5, No.1).* Development Assistance Committee of the Organization for Economic Co-operation and Development. Paris, France: OECD Publications.

———. 2002. *The Development Assistance Committee Journal of Development Co-Operation 2001 Report (Vol.3, No. 1).* Paris, France: OECD Publications.

———. 2000. *The Development Assistance Committee Journal of Development Co-Operation 1999 Report.* Paris, France: OECD Publications.

———. 1996. *The Development Assistance Committee Journal of Development Co-Operation 1996 Report.* Paris, France: OECD Publications.

Osguthorpe, J.D. and Hadley J.A. 1999. Rhinosinusitis: Current Concepts in Evaluation and Management. *Medical Clinics of North America.* 83(1):27–41.

Overholser, G. 2001. The Pay Gap between CEOs and Us. *The Boston Globe.* June 10.

Overseas Development Institute. 2002. HPG Briefing: Trends in US Humanitarian Policy. Available online at www.odi.org.uk/hpg/papers/hpgbrief3.pdf.

Oxfam. 2002a. Rigged Rules and Double Standards: Trade, Globalization and the Fight Against Poverty. *Oxfam/Make Trade Fair.* Available online at www.oxfamamerica.org/pdfs/rigged_rules_report_summary.pdf.

———. 2002b. Mugged, Poverty in Your Coffee Cup. *Oxfam/Make Trade Fair.* Available online at www.oxfamamerica.org/newsandpublications/publications/research_reports/mugged.

Pappas, G. et al. 1993. The Increasing Disparity in Mortality Between Socioeconomic Groups in the United States, 1960 and 1986. *New England Journal of Medicine.* 329(15):103–109.

Partners In Health. 2002. Library: DOTS-Plus Handbook. Available online at www.pih.org/library/books/MDRTBguide.htm.

Patsilelis, C. 1995. Review of Stephen Ambrose's *D-Day.* (Back cover of book.) New York, NY: Simon and Schuster.

Pelletier, D.L. et al. 1993. Epidemiological Evidence for a Potentiating Effect of Malnutrition on Child Mortality. *American Journal of Public Health.* 83(8):1130–1133.

Perkins, J. 2004. *Confessions of an Economic Hit Man.* San Francisco, Calif: Berrett-Koehler Publishers.

Peterson, E.D. et al. 1994. Racial Variation in Cardiac Procedure: Use and Survival Following Acute Myocardial Infarction in the Department of Veterans Affairs. *JAMA.* 271(15):1175–1180.

Physicians for Human Rights. 2004. Physicians for Human Rights Commends Senator Frist for Introducing Legislation to Help Eliminate Racial and Ethnic Disparities in the Quality of US Health Care. Available online at www.prusa.org/research/.domestic/race/race_report/press_release_03.html.

"Playing Politics with Population." 1999. *The Boston Globe.* August 18.

"Poor, Rich Face Off at Cancun Trade Talks." 2003. *The New York Times.* September 9.

Power, S. 2003. *A Problem from Hell: America in the Age of Genocide.* London, England: Flamingo Press.

Program on International Policy Attitudes (PIPA). 2001. Americans on Foreign Aid and World Hunger, a Study of U.S. Public Attitudes. Available online at www.pipa.org/OnlineReports/BFW/toc.html.

Prothrow-Stith, D. 1991. *Deadly Consequences, How Violence is Destroying Our Teenage Population and a Plan to Begin Solving the Problem.* New York, NY: HarperCollins.

Radelet, S. 2003. *Challenging Foreign Aid: A Policymaker's Guide to the Millennium Challenge Account.* Washington, DC: Institute for International Economics.

"Raising the Barricades, If the Economy Falters, Free Trade Will Suffer." 2003. *The Economist.* September 18.

RAND Corporation. 2000. Americans Lack Knowledge—But Not Concern—About World Population Issues. RAND News Release. Available online at www.rand.org.

Randel, J. et al. 2002. *The Reality of AID 2002: An Independent Review of Poverty Reduction and International Development Assistance.* Manila: IBON Books.

"Rapid Health Response, Assessment, and Surveillance After a Tsunami—Thailand, 2004–2005." 2005. *Massachusetts Morbidity and Mortality Report.* 54(3).

Redlener, I. 1994. Healthcare for the Homeless—Lessons from the Frontline,. *New England Journal of Medicine.* 331:327–328.

"Reneging on Food Aid." 2004. *The Boston Globe.* December 26.

Revkin, A. 2005. The Future of Calamity. *The New York Times.* January 2.

Rich, B. 1994. World Bank/ IMF: 50 Years is Enough. In: *50 Years is Enough: The Case Against the World Bank and The International Monetary Fund* (Danaher K., ed). Boston, Mass: South End Press.

Robey, B. et al. 1993. The Fertility Decline in Developing Countries. *Scientific American.* 269(6):60–67.

Rocha, J. 2000. Analysis: Brazil's Racial Democracy. BBC News. April 19.

Rosenberg, N. 1994. How the Developed Countries Became Rich. Cambridge, Mass: American Academy of Arts and Sciences.

Rosenberg, T. 2002. Have Not: A Way to Make Globalization Work for Everybody Else. *The New York Times Magazine.* August 18.

Sachs, J. 2005a. *The End of Poverty: Economic Possibilities For Our Time.* New York, NY: The Penguin Press.

———. 2005b. The Development Challenge. *Foreign Affairs.* 84(2).

———. 2003. A Better Use for Our $87b. *The Boston Globe.* September 13.

———. 2002. Weapons of Mass Salvation. *The Economist.* October 24.

———. 2001a. The Strategic Significance of Global Inequality. *Washington Quarterly*. Summer.

———. 2001b. *Macroeconomics and Health: Investing in Health for Economic Development, Report of the Commission on Macroeconomics and Health*. Geneva, Switzerland: World Health Organization.

———. 2001c. What's Good for the Poor is Good for America. *The Economist*. 12 July.

———. 2001d. The Geography of Poverty and Wealth. *Scientific American*. March.

Sachs, S. and Miller, J. 2004. Under Eye of the UN: Billions for Hussein in Oil-for-Food Plan. *The New York Times*. August 13.

Safire, W. 2004. My Son, My Son. *The New York Times*. November 29.

Sahagun, L. 1997. Violent Crime Besieges Reservations. *The Boston Globe*. November 23.

Salant, J. 2002. 43% of Incoming Freshman Congressmen are Millionaires. *The Boston Globe*. December 25.

Schweitzer, A. 1949a. *Out of My Life and Thought: An Autobiography*. New York, NY: Henry Holt and Co.

———. 1949b. *The Philosophy of Civilization*. New York, NY: Prometheus Books.

———. 1949c. *Memoirs of Childhood and Youth*. New York, NY: Macmillan Co.

———. 1948a. *The Psychiatric Study of Jesus*. Boston, Mass: Beacon Press.

———. 1948b. *On the Edge of the Primeval Forest*. New York, NY: Macmillan Co.

———. 1939. *Christianity and the Religions of the World*. London, England: Allan & Unwin.

———. 1933. *Out of My Life and Thought: An Autobiography*. Baltimore, Md: Johns Hopkins University Press.

———. 1906. *The Quest of the Historical Jesus*. Frankfurt, Germany: JCB Mohr.

Sen, A. 1999. *Development as Freedom*. New York, NY: Random House.

———. 1993. The Economics of Life and Death. *Scientific American*. March.

Sengupta, S. 2002. In Bombay, Public Indignity is Poverty's Partner. *New York Times*. February 9.

Sennott, C.M. 1996. A Special Report: Armed for Profit, the Selling of US Weapons. *The Boston Globe*. February 11.

Shapiro, I. 2000. Trends in US Development Aid and the Current Budget Debate. Center on Policy and Budget Priorities. Available online at www.cbpp.org/4-25-00bud.htm.

Shatz, A. 2002 Mission Impossible. *The Boston Globe*. October 20.

Shilts, R. 1987. *And the Band Played On: Politics, People, and the AIDS Epidemic*. New York, NY: St Martin's Press.

Sidel, V.W. 1988. The Arms Race as a Threat to Health. *Lancet*. 2(8608):442–444.

Sider, R.J. 1997. Rich Christians in an Age of Hunger, Moving from Affluence to Generosity. Dallas, Texas: Word Publishers.

Sides, H. 2002. *Ghost Soldiers*. New York, NY: Anchor Books.

Singer, R. 2002. O'Neill, Bono Decry AIDS Funds Use. *The Boston Globe*. May 25.

Singh, J.A. 2003. Is Donor Aid to Iraq Fair? *Lancet*. 362(9396):1672–1673.

"Sins of the Secular Missions." 2000. *The Economist*. January 29.

Sivard, R.L. 1996. World Military and Social Expenditures 1996. 16th ed. Washington DC: World Priorities.

60 Minutes. 1996. Jeffrey Wigand, PhD. *60 Minutes* (CBS). February 4. Available online at www.jeffreywigand.com/insider/60minutes.html.

Skocpol, T. 1996. *Boomerang,: Clinton's Health Security Effort and the Turn Against Government in US Politics*. New York, NY: W.W. Norton.

"Slavery and Slave Redemption in the Sudan." 2005. Human Rights Watch Backgrounder. Available online at www.hrw.org/backgrounder/africa/sudanupdate.htm.

"Slavery Returns with War in Sudan, Arab Traders Prey on Southern Tribe." 1998. *The Boston Globe.* February 8.

Smedley, B.D. et al. 2001. Unequal Treatment: Confronting Racial and Ethnic Disparities in Health Care. The Institute of Medicine. Available to online at www.nap.edu.

Solomon, D. 2004. Taking Religious Liberties. *The New York Times Magazine.* April 4.

Sontag, D. 2004. Early Tests for US in Its Global Fight on AIDS. *The New York Times.* July 14.

"Special Report: The United Nations, Fighting for Survival." 2004. *The Economist.* November 20.

Starr, P. 1982. *The Social Transformation of American Medicine.* New York, NY: Harper Collins.

Stephenson, J. 2002. Bangladesh Arsenic Water Crisis. *JAMA.* 288(14):1708.

Stevenson, R.W. 2002. Stars of Rock and Heavy Policy Seek Answers to Africa's Poverty. *The New York Times.* May 22.

Stohl, R. 2003. Control Arms Campaign Launch. Center for Defense Information, a speech delivered at The Washington Club. October 9, 2003. Available online at www.cdi.org.

Stolberg, S.G. 2002. With Convert's Zeal, Congress Awakens to AIDS. *The New York Times.* May 12.

Stover, E. et al. 1994. The Medical and Social Consequences of Land Mines in Cambodia. *JAMA.* 272(5):331–336.

Strickland, T.G. 2000. *Hunter's Tropical Medicine and Emerging Infectious Diseases.* 8th ed. Philadelphia, Pa: W.B. Saunders Co.

Strom, S. 2005. Gates Charity Is Doubling Vaccination Gift. *The New York Times.* January 25.

Sublett, R. 1994. Opening remarks. *Kellogg National Fellowship Program.* Chicago, Ill.

Swarns, R. 2002. Broad Accord Reached at Global Environmental Meeting. *The New York Times.* September 4.

Taylor, A. 1998. Violations of the International Code of Marketing of Breast Milk Substitutes: Prevalence in Four Countries. *British Medical Journal.* 316(7138):1117–1122.

"The Cancun Challenge." 2003. *The Economist.* September 6.

"The Case Against the Prosecution." 2004. *The Economist.* February 28.

"The Cost of AIDS: An Imprecise Catastrophe." 2004. *The Economist.* May 20.

The Economist. 2005. *Pocket World in Figures 2005 Edition.* London, England: Profile Books.

———. 2003. *Pocket World in Figures 2003 Edition.* London, England: Profile Books.

"The *Forbes* 400." 2001. *Forbes.* October 8.

"The Global Fund, Weaving a Safety Net." 2005. *The Economist.* September 10.

"The Greatest Man in the World." 1947. *Life.* October 6.

"The Great Flood Begins." 2003. *The Economist.* June 5.

"The Human Toll of World War II." 1995. *The Boston Globe.* August 14.

The National Priorities Project. 2005. The War in Iraq Costs. Available online at http://costofwar.com.

"The Non-Governmental Order." 1999. *The Economist.* December 9.

"The Other War: George Bush' Pledge of More Money to Fight AIDS Should be Welcomed." 2003. *The Economist.* January 30.

"The Right Fix?" 2003. *The Economist.* August 29.

"The United Nations: A Winning Recipe for Reform?" 2004. *The Economist.* July 24.

"The View from the Slums." 2002. *The Economist.* June 27.

The White House. 2005. President Discusses Hurricane Relief in Address to the Nation. Available online at www.whitehouse.gov.

The World Commission on Dams. 2001. Dams and Development: A New Framework for Decision-Making. Available online at www.dams.org/report/contents.htm.

"The World's View of Multinationals." 2000. *The Economist.* January 27.

Thomas, L. 1983. *The Youngest Science.* New York, NY: Penguin Books.

Thompson, G. and Faith, N. 2005 For Honduras and Iran, World's Aid Evaporated. *The New York Times.* January 11.

Tisch, S.J. and Wallace, M.B. 1994. *Dilemmas of Developmental Assistance: The What, Why, and Who of Foreign Aid.* Boulder, Colo: Westview Press.

Transparency International. 2004. Global Corruption Report 2004. Available online at www.globalcorruptionreport.org/download/gcr2004/Highlights_from_the_GCR_2 04_FINAL.pdf.

———. 2003. Transparency International Corruption Perceptions Index 2003. Available online at www.transparency.org/pressreleases_archive/2003/dnld/ cpi2003.pressrelease.en.pdf.

Traub, J. 2005. The Statesman: Why, and How, Bono Matters. *The New York Times.* September 18.

Tsui A.O. et al. 1997. *Reproductive Health in Developing Countries: Expanding Dimensions, Building Solutions.* Washington, DC: The National Academies Press.

"Turner Pays US Dues; UN Budget Deal Goes Through." 2000. *NewsMax.com Wires.* December 23. Available online at www.newsmax.com/archives/articles/ 2000/12/22/203525.shtml.

Ubelaker, D.H. 1999. The Impact of Disease: Two Worlds Meet. *Perspectives in Health.* 4(1)14–17.

UNAIDS. 2004. AIDS epidemic update, December 2003. *Joint United Nations Programme on HIV/AIDS.* Available online at www.unaids.org/Unaids/EN/ Resources/ Publications/corporate+publications/aids+epidemic+update+-+december+2003.asp.

Unger, C. 2004 *House of Bush, House of Saud: The Secret Relationship Between the World's Two Most Powerful Dynasties.* New York, NY: Scribner.

UNICEF. 2004. Child Work. Available online at www.childinfo.org/eddb/work/ index.htm.

———. 2002. UNICEF says clean water is key to building a world truly fit for children. Available online at www.unicef.org/newsline/02ma10wssd.htm.

———. 2001. State of the World's Children 2001. Available online at www.unicef. org/sowc01/toc.htm.

———. 1998. State of the World's Children: Focus on Nutrition. Available online at www.unicef.org/sowc98/.

———. 1997a. Statistical Annex. Available online at www.unicef-icdc.org/publications/ pdf/monee6/annex.pdf.

———. 1997b. State of the World's Children: Focus on Child Labor. Available online at www.unicef.org/sowc97/report/summary.htm.

United Nations. 2003. The State of the World Population 2002: People, Poverty and Possibilities—Overview. UN Population Fund Annual Report for 2002. Available online at www.unfpa.org/swp/2002/english/ch1/index.htm.

————.2002a. Ensuring Reproductive Health and Rights Would Go a Long Way in Overcoming Poverty, New Report Says. United Nations Population Fund. Available online at www.unfpa.org/news/2002/pressroom/swp2002pr1.htm.

————. 2002b. Fact Sheet on Water. United Nations World Summit on Sustainable Development, Johannesburg. Available online at www.un.org/jsummit/html/media_info/factsheets.html.

————. 2002c. Realizing the Vision: The Global Fund to Fight AIDS, Tuberculosis, and Malaria. Cambridge, Mass: United Nations Association of Greater Boston, American Academy of Arts and Sciences. Summary review available online at www.globalhealth.org/publications/article.php3?id=775.

United Nations Development Program (UNDP). 2005 *Human Development Report 2005*. New York, NY: Oxford University Press.

————. 2003 *Human Development Report 2003*. New York, NY: Oxford University Press.

————. 2002. *Human Development Report, 2002*. New York, NY: Oxford University Press.

————. 2001. *Human Development Report, 2001*. New York, NY: Oxford University Press.

————. 2000. *Human Development Report, 2000*. New York, NY: Oxford University Press.

————. 1999. *Human Development Report, 1999*. New York, NY: Oxford University Press.

————. 1998. *Human Development Report, 1998*. New York, NY: Oxford University Press.

————. 1997. *Human Development Report, 1997*. New York, NY: Oxford University Press.

————. 1996. *Human Development Report, 1996*. New York, NY: Oxford University Press.

————. 1995. *Human Development Report, 1995*. New York, NY: Oxford University Press.

————. 1994. *Human Development Report, 1994*. New York, NY: Oxford University Press.

US Agency for International Development (USAID). 2003. Foreign Aid in the National Interest, Promoting Freedom, Security and Opportunity. Washington, DC: USAID.

US Bureau of Economic Analysis. 2004. Growth Moderates in Fourth Quarter but is Up for the Year. Available online at www.bea.gov/bea/newsrelarchive/2004/gdp403a_fax.pdf.

US Congress. 1987. House of Representatives. H.R. 3669, A Bill to Amend the Public Health Service Act to Establish an International Health Corps. 100th Congress, 1st session.

US Department of State. 2005. Department of State Overview/FY 2005 International Affairs Summary. Available online at http://usinfo.state.gov/usa/infousa/trade/files/98-916.pdf.

————. 2004. The President's Emergency Plan for AIDS Relief: Five-Year Strategy. Available online at www.state.gov/s/gac/rl/fs/2004/29706.htm.

Vaccarino, V. et al. 2005. Sex and Racial Differences in the Management of Acute Myocardial Infarction: 1994 through 2002. *New England Journal of Medicine.* 353:671–682.

Vidal, J. 2003. Farmer Commits Suicide at Protests. *The Guardian.* September 11.

Vogel, G. 2003. 2003 Nobel Prizes: Physicists Honored for Their Medical Insights. *Science.* 302(5644):382–383.

Watkins, K. 1995. *The Oxfam Poverty Report.* Oxford, England: Oxfam.

Werner D. and Sanders D. 1997. *Questioning the Solution: The Politics of Primary Health Care and Child Survival, With an In-Depth Critique of Oral Rehydration Therapy.* Palo Alto, Calif: Healthrights Press.

West, C. 1994. *Race Matters.* New York, NY: Vintage Books.

"What's the Charity Doing with Your Money?" 2002. *Forbes.* Available online at www.forbesimg.com/downloads/pdf/invguide03.pdf.

"What's the Tip on $22,000? Ask Table for Three." 1997. *The Boston Globe.* November 18.

"What the President Giveth. . . ." 2002. *The Economist.* March 28.

Whitehead, M. et al. 1992. *Inequalities in Health: The Black Report and the Health Divide.* New York, NY: Penguin Books.

Whitelaw, K. 1997. Good works, Evil Results: When Aid Workers Become the Bait—or the Targets. *US News & World Report.* May 26.

Wider, J. 2002. International Bank Lending, Water Flowing Uphill? UNU World Institute for Development Economic Research. Available online at www.wider.unu.edu/publications/dps/dps2002/dp2002-42.pdf.

Wilkinson, R.G. 1994a. Divided We Fall. *British Medical Journal.* 308(6937):1113–1114.

———. 1994b. The Epidemiological Transition: From Material Scarcity to Social Disadvantage? *Daedalus.* Fall.

———. 1992a. National Mortality Rates: the Impact of Inequality? *American Journal of Public Health.* 82(8):1082–1084

———. 1992b. Income Distribution and Life Expectancy. *British Medical Journal.* 304(6820):165–168.

Willard, A. 2003. World Bank Poll Finds Bank Arrogant, Tied to US. *Reuters.* June 4.

Williams, T. 2005 Bush Appoints Bolton as UN Envoy, Bypassing Senate. *The New York Times.* August 1.

Wilson, W.J. 1996. *When Work Disappears.* New York, NY: Alfred A. Knopf.

Wolf, E.R. 1982. *Europe and the People Without History.* Berkeley, Calif: University of California Press.

Woods, E. 2005 Aid That Doesn't Deliver. Foreign Policy in Focus. Available online at www.fpif.org.

Woolner, A. 2004. Big Tobacco Whines for Sympathy. *The Week.* October 8.

World Bank Group. 2004a. Annual Report 2004. Available online at www.worldbank. org/annualreport/2004/lending.html.

———. 2004b. A Changing World Bank. Available online at http://web.worldbank.org.

———. 1999a. The HIPC Debt Initiative. Available online at www.worldbank.org/ hipc/about/hipcbr/hipcbr.htm.

———. 1999b. "Annual Report 1999." Available online at www.worldbank.org/html/ extpb/annrep99/develop7.htm.

———. 1993. *World Development Report 1993: Investing in Health.* New York, NY: Oxford University Press.

"World Bank's Cure for Donor Fatigue" 1993. *Lancet.* 342(8863):63–64.

"Worldbeater, Inc." 1997. *The Economist.* November 20.

World Health Organization (WHO). 2004. Tuberculosis. Available online at www. who.int/tb/en.

———. 2002a. World Report on Violence and Health. Geneva, Switzerland: WHO Press.

———. 2002b. Basic Facts on TB. WHO/The Stop TB Partnership. Available online at www.stoptb.org/world.tb.day/WTBD_2002/Basicfacts.pdf.

———. 1999. *The World Health Report 1999, Making a Difference.* Geneva, Switzerland: WHO Press.

———. 1998. *The World Health Report 1998, Life In The 21st Century: A Vision For All.* Geneva, Switzerland: WHO Press.

———. 1997. *Polio, The Beginning of the End.* Geneva, Switzerland: WHO Press.

———. 1995. *The World Health Report 1995: Bridging the Gaps.* Geneva, Switzerland: WHO Press.

Wright, T. 1997. *The Original Jesus: The Life and Vision of a Revolutionary.* Grand Rapids, Mich: William B. Eerdman's Publishing Company.

"Wrong Way Round." 2005. *The Economist.* June 27.

Zakaria, F. 2003. *The Future of Freedom:, Illiberal Democracy at Home and Abroad.* New York, NY: Norton Press.

Zinsser, H. 1934. *Rats, Lice, and History.* Boston, Mass: Little, Brown and Co.

Index

About the Author

Edward O'Neil Jr, MD, is a practicing emergency physician at Caritas
St Elizabeth's Medical Center in Boston and an assistant professor of emergency medicine at Tufts University School of Medicine. Dr O'Neil is an alumnus of the W.K. Kellogg National Leadership Program and is the founder and
president of Omni Med (www.omnimed.org), a nongovernmental organization founded in 1998 that runs innovative, cooperatively designed programs
emphasizing health volunteerism and ethical leadership in Belize, Kenya,
Thailand, and Guyana. Since its inception, volunteer health providers have
made over 100 trips abroad–mostly educational–through its various programs. Omni Med was founded on the philosophy that *all* people have a
right to health and quality health care, and that all health professionals, by
their very involvement in the profession, share an ethical imperative to make
quality health care broadly accessible to all people, regardless of their nationality or income. For a number of years prior to and during medical training,
Dr O'Neil played piano professionally in Washington D.C. and Boston, as
well as during travels through the United States, Europe, Asia, and Africa.
He and his wife, Judy, live in Newton, Massachusetts with their three
children, James, Michaela, and Sean.